Cataract Surgery: Advanced Techniques

Cataract Surgery: Advanced Techniques

Editor: Lorenzo Fernandez

FOSTER ACADEMICS
www.fosteracademics.com

www.fosteracademics.com

FOSTER
ACADEMICS

Cataloging-in-Publication Data

Cataloging-in-Publication Data

Cataract surgery : advanced techniques / edited by Lorenzo Fernandez.
p. cm.
Includes bibliographical references and index.
ISBN 978-1-63242-754-0
1. Cataract--Surgery. 2. Cataract--Surgery--Technique. 3. Cataract--Surgery--Complications.
I. Fernandez, Lorenzo.
RE451 .C38 2019
617.742--dc23

Foster Academics,
118-35 Queens Blvd., Suite 400,
Forest Hills, NY 11375, USA

ISBN 978-1-63242-754-0 (Hardback)

Printed and bound in China.

Contents

Preface

The main aim of this book is to educate learners and enhance their research focus by presenting diverse topics covering this vast field. This is an advanced book which compiles significant studies by distinguished experts in the area of analysis. This book addresses successive solutions to the challenges arising in the area of application, along with it; the book provides scope for future developments.

A cataract surgery is a kind of surgery which involves the removal of the natural lens of the eye, which has developed an opacification. It is replaced with an intraocular lens (IOL). Two of the most common cataract surgery procedures include phacoemulsification (phaco) and extracapsular cataract extraction (ECCE). A machine having an ultrasonic handpiece equipped with a titanium or steel tip is used while performing phacoemulsification. In the process of extracapsular cataract extraction, almost the entire natural lens is removed but the elastic lens capsule is left intact to allow the implantation of an intraocular lens. The ever growing need of advanced technology is the reason that has fueled the research in the field of cataract surgery in recent times. This book explores all the important aspects of cataract surgery in the present day scenario. Doctors, ophthalmologists, researchers and students actively engaged in this field will find this book full of crucial and unexplored concepts.

It was a great honour to edit this book, though there were challenges, as it involved a lot of communication and networking between me and the editorial team. However, the end result was this all-inclusive book covering diverse themes in the field.

Finally, it is important to acknowledge the efforts of the contributors for their excellent chapters, through which a wide variety of issues have been addressed. I would also like to thank my colleagues for their valuable feedback during the making of this book.

Editor

1

Prevalence of and Risk Factors for Age-Related and Anterior Polar Cataracts in a Korean Population

Kyung-Sun Na[1,3,4], Yong-Gyu Park[2], Kyungdo Han[2], Jee Won Mok[3], Choun-Ki Joo[1]*

1 Department of Ophthalmology and Visual Science, Seoul St. Mary's Hospital, College of Medicine, The Catholic University of Korea, Seoul, Korea, **2** Department of Biostatistics, The Catholic University of Korea, Seoul, Korea, **3** Catholic Institutes of Visual Science, The Catholic University of Korea, Seoul, Korea, **4** Department of Health Promotion Center, Seoul St. Mary's Hospital, College of Medicine, The Catholic University of Korea, Seoul, Korea

Abstract

Objective: To investigate the potential risk factors associated with nuclear, cortical, posterior subcapsular, and anterior polar cataracts (APC) in the Korean population.

Research Design and Methods: This was a population-based, cross-sectional study of 7992 adults (over 40 years of age) from the data of the fourth annual Korea National Health and Nutrition Examination Survey, performed from 2007 to 2009. The presence of lens opacity was examined by slit-lamp biomicroscopy and evaluated according to LOCS II standard photographs. The subtype of cataract present, including nuclear, cortical, posterior subcapsular, and anterior polar cataracts, was noted. Multivariable adjusted logistic regression analysis was conducted to examine the odds ratio (OR) and 95% confidence interval (CI) for association of each specific type of cataract with age, sex, health examination, and medical history.

Results: The prevalence of nuclear, cortical, and posterior subcapsular cataract increased gradually with increasing age. However, the prevalence of APC peaked in the 50- to 59-year-old subjects. All types of cataract except for APCs were more prevalent in women. Oral steroid use was associated with a lower risk of APC.

Conclusions: These findings showed the unique characteristics of APC in the Korean population.

Editor: Usha P. Andley, Washington University, United States of America

Funding: This study was funded by the National Research of Korea (2011-0027157), Seoul, Korea. The funders had no role in study design, data collection and analysis, decision to publish, or preparation of the manuscript.

Competing Interests: The authors have declared that no competing interests exist.

* Email: ckjoo@catholic.ac.kr

Introduction

Cataracts are the principal cause of blindness and visual impairment worldwide, making it necessary from the public health standpoint to identify risk factors for their development and progression [1–3]. Studies on the prevalence of and risk factors for cataracts have been conducted mainly in white European-derived populations in the United States, Australia, and Europe [4–11]. Less is known about populations of African, Indian, or East Asian descent [3,12–15].

Anterior polar cataract generally refers to the congenital type of capsulolenticular cataract seen in Western countries and has been reported to be related to microphthalmia, aniridia, and bilateral retinoblastoma [2]. However, there is a unique type of cataract with focal opacity at the anterior capsulolenticular area that develops in early adulthood in otherwise healthy Korean patients (Fig. 1(A), (B), and (C)). APC is not well documented even in other Asian countries and is considered unique to Koreans. Previously, we conducted a hospital-based study showing that the prevalence of APC in our patients was 6.02%, and male predominated [16]. Until very recently, Korea was largely considered to be a homogenous, racially intolerant country with little or no experience with large-scale immigration. We have previously shown that the cataractous lens epithelial cells (LECs) of anterior subcapsular cataracts are transdifferentiated into spindle-shaped fibroblast-like cells without cellular junctions and are embedded within a fibrillar meshwork mass [17]. Lens epithelial cells in the anterior subcapsular area fail to migrate to the equatorial area, resulting in the accumulation of several layers of proliferating cells in the anterior subcapsular area. This change is different from the changes in lens fiber proteins in other types of cataracts.

In this study, we aimed to elucidate the prevalence of and risk factors for non-age related anterior polar cataracts in the absence of any general abnormality and those of age-related cataracts, including nuclear and cortical cataracts.

Materials and Methods

Study Subjects

This cross-sectional study included a representative sample of the data gathered in the fourth Korea National Health and Nutrition Examination Survey (KNHANES IV), which was performed from 2007 to 2009 by the Division of Chronic Disease Surveillance under the Korea Centers for Disease Control and Prevention.

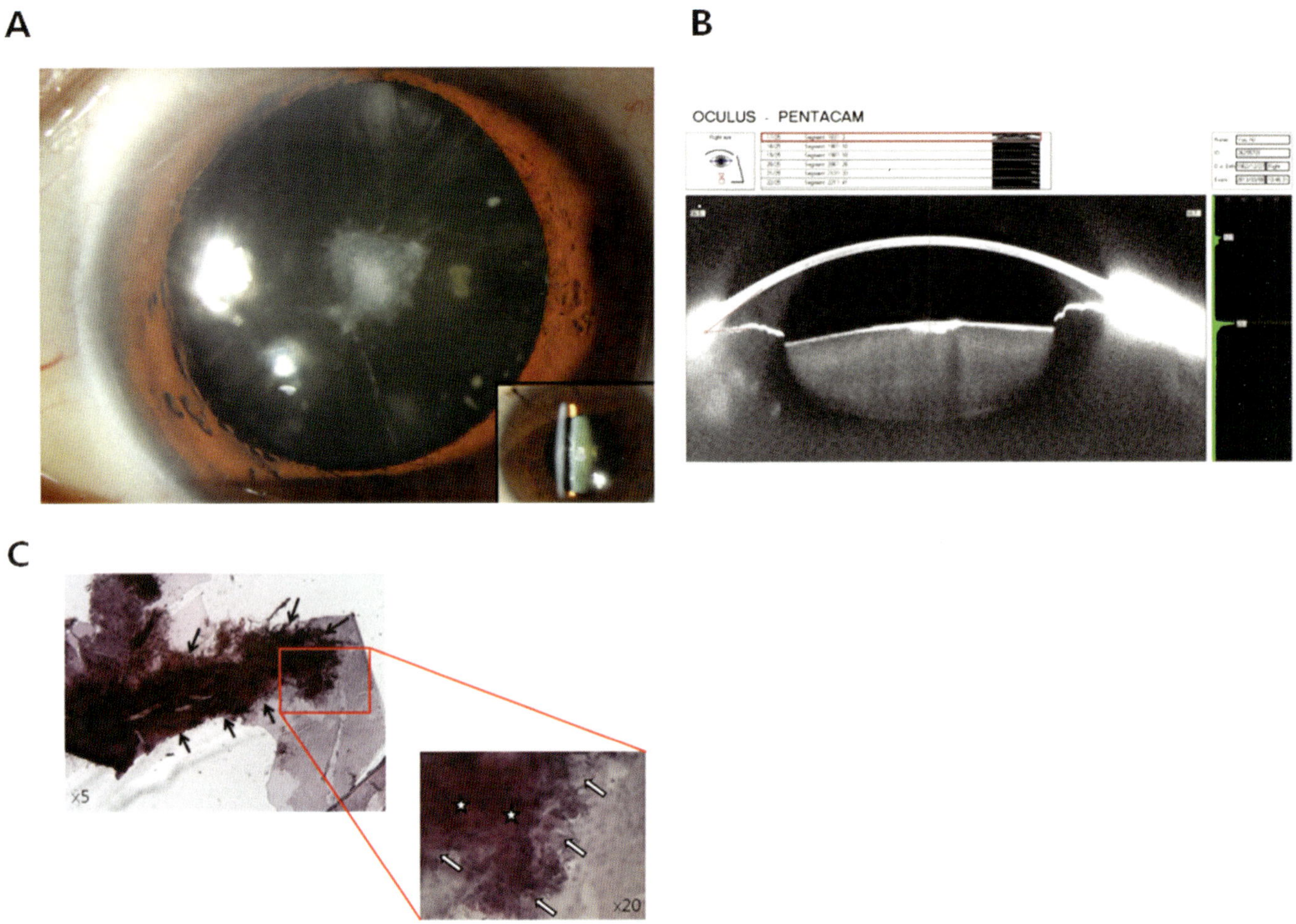

Figure 1. Fifty-year-old man showed findings of anterior polar cataract. (A) Slit-lamp examination demonstrates the form of white-grey opacity appearing under the central part of the anterior lens capsule. (B) Sheimpflug-measured lens density showing focal anterior polar opacity. (C) Light microscopy of the anterior capsule following cataract surgery of anterior polar cataract. Multilamellar arrangement and isolated aggregations of collagenous materials are present (arrows). High-power image shows proliferative changes of the lens epithelial cells (open arrows) and increased collagenous aggregations (stars).

The sampling units were households selected through a stratified, multistage, probability sampling, based on geographic area, sex, and age group, of household registries. Information was collected from stratified multistage probability samples of Korean households representing the noninstitutionalized civilian population. The survey was composed of 3 parts, that is, a health interview survey, a health examination survey, and a nutrition survey, and was a nationwide representative study of noninstitutionalized civilians, involving a stratified, multistage, probability-sampling design with a rolling survey sampling model. Sampling units were defined based on household unit data from the 2005 National Census Registry, including those for geographic area, sex, and age.

Among 25250 individuals who completed all surveys, total 19386 (76.8%) had an ophthalmic examination. Of the 8801 subjects, who were older than 40 years old, 416 were bilaterally pseudophakic or aphakic; and 393 had mixed-type cataracts. The remaining 5242 free of cataract and 2750 with cataract were included in this study. Institutional Review Board/Ethics Committee approvals for the study were obtained from the Catholic University of Korea in accordance with the Declaration of Helsinki. The data are publicly available from the Korean Centers for Disease Control and Prevention [18].

Procedures

Questionnaires were used to collect demographic information, smoking history, educational status, weight change after the age of 20 years (gain or loss), daily sunlight exposure, alcohol consumption, sleep duration, stress level, medical history, and any use of prescription drugs or nonprescription medication. Smoking behavior was categorized as current smoker, ex-smoker, or nonsmoker. Alcohol-consumption behavior was classified as nondrinker, mild-to-moderate drinker (1.0–30.0 g alcohol/day), or heavy drinker (>30.0 g alcohol/day) after conversion of the average frequency and amount of alcoholic beverages consumed into the amount of pre-alcohol (in grams) consumed per day. Psychological stress level was investigated according to the subjective cognitive complaints by the questionnaires.

Waist circumference was measured to the nearest 0.1 cm in a horizontal plane at the level of the midpoint between the iliac crest and the costal margin at the end of a normal expiration. The body mass index (BMI) was calculated as the individual's weight in kilograms divided by the square of the individual's height in

Table 1. Baseline characteristics of study participants.

	Nuclear (n = 1783)	Cortical (n = 807)	PSC (n = 56)	APC (n = 104)
Age				
40–49	13.8(0.6)	15.5(0.6)	16.5(0.6)	16.6(0.6)
50–59	14.9(0.6)	17.6(0.6)	18.7(0.6)	28.4(0.7)
60–69	28.7(0.8)	28.6(0.8)	28.5(0.7)	18.5(0.6)
≥70	42.6(1.2)	38.2(1.1)	36.3(1.1)	36.5(1.1)
Sex				
Male	48.2(0.7)	48.0(0.6)	47.9(0.6)	52.2(0.6)
Smoke				
Never	77.4(0.7)	77.3(0.6)	77.6(0.6)	77.6(0.6)
Current	22.6(0.7)	22.7(0.6)	22.4(0.6)	22.4(0.6)
Education				
High school to college graduate	31.6(1.9)	27.9(2.8)	39.9(10.1)	37.4(7.0)
Weight change[†]				
Gain>10 kg	0.5(0.2)	0.4(0.4)	.	.
Gain≤10 kg	9.9(0.9)	11.7(1.5)	11.1(5.3)	10.1(3.2)
No change	72.7(1.3)	71.7(2.1)	68.5(7.1)	66.8(5.8)
Loss≤10 kg	16.3(1.1)	15.6(1.6)	20.5(6.4)	23.1(4.5)
Loss >10 kg	0.5(0.1)	0.6(0.3)	.	.
Daily sunlight exposure				
More than 6 hours	35.5(2.1)	41.5(3.8)	32.5(8.4)	48.2(8.7)
Alcohol[‡]				
Never drinker	40.5(1.6)	39.6(2.2)	32.4(8.1)	44.9(4.5)
Mild to Moderate drinker	50.3(1.6)	50.5(2.4)	65.6(8.6)	44.9(4.9)
Heavy drinker	9.2(1.1)	9.8(1.4)	2.0(1.5)	10.1(3.3)
Daily sleep				
4 hours or less	3.2(0.5)	2.5(0.6)	4.7(3.0)	0.6(0.6)
4–6 hours	20.8(1.2)	18.1(1.6)	24.1(7.3)	17.0(4.1)
More than 6 hours	75.9(1.3)	79.4(1.6)	71.2(7.7)	82.4(4.1)
Stress level				
Excessive	6.3(0.7)	6.1(1.0)	4.0(4.0)	7.3(2.8)
Much	20.5(1.1)	20.5(1.7)	30.2(7.8)	12.6(3.7)
Frequent	50.3(1.6)	51.6(2.1)	40.3(8.6)	62.3(5.7)
Rare to never	23.0(1.3)	21.7(1.9)	25.5(7.3)	17.8(4)
BMI				
≥25 kg/m^2	34.3(2.1)	36.3(1.4)	45.2(5.3)	34.6(8.3)
Waist circumference				
≥90 cm in male, ≥80 cm in female	40.0(2.5)	48.4(1.6)	45.9(5.9)	43.1(8.4)
Estrogen use (women only)				
Yes	12.6(1.4)	12.7(1.9)	11.1(7.1)	6.9(3.0)
Steroid use				
Yes	77.4(2.2)	80.3(3.1)	90.5(6.7)	56.3(10.6)
NSAIDs use				
Yes	66.3(4.7)	63.3(7.7)	59.6(27.4)	54.7(14.5)
Hypertension				
Yes	38.1(1.6)	36.4(2.0)	31.9(7.4)	38.1(5.6)
Diabetes				
Yes	15.7(1)	12.7(1.4)	26.7(7.5)	9.4(2.9)
Vitamin use				

Table 1. Cont.

	Nuclear (n = 1783)	Cortical (n = 807)	PSC (n = 56)	APC (n = 104)
Yes	80.4(1.3)	81.9(2.2)	84.9(8.7)	70.6(5.8)

Data are expressed as percentage (SE).
PSC = posterior subcapsular opacity; APC = anterior polar cataract; BMI = body mass index; NSAIDs = nonsteroidal anti-inflammatory drugs.
†Weight change after the age of 20 years.
‡Classified as nondrinker, mild-to-moderate drinker (1.0–30.0 grams alcohol/day), or heavy drinker (>30.0 grams alcohol/day) after conversion of the average frequency and amount of alcoholic beverages consumed into the amount of pre-alcohol (in grams) consumed per day.

meters. The BMI was grouped into 2 categories, that is, normal (< 25.0 kg/m^2) and overweight (≥25.0 kg/m).

Systemic hypertension was defined as a measured systolic blood pressure >160 mm Hg and/or a diastolic blood pressure > 90 mm Hg or current use of systemic antihypertensive drugs. Diabetes was defined as a measured fasting blood sugar level of > 126 mg/dL or current use of antidiabetic medication. Peripheral blood was obtained after fasting for a minimum of 8 hours.

Definition of Cataract

Lens opacity was diagnosed by trained ophthalmologists by using the Lens Opacity Classification System (LOCS) II system [19]. The Lens Opacities Classification System II (LOCS II) was used to classify opacities until into 7 cortical (C0, Ctr, CI, CII, CIII, CIV, CV), 5 nuclear (NO, NI, NII, NIII, NIV), and 5 PSC (P0, PI, PII, PIII, PIV) grades of increasing severity, according to photographic standards. Aphakia or pseudophakia were also documented even though excluded in the current study. The pupils were dilated with 1% tropicamide/2.5% phenylephrine hydrochloride eye drops, and the presence of lens opacity was examined by slit-lamp biomicroscopy and evaluated according to LOCS II standard photographs. The severity or grade of lens opacity was not recorded, and only the subtype of cataract present, including nuclear, cortical, posterior subcapsular, and anterior polar cataracts, was noted.

The definitions of lens opacities used in this study were similar to those used in the previous study [20,21]. Nuclear, cortical, posterior subcapsular cataract (PSC), and APC cataracts were recorded in individuals with the same single type of opacity present in both eyes. They were defined in individuals with only a single type opacity with a LOCS II≥2, presented between both eyes. If a participant had unilateral lens extraction, the contralateral phakic eye was used to define the lens opacity type in that individual. Subjects with mixed-type opacities or bilateral lens extraction were excluded.

Histological Examination of Anterior Capsule

The extracted anterior capsules were fixed for 10 min in 4% formaldehyde in PBS and permeabilized in PBS containing 0.5% Triton X-100, also for 10 min. The specimens were stained with hematoxilin and eosin. Images were captured and analyzed with light microscope.

Statistical Analysis

The data are expressed as numbers and percentages (categorical) or the mean ± standard error (continuous). Multivariable adjusted logistic regression analysis was conducted to examine the odds ratio (OR) and 95% confidence interval (CI) for association of each specific type of cataract with age, sex, smoking history, education, weight change, sunlight exposure, alcohol consumption, sleep duration, stress level, BMI, waist circumference, estrogen use (women only), NSAID use, other anti-inflammatory medication use, vitamin use, hypertension, and diabetes. Age and sex were used as covariates for calculating the adjusted OR.

Because the KNHANES III included weights to compensate for the complex sampling design and to allow approximations of the Korean population, weighted analyses were performed with the SAS software. All statistical analyses were performed with the SAS (version 9.2; SAS Institute, Cary, NC, USA) survey procedure to account for the complex sampling design and provide nationally representative prevalence estimates. A P value<0.05 was considered statistically significant.

Results

Baseline Characteristics

The clinical characteristics of the study participants are presented in Table 1. The numbers of participants analyzed were 1783, 807, 56, and 104 for subjects with nuclear cataracts, cortical cataracts, PSCs, and APCs, respectively.

The prevalence of age-related cataracts, including nuclear cataract, cortical cataract, and PSC increased gradually with increasing age. However, the prevalence of APC peaked in the 50- to 59-year-old subjects.(Fig. 2(A),(B)) All types of cataract except for APCs were more prevalent in women; the incidence of APC was greater in men than in women (1.12% vs. 0.96%). The incidence of APC was relatively lower in subjects using estrogen (woman only) or NSAIDs. Diabetes was more frequent in subjects with PSCs than in those with other types of cataracts.

Significant Associations with Cataracts

Table 2 demonstrates the results of logistic regression models that evaluated the associations of various baseline factors with the presence of nuclear cataracts, cortical cataracts, PSCs, and APCs.

Nuclear cataracts

The prevalence of definite nuclear cataract increased significantly with increasing age. The factors associated with increased likelihood of nuclear cataract were low educational level (middle school or less) (OR, 2.41; 95% CI, 2.01–2.88; p<.0001), mild weight loss less than 10 kg since 20 years of age (OR, 1.19; 95% CI, 1.00–1.42; p<.0001), sunlight exposure greater than 6 hours (OR, 1.27; 95% CI, 1.06–1.51; p = 0.0089), sleep duration 4–6 hours (OR, 1.62; 95% CI, 1.38–1.91; p<.0001), hypertension (OR, 1.97; 95% CI, 1.67–2.31; p<.0001), and diabetes (OR, 1.99; 95% CI, 1.60–2.48;p<.0001) after adjustment for age and gender. The factors associated with decreased likelihood of nuclear cataract were a waist circumference of ≥90 cm (men) or ≥ 80 cm (women) (OR, 0.71; 95% CI, 0.62–0.82; p<.0001) and estrogen use in women (OR, 0.76; 95% CI, 0.59–0.99; p = 0.0426).

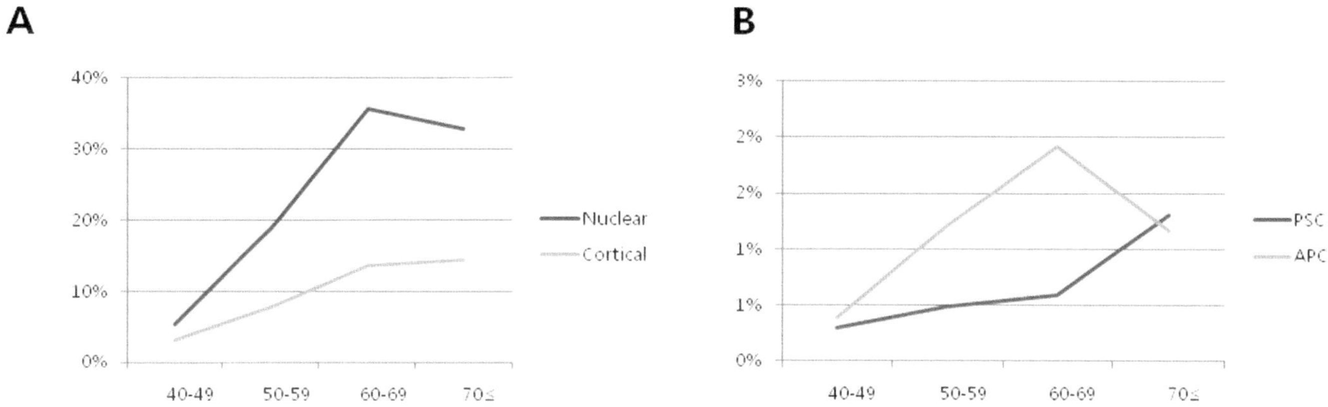

Figure 2. Linear graphs showing age distribution of cataract. (A) Age distribution of nuclear cataract and cortical cataract in Korean population. Both types of cataract show a highest incidence at the age of 60–69. (B) Age distribution of posterior subcapsular cataract (PSC) and anterior polar cataract (APC). PSC shows a gradual increase according to age, and APC present a highest peak at the age of 50–59. * PSC = posterior subcapsular opacity; APC = anterior polar cataract.

Cortical cataracts

Cortical cataracts were associated with increasing age. A higher risk for cortical cataract was associated with lower educational level (OR, 2.63; 95% CI, 1.99–3.48; $p<.0001$), sunlight exposure greater than 6 hours (OR, 1.63; 95% CI, 1.20–2.20; $p = 0.0015$), and waist circumference ≥90 cm (men) or ≥80 cm (women) was associated with higher risk (OR, 1.25; 95% CI, 1.00–1.55; $p = 0.0439$) after adjustment for age and gender.

Posterior subcapsular cataracts

Higher risk was associated with increasing age but was only statistically significant for the ≥70 years age group (OR, 4.36; 95% CI, 1.28–14.78; $p<.0001$). An increased risk of PSC was also associated with diabetes (OR, 3.16; 95% CI, 1.47–6.78; $p = 0.0031$).

Anterior polar cataracts

The highest odds ratios were for the 50–59 years age group (OR, 4.94 ; 95% CI, 2.12–11.5, reference category 40–49 years; $p = 0.0008$). Oral steroid use was associated with a lower risk for APC (OR, 0.37; 95% CI, 0.17–0.84; $p = 0.0171$).

Discussion

Increasing age was a significant risk factor for nuclear cataract, cortical cataract, and PSC, which is consistent with previous reports [2,7,12,15,20,21]. In contrast to the results for other types of cataracts, the prevalence of and odds ratio for APCs were highest in the 50–59-year-old age group, suggesting that these cataracts develop during early adulthood; therefore, age may not be a significant factor in the pathogenesis of APC. This population-based study showed an APC prevalence of 3.78% among all participants, which broke down to 0.4%, 1.9%, 1.2%, and 1.2% in the 40–49-, 50–59-, 60–69-, and ≥70-year-old age groups, respectively. As APC is more likely to develop in early adulthood, the patients themselves may more readily detect the visual impairment and may therefore be more likely to seek early cataract surgery than patients with age-related cataracts.

We previously reported in a hospital-based study that 6.02% of all cataracts were APCs and that 87% of APCs were in men [16]. The differences in prevalence between the studies may result from the participant selection. The previous, hospital-based study was a chart review of the patients who underwent cataract surgery, while the present study was a cross-sectional investigation of the normal population. Men with APC have a greater tendency to undergo early surgical intervention than women because men are more socially active in Korea. Other explanation may be possible that since there was Korean war from 1950 to 1953, Koreans (especially, mothers and their babies) might underwent unusual experiences including nutrition, chemical exposures, and psychiatric stress. Still, the gender differences could not be solved if they were exposed as the same environment.

Diabetes was associated with a significantly higher risk for nuclear cataract and PSC. In contrast to the results of the AREDS study [7], cortical cataract was not significantly associated with diabetes in the current study. The Blue Mountains study confirmed diabetes as a risk factor for nuclear cataract and implicated impaired fasting glucose as a possible risk factor for cortical cataract [22]. Our results support the latter study. We also found that hypertension was associated with an increased risk of nuclear cataract. The results for hypertension regarding the cataract prevalence are inconsistent. The Blue Mountain Eye Study [22] reported a relationship between blood pressure and having cataract surgery and the Los Angeles Latino Eye Study [21] showed that systolic blood pressure to be an independent risk factor for PSC. The varying effect of different antihypertensive medications may be a confounding factor in all of these observational investigations and further prospective studies would be needed.

Our results revealed an increased risk for PSCs but a reduced risk for APCs in systemic steroid users. There is a possibility of an inflammatory etiology of APC since systemic steroids are primarily used for inflammatory activities. While the association between hormonal replacement therapy (HRT) and cataract development is inconsistent [7,23], this study showed a lower risk for nuclear cataracts in estrogen users and a non-significant tendency toward an increased risk for APCs. Estrogens have antioxidant properties, but the possible protective effect of estrogen may be more associated with endogenous estrogen. Exogenous estrogen in the form of hormone replacement therapy should not be regarded as a physiologic substitute and could have other effects.

The current study revealed that vitamin use significantly reduced the risk for APC, but not for other types of cataracts, after adjustment for age and gender. Most of the large prospective studies investigated the effect of Centrum [7,24], which contains a broad spectrum of vitamins and minerals, while our results are

Table 2. Odds ratio (95% CI) on multivariate analysis for different cataract subtypes (nuclear, cortical, PSC, and APC) in Korean.

	Nuclear (n = 1783)		Cortical (n = 807)		PSC (n = 56)		APC (n = 104)	
	MODEL1[†]	MODEL2[‡]	MODEL1	MODEL2	MODEL1	MODEL2	MODEL1	MODEL2
	OR(95% CI)	OR(95% CI)	OR(95% CI)	OR(95% CI)	OR(95% CI)	OR(95% CI)	OR(95% CI)	OR(95% CI)
Age								
40–49	1	1	1	1	1	1	1	1
50–59	4.19(3.12–5.63)*	4.19(3.12–5.63)*	2.57(1.84–3.60)*	2.57(1.84–3.60)*	1.61(0.45–5.77)	1.61(0.45–5.76)	4.94(2.12–11.5)*	4.98(2.13–11.62)*
60–69	10.01(7.18–13.96)*	10.02(7.19–13.97)*	4.75(3.29–6.86)*	4.76(3.29–6.87)*	1.96(0.57–6.74)	1.95(0.58–6.59)	3.11(1.25–7.72)*	3.12(1.26–7.73)*
70+	8.82(6.28–12.38)*	8.85(6.31–12.43)*	5.10(3.49–7.44)*	5.11(3.51–7.46)*	4.36(1.28–14.78)*	4.30(1.32–14.02)*	2.98(1.23–7.24)*	3.06(1.25–7.51)*
Sex								
Male	0.92(0.81–1.04)	1.07(0.94–1.22)	0.94(0.79–1.11)	1.05(0.89–1.25)	0.82(0.44–1.52)	0.9(0.51–1.60)	1.17(0.77–1.76)	1.27(0.83–1.92)
Smoke								
Never	1	1	1	1	1	1	1	1
Current smoker	0.92(0.77–1.08)	1.14(0.95–1.38)	0.76(0.62–0.94)	0.86(0.68–1.09)	0.42(0.14–1.24)	0.46(0.14–1.49)	0.89(0.47–1.71)	0.89(0.45–1.77)
Education								
Middle school or less	2.41(2.01–2.88)*	1.24(1.01–1.53)*	2.63(1.99–3.48)*	1.75(1.28–2.40)*	1.43(0.63–3.26)	0.81(0.41–1.59)	1.59(0.89–2.86)	1.19(0.54–2.63)
Weight change[Φ]								
Gain>10 kg	0.72(0.34–1.54)	0.95(0.43–2.11)	0.5(0.07–3.72)	0.61(0.08–4.79)	.	.	.	.
Gain≤10 kg	0.64(0.52–0.79)*	0.91(0.74–1.13)	0.81(0.6–1.11)	1.08(0.79–1.47)	0.82(0.29–2.32)	1.01(0.34–2.98)	0.76(0.37–1.58)	0.93(0.43–2.03)
No change	1	1	1	1	1	1	1	1
Loss≤10 kg	1.19(1.00–1.42)*	1.08(0.90–1.30)	1.13(0.87–1.45)	1.04(0.80–1.35)	1.53(0.72–3.27)	1.44(0.69–2.99)	1.78(1.03–3.07)	1.68(0.98–2.89)
Loss >10 kg	0.58(0.30–1.12)	0.43(0.22–0.84)*	0.81(0.28–2.28)	0.67(0.22–2.01)	.	.	.	.
Daily sunlight exposure								
More than 6 hours	1.27(1.06–1.51)*	1.07(0.88–1.30)	1.63(1.20–2.20)*	1.48(1.10–2.00)*	1.05(0.50–2.21)	0.98(0.46–2.08)	2.04(1.05–4.00)*	1.86(0.92–3.76)
Alcohol[§]								
Mild to moderate drinker	0.66(0.57–0.76)*	1.09(0.93–1.28)	0.71(0.58–0.87)*	1.06(0.85–1.33)	1.17(0.56–2.43)	1.71(0.74–3.96)	0.57(0.39–0.85)*	0.67(0.42–1.05)
Heavy drinker	0.68(0.51–0.91)*	1.23(0.9–1.69)	0.79(0.58–1.07)*	1.26(0.89–1.76)	0.2(0.05–0.86)*	0.32(0.06–1.62)	0.73(0.35–1.49)*	0.78(0.34–1.78)
Daily sleep hour								
4 hours or less	2.52(1.76–3.62)*	1.37(0.94–1.99)	1.53(0.91–2.59)	0.94(0.55–1.60)	3.08(0.82–11.56)	2.06(0.55–7.73)	0.35(0.05–2.64)	0.25(0.03–1.89)
4–6 hours	1.62(1.38–1.91)*	1.26(1.06–1.50)*	1.24(0.99–1.55)	1.00(0.79–1.25)	1.81(0.81–4.01)	1.52(0.71–3.27)	1.10(0.63–1.93)*	0.96(0.55–1.68)
More than 6 hours	1	1	1	1	1	1	1	1
Stress level								
Excessive	1.00(0.75–1.33)	1.41(1.05–1.91)*	1.04(0.67–1.60)	1.35(0.85–2.13)	0.58(0.07–4.62)	0.70(0.09–5.37)	1.50(0.61–3.71)	1.85(0.72–4.71)
Much	0.70(0.57–0.86)	1.15(0.93–1.43)	0.78(0.59–1.02)	1.15(0.86–1.54)	1.00(0.41–2.43)	1.35(0.55–3.33)	0.59(0.29–1.21)	0.81(0.38–1.70)
Frequent	0.69(0.58–0.83)	1.14(0.94–1.38)	0.80(0.63–1.01)	1.17(0.91–1.51)	0.54(0.23–1.26)	0.73(0.33–1.61)	1.20(0.67–2.12)	1.60(0.86–2.96)
Rare to never	1	1	1	1	1	1	1	1
BMI								

Table 2. Cont.

	Nuclear (n = 1783)		Cortical (n = 807)		PSC (n = 56)		APC (n = 104)	
	MODEL1[†]	MODEL2[‡]	MODEL1	MODEL2	MODEL1	MODEL2	MODEL1	MODEL2
	OR(95% CI)	OR(95% CI)	OR(95% CI)	OR(95% CI)	OR(95% CI)	OR(95% CI)	OR(95% CI)	OR(95% CI)
≥25 kg/m^2	1.01(0.88–1.67)	1.08(0.94–1.25)	0.921(0.76–1.11)	0.97(0.79–1.17)	0.94(0.46–1.93)	0.98(0.48–1.98)	1.47(0.97–2.24)	1.53(0.99–2.36)
Waist circumference								
≥90 cm in male, ≥80 cm in female	0.71(0.62–0.82)*	0.81(0.70–0.94)*	1.08(0.87–1.34)	1.25(1.00–1.55)*	0.95(0.49–1.84)	1.10(0.61–1.97)	0.84(0.53–1.35)	0.87(0.54–1.40)
Estrogen use (women only)								
Yes	0.76(0.59–0.99)*	0.70(0.54–0.91)*	0.79(0.54–1.14)	0.74(0.51–1.06)	0.94(0.23–3.91)	0.77(0.19–3.21)	1.59(0.62–4.04)	1.52(0.59–3.93)
Steroid use								
Yes	1.06(0.79–1.42)	0.96(0.71–1.28)	1.28(0.86–1.91)	1.19(0.78–1.80)	2.95(1.64–13.52)*	2.72(1.57–12.96)*	0.39(0.16–0.93)*	0.37(0.17–0.84)*
NSAIDs use								
Yes	0.96(0.60–1.54)	1.04(0.64–1.70)	0.84(0.43–1.64)	0.88(0.44–1.73)	0.72(0.08–6.73)	0.81(0.09–7.17)	0.59(0.19–1.88)	0.64(0.20–2.04)
Hypertension								
Yes	1.97(1.67–2.31)*	1.21(1.03–1.43)*	1.60(1.33–1.92)*	1.11(0.90–1.37)	1.24(0.63–2.41)	0.84(0.39–1.82)	1.64(1.02–2.62)*	1.30(0.8–2.12)
Diabetes								
Yes	1.99(1.60–2.48)*	1.47(1.15–1.87)*	1.29(0.99–1.66)	1.00(0.77–1.32)	3.16(1.47–6.78)*	2.60(1.19–5.68)*	0.89(0.46–1.74)	0.74(0.39–1.43)
Vitamin use								
Yes	0.99(0.83–1.19)	0.95(0.79–1.14)	1.10(0.81–1.49)	1.07(0.79–1.45)	1.36(0.36–5.18)	1.33(0.35–5.06)	0.58(0.33–1.00)	0.55(0.31–0.95)*

PSC = posterior subcapsular opacity; APC = anterior polar cataract; OR = odds ratio; CI = confidential interval; BMI = body mass index; NSAIDs = nonsteroidal anti-inflammatory drugs.
[†]Model1 = no adjustment.
[‡]Model2 = adjusted for age and sex.
* Statistically significant.
[Φ]Weight change after the age of 20 years.
[§]Classified as nondrinker, mild-to-moderate drinker (1.0–30.0 g alcohol/day), or heavy drinker (>30.0 g alcohol/day) after conversion of the average frequency and amount of alcoholic beverages consumed into the amount of pre-alcohol (in grams) consumed per day.

based on a survey of general vitamin use [7]. Identification of the components of Centrum that contribute to its protective effect against nuclear cataracts remains an area of active investigation.

Our study has some potential limitations. The KNHANES data were not collected for ophthalmologic evaluation, and much of the information is based on self-reporting. The information on smoking history, sunlight exposure, stress level, alcohol consumption, and medication use may therefore be biased. Recall bias may also confound the reporting of weight change since the age of 20 years. And although this study used photographic standards according to LOCS II classification, the gradings of the lens opacities were not investigated. We used the cut-off values for defining cataracts and this may be a weak point evaluating associated factors of cataracts. However, the strength of this study is that there have been few studies in high income Asian countries which would be interesting to compare to low and middle income Asian countries where the prevalence of cataracts were shown to be high. Also, the anthropometric measurements and diabetes and hypertension diagnoses in the current study were made by trained examiners and physicians, while many of the previous studies based this information on self-reporting. Finally, as Koreans have relatively uniform genetic and environmental influences, including a single race, climate, and food culture, the results may be more consistent than those of other large, population-based studies. Moreover, the exceptionally high prevalence of anterior polar cataract (APC) in the Korean population warrants a national data study to advance scientific knowledge and identify possible racial differences. Further studies on immigrants to Korea may provide a clue to the environmental and genetic contributors to the pathogenesis of APC.

Author Contributions

Conceived and designed the experiments: KSN. Performed the experiments: KSN CKJ. Analyzed the data: JWM CKJ. Contributed reagents/materials/analysis tools: KH YGP. Wrote the paper: KSN.

References

1. Taylor HR (1999) Epidemiology of age-related cataract. Eye (Lond) 13 (Pt 3b): 445–448.
2. West SK, Valmadrid CT (1995) Epidemiology of risk factors for age-related cataract. Surv Ophthalmol 39: 323–334.
3. Nirmalan PK, Robin AL, Katz J, Tielsch JM, Thulasiraj RD, et al. (2004) Risk factors for age related cataract in a rural population of southern India: the Aravind Comprehensive Eye Study. Br J Ophthalmol 88: 989–994.
4. Mares JA, Voland R, Adler R, Tinker L, Millen AE, et al. (2010) Healthy diets and the subsequent prevalence of nuclear cataract in women. Arch Ophthalmol 128: 738–749.
5. Landers J, Henderson T, Craig J (2010) Prevalence and associations of cataract in indigenous Australians within central Australia: the Central Australian Ocular Health Study. Clin Experiment Ophthalmol 38: 387–392.
6. (2001) Risk factors associated with age-related nuclear and cortical cataract : a case-control study in the Age-Related Eye Disease Study, AREDS Report No. 5. Ophthalmology 108: 1400–1408.
7. Chang JR, Koo E, Agrón E, Hallak J, Clemons T, et al. (2011) Risk factors associated with incident cataracts and cataract surgery in the Age-related Eye Disease Study (AREDS): AREDS report number 32. Ophthalmology 118: 2113–2119.
8. Graw J, Welzl G, Ahmad N, Klopp N, Heier M, et al. (2011) The KORA Eye Study: a population-based study on eye diseases in Southern Germany (KORA F4). Invest Ophthalmol Vis Sci 52: 7778–7786.
9. Hirvelä H, Luukinen H, Laatikainen L (1995) Prevalence and risk factors of lens opacities in the elderly in Finland. A population-based study. Ophthalmology 102: 108–117.
10. McCarty CA, Mukesh BN, Fu CL, Taylor HR (1999) The epidemiology of cataract in Australia. Am J Ophthalmol 128: 446–465.
11. Delcourt C, Cristol J-P, Tessier F, Leger CL, Michel F, et al. (2000) Risk factors for cortical, nuclear, and posterior subcapsular cataracts: the POLA study. Am J epidemiol 151:497–504.
12. Zhang JS, Xu L, Wang YX, You QS, Wang JD, et al. (2011) Five-year incidence of age-related cataract and cataract surgery in the adult population of greater Beijing: the Beijing Eye Study. Ophthalmology 118: 711–718.
13. Vashist P, Talwar B, Gogoi M, Maraini G, Camparini M, et al. (2011) Prevalence of cataract in an older population in India: the India study of age-related eye disease. Ophthalmology 118: 272–278, e1–2.
14. Wu R, Wang JJ, Mitchell P, Lamoureux EL, Zheng Y, et al. (2010) Smoking, socioeconomic factors, and age-related cataract: The Singapore Malay Eye study. Arch Ophthalmol 128: 1029–1035.
15. Foster PJ, Wong TY, Machin D, Johnson GJ, Seah SK (2003) Risk factors for nuclear, cortical and posterior subcapsular cataracts in the Chinese population of Singapore: the Tanjong Pagar Survey. Br J Ophthalmol 87: 1112–1120.
16. Kim H, Joo CK (2008) The prevalence and demographic characteristics of anterior polar cataract in a hospital-based study in Korea. Korean J Ophthalmol 22: 77–80.
17. Joo CK, Lee EH, Kim JC, Kim YH, Lee JH, et al. (1999) Degeneration and transdifferentiation of human lens epithelial cells in nuclear and anterior polar cataracts. J Cataract Refract Surg 25: 652–658.
18. Korea Centers for Disease Control and Prevention Korean National Health and Nutrition Examination Survey. Available: http://knhanes.cdc.go.kr. Accessed 2010 Sep 3.
19. Chylack LT Jr, Leske MC, McCarthy D, Khu P, Kashiwagi T, et al. (1989) Lens opacities classification system II (LOCS II). Arch Ophthalmol 107: 991–997.
20. Leske MC, Connell AM, Wu SY, Hyman L, Schachat A (1997) Prevalence of lens opacities in the Barbados Eye Study. Arch Ophthalmol 115: 105–111.
21. Richter GM, Torres M, Choudhury F, Azen SP, Varma R (2012) Risk factors for cortical, nuclear, posterior subcapsular, and mixed lens opacities: the Los Angeles Latino Eye Study. Ophthalmology 119: 547–554.
22. Tan JS, Wang JJ, Mitchell P (2008) Influence of diabetes and cardiovascular disease on the long-term incidence of cataract: the Blue Mountains eye study. Ophthalmic Epidemiol 15: 317–327.
23. Lindblad BE, Håkansson N, Philipson B, Wolk A (2010) Hormone replacement therapy in relation to risk of cataract extraction: a prospective study of women. Ophthalmology 117: 424–430.
24. Maraini G, Williams SL, Sperduto RD, Ferris F, Milton RC, et al. (2008) A randomized, double-masked, placebo-controlled clinical trial of multivitamin supplementation for age-related lens opacities. Clinical trial of nutritional supplements and age-related cataract report no. 3. Ophthalmology 115: 559–607, e1.

2

αA Crystallin May Protect against Geographic Atrophy—Meta-Analysis of Cataract vs. Cataract Surgery for Geographic Atrophy and Experimental Studies

Peng Zhou[1¶], Hong-Fei Ye[1¶], Yong-Xiang Jiang[1], Jin Yang[1], Xiang-Jia Zhu[1], Xing-Huai Sun[1], Yi Luo[1], Guo-Rui Dou[2], Yu-Sheng Wang[2], Yi Lu[1]*

1 Department of Ophthalmology, Eye and ENT Hospital of Fudan University, Shanghai, People's Republic of China, **2** Department of Ophthalmology, Xijing Hospital, Fourth Military Medical University, Xi'an, People's Republic of China

Abstract

Background: Cataract and geographic atrophy (GA, also called advanced "dry" age-related macular degeneration) are the two major causes of visual impairment in the developed world. The association between cataract surgery and the development of GA was controversial in previous studies.

Methods/Principal Findings: We performed a meta-analysis by pooling the current evidence in literature and found that cataract is associated with an increased risk of geographic atrophy with a summary odds ratio (OR) of 3.75 (95% CI: 95% CI: 1.84–7.62). However, cataract surgery is not associated with the risk of geographic atrophy (polled OR = 3.23, 95% CI: 0.63–16.47). Further experiments were performed to analyze how the αA-crystallin, the major component of the lens, influences the development of GA in a mouse model. We found that theαA-crystallin mRNA and protein expression increased after oxidative stress induced by $NaIO_3$ in immunohistochemistry of retinal section and western blot of posterior eyecups. Both functional and histopathological evidence confirmed that GA is more severe in αA-crystallin knockout mice compared to wild-type mice.

Conclusions: Therefore, αA-crystallin may protect against geographic atrophy. This study provides a better understanding of the relationship between cataract, cataract surgery, and GA.

Editor: Demetrios Vavvas, Massachusetts Eye & Ear Infirmary, Harvard Medical School, United States of America

Funding: This research was supported by grant from the National Basic Research Program of China (973 Program) No. 2011CB510200, National Natural Science Foundation of China (NSFC) No. 81070740 and No. 81070717. The funders had no role in study design, data collection and analysis, decision to publish, or preparation of the manuscript.

Competing Interests: The authors have declared that no competing interests exist.

* E-mail: luyi0705@yahoo.com.cn

¶ These authors contributed equally to this work.

Introduction

Cataract and age-related macular degeneration (AMD) are the two major causes of visual impairment in the developed world [1]. Cataract is a clouding that develops in the crystalline lens of the eye. Cataract surgery is currently one of the most frequently performed and successful surgical procedures [2]. Advanced AMD has two major subtypes: geographic atrophy (GA, also called advanced "dry" AMD) and choroidal neovascularization (also called "wet" AMD) [3]. Geographic atrophy [4–6] is characterized by confluent areas of cell death in photoreceptors and retinal pigment epithelium, is bilateral in more than half of patients, and is responsible for 10% of the cases of legal blindness resulting from age-related macular degeneration. Both cataract and GA are strongly age related.

The association between cataract surgery and the development of GA was controversial in previous studies. In the Beaver Dam Eye Study (BDES) [7], a positive cross-sectional association was found between cataract surgery and GA. The association was consistent with findings in the Los Angeles Latino Eye Study (LALES) [8], but not with findings in the Blue Mountains Eye Study (BMES) [9] or the Age-related Eye Disease Study (AREDS) [10]. However, the positive association between cataracts and GA was consistent in the Beaver Dam Eye Study [7] and LALES [8].

The pathogenesis of the association between cataract surgery and GA is less clear. The previous hypothesis is that cataract removal results in increased risk because the cataract, a barrier to ultraviolet radiation, has been removed [11]. Based on this hypothesis, in theory, the prevalence of GA should be decreased in patients with cataract. However, the truth is that the prevalence of GA is higher in patients with cataract than the control. Therefore, this hypothesis is not sufficient to explain the clinical phenomenon.

One common change involving cataracts and cataract surgery has been neglected: the change of α-crystallins, which are the major protein of lens. The α-crystallins are small heat shock proteins which play central roles in maintaining lens transparency and refractive properties [12]. The discovery in 1992 that these proteins possess chaperone-like activity has led most researchers to focus on the ability of α-crystallins to prevent protein aggregation in vitro. While the ability of α-crystallins to efficiently trap aggregation-prone denatured proteins in vitro is thought to delay the development of age-related cataracts in vivo, α-crystallins have additional functions which may also contribute to cataract pathology. In addition to chaperone activity, α-crystallins are known to protect cells from stress-induced apoptosis, regulate cell growth, and enhance genomic stability [13]. They also physically and functionally interact with both the cell membrane and cytoskeleton. Functional changes in α-crystallin have been shown to modify membrane and cell-cell interactions and lead to lens cell pathology in vivo [14].

Because most studies on geographic atrophy and cataract surgery or cataracts had relatively small sample sizes, we combined pieces of evidence from the published literature for a meta-analysis. In this study, we preformed a meta-analysis focusing on the association between GA and cataracts or cataract surgery. Furthermore, the function of α-crystallins was studied in a GA animal model to investigate its role in the development of GA.

Materials and Methods

Meta-analysis

This meta-analysis followed the PISMA statement guidelines. [15] The meta-analysis of the association between GA and cataract or cataract surgery was performed as we have described previously [16]. In brief, relevant studies were selected by searching PubMed and Web of Science database (updated to December 5, 2011) using the following search terms: ("cataract" OR "cataract surgery") AND ("age-related macular degeneration" OR "geographic atrophy") with the limit "humans". All the resulting studies were retrieved, and their references were checked for other relevant publications. Review articles were also searched to find additional eligible studies. Only studies published in English with full-text articles were included in this meta-analysis. We did not define any minimum number of patients for a study to be included in the meta-analysis. For overlapping studies, only the one with the latest published was included.The identified articles were read carefully and assessed independently by two of the authors (Zhou, P and Lu, Y), and any discrepancies in their eligibility were adjudicated by Sun, XH.

The inclusion criteria were: (1) evaluating the association between the cataract and risk of geographic atrophy; (2) evaluating the association between the cataract surgery and risk of geographic atrophy; and (3) with sufficient available data to estimate an OR with its 95% CI. The included studies had to meet [(1)+(3)] or [(2)+(3)] of the above-mentioned criteria. Any study with internally inconsistent data was excluded. The following variables were extracted from each study, if available: first author's surname, publication year, numbers of cases and controls, and numbers of cases and controls in different groups whenever possible. Information was carefully and independently extracted from all the eligible publications by two of the authors (Zhou, P and Lu, Y). Disagreement was resolved by discussion between the authors. If they could not reach a consensus, another investigator (Sun, XH) adjudicated over the disagreements. (Figure S1, Table S1)

ORs and their 95% CIs were obtained directly or calculated from the data given in the articles. A random- or a fixed-effects model was used to calculate the pooled effect estimates in the presence ($P<0.10$) or absence ($P>0.10$) of heterogeneity, respectively. The potential publication bias was examined visually in a funnel plot of log [OR] against its standard error (SE), and the degree of asymmetry was tested using Egger's test ($P<0.05$ considered to be statistically significant). We conducted influence analysis by omitting each study to find potential outliers. All of the statistical analyses were performed using Stata/SE version 11.0 (Stata Corporation, College Station, TX).

Animals

The 129S6/SvEvTac wild-type mice were purchased from Chinese Scientific Academy (Shanghai, China), while the αA-crystallin knockout mice in 129S6/SvEvTac background [17] were obtained from the National Eye Institute. Mice between 6 and 8 weeks old were fed the standard laboratory chow in an air-conditioned room equipped with a 12-hour light/12-hour dark cycle. All procedures were performed in compliance with the Fudan University Institutional Animal Care and Use Committee's approved protocols and the ARVO Statement for the Use of Animals in Ophthalmic and Vision Research.

Chemical formulation and experimental procedure

Mice were briefly restrained. Sodium iodate ($NaIO_3$; Sigma, St. Louis, MO) was diluted with Phosphate buffered saline (PBS) solution and 20 mg/kg body weight of $NaIO_3$ was injected through the tail vein. [18] Animals injected with equivalent volumes of PBS solution served as controls. Electroretinography and fundus photographs were assessed at 21 days post injection. After the tests were made, mice were euthanized with CO_2 and their eyes processed for histology.

Experimental groups

The mice were divided into four groups: control wild type (PBS-treated WT), $NaIO_3$-treated wild type ($NaIO_3$-treated WT), control αA-crystallin knockout mice (PBS-treated αA−/−), and $NaIO_3$-treated αA-crystallin knockout mice ($NaIO_3$-treated αA−/−). Each group consisted of seven mice in the age range of 6–8 weeks.

Electroretinography (ERG)

Mice were dark-adapted overnight and anesthetized by intraperitoneal injection of ketamine (100 mg/kg body weight) and xylazine (10 mg/kg body weight). Pupils were dilated with topical administration of 2.5% phenylephrine containing 0.5% tropicamide, and the cornea was anesthetized with 0.5% proparacaine. Scotopic ERGs were measured from dark-adapted mice using a low-intensity stimulus, and mesopic ERGs were measured using a non-attenuated light stimulus. To measure cone responses, a 6 lux white background light was delivered through the other arm of the coaxial cable to suppress rod responses, and a non-attenuated light stimulus was applied. The a-wave amplitude was measured from the baseline to the trough of the a-wave, while b-wave amplitude was measured from the trough of the a-wave to the peak of the b-wave.

Histopathologic analysis

For histopathologic analysis, eyes were enucleated, and the anterior poles were removed. The remaining eyecups were snap-frozen in tissue-freezing medium (Triangle Biomedical Sciences, Durham, NC). Sections (8 μm) were stained with hematoxylin and eosin (H&E) to assess the histopathologic changes of retina.

Western blot analysis

The western blot was performed as described previously. [19,20] Lysed posterior eyecups, including retina and RPE, were centrifuged at 11,000 g for 20 minutes. Supernatants were collected, and proteins were resolved on Tris-HCl 10% polyacrylamide gels (Ready Gel; Bio-Rad, Hercules, CA) at 120 V. The proteins were transferred to PVDF blotting membrane (Millipore, Bedford, MA). The membranes were probed with antibody for αA-crystallin (Stressgen, San Diego, CA) and GAPDH (Millipore) at 1:1,000 dilution. Membranes were washed and incubated with a horseradish peroxidase (HRP)-conjugated secondary antibody (1:3,000, Vector Laboratories, Burlingame, CA) for 30 min at room temperature. Images were developed by adding ECL chemiluminescence detection solution (Amersham Pharmacia Biotech, Cleveland, OH).

Immunohistochemistry

Immunohistochemical stains were performed on freezing tissue sections. After blocking with 20% normal donkey serum for 30 minutes, slides were probed overnight at 4°C with primary αA-crystallin antibody (Stressgen, San Diego, CA) diluted into blocking solution. Slides were incubated with biotinylated goat anti-rabbit immunoglobulin Ig G (1:500) for 1 h at room temperature. The signal was detected using streptavidin-conjugated horseradish peroxidase and peroxidase activity was visualized with diaminobenzidine/H2O2 (Vector Laboratories, Burlingame, CA). After color development, slides were counterstained with hematoxylin.

Reverse transcription PCR and relative quantitative real-time PCR

The reverse transcription PCR (RT-PCRwas performed as described previously. [16] Total RNA was isolated using a TRIzol reagent (Invitrogen, Carlsbad, CA, USA). The first strand of cDNA was synthesized with 1 µg of total RNA, oligo(dT) primer and AMV reverse transcriptase (Promega, Madison, WI, USA). The primers used in RT-PCR were as follows: CRYAA forward: 5′- TTTTGAGTATGACCTGCTGCC - 3′, reverse: 5′-TGGAACTCACGGGAAATGTAG -3′; GAPDH, forward: 5′-GAAGGTGAAGGTCGGAGTC -3′, reverse: 5′- GAA-GATGGTGATGGGATTTC -3′. [21] The specificity of the PCR amplification products was checked by performing dissociation melting-curve analysis and by 1% agarose gel electrophoresis. Quantification analysis of CRYAA mRNA was normalized with a housekeeping gene, GAPDH, as an internal control.

Isolation of primary cultured RPE cells from mice

Primary cultured RPE cells were isolated from knockout mice as previously described. [22] The cornea, lens, vitreous, and retina were removed from eyes soaked in phosphate buffered saline (PBS) containing 5% penicillin/streptomycin (Sigma). The choroid/sclera tissue was then placed into a 2% dispase solution in PBS for 20 min at 37°C. After the incubation, the tissue was rapidly pipetted up and down for 30 s. The dispase solution containing the RPE cells was passed through a 70 µ filter followed by a 40 µ filter after which the cells were spun down and resuspended in Ham's F-12 Media (Cellgro, Herndon, VA) containing at least 25% fetal bovine serum (FBS; Irvine Scientific, Santa Ana, CA). The RPE were then grown on laminin coated plates (Becton Dickinson and Company, Franklin Lakes, NJ).

Detection of ROS Production

To determine the compartmentalized accumulation of reactive oxygen species (ROS), cells on an eight-well Lab-TekTM chamber were stained with carboxy-H2-DCFDA (Molecular Probes; 5 µM for 1 h at 37°C), and rapidly evaluated by confocal microscopy (LSM510, Zeiss, Thornwood, NY, USA). A green color is observed when ROS accumulated. Nucleus were stained with propidium Iodide (PI) as red fluorescence.

Statistics

All experiments were repeated at least three times. Values in the figures were expressed as means ± SE. Statistical analyses were performed with Student's *t* test. Values in the figures are expressed as means±SE. Values of $P<0.05$ were considered statistically significant.

Results

Meta-analysis shows that cataract, not cataract surgery, is associated with an increased risk of geographic atrophy

We performed a meta-analysis focusing on the relationship between geographic atrophy and cataract or cataract surgery. There were four published articles [7–10] investigating the association between cataract surgery and geographic atrophy risk (Figure S1). Two studies investigated the association between cataract and geographic atrophy risk [7,8] (Figure S1). Table 1 lists the main characteristics of relevant studies.

Positive association between cataract and risk of geographic atrophy was found (polled OR = 3.75, 95% CI: 1.84–7.62, $P = <0.001$). However, no significant association between cataract

Table 1. Characteristics of studies included in meta-analysis.

No.	Year	First Author	Studies	Cataract surgery				Cataract			
				surgery		control		cataract		control	
				(n = 988)		(n = 21,918)		(n = 1,969)		(n = 12,924)	
				GA	No GA	GA	No GA	GA	No GA	GA	No GA
1	2002	Klein	BDES	3	94	17	3328	8	562	11	2718
2	2006	Cugati	BMES	4	128	51	2271	N.A.	N.A.	N.A.	N.A.
3	2008	Chew	AREDS	14	525	205	5383	N.A.	N.A.	N.A.	N.A.
4	2010	Fraser-Bell	LALES	4	216	9	10654	5	1394	8	9287

BDES = Beaver Dam Eye Study;
LALES = Los Angeles Latino Eye Study;
BMES = Blue Mountains Eye Study;
AREDS = Age-related Eye Disease Study;
N.A. = not available.

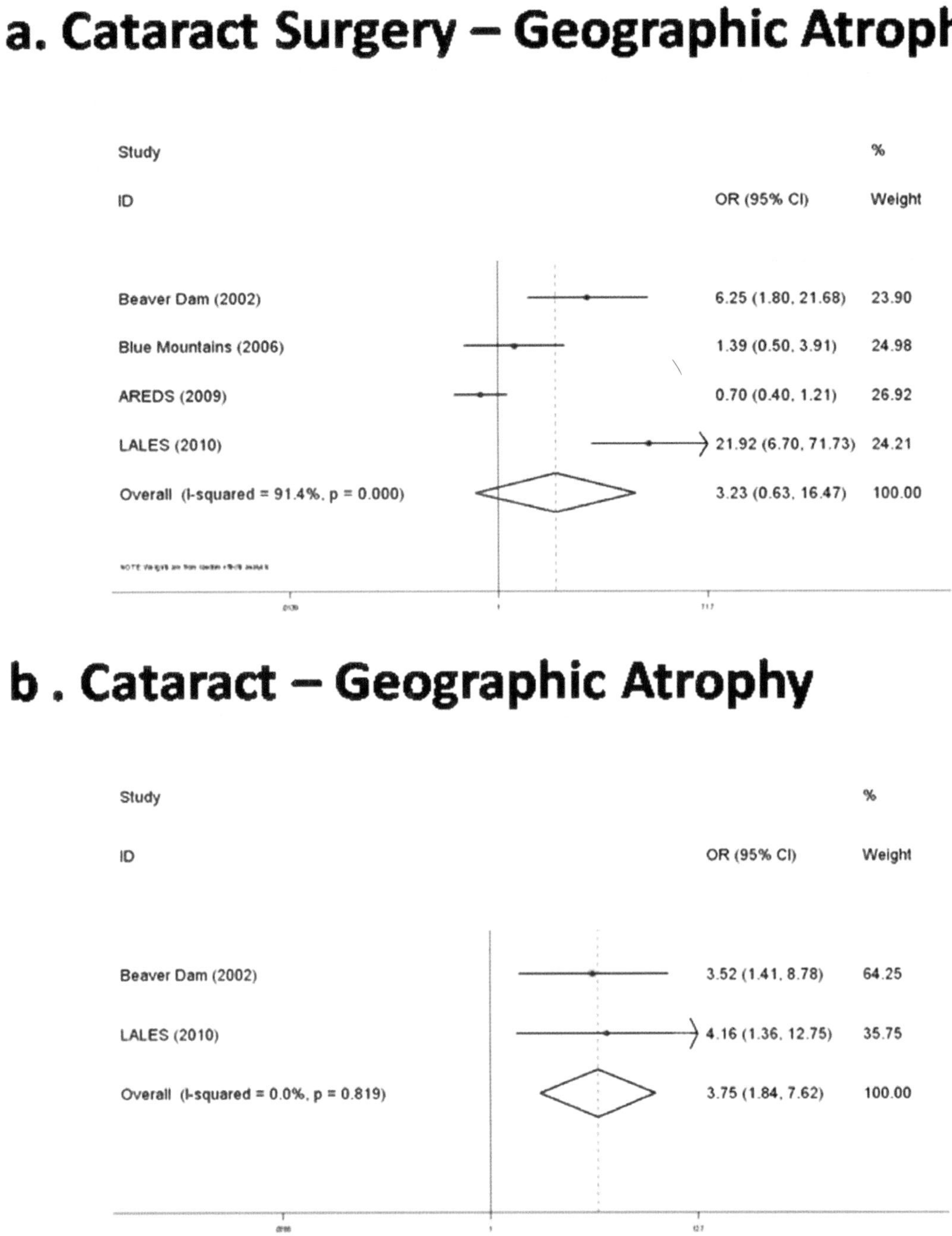

Figure 1. The forest plot of meta-analysis. Each study is shown by the point estimate of the odds ratio (OR) (the size of the square is proportional to the weight of each study) and the 95% confidence interval (CI) for the OR (extending lines). a. the association of cataract surgery with geographic atrophy; b. the association of cataract with geographic atrophy. LALES = Los Angeles Latino Eye Study; BMES = Blue Mountains Eye Study; AREDS = Age-related Eye Disease Study.

surgery and risk of geographic atrophy was found (polled OR = 3.23, 95% CI: 0.63–16.47, $P = 0.159$). (Figure 1, Table 2).

Reduced ERG amplitudes in $NaIO_3$-treated αA-crystallin knockout mice

To determine whether the absence of αA-crystallin had an effect on the retinal function of $NaIO_3$-induced retinal degeneration, we compared mesopic (mixed rod and cone) ERG responses of the four groups of mice (PBS-treated WT, $NaIO_3$-treated WT, PBS-treated αA−/−, and $NaIO_3$-treated αA−/−) at the end of 3 weeks. Significant differences were observed in the ERGs of $NaIO_3$-treated αA−/− mice compared with the PBS-treated αA−/− mice (Figure 2). No significant differences were found between the ERGs of the $NaIO_3$-treated and control in wild-type mice.

The amplitudes of a-wave of the ERG of $NaIO_3$-treated αA−/− mice decreased by 78.11% of that of PBS-treated αA−/−

Table 2. Pooled ORs of TLR3 1234C>T in different genetic models.

	Ph	Polling Model	Polled OR (95%CI)	*P*
Cataract surgery - GA	<0.001	Random M-H	3.23 (0.63–16.47)	0.159
Cataract - GA	0.819	Fixed M-H	3.75 (1.84–7.62)	<0.001

Ph = *P* value of *Q* test for heterogeneity test;
OR = odds ratio;
CI = confidence interval.
M-H = Mantel-Haenszel.

mice. The amplitudes of b-wave of the ERG of $NaIO_3$-treated αA−/− mice decreased by 60.26%, compared with that of PBS-treated αA−/− mice. Generally speaking, a-wave of ERG demonstrates the function of the outer layer of the retina, while b-wave shows that of the inner layer. The ERG results suggested that the function of the outer layer of retina was more suppressed than that of the inner layer.

Histopathological evidence for accelerated $NaIO_3$-induced degeneration in αA-crystallin knockout mice

Retinas from αA-crystallin knockout mice revealed more severe degeneration from $NaIO_3$ injection as compared to wild-type retinas. An assessment of the extent of retinal damage by $NaIO_3$ was made by counting the number of nuclei in the inner nuclear layer, outer nuclear layer, and ganglion cell layer of wild type and

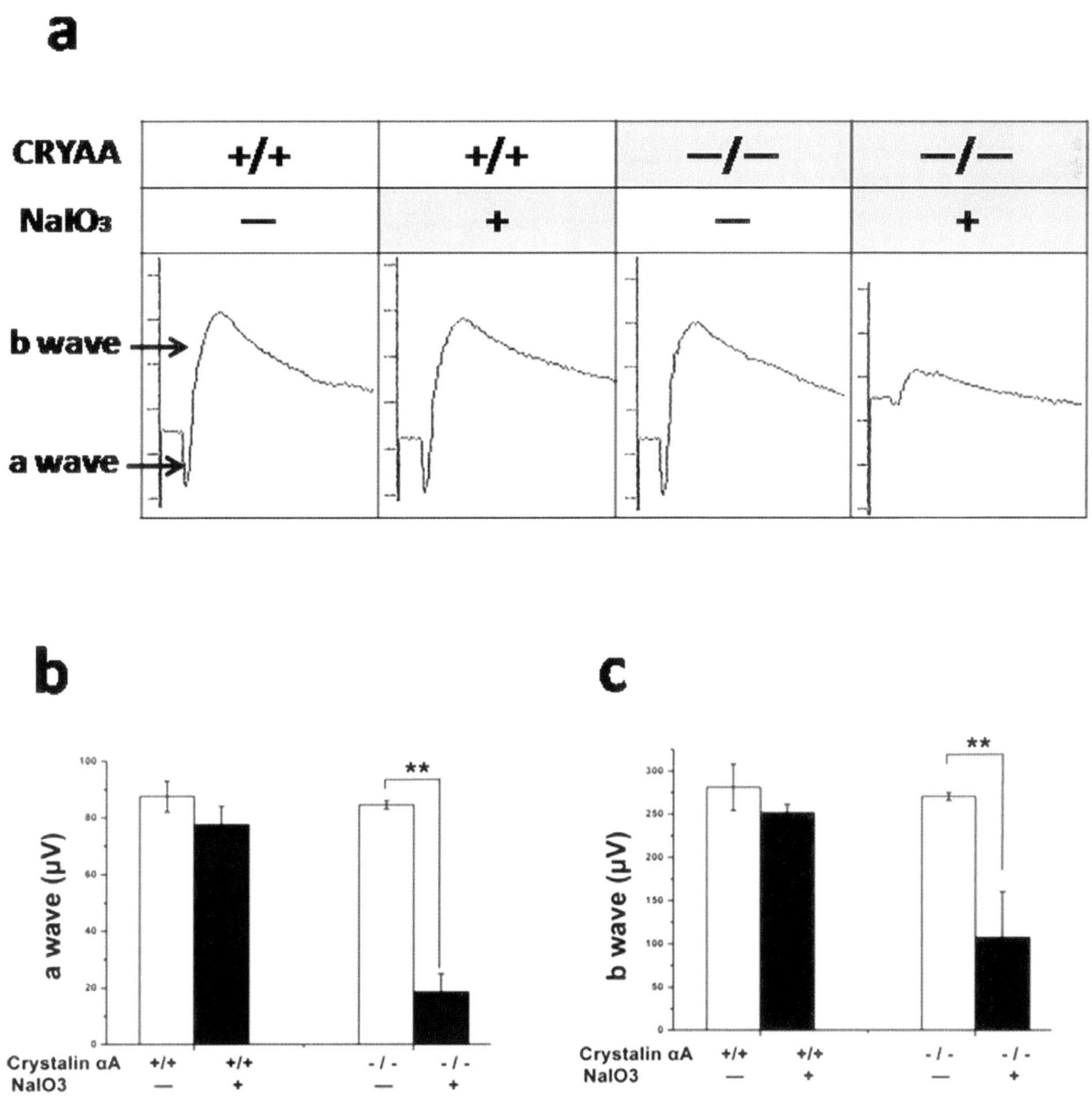

Figure 2. Reduced ERG amplitudes in $NaIO_3$-treated αA-crystallin knockout mice. The amplitudes of a-wave of the ERG of $NaIO_3$-treated αA−/− mice decreased to 21.89% of that of PBS-treated αA−/− mice. The amplitudes of b-wave of the ERG of $NaIO_3$-treated αA−/− mice decreased by 60.26%, compared with that of PBS-treated αA−/− mice. Data are mean ± SEM, n = 5/group, $^{**}P<0.01$.

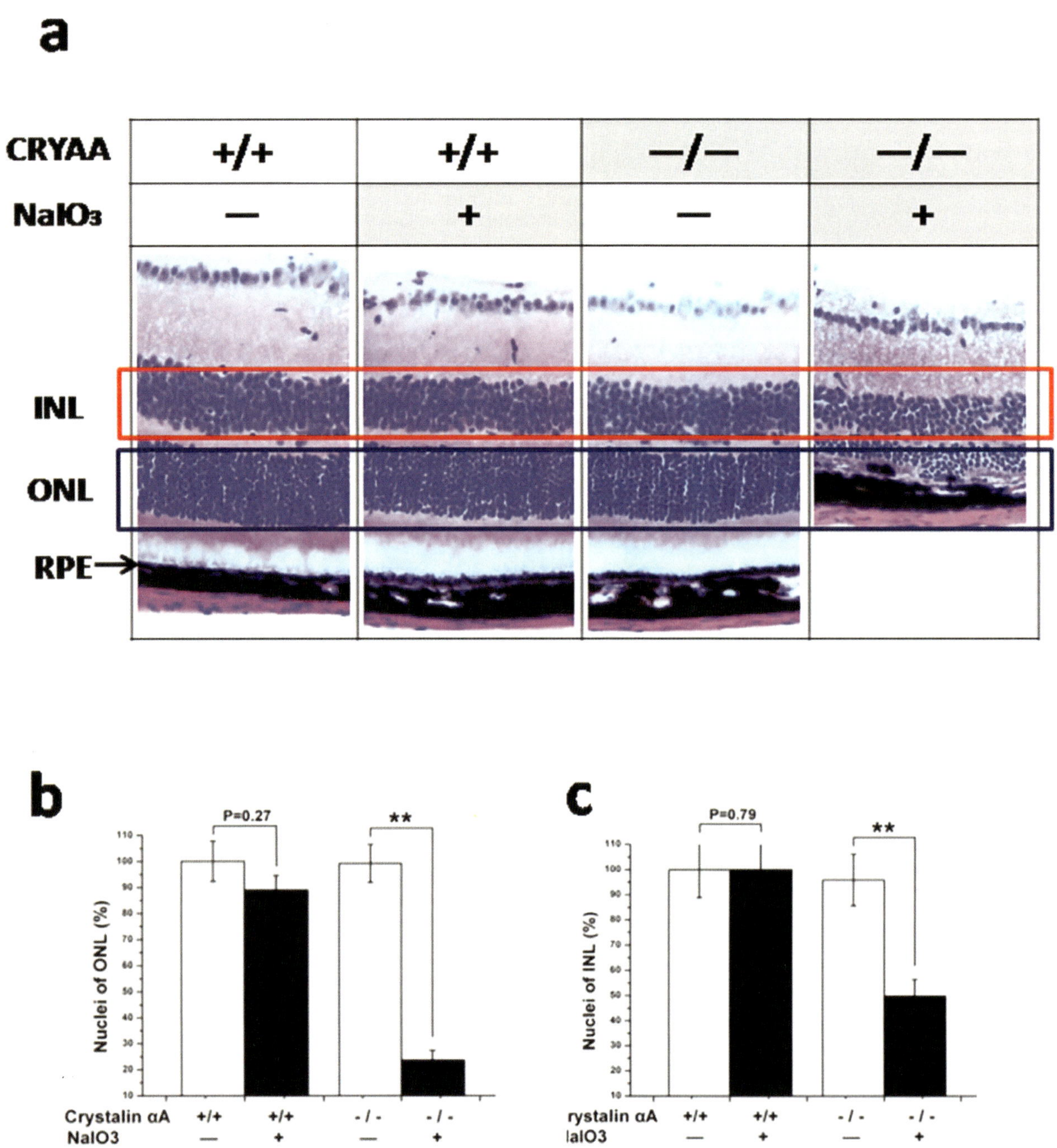

Figure 3. Histopathological evidence for accelerated $NaIO_3$-induced degeneration in αA-crystallin knockout mice. Retinas from αA-crystallin knockout mice revealed more severe degeneration from $NaIO_3$ injection as compared to wild-type retinas. The loss of nuclei was more prominent in αA-crystallin knockout retina vs. that of wild type. The decrease in the number of nuclei per unit area was statistically significant with $NaIO_3$ injection only in the outer nuclear layer of the crystallin knockout mice. No significant differences of nuclei numbers were found between the $NaIO_3$-injected and PBS-injected in wild-type mice. The RPE layers were discontinuous and damaged in αA-crystallin knockout mice with $NaIO_3$ injection, while they were continuous in wild-type mice. CRYAA = αA-crystallin; INL = inner nuclear layer; ONL = outer nuclear layer; RPE = retinal pigmental epithelium; **$P<0.01$.

αA-crystallin knockout retinas. This semi-quantitative analysis revealed that the loss of nuclei was more prominent at 3 weeks post injection of $NaIO_3$ in αA-crystallin knockout retina vs. that of wild type. The decrease in the number of nuclei per unit area was statistically significant ($p<0.01$) with $NaIO_3$ injection only in the outer nuclear layer of the crystallin knockout mice. No significant differences of nuclei numbers were found between the $NaIO_3$-injected and PBS-injected in wild-type mice (Figure 3).

The RPE layers were discontinuous and damaged in αA-crystallin knockout mice with $NaIO_3$ injection, while they were continuous in wild type mice.

Increased αA-crystallin expression after $NaIO_3$ treatment

Immunohistochemistry staining showed that αA-crystallin in retina increased after $NaIO_3$ treatment. (Figure 4a) Protein expression of αA-crystallin of mice eye cup after $NaIO_3$ treatment

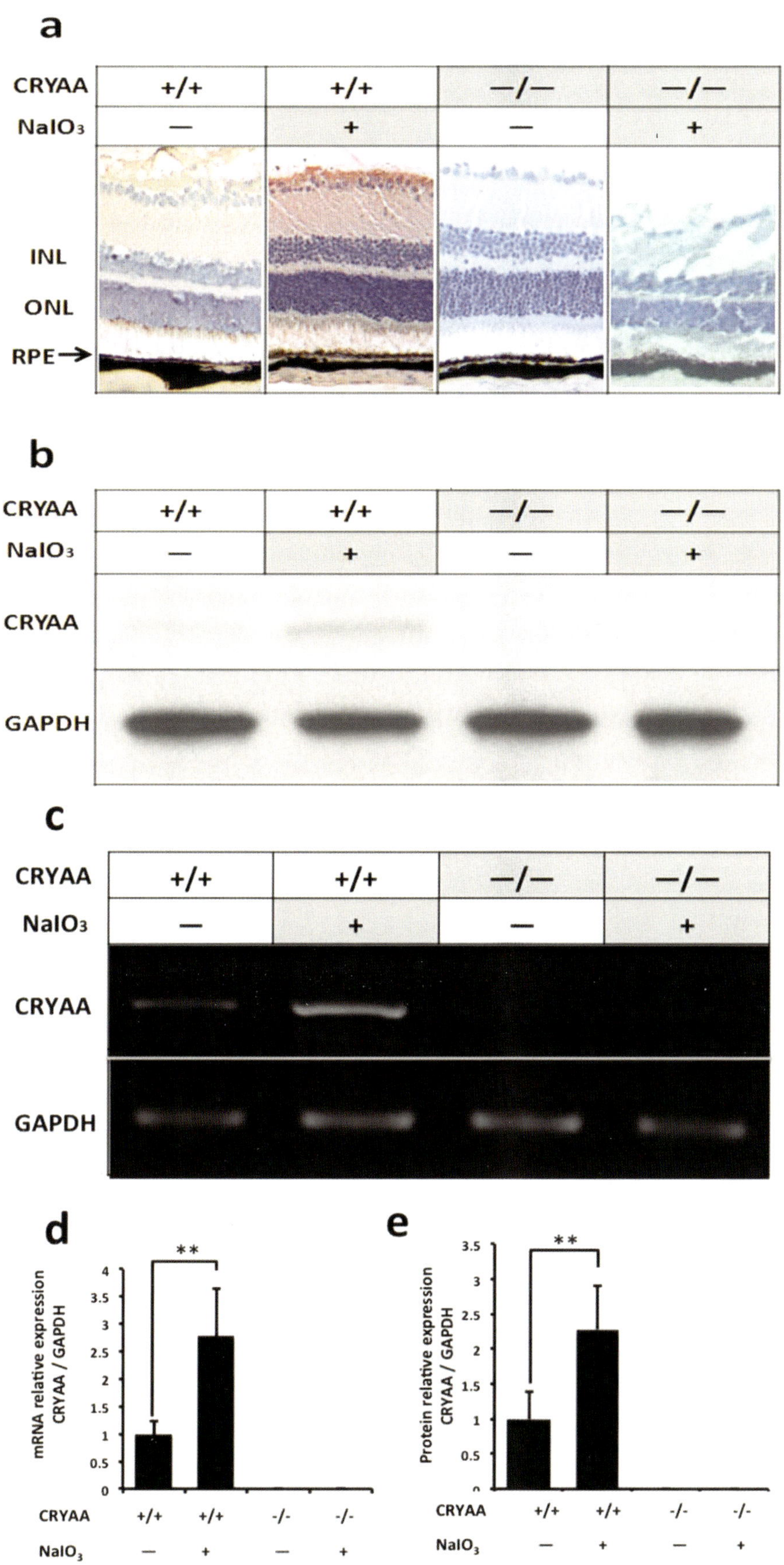
a
CRYAA
+/+
+/+
—/—
—/—
NaIO3
—
+
—
+
INL
ONL
RPE
b
CRYAA
+/+
+/+
—/—
—/—
NaIO3
—
+
—
+
CRYAA
GAPDH
c
CRYAA
+/+
+/+
—/—
—/—
NaIO3
—
+
—
+
CRYAA
GAPDH
d
mRNA relative expression CRYAA / GAPDH
**
CRYAA +/+ +/+ -/- -/-
NaIO3 — + — +
e
Protein relative expression CRYAA / GAPDH
**
CRYAA +/+ +/+ -/- -/-
NaIO3 — + — +

Figure 4. Increased αA-crystallin expression after $NaIO_3$ treatment. Immunohistochemistry staining showed that αA-crystallin in retina increased after $NaIO_3$ treatment. Protein expression of αA-crystallin of mice eye cup after $NaIO_3$ treatment was examined by Western blot analysis. αA-crystallin prtein increased to 2.28±0.62 times comparing to control ($p<0.01$), while mRNA increased 2.79±0.86 times comparing to control ($p<0.01$). No αA-crystallin was detected in αA-crystallin knockout mice. CRYAA = αA-crystallin, **P<0.01.

was examined by Western blot analysis. αA-crystallin increased to 2.28±0.62 times comparing to control ($p<0.01$). No αA-crystallin protein was detected in αA-crystallin knockout mice. (Figure 4b, d) mRNA expression of αA-crystallin of mice eye cup after $NaIO_3$ treatment was examined by RT-PCR analysis. αA-crystallin increased to 2.79±0.86 times comparing to control ($p<0.01$). No αA-crystallin mRNA was detected in αA-crystallin knockout mice. (Figure 4c, e) All experiments were repeated at least three times.

Increased accumulation of ROS in CRYAA −/− RPE cells

Primary cultured RPE cells was isolated from knockout mice and treated with $NaIO_3$. Figure 5 shows confocal images of ROS accumulation in RPE cells. The accumulation of ROS was much stronger in RPE cells from αA-crystallin knock our mice than that from wild type mice. These results show that knock out αA-crystallin results in increased accumulation of ROS in RPE cells treated with $NaIO_3$.

Discussion

The meta-analysis shows that cataract, not cataract surgery, is associated with an increased risk of geographic atrophy. Further experiments found that αA-crystallin may play an important role in this association.

Only a small number of publications could be included in the meta-analysis. The overall scientific level of evidence of these articles was not high. There were no trials at the highest level of evidence, which are randomized controlled trials (RCT). It needs to be mentioned that randomizing patients to not undergo cataract surgery when their vision is poor enough to affect their daily life would neither be ethical nor practicable. Thus, observational cohort studies and non-randomized clinical trials are probably the best possible evidence. Both are rated as a level 2 on the five-step hierarchy of levels of evidence for medical studies [23].

The results of our meta-analysis is not consistent with previous theory that increased risk or progression of GA (dry age-related macular degeneration) after cataract surgery is related to the increased exposure of the retina to short-wavelength light [11,24,25]. However, the meta-analysis of 22,906 patients did not find significant association between cataract surgery and GA. Instead, we found that cataract is associated with an increased risk of geographic atrophy. That means that the risk of GA increased in cataract patients, although they had cataract as a barrier to short-wavelength light. Therefore, the short-wavelength light damage theory is not sufficient to explain our meta-analysis findings.

αA-Crystallin, which is a member of the small heat shock protein (sHSP also known as the HSP20) family, plays an important neuroprotection function in retina. [22,26–28] We analyzed cataracts and cataract surgery, and found that they have a common change: the crystallins in the lens. Cataracts cause crystallins to degenerate, and cataract surgery removes the lens, the largest bank of crystallins from the eyes. Furthermore, experiments were performed to analyze the effect of αA-crystallin on GA in a mouse model. We found that αA-crystallin expression increased after oxidative stress induced by NaIO3. Both functional and histopathological evidence confirmed that GA is more severe in αA-crystallin knockout mice compared with wild-type mice.

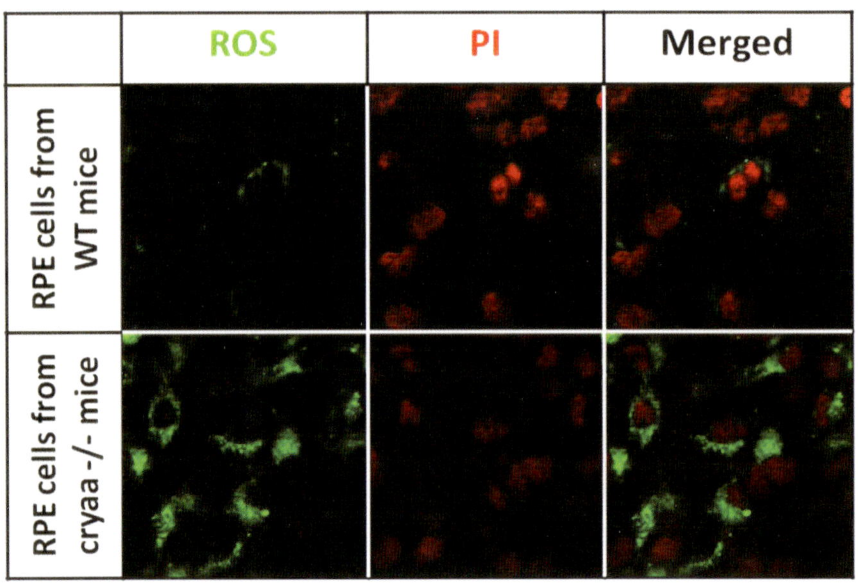

Figure 5. Increased accumulation of ROS in CRYAA −/− RPE cells. Primary cultured RPE cells was isolated from knockout mice and treated with NaIO3. Confocal images show ROS accumulation in RPE cells. The accumulation of ROS was much stronger in RPE cells from αA-crystallin knock our mice than that from wild type mice. These results show that knock out αA-crystallin results in increased accumulation of ROS in RPE cells treated with NaIO3.

Dry AMD is a challenging disease to study because of its complex genetics, late onset, and confounding environmental risk factors. As with other human diseases, finding a model system for AMD has been a demanding task. The pathology of dry AMD consists of degeneration of photoreceptors and the RPE, lipofuscin accumulation, and drusen formation. Genetically engineered mice have been used for generating models that simulate human AMD features. However, most mice develop retinal lesions at an older age (6–24 months). [29] Furthermore, there is no CRYAA −/− genetically engineered dry AMD mice. Therefore, we tried to find another way to mimic the dry AMD. Oxidative stress plays an important role in the pathogenesis of dry AMD. [30] NaIO3 can induce oxidative stress. NaIO3 damages mostly the central pole of the retina in low dose. Such a pathological phenomenon resembles those observed in dry AMD in their clinical course that initially involve the central part of the retina and spread gradually. Therefore, chemical damage induced by NaIO3 mimics dry AMD in humans and may serve as a model useful for studying retinal damage. [31] Therefore, we selected this model in our study.

The association of cataract with an increased risk of geographic atrophy can be explained by our findings. The pathogenesis of cataract is the degeneration of crystallins [32]. αA-crystallin is the major protein of the lens [17]. Neal's study showed that the concentration of alpha-A crystallins in vitreous is decreased in cataract patients. [33] After having cataract, the αA-crystallin degenerates. The total of active αA-crystallin decreases. Therefore, those people with cataract are more susceptible to have GA compared with people without cataract in the same dose of oxidative stress.

The phenomenon that cataract surgery is not associated with an increased risk of geographic atrophy can also be explained by our findings. Neal et. al reported that the concentration of αA-crystallin in vitreous is increased after cataract surgery [33]. Increased αA-crystallin may protect retina from GA. The protective αA-crystallins is produced by "after cataract". Over the year, many patients who have an uncomplicated routine cataract surgery will developed a clouding or a thickening of a natural membrane in the eye which sits just behind the lens implant, called the posterior lens capsule. This has been referred to as "after-cataract" or a secondary capsular opacification. The "after cataract" will produce new αA-crystallins and leak into vitreous.

In this study, ERG findings, the a-wave amplitude decreased more than that of b-wave in knockout mice exposed to oxidative stress. This suggests that the function of the outer retina was more suppressed than the inner, in relation to controls. However, only outer retinal atrophy was seen in histopathological findings. This phenomenon may because that the changes of function are earlier than that of anatomy. [34] ERG may be a better test to evaluate the retinal response to oxidative stress damage.

Some limitations of this meta-analysis should be acknowledged. First, this study involves two subjects, human patients with unknown genetic background and mice with clear genetic defects. However, there is not a sub-population of human subjects with congenital aA-Crystallin defects, which may share similarity to the aA-crystallin KO mice and contribute the correlations between lens and retina degenerating defects.

We put forward a hypothesis that the eye has an oxidation/anti-oxidation homeostasis. αA-crystallin is an important anti-oxidation factor. In young people, the αA-crystallin is sufficient to fend off oxidative stress damage, so their eyes do not have GA. When people have cataracts, the degenerative αA-crystallin cannot protect against oxidative stress damage, and they get GA. After cataract surgery, the concentration of αA-crystallin increases in the vitreous, and those eyes have more anti-oxidation factors. They are less likely to have GA than those who did not have cataract surgeries.

Supporting Information

Figure S1 Flow diagram of papers accepted and rejected during selection procedure. Five - hundred-seventy-seven potentially relevant studies were identified from the PubMed and Web of Science database of which 6 were eligible for our review.

Table S1 Checklist of items to include when reporting a systematic review or meta-analysis.

Author Contributions

Conceived and designed the experiments: YL PZ YSW. Performed the experiments: PZ HFY YXJ JY XJZ GRD. Analyzed the data: XHS YL. Contributed reagents/materials/analysis tools: PZ. Wrote the paper: PZ.

References

1. Chang JR, Koo E, Agron E, Hallak J, Clemons T, et al. (2011) Risk Factors Associated with Incident Cataracts and Cataract Surgery in the Age-Related Eye Disease Study (AREDS): AREDS Report Number 32. Ophthalmology 118: 2113–2119.
2. Meekins LC, Afshari NA (2011) Ever-evolving technological advances in cataract surgery: can perfection be achieved? Curr Opin Ophthalmol.
3. Yang Z, Stratton C, Francis PJ, Kleinman ME, Tan PL, et al. (2008) Toll-like receptor 3 and geographic atrophy in age-related macular degeneration. N Engl J Med 359: 1456–1463.
4. Ferris FL 3rd, Fine SL, Hyman L (1984) Age-related macular degeneration and blindness due to neovascular maculopathy. Arch Ophthalmol 102: 1640–1642.
5. Hyman LG, Lilienfeld AM, Ferris FL 3rd, Fine SL (1983) Senile macular degeneration: a case-control study. Am J Epidemiol 118: 213–227.
6. Sarks JP, Sarks SH, Killingsworth MC (1988) Evolution of geographic atrophy of the retinal pigment epithelium. Eye (Lond) 2 (Pt 5): 552–577.
7. Klein R, Klein BE, Wong TY, Tomany SC, Cruickshanks KJ (2002) The association of cataract and cataract surgery with the long-term incidence of age-related maculopathy: the Beaver Dam eye study. Arch Ophthalmol 120: 1551–1558.
8. Fraser-Bell S, Choudhury F, Klein R, Azen S, Varma R (2010) Ocular risk factors for age-related macular degeneration: the Los Angeles Latino Eye Study. Am J Ophthalmol 149: 735–740.
9. Cugati S, Mitchell P, Rochtchina E, Tan AG, Smith W, et al. (2006) Cataract surgery and the 10-year incidence of age-related maculopathy: the Blue Mountains Eye Study. Ophthalmology 113: 2020–2025.
10. Chew EY, Sperduto RD, Milton RC, Clemons TE, Gensler GR, et al. (2009) Risk of advanced age-related macular degeneration after cataract surgery in the Age-Related Eye Disease Study: AREDS report 25. Ophthalmology 116: 297–303.
11. Patel JI (2007) Is cataract surgery a risk factor for progression of macular degeneration? Curr Opin Ophthalmol 18: 9–12.
12. Maulucci G, Papi M, Arcovito G, De Spirito M (2011) The thermal structural transition of alpha-crystallin inhibits the heat induced self-aggregation. PLoS One 6: e18906.
13. Derham BK, Harding JJ (1999) Alpha-crystallin as a molecular chaperone. Prog Retin Eye Res 18: 463–509.
14. Andley UP (2009) Effects of alpha-crystallin on lens cell function and cataract pathology. Curr Mol Med 9: 887–892.
15. Liberati A, Altman DG, Tetzlaff J, Mulrow C, Gotzsche PC, et al. (2009) The PRISMA statement for reporting systematic reviews and meta-analyses of studies that evaluate health care interventions: explanation and elaboration. PLoS Med 6: e1000100.
16. Zhou P, Fan L, Yu KD, Zhao MW, Li XX (2011) Toll-like receptor 3 C1234T may protect against geographic atrophy through decreased dsRNA binding capacity. FASEB J 25: 3489–3495.
17. Brady JP, Garland D, Duglas-Tabor Y, Robison WG Jr, Groome A, et al. (1997) Targeted disruption of the mouse alpha A-crystallin gene induces cataract and cytoplasmic inclusion bodies containing the small heat shock protein alpha B-crystallin. Proc Natl Acad Sci U S A 94: 884–889.

18. Kiuchi K, Yoshizawa K, Shikata N, Moriguchi K, Tsubura A (2002) Morphologic characteristics of retinal degeneration induced by sodium iodate in mice. Curr Eye Res 25: 373–379.
19. Zhou P, Lu Y, Sun XH (2011) Zebularine suppresses TGF-beta-induced lens epithelial cell-myofibroblast transdifferentiation by inhibiting MeCP2. Mol Vis 17: 2717–2723.
20. Zhou P, Lu Y, Sun XH (2012) Effects of a novel DNA methyltransferase inhibitor Zebularine on human lens epithelial cells. Mol Vis 18: 22–28.
21. Zhou P, Zhao MW, Li XX, Yu WZ, Bian ZM (2007) siRNA targeting mammalian target of rapamycin (mTOR) attenuates experimental proliferative vitreoretinopathy. Curr Eye Res 32: 973–984.
22. Yaung J, Jin M, Barron E, Spee C, Wawrousek EF, et al. (2007) alpha-Crystallin distribution in retinal pigment epithelium and effect of gene knockouts on sensitivity to oxidative stress. Mol Vis 13: 566–577.
23. Bockelbrink A, Roll S, Ruether K, Rasch A, Greiner W, et al. (2008) Cataract surgery and the development or progression of age-related macular degeneration: a systematic review. Surv Ophthalmol 53: 359–367.
24. Nolan JM, O'Reilly P, Loughman J, Stack J, Loane E, et al. (2009) Augmentation of macular pigment following implantation of blue light-filtering intraocular lenses at the time of cataract surgery. Invest Ophthalmol Vis Sci 50: 4777–4785.
25. Algvere PV, Marshall J, Seregard S (2006) Age-related maculopathy and the impact of blue light hazard. Acta Ophthalmol Scand 84: 4–15.
26. Kase S, He S, Sonoda S, Kitamura M, Spee C, et al. (2010) alphaB-crystallin regulation of angiogenesis by modulation of VEGF. Blood 115: 3398–3406.
27. Rao NA, Saraswathy S, Wu GS, Katselis GS, Wawrousek EF, et al. (2008) Elevated retina-specific expression of the small heat shock protein, alphaA-crystallin, is associated with photoreceptor protection in experimental uveitis. Invest Ophthalmol Vis Sci 49: 1161–1171.
28. Yaung J, Kannan R, Wawrousek EF, Spee C, Sreekumar PG, et al. (2008) Exacerbation of retinal degeneration in the absence of alpha crystallins in an in vivo model of chemically induced hypoxia. Exp Eye Res 86: 355–365.
29. Ramkumar HL, Zhang J, Chan CC (2010) Retinal ultrastructure of murine models of dry age-related macular degeneration (AMD). Prog Retin Eye Res 29: 169–190.
30. Cai X, McGinnis JF (2012) Oxidative stress: the achilles' heel of neurodegenerative diseases of the retina. Front Biosci 17: 1976–1995.
31. Machalinska A, Lubinski W, Klos P, Kawa M, Baumert B, et al. (2010) Sodium iodate selectively injuries the posterior pole of the retina in a dose-dependent manner: morphological and electrophysiological study. Neurochem Res 35: 1819–1827.
32. Michael R, Bron AJ (2011) The ageing lens and cataract: a model of normal and pathological ageing. Philos Trans R Soc Lond B Biol Sci 366: 1278–1292.
33. Neal RE, Bettelheim FA, Lin C, Winn KC, Garland DL, et al. (2005) Alterations in human vitreous humour following cataract extraction. Exp Eye Res 80: 337–347.
34. Franco LM, Zulliger R, Wolf-Schnurrbusch UE, Katagiri Y, Kaplan HJ, et al. (2009) Decreased visual function after patchy loss of retinal pigment epithelium induced by low-dose sodium iodate. Invest Ophthalmol Vis Sci 50: 4004–4010.

3

Does Cataract Surgery Alleviate Poverty? Evidence from a Multi-Centre Intervention Study Conducted in Kenya, the Philippines and Bangladesh

Hannah Kuper[1]*, Sarah Polack[2], Wanjiku Mathenge[2], Cristina Eusebio[3], Zakia Wadud[4], Mamunur Rashid[5], Allen Foster[2]

1 Department of Epidemiology and Population Health, London School of Hygiene and Tropical Medicine, London, United Kingdom, **2** Department of Infectious and Tropical Diseases, London School of Hygiene & Tropical Medicine, London, United Kingdom, **3** Cataract Foundation of the Philippines, Bacolod, Negros Occidental, Philippines, **4** Child Sight Foundation, Dhaka, Bangladesh, **5** CSS Rawm Hospital, Khulna, Bangladesh

Abstract

Background: Poverty and blindness are believed to be intimately linked, but empirical data supporting this purported relationship are sparse. The objective of this study is to assess whether there is a reduction in poverty after cataract surgery among visually impaired cases.

Methodology/Principal Findings: A multi-centre intervention study was conducted in three countries (Kenya, Philippines, Bangladesh). Poverty data (household per capita expenditure – PCE, asset ownership and self-rated wealth) were collected from cases aged ≥50 years who were visually impaired due to cataract (visual acuity<6/24 in the better eye) and age-sex matched controls with normal vision. Cases were offered free/subsidised cataract surgery. Approximately one year later participants were re-interviewed about poverty. 466 cases and 436 controls were examined at both baseline and follow-up (Follow up rate: 78% for cases, 81% for controls), of which 263 cases had undergone cataract surgery ("operated cases"). At baseline, operated cases were poorer compared to controls in terms of PCE (Kenya: $22 versus £35 p = 0.02, Bangladesh: $16 vs $24 p = 0.004, Philippines: $24 vs 32 p = 0.0007), assets and self-rated wealth. By follow-up PCE had increased significantly among operated cases in each of the three settings to the level of controls (Kenya: $30 versus £36 p = 0.49, Bangladesh: $23 vs $23 p = 0.20, Philippines: $45 vs $36 p = 0.68). There were smaller increases in self-rated wealth and no changes in assets. Changes in PCE were apparent in different socio-demographic and ocular groups. The largest PCE increases were apparent among the cases that were poorest at baseline.

Conclusions/Significance: This study showed that cataract surgery can contribute to poverty alleviation, particularly among the most vulnerable members of society. This study highlights the need for increased provision of cataract surgery to poor people and shows that a focus on blindness may help to alleviate poverty and achieve the Millennium Development Goals.

Editor: Marie-Louise Newell, University of KwaZulu Natal, South Africa

Funding: This study was funded by grants from three international eye care charities: CBM (Christian Blind Mission - http://www.cbmi.org/), SightSavers International (http://www.sightsavers.org/default.html) and Orbis international (http://www.orbis.org/). Representatives from these organisations were part of the steering committee for the study, which gave guidance towards conduct of the study. Professor Allen Foster is president of CBM, but other organisations were not involved in preparing the manuscript, the data collection, data analysis or the decision to publish.

Competing Interests: Professor Allen Foster is president of CBM, but other organisations were not involved in preparing the manuscript, the data collection, data analysis or the decision to publish. Professor Allen Foster was involved in this study in his position as Director of the International Centre for Eye Health at the London School of Hygiene & Tropical Medicine. At the time of the study Professor Foster was also the Medical Advisor to CBM. In January 2006, two years into the study, Professor Foster was appointed president of CBM. He contributed to the conception of the study question, study design and critically reviewed the draft of the article. He was not involved in the data collection, data analysis or interpretation of results.

* E-mail: hannah.kuper@lshtm.ac.uk

Introduction

Poverty and blindness are believed to be intimately linked, with poverty predisposing to blindness, and blindness exacerbating poverty by limiting employment opportunities, or by incurring treatment cost. However, empirical data supporting these claims are sparse, particularly for low and middle income countries (LMICs) [1–3], and few data are available showing the impact of measures to alleviate blindness on poverty reduction [4]. This information is needed urgently as improvements in health and reductions in poverty are central to the achievement of the Millennium Development Goals (MDG).

Cataract is the leading cause of blindness globally, affecting almost 18 million people [5]. Cataract surgery is a relatively cheap and highly cost-effective intervention, even in LMICs [6]. However, competing financial demands limits the allocation of funds to cataract surgery both at the national and individual level, so that poor people may be less likely to have their cataract treated. Blindness may also exacerbate poverty by reducing opportunities of the individual or their families to engage in income generating activities [4]. Consequently, cataract blindness is markedly more prevalent in LMICs [5], and may be more common among poor people within countries [1–3], although data are sparse. This relationship with poverty is also evident for disability in general [7], although few studies have attempted to unravel the nature of the relationship between poverty and cataract or other types of disability through empirical data.

The Cataract Impact Study was undertaken to assess the impact of cataract visual impairment and cataract surgery on poverty, activities and quality of life in three low income countries [8–11]. Our baseline analyses showed that cases visually impaired from cataract were significantly poorer, less likely to be involved in productive activities and had worse quality of life than controls with normal vision in Kenya, the Philippines and Bangladesh [8–11]. At follow-up the cases who had undergone cataract surgery had significantly improved quality of life [12], were significantly more likely to participate in productive activities and received less assistance from caregivers [13]. We hypothesise that these changes would have resulted in reduced poverty among the operated cases at follow-up. The aim of the current analysis is to assess the impact of cataract surgery on poverty among cases with cataract in these three settings.

Methods

Ethics statement

Informed signed or thumb-printed consent was obtained from all cases and controls. All cases with operable cataract were referred for surgery. Ethical approval was obtained from the ethics committees of the London School of Hygiene & Tropical Medicine, the Kenya Medical Research Institute, the Bangladesh Medical Research Council and the University of St. La Salle, Bacolod, Philippines.

Study overview

The 'Cataract Impact Study' was a longitudinal intervention study conducted in Kenya (Nakuru district), Bangladesh (Satkhira district) and the Philippines (Negros Island and Antique district) [8–13]. At baseline cases with visual impairment from cataract and controls without visual impairment were identified and interviewed about time-use, health related quality of life and poverty. All cases were offered free or subsidized surgery. Approximately one year later cases and controls were re-traced, re-examined and re-interviewed. This paper presents the findings from the poverty data.

Participants

Sample size calculations were powered to detect a 30% improvement in per capita expenditure one year after cataract surgery, with an alpha of 0.05 and 80% power and necessitated a sample of 100 cases examined at baseline and follow-up in each country. A total of 180 cases were required at baseline in each country, assuming that 75% of cases underwent surgery and 75% were followed at one year.

Cases and controls were identified primarily through population-based blindness surveys undertaken at baseline [14–16]. Clusters of 50 people aged ≥50 years were selected through probability-proportionate to size sampling, using either the census (Philippines and Bangladesh) or electoral role (Kenya) as the sampling frame. Households within clusters were selected through a modification of compact segment sampling, whereby a map was drawn of the enumeration area which was divided into segments each including approximately 50 people aged ≥50 years and one segment was chosen at random [17]. Households in the segment were included sequentially until 50 people aged ≥50 years were identified. The surveys included 3503 (93% response rate) people aged ≥50 years in Kenya, 4868 (92%) in Bangladesh, 2774 (76%) in Negros and 3177 (83%) in Antique.

All people aged ≥50 years underwent visual acuity (VA) testing and ophthalmic examination. VA was measured in full daylight with available spectacle correction with a Snellen tumbling "E" chart using optotype size 6/18 (20/60) on one side and size 6/60 (20/200) on the other side at 6 or 3 metre distance. If the VA was <6/18 in either eye then pinhole vision was also measured. Participants with pinhole vision <6/18 but >6/60 in the better eye due to age-related cataract were given a second VA test using an 'E' of size 6/24. The ophthalmologist examined all eyes with a presenting VA<6/18 with a torch, direct ophthalmoscope and/or portable slit lamp.

Cases were invited for participation if they had pinhole VA <6/24 in the better eye due to cataract, as diagnosed by an ophthalmologist. One (or up to two in Bangladesh) age- sex-cluster-matched controls without visual impairment (presenting VA>6/18 in better eye) were selected per case from the eligible adults examined in the same cluster. During the survey the eligible controls in each cluster were listed by gender and age group (50–54, 55–59, 65–69 and ≥70 years). When a case was identified, one control (or up to two in Bangladesh) of the same gender and age group was selected at random for inclusion by drawing lots. If there were no matching control at that time then the next eligible control identified in the cluster was recruited. Cases and controls who were significantly communication impaired (e.g. deaf) were excluded (<5 per country).

Due to logistical and time constraints, additional cases were identified in each setting through community-based case detection. In Kenya and Negros (Philippines) additional clusters were selected using probability proportionate to size sampling after completion of the population based-survey. These clusters were visited in advance and asked that all people aged ≥50 years with eyesight problems come to a central point on a specified day and that people unable to attend (e.g. due to blindness or physical disability) be noted. All people attending the central point and those unable to leave their households underwent an eye examination using the procedures described above. People who met the case definition were invited to participate in the study and were interviewed in their homes. In Bangladesh and Antique (Philippines), case finding was conducted simultaneously with the survey so that age- gender matched controls were also included for these cases. In each cluster the teams asked to be taken to a community member with eye problems living within the boundaries of the cluster but outside the selected segment. The ophthalmologist conducted the ophthalmic examination at the household to identify eligible cases.

Intervention

In Kenya and Bangladesh all cases were offered free cataract surgery at the local hospital, with free transport. In the Philippines, patients were referred for surgery which was subsidised for patients who could not afford the fee. "Operated cases" were those who accepted the surgery while "un-operated cases" did not.

Data collection

Baseline surveys were conducted between January 2005 and May 2006. Follow up surveys were undertaken approximately one year later, during the same climatic season as the baseline. Interviews were conducted in respondents' own homes by trained interviewers who were regularly observed by supervisors.

Measures of poverty

The person primarily responsible for household finances was interviewed to assess poverty as measured through (a) household PCE to indicate consumption, (b) asset ownership and (c) self rated wealth:

a) PCE: the household informant was asked to recall the monetary value of food that was purchased, consumed from home production, received as payment in kind or as gifts over the last month by all household members (not including those away) [18]. They were also questioned about expenditure on education, health, household and personal items and rent paid (or rental equivalent for home owners). Consumption was assessed over the previous one week period for frequently consumed items, and this was scaled up to estimate monthly consumption. The amount consumed over the previous month was assessed for items that were consumed more rarely. In total, 85 items were included in the questionnaire in Kenya, 90 in the Philippines and 79 in Bangladesh. The consumption on all items was summed to calculate total monthly household consumption, and this was converted to US dollars at the average exchange rate between baseline and follow-up ($1 = 74 shillings, 67 taka, 51 peso). PCE was calculated by dividing total monthly household consumption by the number of household members.

b) Asset ownership: The informant was also asked about the number and type of context-specific assets owned by the household, including furniture items, electrical equipment, cattle and vehicles. Information was collected on household characteristics (e.g. building material of the floor, roof and walls, type of toilet and the number of rooms). This information was used to derive a relative index of household assets using Principle Components Analysis (PCA) [19].

c) Self-rated wealth: participants were asked *"On a scale of 1 to 10, how well-off do you think your household is in relation to the other households in the village?"*.

Covariates

Cases and controls were interviewed about standard socio-demographic indicators, including household composition, education, and employment. They were also asked about, self-rated health (ranking their "health state today" on a scale of 1–100), and time-use as described in detail elsewhere [10,13,20].

Questionnaire development and training

The questionnaires were translated into the local languages (3 in Kenya, 3 in the Philippines and 1 in Bangladesh) and back-translated by independent translators who also commented on appropriateness of language used. The questionnaire was reviewed and pilot tested in each setting and small modifications were made, where appropriate, to ensure local understanding. Interviewers were trained for one week at baseline and at follow-up.

Statistical analysis

Data on household expenditure were cleaned, excluding gross outliers and imputing rental equivalents based on household characteristics and non-rent expenditure where these estimates were missing or unreasonably low (<$1 per month – 34 in total). PCE and asset scores were divided into quartiles for each country, based on the distribution of the data for the cases and controls combined. All data analyses were restricted to participants with both baseline and follow-up data and were conducted for each country separately.

The following analyses were undertaken:

a) Comparison of socio-demographic characteristics between cases and controls: The baseline socio-demographic characteristics of operated cases and controls were compared calculating p-values through t-test for continuous variables and chi-square for discrete variables (or exact test if cell count<5). We also compared characteristics of un-operated cases to operated cases.

b) Assessment of differences in poverty between cases and controls: We compared both baseline and follow up scores for PCE, assets and self-rated wealth between operated cases and controls using the t-test for log-transformed PCE scores and assets, and the Mann-Witney test for household rank. We also compared scores of un-operated cases to operated cases.

c) Assessment of change in poverty over time: We compared baseline and follow-up scores for the three poverty variables separately for operated cases, un-operated cases and operated controls, calculating paired t-test derived p-values for PCE (all countries) and assets (Bangladesh and Philippines), and

Table 1. Follow-up by country for operated cases, controls and un-operated cases.

Country	Participant type	Total at Baseline (N)	Examined at follow-up (%)	Reasons for loss to follow-up (%)		
				Lost	Died	Refused/unable to communicate
Kenya	Operated cases	82	65 (79%)	9 (53%)	8 (47%)	0 (0%)
	Controls	75	56 (75%)	16 (84%)	3 (16%)	0 (0%)
	Un-operated cases	60	40 (67%)	12 (60%)	7 (35%)	1 (5%)
Bangladesh	Operated cases	117	99 (85%)	11 (61%)	6 (33%)	1 (6%)
	Controls	280	223 (80%)	46 (81%)	10 (18%)	1 (2%)
	Un-operated cases	100	70 (70%)	20 (67%)	7 (23%)	3 (10%)
Philippines	Operated cases	113	99 (88%)	7 (50%)	7 (50%)	0 (0%)
	Controls	182	157 (86%)	18 (72%)	6 (24%)	1 (4%)
	Un-operated cases	127	93 (73%)	12 (35%)	20 (59%)	2 (6%)

Table 2. Baseline demographic characteristics of cases and controls examined at baseline and follow-up.

Variable	Kenya					Bangladesh					Philippines				
	Operated cases (n = 65)	Unoperated Cases (n = 39)	Controls (n = 55)	P-value operated vs un-operated cases	P-value operated cases vs controls	Operated cases (n = 99)	Unoperated Cases (n = 67)	Controls (n = 221)	P-value operated vs un-operated cases	P-value operated cases vs controls	Operated cases (n = 99)	Unoperated Cases (n = 92)	Controls (n = 152)	P-value operated vs un-operated cases	P-value operated cases vs controls
Mean age (95% CI)	78 (75–80)	82 (79–84)	75 (73–78)	0.03	0.15	71 (69–73)	75 (72–77)	69 (68–70)	0.04	0.03	72 (70–73)	77 (75–78)	71 (70–73)	0.0002	0.85
Female	49%	64%	51%	0.14	0.85	53%	72%	57%	0.01	0.46	62%	70%	56%	0.25	0.37
Married	56%	28%	61%	0.007	0.54	48%	32%	58%	0.03	0.12	45%	46%	56%	0.92	0.09
Literate	29%	31%	56%	0.87	0.003	8%	9%	28%	0.84	<0.0001	15%	22%	12%	0.24	0.44
Job	0%	0%	7%	NA	0.01*	6%	12%	18%	0.18	0.006	9%	3%	17%	0.14*	0.09
Mean self-rated health (95% CI)	50 (45–54)	52 (46–57)	58 (53–63)	0.62	0.04	50 (45–55)	42 (37–47)	59 (56–62)	0.04	0.0006	53 (51–56)	49 (47–52)	62 (59–65)	0.05	<0.0001
Pre op VA															
Normal	0	0	100%	0.008	NA	0	0	100%	0.69	NA	0	0	100%	0.18	NA
VI	40%	56%				29%	22%				26%	34%			
SVI	18%	33%				16%	21%				21%	14%			
Blind	18%	3%				12%	15%				24%	31%			
PL	23%	8%				42%	42%			29%	20%				

*Fisher's exact test.

Wilcoxon signed rank test for household rank and assets scores in Kenya (these data were skewed and could not be transformed).

d) Multivariate analyses comparing poverty in operated cases and controls: Logistic regression analyses were undertaken, separately for each country, comparing operated cases and controls for the three poverty variables divided into quartiles at both baseline and at follow-up, adjusting analyses for the matching variables (age, sex and location, and study site in the Philippines). Analyses were additionally adjusted for social support indicators (marital status and household size), self-rated health and markers of early life poverty (school attendance and literacy), as potential confounders.

e) Identification of predictors of change in PCE among operated cases: We compared the mean change in PCE between baseline and follow-up among operated cases stratified by socio-demographic and ocular groups, calculating t-test derived p-values for comparing log PCE values for baseline and follow-up and comparing change between the groups. We also compared the mean allocation to different expenditure categories (e.g. food, education health etc) at baseline and at follow-up among operated cases.

Results

At baseline we included 142 cases and 75 controls in Kenya, 217 cases and 280 controls in Bangladesh and 240 cases and 182 controls in the Philippines (Table 1). Uptake of surgery among cases was consistently low (Kenya: 58%, Bangladesh: 54%, Philippines: 47%). Follow-up rates were high, particularly for the operated cases (>79%) and controls (>75%). Overall, 62% of loss to follow-up was due to drop-out, 34% due to death, and 4% due to refusal/inability to communicate. Operated cases, un-operated cases and controls lost to follow-up did not differ systematically from those included in terms of socio-demographic characteristics (data not shown).

More of the cases observed at baseline and follow-up were identified from the population-based survey (Kenya = 60, Bangladesh = 125, Philippines = 113), than through population based case finding (Kenya = 44, Bangladesh = 41, Philippines = 78). In Kenya and the Philippines there was no difference between these two case types in socio-demographic characteristics (age, sex, marital status, literacy, job, VA). In Bangladesh RAAB cases were significantly older and had better VA. All controls were identified through the population-based survey.

Comparison of baseline socio-demographic characteristics

Operated cases and controls were broadly similar in age, sex and marital status in the three countries, although operated cases were slightly older than controls in Bangladesh (Table 2). Controls were far more likely to have a job at baseline than cases and to be literate, except in the Philippines. Baseline self-rated health was consistently higher among controls compared to operated cases. Operated cases were also compared to un-operated cases. The un-operated cases were older. In Bangladesh the un-operated cases were more likely to be female and in Kenya and Bangladesh they were less likely to be married than operated cases, but they were similar in terms of job status and literacy. Baseline self-rated health

Table 3. Comparison of PCE, assets and household rank at baseline and follow up for operated cases and controls.

Poverty measures	Mean scores (95% CI)	Kenya			Bangladesh			Philippines		
		Operated cases (n = 65)	Controls (n = 56)	p-value operated cases versus controls	Operated cases (n = 99)	Controls (n = 222)	p-value operated cases versus controls	Operated cases (n = 99)	Controls (n = 152)	p-value operated cases versus controls
PCE ($)	Baseline	22 (18–26)	35 (24–46)	0.02	16 (12–21)	24 (16–33)	0.004	24 (19–28)	32 (27–38)	0.0007
	Follow-up	30 (22–37)	36 (22–51)	0.49	23 (18–28)	23 (21–24)	0.20	45 (28–62)	36 (30–42)	0.68
	Change (95% CI)	8 (0–15)	1 (−6–9)		7 (1–12)	−2 (−10–7)		21 (4–38)	3 (−4–10)	
	p-value for change	0.07	0.71		<0.0001	<0.0001		<0.0001	0.22	
Assets	Baseline	−0.8 (−1.2–−0.3)	0.5 (−0.3–1.3)	0.004	−0.7 (−1.1–−0.2)	0.2 (−0.1–0.6)	0.003	−0.2 (−0.7–0.3)	0.3 (−0.2–0.7)	0.14
	Follow-up	−0.8 (−1.2–−0.4)	0.2 (−0.5–1.0)	0.02	−0.7 (−1.1–−0.2)	0.2 (−0.1–0.5)	0.002	−0.1 (−0.6–0.4)	0.4 (0–0.8)	0.16
	Change (95% CI)	0 (−0.2–0.3)	−0.3 (−0.5–0)		0.03 (−0.1–0.2)	0 (−0.1–0.1)		0.1 (−0.2–0.5)	0.1 (−0.1–0.3)	
	p-value for change	0.36	0.05		0.81	0.96		0.47	0.35	
Household rank	Baseline	3.4 (3.1–3.8)	4.9 (4.4–5.4)	<0.0001	3.8 (3.4–4.2)	4.5 (4.2–4.8)	0.003	4.1 (3.8–4.4)	4.3 (4.0–4.6)	0.31
	Follow-up	4.1 (3.7–4.5)	4.8 (4.3–5.3)	0.05	3.9 (3.5–4.3)	4.4 (4.1–4.6)	0.02	4.6 (4.3–4.9)	4.6 (4.3–4.9)	0.83
	Change (95% CI)	0.7 (0.2–1.1)	−0.1 (−0.7–0.5)		0.1 (−0.2–0.4)	−0.1 (−0.4–0.1)		0.5 (0.1–0.9)	0.3 (−0.3–0.5)	
	p-value for change	0.005	0.80		0.64	0.61		0.007	0.08	

was lower for un-operated cases compared to operated cases in Bangladesh and the Philippines, and in Kenya the operated cases had poorer baseline vision than un-operated cases.

Assessment of differences in poverty between cases and controls and change over time

Both cases and controls were generally poor at baseline and remained so at follow-up, with daily PCE averaging \$0.53–\$1.50 per person. At baseline, operated cases had significantly lower PCE compared to controls in all three countries (Table 3). At follow up, average PCE had increased among operated cases by \$8 in Kenya (36%, $p = 0.07$), \$7 in Bangladesh (44%, $p < 0.0001$) and \$21 in the Philippines (88%, $p < 0.0001$) and was no longer significantly lower than among controls.

Baseline mean asset scores were also poorer among operated cases than controls in each country (Kenya: −0.8 vs 0.5; Bangladesh; −0.7 vs 0.2), although this was non-significant in the Philippines (−0.2 vs 0.3). There was virtually no change in asset scores among either operated cases or controls between baseline and follow-up, so that controls retained higher asset scores in Kenya and Bangladesh.

Household rank was significantly lower among operated cases than controls at baseline in Kenya (3.4 vs 4.9) and Bangladesh (3.8 vs 4.5), but not in the Philippines (4.1 vs 4.3). At follow up, household rank had increased significantly among operated cases in Kenya and the Philippines compared to baseline, but remained significantly lower than controls in both Kenya and Bangladesh and no different in the Philippines.

PCE, assets and household rank remained broadly similar between baseline and follow-up among controls.

Un-operated cases were similar to operated cases at baseline in terms of PCE (Kenya \$20.2, $p = 0.59$; Bangladesh \$19.5, $p = 0.35$, Philippines \$27.3, $p = 0.25$) assets (−1.0, $p = 0.58$; −0.21, $p = 0.29$; −0.3, $p = 0.76$) and household rank (3.2, $p = 0.46$; 4.1, $p = 0.38$; 4.0, $p = 0.68$). There were significant, though generally smaller, increases in PCE among un-operated cases between baseline and follow up in Kenya (\$8 increase, 95% CI = \$0–17 $p = 0.05$), Bangladesh (\$3, −\$2–\$8 $p = 0.02$) and the Philippines (\$7, \$0–14 $p = 0.01$). There was generally no change at follow-up in assets (Kenya: −0.8, Philippines −0.6) or self-rated wealth (Kenya: 3.7; Bangladesh: 4.0, Philippines: 4.2), and only the increase for assets in Bangladesh reached statistical significance (0.3 points, 0.1–0.6 $p = 0.01$).

Multivariate analyses of the association between poverty and case/control status at baseline and follow-up

We divided poverty indicator scores into quartiles to allow a comparison of operated cases and controls with adjustment for potential confounders. At baseline, operated cases were significantly more likely than controls to be in the poorest quartile of PCE in Kenya (OR = 3.3, 95% CI = 1.0–10.8), Bangladesh (3.2, 1.5–6.6) and the Philippines (4.4, 1.9–10.0), and there was a significant trend of association between falling PCE and case status (Table 4). At follow up, these differences were no longer statistically significant in Kenya (1.1, 0.3–3.2) and the Philippines (1.1, 0.5–2.4) and were weakened in Bangladesh (2.2, 1.1–4.5). Similarly, at baseline operated cases were much more likely than controls to be in the poorest quartile for asset ownership and household rank. The associations between case status and asset ownership or household rank were weaker at follow-up, particu-

Table 4. Multivariable analyses for the comparison of poverty variables at baseline and follow-up among operated cases and controls.

Poverty measures	Quartiles	Kenya		Bangladesh		Philippines	
		Baseline	Follow-up	Baseline	Follow-up	Baseline	Follow-up
		OR (95% CI) adjusted for age, sex and location	OR (95% CI) adjusted for age, sex and location	OR (95% CI) adjusted for age, sex and location	OR (95% CI) adjusted for age, sex and location	OR (95% CI) adjusted for age, sex, location and province	OR (95% CI) adjusted for age, sex, location and province
Per capita expenditure	1 (lowest)	3.3 (1.0–10.8)	1.1 (0.3–3.2)	3.2 (1.5–6.6)	2.2 (1.1–4.5)	4.4 (1.9–10.0)	1.1 (0.5–2.4)
	2	3.5 (1.1–11.5)	0.6 (0.2–1.9)	1.7 (0.8–3.5)	1.1 (0.5–2.1)	4.4 (1.9–10.2)	0.8 (0.4–1.7)
	3	1.1 (0.4–3.4)	1.5 (0.5–4.4)	1.7 (0.8–3.7)	1.1 (0.5–2.2)	1.7 (0.7–3.8)	0.6 (0.3–1.3)
	4 (highest)	Baseline	Baseline	Baseline	Baseline	Baseline	Baseline
	P for trend	0.01	0.69	0.003	0.03	<0.0001	0.66
Assets	1 (lowest)	4.7 (1.4–16.6)	2.6 (0.8–8.6)	3.0 (1.4–6.2)	2.2 (1.1–4.5)	1.7 (0.7–3.8)	1.7 (0.8–3.9)
	2	4.3 (1.3–14.4)	3.8 (1.1–13.5)	2.1 (1.0–4.4)	1.6 (0.8–3.3)	2.2 (1.0–5.0)	1.6 (0.7–3.5)
	3	3.2 (1.0–10.6)	2.2 (0.7–7.1)	1.7 (0.8–3.5)	1.0 (0.5–2.1)	2.2 (1.0–4.8)	1.6 (0.7–3.4)
	4 (highest)	Baseline	Baseline	Baseline	Baseline	Baseline	Baseline
	P for trend	0.01	0.11	0.003	0.01	0.23	0.20
Household rank	1 (lowest)	11.2 (2.6–48.3)	2.2 (0.6–8.3)	3.0 (1.4–6.4)	2.4 (1.1–5.2)	2.1 (0.8–5.9)	0.9 (0.4–2.1)
	2	8.4 (2.2–32.1)	4.4 (1.4–13.9)	2.1 (1.0–4.3)	1.5 (0.8–3.1)	2.7 (0.9–7.8)	1.5 (0.7–3.4)
	3	2.8 (0.7–10.8)	3.6 (1.2–11.1)	1.6 (0.7–3.4)	1.5 (0.7–3.3)	1.2 (0.5–3.2)	0.8 (0.3–1.6)
	4 (highest)	Baseline	Baseline	Baseline	Baseline	Baseline	Baseline
	P for trend	0.0002	0.13	0.003	0.04	0.05	0.73

larly in Kenya and the Philippines. For all measures of poverty, the trends of level of poverty in relation to case status remained statistically significant in Bangladesh at follow-up but not in Kenya or the Philippines. Additional adjustment for marital status, household size, baseline self rated health, school attendance and literacy weakened the associations at baseline, though they generally remained strong and statistically significant, and did not change the follow-up associations (data not shown).

Operated cases were also compared to un-operated cases for the three poverty indicators at baseline and follow-up (Table 5). In Kenya, there was no difference between operated and un-operated cases in PCE or assets at either baseline or follow-up. At baseline, there was no difference in household rank, but at follow-up the operated cases were less likely to be in the poorest quartiles of household rank compared to the un-operated cases. In Bangladesh, the operated cases were somewhat poorer than the un-operated cases at baseline in terms of PCE, but this association disappeared at follow-up. Assets and household rank did not differ between operated and un-operated cases, either at baseline or follow-up. In the Philippines the operated and un-operated cases were similar at baseline for all three poverty measures. At follow-up, the operated cases were less likely than the un-operated cases to be in the poorest quartiles for each of the three measures.

Predictors of change among operated cases

Predictors of change in PCE from baseline to follow-up were assessed among the operated cases (Table 6). There was no evidence for significant difference in change in PCE by any of the variables assessed, but some consistent trends were apparent. Improvements in PCE were larger among those <75 years compared to older participants in Bangladesh and the Philippines, and increases were larger among women than men in Kenya and the Philippines. Increases in PCE were consistently larger among unmarried than married people in all three countries. In the Philippines the increase in PCE was most apparent among people with high self-rated health or better baseline VA at baseline, while this was not apparent in Kenya and Bangladesh. No consistent trends were apparent for the change in PCE by outcome VA or number of eyes operated. In each setting the largest proportional increase in PCE was apparent among those in the poorer half of PCE at baseline compared to those above the median for PCE (Kenya: 158% increase in PCE versus 4% increase, Bangladesh: 94% versus 12%, Philippines: 116% versus 73%) (Figure 1).

We also explored how PCE was allocated and how this allocation changed over time. The largest proportion of PCE was spent on food both at baseline and at follow-up in all three countries. In the wealthier operated cases (i.e. above the median PCE at baseline) the largest increase in expenditure from baseline to follow up was on non-food items, so that the proportion of expenditure on food fell. In contrast among the poorer half (below the median PCE at baseline) most of the increased spending was on food items. As a result, at follow up there was little difference in expenditure on food between the poorer and wealthier operated cases.

Table 5. Multivariable analyses for the comparison of poverty variables at baseline and follow-up among operated cases and unoperated cases.

Poverty measures		Quartiles	Kenya		Bangladesh		Philippines
		Baseline	Follow-up	Baseline	Follow-up	Baseline	Follow-up
		OR (95% CI) adjusted for age, sex and location	OR (95% CI) adjusted for age, sex and location	OR (95% CI) adjusted for age, sex and location	OR (95% CI) adjusted for age, sex and location	OR (95% CI) adjusted for age, sex, location and province	OR (95% CI) adjusted for age, sex, location and province
Per capita expenditure	1 (lowest)	0.8 (0.3–2.6)	0.8 (0.3–2.2)	2.5 (1.0–6.3)	0.8 (0.3–2.0)	1.3 (0.5–3.0)	0.5 (0.2–1.2)
	2	0.6 (0.2–1.8)	0.7 (0.2–2.0)	1.9 (0.7–5.0)	0.6 (0.2–1.7)	1.8 (0.7–4.3)	0.5 (0.2–1.3)
	3	1.4 (0.4–4.7)	1.8 (0.5–5.9)	1.8 (0.7–4.8)	0.5 (0.2–1.3)	2.3 (0.8–6.2)	0.4 (0.2–0.9)
	4 (highest)	Baseline	Baseline	Baseline	Baseline	Baseline	Baseline
	P for trend	0.48	0.35	0.08	0.95	0.87	0.24
Assets	1 (lowest)	0.8 (0.3–2.6)	0.9 (0.3–2.9)	1.1 (0.4–2.8)	1.0 (0.4–2.5)	0.6 (0.2–1.6)	0.4 (0.2–1.1)
	2	1.6 (0.4–6.1)	0.9 (0.3–2.9)	0.9 (0.3–2.3)	1.0 (0.4–2.6)	0.8 (0.3–2.0)	0.6 (0.2–1.4)
	3	2.1 (0.6–7.6)	1.9 (0.5–6.5)	2.0 (0.7–5.8)	1.5 (0.5–4.3)	1.2 (0.5–2.9)	0.6 (0.2–1.5)
	4 (highest)	Baseline	Baseline	Baseline	Baseline	Baseline	Baseline
	P for trend	0.37	0.52	0.62	0.78	0.22	0.09
Household rank	1 (lowest)	0.7 (0.1–4.2)	0.4 (0.1–1.8)	1.4 (0.5–3.5)	0.7 (0.3–2.0)	0.8 (0.3–2.5)	0.4 (0.2–1.1)
	2	1.2 (0.2–7.1)	0.5 (0.2–1.8)	2.1 (0.7–5.8)	1.8 (0.7–5.0)	0.9 (0.3–3.0)	1.0 (0.4–2.6)
	3	1.8 (0.3–12.9)	1.7 (0.4–6.4)	1.1 (0.4–3.0)	1.4 (0.4–4.2)	1.2 (0.4–3.5)	1.1 (0.4–2.6)
	4 (highest)	Baseline	Baseline	Baseline	Baseline	Baseline	Baseline
	P for trend	0.22	0.05	0.37	0.58	0.40	0.05

Table 6. Predictors of change in PCE between baseline and follow-up among operated cases.

		Kenya				Bangladesh				Philippines			
		N	Baseline mean PCE (95% CI)	Follow up mean PCE (95% CI)	Mean change (95% CI)	N	Baseline mean PCE (95% CI)	Follow up mean PCE (95% CI)	Mean change (95% CI)	N	Baseline mean PCE (95% CI)	Follow up mean PCE (95% CI)	Mean change (95% CI)
Age	≤75	27	24 (17–32)	32 (22–43)	8 (−3–20)	64	15 (13–17)	23 (17–29)	8 (2–14)	56	20 (17–22)	43 (15–72)	24 (−5–52)
	>75	38	20 (15–26)	27 (17–37)	7 (−3–17)	35	19 (7–31)	23 (14–31)	4 (−8–16)	43	29 (19–38)	47 (33–60)	18 (3–33)
	p-value		0.34	0.30	0.88		0.92	0.80	0.51		0.11	0.03	0.72
Sex	Male	33	20 (15–24)	22 (17–27)	2 (−4–8)	47	18 (9–27)	25 (18–31)	7 (−3–16)	38	21 (16–25)	34 (22–47)	14 (3–25)
	Female	32	24 (16–32)	38 (24–51)	13 (0–27)	52	15 (12–18)	22 (15–28)	7 (0–13)	61	26 (19–32)	51 (25–78)	25 (−2–53)
	p-value		0.48	0.13	0.12		0.83	0.30	0.99		0.28	0.27	0.41
Married	Yes	35	20 (14–26)	24 (15–34)	4 (−8–16)	48	20 (11–28)	23 (18–27)	4 (−5–11)	43	22 (19–26)	35 (24–46)	13 (3–23)
	No	28	23 (16–30)	35 (24–46)	12 (3–21)	51	13 (11–15)	23 (15–31)	10 (2–18)	53	25 (17–33)	53 (23–84)	28 (−3–60)
	p-value		0.30	0.10	0.26		0.09	0.29	0.24		0.53	0.50	0.35
Literate	Yes	19	25 (18–32)	28 (19–36)	3 (−7–12)	8	17 (13–21)	25 (19–32)	8 (0–16)	84	24 (19–30)	49 (29–68)	24 (4–44)
	No	46	21 (15–26)	30 (21–40)	10 (0–19)	91	16 (12–21)	23 (18–28)	6 (0–13)	15	19 (15–24)	23 (13–33)	3 (−8–15)
	p-value		0.15	0.58	0.30		0.24	0.01	0.68		0.56	0.04	0.07
Baseline self-rated health	<median	19	17 (13–20)	24 (15–33)	8 (1–14)	47	15 (12–19)	23 (16–29)	8 (1–14)	59	25 (18–32)	33 (26–41)	8 (−1–18)
	≥median	46	24 (18–30)	32 (22–41)	7 (−2–17)	52	18 (10–26)	23 (16–30)	5 (−4–15)	40	22 (18–26)	62 (21–103)	40 (0–80)
	p-value		0.23	0.45	0.98		0.69	0.71	0.66		0.72	0.18	0.13
Baseline PCE	<median	28	10 (9–11)	26 (12–39)	16 (3–29)	59	9 (9–10)	18 (13–23)	9 (4–14)	61	14 (13–16)	31 (24–38)	17 (10–24)
	≥median	37	31 (25–37)	33 (24–41)	1 (−7–9)	40	27 (17–37)	30 (21–39)	3 (−9–16)	38	39 (29–49)	67 (24–110)	28 (−16–73)
	p-value		<0.0001	0.03	0.05		<0.001	0.0003	0.40		<0.0001	0.002	0.60
Baseline VA	MVI/SVI	38	20 (15–27)	28 (21–36)	8 (1–15)	45	15 (12–18)	20 (17–23)	5 (2–9)	47	24 (15–33)	53 (19–87)	29 (−6–64)
	Blind	27	24 (17–32)	31 (17–45)	7 (−8–22)	54	18 (10–25)	25 (17–34)	8 (−2–18)	52	23 (19–27)	37 (26–48)	14 (4–24)
	p-value		0.22	0.96	0.90		0.77	0.89	0.66		0.45	0.59	0.41
Outcome VA	6/6–6/18	41	25 (19–32)	33 (22–44)	8 (−3–19)	83	17 (12–22)	22 (17–26)	5 (−1–11)	71	24 (18–30)	47 (23–70)	23 (−1–47)
	<6/18	24	16 (13–20)	24 (17–31)	7 (0–14)	16	14 (10–17)	29 (10–48)	16 (−3–34)	28	23 (18–29)	40 (28–51)	16 (5–28)
	p-value		0.11	0.40	0.95		0.65	0.43	0.17		0.58	0.51	0.62
Eyes operated	1	44	21 (16–25)	27 (20–35)	7 (0–13)	75	14 (12–16)	23 (17–29)	9 (3–15)	67	24 (18–31)	36 (27–44)	11 (2–21)
	2	21	25 (15–34)	34 (17–50)	9 (−10–29)	24	24 (7–41)	23 (16–30)	−1 (−16–14)	30	21 (17–26)	66 (12–120)	45 (−9–99)
	p-value		0.56	0.37	0.80		0.11	0.66	0.21		0.66	0.36	0.22

Discussion

This intervention study conducted in Kenya, Bangladesh and the Philippines showed that one year after cataract surgery PCE increased significantly among operated cases so that it was no longer lower than controls, while assets remained largely unchanged and self-rated wealth improved in Kenya and the Philippines. Overall PCE increased between 36% and 88% in the three countries. These gains were apparent in different socio-demographic and ophthalmic groups, and did not vary by ophthalmic characteristics. Gains in PCE were most noticeable in the most vulnerable groups, that is, those who were poorer, older, female or unmarried.

These data can provide further insight into the association between poverty and cataract. In this study, cases had lower levels of education than controls and thereby potentially more early life poverty. In addition, cost was cited as the main barrier to uptake of cataract surgery in this study [14–16], as it is in other studies [21]. This confirms the "selection effect" whereby poorer people are more likely to become blind because they are less likely to have their cataract treated [22]. Together, these data suggest that poverty causes blindness.

The data also suggest that cataract blindness may cause poverty. In this study the association between poverty and cataract at baseline persisted after adjustment for health, markers of early-life wealth (e.g. education) and social support, potentially suggesting an additional direct effect of cataract on poverty. One possible explanatory route for cases being poorer than controls at baseline is the impact of visual impairment on productivity. A companion paper from this study showed that cases were less likely to participate in productive activities (i.e. paid work and non-market activities) compared to controls at baseline [10]. Cataract blindness may also have resulted in restrictions of productivity of other household members as almost half of cases in Bangladesh and a quarter of cases in Kenya and the Philippines reported receiving assistance from household members at baseline (compared to <10% of controls) [10]. Furthermore, the time-use data suggested that after surgery the operated cases were significantly more likely to be involved in productive activities and spent on average 1–2 hours more on these activities in each setting. At the

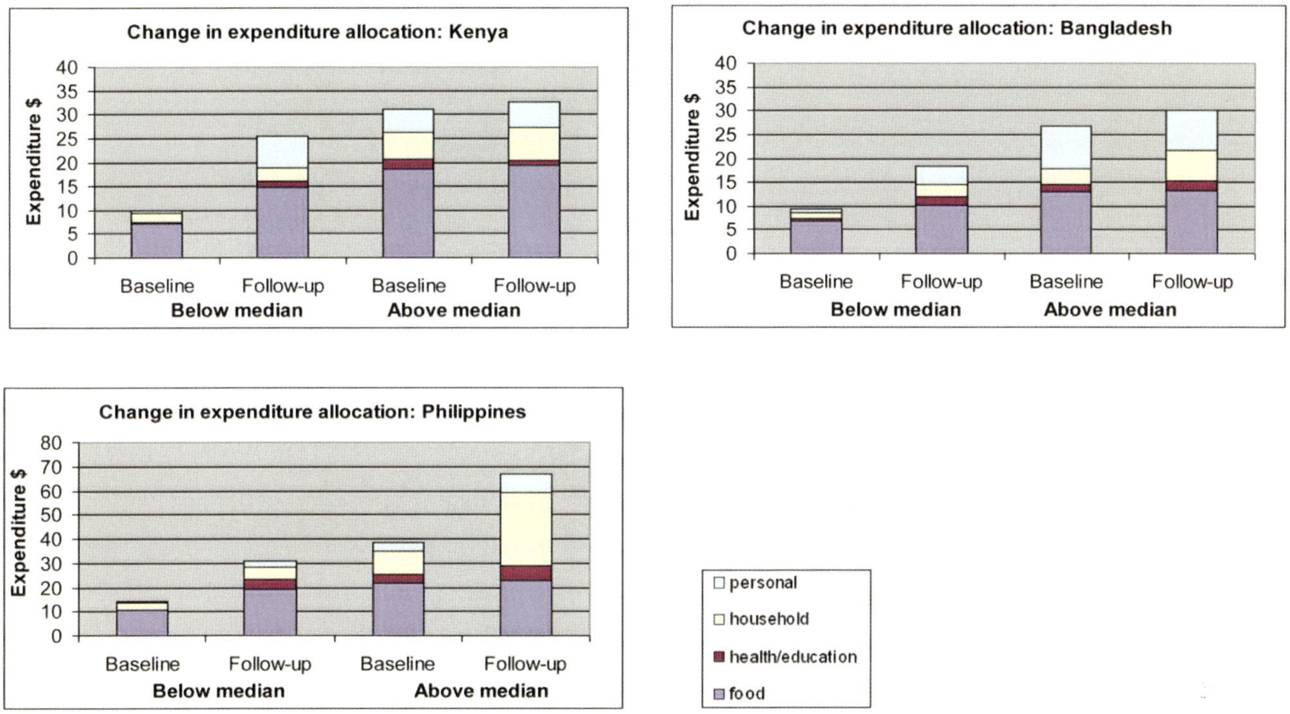

Figure 1. Change in allocation of expenses between baseline and follow-up among operated cases.

same time the frequency of reported assistance with activities more than halved in each setting [12]. The increase in PCE and consequent reduction in poverty that was evident after cataract surgery could therefore potentially be explained by increases in productivity of cases after surgery. This lends empirical support to the argument that blindness contributes to poverty and provides further evidence for the cyclical link between poverty and disability.

Other studies, though sparse, are consistent with our findings. The cross-sectional association between poverty and blindness has also been demonstrated in Pakistan [2], India [1], and Cambodia [3]. Longitudinal studies have demonstrated a reduction in employment and productivity associated with the onset of disability and that this is reversed if disability is alleviated [22]. A survey of patients in India also demonstrated the impact of blindness on loss of jobs, and found that most people who had lost their job as a result of blindness subsequently regained employment after cataract surgery, with consequent increased productivity [4]. The selection effect, whereby poor people are more likely to become disabled was clearly demonstrated using longitudinal data in the UK [22], and in Ireland [23].

There were a number of limitations to the study. Recall bias was possible since operated cases were generally very satisfied with their surgery. However, smaller changes were seen for asset scores or self-rated wealth, the latter being arguably the most subjective and therefore vulnerable to recall bias. Furthermore, the change in allocation of expenditure followed a meaningful pattern as expenditure on food did not increase among households that were richer at baseline, whereas expenditure on food increased among the poorer households. This supports Engel's law that states that as income rises the proportion of income spent on food falls [24], so that we would expect to see greater gains in expenditure on food among the poorer compared to the wealthier households as was the case in this study. PCE among controls was similar at baseline and follow-up providing support for cataract surgery being the key causal factor in the changes among operated cases.

Improvements in PCE at follow-up were observed among un-operated cases despite having received no intervention. The increase in PCE was of a similar magnitude in Kenya for the two case types, in Bangladesh it was about half the amount for the un-operated cases as for the operated cases, and in the Philippines it was about one third of the level in the un-operated cases as in the operated cases. The multivariable analyses showed few differences for poverty variables between operated and un-operated cases at baseline or follow-up in Kenya, while in Bangladesh and the Philippines there was some indication that the operated cases received benefits by follow-up in terms of PCE increases compared to the un-operated cases. However, the sample size was not powered to detect differences between operated and un-operated cases. It is not clear why PCE increased among un-operated cases, and similar changes were not observed in vision-related or generic quality of life [12], or participation in productive activities [13]. One possible explanation is that the household members of the un-operated cases, and the cases themselves, adapted over time so that the productivity constraints on the carer(s) was reduced.

PCE showed a greater change after surgery compared to the other measures of poverty (assets and self-rated wealth). PCE is a short-term measure of wealth and can change rapidly as the circumstances of the household change (e.g. a member becomes involved in paid employment or is able to cultivate land). In contrast, assets and self-rated wealth are longer term measures of poverty, as it takes time to accumulate assets or to alter perception of household wealth. Assets and self-perceived wealth are therefore less responsive to change compared to PCE and therefore one year of follow-up may have been insufficient to observe an impact of cataract surgery on these measures.

We did not consider economies of scale or use equivalence scales, because there is no widely accepted alternative to the simple equal-sharing convention. However, the majority of expenditure was on food which does not allow for economies of scale and the case and control households were of similar sizes in the three settings [11]. We only measured economic poverty, and did not consider social participation or inclusion or other aspects of wellbeing, although quality of life and activities are subjects of other analyses from this study [8–10].

Finally, the uptake of surgery was lower than anticipated. As a consequence there are concerns that we had insufficient power to detect the associations (particularly in Kenya). There were few differences in poverty or socio-demographic characteristics between operated and un-operated cases limiting the potential impact on external validity. The exception was that un-operated cases were older than the operated cases. It is therefore possible that if more of the un-operated cases had undergone surgery and been included at the follow up, average increases in PCE may have been slightly smaller. We also had to include two different case types although, the socio-demographic characteristics of cases identified through the RAAB was very similar to those identified through population-based case finding indicating that this would have contributed little to selection bias.

In terms of strengths, this was the first study to assess longitudinally the impact of cataract surgery on poverty in LMICs. It was large and allowed comparisons across three international settings. We selected population-based cases rather than cases presenting at the clinic in order to reduce selection bias and improve generalisability of our findings. We used the same standard questionnaires at baseline and follow-up in the three settings. We assessed poverty using three complementary indices, which included short-term measure which is responsive to change (PCE), as well as long-term measures (asset) and self-perceptions of wealth. PCE is generally believed to be a good indicator of current standard of living, and is more accurately recalled than income [7].

In conclusion, this study showed for the first time that cataract surgery can contribute to poverty alleviation, particularly among the most vulnerable members of society. Almost all our participants were living on less than $1 per day, and so are target of the first MDG. This study provides strength to the argument that a focus on blindness and potentially disability more broadly is an important step in achieving the MDGs.

Acknowledgments

We would like to thank the many field workers, doctors, office managers, data entry clerks, drivers, and helpers who made this study possible. We are particularly grateful to all the study participants for giving their time so generously.

Author Contributions

Conceived and designed the experiments: HK SP AF. Performed the experiments: HK, SP, CE, WM, MR, ZW. Analyzed the data: HK. Wrote the paper: HK. SP responsible for data management.

References

1. Dandona L, Dandona R, Srinivas M, Giridhar P, Vilas K, et al. (2001) Blindness in the Indian state of Andhra Pradesh. Invest Ophthalmol Vis Sci 42: 908–916.
2. Gilbert CE, Shah SP, Jadoon MZ, Bourne R, Dineen B, et al. (2008) Poverty and blindness in Pakistan: results from the Pakistan national blindness and visual impairment survey. Bmj 336: 29–32.
3. Zimmer Z (2008) Poverty, wealth inequality and health among older adults in rural Cambodia. Soc Sci Med 66: 57–71.
4. Javitt JC (1993) Cataract. In: Jamison DT, Mosley WH, Measham AR, Bobadilla JL, eds. Disease control priorities in developing countries. New York: Oxford University Press.
5. Resnikoff S, Pascolini D, Mariotti SP, Pokharel GP (2008) Global magnitude of visual impairment caused by uncorrected refractive errors in 2004. Bull World Health Organ 86: 63–70.
6. Baltussen R, Sylla M, Mariotti SP (2004) Cost-effectiveness analysis of cataract surgery: a global and regional analysis. Bull World Health Organ 82: 338–345.
7. Braithwaite J, Mont D (2009) Disability and poverty: a survey of World Bank Poverty Assessments and implications. European Journal of Disability Research 3: 219–232.
8. Polack S, Kuper H, Mathenge W, Fletcher A, Foster A (2007) Cataract visual impairment and quality of life in a Kenyan population. Br J Ophthalmol 91: 927–932.
9. Polack S, Kuper H, Wadud Z, Fletcher A, Foster A (2008) Quality of life and visual impairment from cataract in Satkhira district, Bangladesh. Br J Ophthalmol 92: 1026–1030.
10. Polack S, Kuper H, Eusebio C, Mathenge W, Wadud Z, et al. (2008) The impact of cataract on time-use: results from a population based case-control study in Kenya, the Philippines and Bangladesh. Ophthalmic Epidemiol 15: 372–382.
11. Kuper H, Polack S, Eusebio C, Mathenge W, Wadud Z, et al. (2008) A case-control study to assess the relationship between poverty and visual impairment from cataract in Kenya, the Philippines, and Bangladesh. PLoS Med 5: e244.
12. Polack S, Eusebio C, Mathenge W, Wadud Z, Mamun R, et al. (In press) The impact of cataract surgery on health related quality of life in Kenya, Bangladesh and The Philippines. Ophthalmic Epidemiol.
13. Polack S, Eusebio C, Mathenge W, Wadud Z, Mamun R, et al. (2010) The impact of cataract surgery on time-use: results from a longitudinal study in Kenya, Bangladesh and The Philippines. PLoS One 5: e10913.
14. Mathenge W, Kuper H, Polack S, Onyango O, Nyaga G, et al. (2007) Rapid Assessment of Avoidable Blindness in Nakuru District, Kenya. Ophthalmology 114: 599–605.
15. Wadud Z, Kuper H, Polack S, Lindfield R, Rashid Akm M, et al. (2006) Rapid Assessment of Avoidable Blindness and Needs Assessment of Cataract Surgical Services in Satkhira District, Bangladesh. Br J Ophthalmol 90: 1225–1229.
16. Eusebio C, Kuper H, Polack S, Enconado J, Tongson N, et al. (2007) Rapid assessment of avoidable blindness in Negros Island and Antique District, Philippines. Br J Ophthalmol 91: 1588–1592.
17. Turner AG, Magnani RJ, Shuaib M (1996) A not quite as quick but much cleaner alternative to the Expanded Programme on Immunization (EPI) Cluster Survey design. Int J Epidemiol 25: 198–203.
18. Grosh M, Glewwe P, eds. Designing household survey questionnaires for developing countries. Lessons from 15 years of the living standards measurement study. Washington, D.C.: World Bank.
19. Filmer D, Pritchett L (2001) Estimating wealth effects without expenditure data - or tears. An application to educational enrollment in states of India. Demography 38: 115–132.
20. Rabin R, de Charro F (2001) EQ-5D: a measure of health status from the EuroQol Group. Ann Med 33: 337–343.
21. Lewallen S, Courtright P (2000) Recognising and reducing barriers to cataract surgery. Journal of community eye health 13: 20–21.
22. Jenkins SP, Rigg JA (2004) Disability and disadvantage: selection, onset, and duration effects. Journal of Social Policy 33: 479–501.
23. Gannon B, Nolan B (2007) The impact of disability transitions on social inclusion. Soc Sci Med 64: 1425–1437.
24. Engel E (1857) Die Productions und Consumptions-verhaltnisse des Königsreiche Sachsen. Zeitschrift des Statistischen Bureaus des Königlich Sächsischen Ministerium des Inneren. pp 8–9.

Prevalence, Causes and Socio-Economic Determinants of Vision Loss in Cape Town, South Africa

Nicky Cockburn[1]*, David Steven[2], Karin Lecuona[1], Francois Joubert[1], Graeme Rogers[1], Colin Cook[1], Sarah Polack[3]

1 Department of Ophthalmology, Groote Schuur Hospital, Cape Town, South Africa, **2** Eerste River Hospital, Cape Town, South Africa, **3** London School of Hygiene and Tropical Medicine, London, United Kingdom

Abstract

Purpose: To estimate the prevalence and causes of blindness and visual impairment in Cape Town, South Africa and to explore socio-economic and demographic predictors of vision loss in this setting.

Methods: A cross sectional population-based survey was conducted in Cape Town. Eighty-two clusters were selected using probability proportionate to size sampling. Within each cluster 35 or 40 people aged 50 years and above were selected using compact segment sampling. Visual acuity of participants was assessed and eyes with a visual acuity less than 6/18 were examined by an ophthalmologist to determine the cause of vision loss. Demographic data (age, gender and education) were collected and a socio-economic status (SES) index was created using principal components analysis.

Results: Out of 3100 eligible people, 2750 (89%) were examined. The sample prevalence of bilateral blindness (presenting visual acuity <3/60) was 1.4% (95% CI 0.9–1.8). Posterior segment diseases accounted for 65% of blindness and cataract was responsible for 27%. The prevalence of vision loss was highest among people over 80 years (odds ratio (OR) 6.9 95% CI 4.6–10.6), those in the poorest SES group (OR 3.9 95% CI 2.2–6.7) and people with no formal education (OR 5.4 95% CI 1.7–16.6). Cataract surgical coverage was 68% in the poorest SES tertile (68%) compared to 93% in the medium and 100% in the highest tertile.

Conclusions: The prevalence of blindness among people ≥50 years in Cape Town was lower than expected and the contribution of posterior segment diseases higher than previously reported in South Africa and Sub Saharan Africa. There were clear socio-economic disparities in prevalence of vision loss and cataract surgical coverage in this setting which need to be addressed in blindness prevention programs.

Editor: Julius Atashili, University of Buea, Cameroon

Funding: This study received funds from the Lions District 401a Sight Foundation. The funder had no role in study design, data collection and analysis, decision to publish, or preparation of the manuscript. No other external funding was received.

Competing Interests: The authors have declared that no competing interests exist.

* E-mail: nicole.cockburn@uct.ac.za

Introduction

Globally there are an estimated 45 million people who are blind, with the highest of prevalence of blindness found in Africa [1,2]. VISION 2020 is a joint initiative between the World Health Organisation (WHO) and the International Agency for the Prevention of blindness which aims to eliminate avoidable blindness by the year 2020 [3]. WHO estimates from 2002 indicate the prevalence of blindness in Sub-Saharan Africa (SSA) is 1% in all ages and 9% among people ≥50 years [1]. However, recent population based surveys suggest that the prevalence of blindness in the region may be considerably lower [4,5,6,7,8,9].

The majority of blindness surveys in SSA are from rural settings [4,5,6,7,9]. Data are lacking from urban, middle income settings such as Cape Town in South Africa. Studies in rural South Africa conducted more than 20 years ago estimated the prevalence of blindness to be between 0.6% and 1.0% [10,11] for all ages and 1.4–3.2% among people aged ≥40 years [12,13] with cataract accounting for 55–59% of blindness [10,11]. However, extrapolating findings from these and other surveys in SSA to Cape Town may not be appropriate given the likely higher proportion of older persons [14], higher prevalence of diabetes [15] and greater availability of ophthalmic services in this urban setting; all factors which influence the epidemiology of vision loss. Reliable, up-to-date data on the prevalence and cause of blindness is needed in Cape Town order to appropriately plan Vision 2020 blindness prevention programmes.

Although vision loss is widely acknowledged to have important demographic and socio-economic determinants, there is relatively limited quantitative research exploring the nature of the association in different settings [16]. Poverty and blindness are thought to be cyclically linked, with poverty increasing the risk of becoming blind [17] and blindness exacerbating poverty through limiting opportunities to engage in income generating activities [18,19] At country level, the prevalence of blindness is higher in poor countries compared to in wealthier countries [1] and within countries, limited data suggest that the poor are more likely to be blind [20,21]. Studies in South Africa have shown that socioeconomic status (SES) is associated with access to [22,23] and satisfaction with [24] health care. However, the role of these factors in vision loss in South Africa is not known. Understanding this association and identifying at risk groups can help to inform the equitable and efficient use of limited eye care resources.

The aim of this study was to estimate the prevalence and causes of blindness and visual impairment in Cape Town and to investigate the relationship between socio economic factors and vision loss.

Methods

Study setting

This survey was undertaken in Cape Town between September and November 2010. Cape Town has a population of approximately 3.7 million [25] 76% of whom have no medical insurance and are dependent on the public sector [26]. There are three public sector tertiary level hospitals (two for adults, 1 for children) and one district level hospital providing eye care in Cape Town. There are 12 ophthalmologists (excluding residents/registrars) working full time in the public sector and considerably more (54) working in the private sector.

Sample-size

The prevalence of blindness in people aged >50 years was estimated to be 3% [4,5,6,7,9]. Allowing a worst acceptable result of 1%, a design effect of 1.5, confidence of 95%, and a 10% non-response rate, a minimum sample size of 3077 was required. In total 77 clusters of 40 people were required for this survey. For logistical reasons we selected 36 clusters of 35 people and 46 clusters of 40 people (total 82 clusters).

Sampling procedure

We used the data from the 2001 census as the sampling frame, updated with expected population growth estimates [25]. Clusters ('small areas') were selected using probability proportionate to size sampling. Two of the selected clusters were considered unsafe for the survey team to visit and were replaced by selecting the next small area listed on the sampling frame. Within clusters, households were selected using compact segment sampling [27,28]. Aerial maps displaying houses, street names and boundaries were obtained for all selected clusters. Based on the housing density, clusters were divided into segments each including approximately 35 or 40 (depending on cluster size) people aged ≥50 years. One of the segments was selected at random by drawing lots, and all eligible people were included sequentially until the required cluster size was achieved. If the target number was not reached then another segment was chosen at random and sampling continued. The survey team visited households door-to-door to identify eligible people. Absentees were re-visited on the same day in the evening. If more than 10% of the cluster were absent after the second visit, the households were re-visited the following Saturday.

Data collected and protocol for ocular examination

A standardised survey form was completed for each eligible person which included data on examination status, presenting and pinhole vision, lens examination, principal cause of visual impairment, history of visual impairment from a relative or neighbour if subject was not available, why cataract operation had not been carried out (in people with VA<6/60 from cataract in either eye) and details about the operation in those who had had cataract surgery.

Visual acuity (VA) was measured with available spectacle correction by a doctor using a tumbling "E" chart, with optotype size 6/18 (20/60) on one side and size 6/60 (20/200) on the other side, at a distance of 6 meters. If VA was <6/18 in either eye pinhole vision was also measured. Blindness was defined as VA<3/60, severe visual impairment (SVI) as VA<6/60–3/60 and visual impairment as VA<6/18–6/60.

The lens status of all participants was assessed by an ophthalmologist using a direct ophthalmoscope in a dark environment. People with pinhole corrected VA<6/18 in either eye underwent further examination by the ophthalmologist using a direct ophthalmoscope to ascertain the cause of vision loss. According to WHO convention the major cause was assigned to the primary disorder or, if there were two existing primary disorders, to the one that is easiest to treat [29]. The pupil was dilated to allow adequate visualisation of the posterior pole if the cause of visual impairment could not be determined by examination with an undilated pupil.

Socioeconomic and demographic variables

Data were collected on age, gender and highest level of education completed. We used a household SES index as a proxy for wealth. Participants were asked about household ownership of 14 durable items [30] and an SES index was created from these variables using principal component analysis [31]. The index was divided into tertiles of wealth from poorest (lowest SES index) to wealthiest (highest SES).

Training

Five teams, each consisting of one ophthalmologist and one or two Community Based Eye Workers received 5 days training. The inter-observer agreement for VA measurement, lens examination and cause of vision loss was assessed and the kappa value was of an acceptable standard (>0.6) for each team.

Data analysis

All data were double entered. Data on prevalence and causes of vision loss and details of cataract surgery were analysed using the automated RAAB data package. Confidence intervals are calculated taking into account the cluster sampling design. Cataract surgical coverage (CSC) was defined as the proportion of people needing cataract surgery who had received it.

For persons this is calculated as:

$$\frac{X+Y}{X+Y+Z} \times 100$$

In which:

X = Number of people with unilateral (pseudo)aphakia and visual impairment from cataract in the other eye

Y = Number of people with bilateral (pseudo)aphakia

Z = Number of people with bilateral visual impairment from cataract

VA before surgery is unknown and therefore these calculations were undertaken assuming, in turn, that only patients with VA<3/60, <6/60 and <6/18 undergo cataract surgery. CSC was also calculated for eyes.

Stata 11 software was used to analyse the association between vision loss (VA<6/18) demographic (age and gender) and socio-economic variables (SES, and education). We used vision loss rather than blindness as the dependent variable because of the small number of people who were blind. Associations between

Table 1. Age and gender distribution of the survey sample and census population.

	Male				Female				Total			
Age	**Sample**		**Census**		**Sample**		**Census**		**Sample**		**Census**	
50–59	464	(45%)	134,296	(52%)	773	(45%)	134138	(44%)	1,237	(45%)	268,434	(48%)
60–69	322	(31%)	78,675	(31%)	494	(29%)	99,909	(33%)	816	(30%)	178,584	(32%)
70–79	178	(17%)	31,948	(13%)	290	(17%)	55,182	(18%)	468	(17%)	87,130	(16%)
80+	68	(7%)	11,336	(4%)	155	(9%)	15,944	(5%)	223	(8%)	27,280	(5%)

age, gender, SES and education were assessed through logistic regression analysis using the svy command in STATA to account for the cluster sampling design. To explore the independent association of SES and education with vision loss a multivariate logistic regression analysis was undertaken including all the variables in the model. We also calculated the cataract surgical rate stratified by the different SES groups.

Ethical considerations

Informed written consent was obtained from all participants. Ethical approval for this work was granted by University of Cape Town Health Sciences Human Ethics Committee (Cape Town, South Africa) and London School of Hygiene and Tropical Medicine (London, UK). All people with ophthalmic conditions requiring treatment or further investigation were referred.

Results

Prevalence and causes of vision loss

Out of 3100 eligible people, 2750 (89%) were examined, 169 (5.5%) were not available, 170 (5.5%) refused and 11 (0.4%) were unable to communicate. The mean age of people who were examined and refused were similar (62.7 years, 95% CI 62.4–63.1 and 63.4 years, 95% CI 61.9–64.8 respectively), while those who were not available were slightly younger (59.1 years, 95% CI 57.8–60.4) and those unable to communicate were older (73.5 years 95% CI 66.8–80.1). The age distribution of the sample was similar to that of the census (table 1), however men were slightly under-represented compared to census data.

The prevalence of bilateral blindness (presenting vision) in the survey sample was 1.4% (95% CI 0.9–1.8), severe visual impairment (SVI) was 0.9% (0.6–1.4) and visual impairment (VI) was 4.9% (4.1–5.7) (table 2).

Posterior segment diseases were the leading cause of blindness (65%) and were responsible for just over a third of SVI (37%) and one fifth of VI (Table 3). Diabetic retinopathy accounted for 8%, 11% and 2% of blindness, SVI and VI respectively and glaucoma for 11%, 7% and 6%. The remaining posterior segment diseases included age related macular degeneration (ARMD), optic atrophy, trauma and macular hole. Cataract was the second leading cause of blindness (27%) and the leading single cause of SVI (37%). Refractive errors were responsible for 22% of SVI and were the leading cause of VI (50%). Phthisis, cataract surgical complications and other corneal scar were rare as causes of vision loss (<4%). Avoidable causes, which include causes that are treatable or preventable (i.e. operated and un-operated cataract, pthysis, refractive error and corneal scar), made up the 35% of all blindness, 63% of SVI and 79% of VI. If adequate diagnostic and treatment services for DR and glaucoma are in place, so that visual impairment from these conditions is also preventable, avoidable causes rise to 54% of blindness, 81% of SVI and 87% of VI.

Extrapolating the data to the age and gender distribution of the population using the census data, it is estimated that are about 6500 people with bilateral blindness in Cape Town, 5000 with SVI and 24,000 with VI. Of these there are an estimated 1150

Table 2. Estimated prevalence of blindness (VA<3/60), severe visual impairment (VA<6/60–3/60) and visual impairment (VA<6/80–6/60) in Cape Town by person and eyes with available correction.

	Male		Female		Total	
VA with available correction	**N**	**Prevalence (95% CI)**	**n**	**Prevalence (95% CI)**	**n**	**Prevalence (95% CI)**
Blind						
Persons	11	1.1% (0.4–1.7)	26	1.5% (0.9–2.1)	37	1.4% (0.9–1.8)
Eyes	94	4.5% (3.5–5.5)	150	4.4% (3.4–5.3)	242	4.4% (3.9–4.9)
Severe visual impairment						
Persons	6	0.6% (0.1–1.0)	21	1.2% (0.7–1.7)	27	0.9% (0.6–1.4)
Eyes	24	1.2% (0.7–1.7)	72	2.1% (1.5–2.7)	96	1.8% (1.4–2.1)
Visual impairment						
Persons	43	4.1% (2.9–5.2)	91	5.3% (4.2–6.4)	134	4.9% (4.1–5.7)
Eyes	122	5.9% (4.8–7.0)	248	7.2% (6.1–8.4)	372	6.8% (6.1–7.4)

CI, Confidence Interval; VA, Visual Acuity;
NB: data for persons refers to VA in the better eye.

Table 3. Principal cause of bilateral blindness (VA<3/60), bilateral severe visual impairment (VA<6/60–3/60) and bilateral visual impairment (VA<6/80–6/60) among persons with available correction.

	Blindness		Severe Visual impairment		Visual impairment	
	n	%	n	%	n	%
Refractive error	0	(0%)	6	(22%)	67	(50%)
Cataract, untreated	10	(27%)	10	(37%)	36	(27%)
Aphakia uncorrected	1	(3%)	0	(0%)	0	(0%)
Cataract surgical complications	0	(0%)	0	(0%)	2	(2%)
Phthisis	1	(3%)	0	(0%)	0	(0%)
Other corneal scar	1	(3%)	1	(3%)	1	(1%)
Avoidable vision loss[a]	**13**	**(35%)**	**17**	**(63%)**	**106**	**(80%)**
Diabetic retinopathy	3	(8%)	3	(11%)	3	(2%)
Glaucoma	4	(11%)	2	(7%)	8	(6%)
Age related macular degeneration	4	(11%)	2	(7%)	2	(2%)
Other posterior segment	13	(35%)	7	(13%)	24	(18%)
Total posterior segment	**24**	(65%)	**11**	**(37%)**	**27**	**(20%)**

VA, Visual Acuity.
[a]Avoidable causes: Cataract (including un-operated cataract and postoperative complications), refractive error, trachoma, and other causes of corneal scars.

people with bilaterally blinding cataract and 14,800 eyes blind from cataract, 1100 people and 3600 eyes with SVI from cataract and 5,600 people and 14,700 eyes VI from cataract. The age and gender adjusted prevalence was 1.2% for blindness, 1.0% for SVI and 4.2% of VI.

Cataract surgical coverage was high for people and eyes, with 96% of people who needed surgery at VA<3/60 having received it, 93% at VA<6/60 and 80% at VA<6/18 (Table 4). Coverage was similar for males and females (Table 4). The majority of surgeries (63%) were undertaken at a private hospital and 35% were at a government hospital. Place of surgery varied by level of socio-economic status: 65% of people in the poorest tertile had surgery at a government facility and 35% at a private facility, while among those in the richest tertile 26% attended a government facility and 74% a private facility (data not shown). Nearly all (98%) cataract surgeries were with intra-ocular lenses (IOLs). Out of all operated eyes, 80% had a good outcome (VA>6/18) with available correction, while 12% had borderline outcome (VA<6/18–6/60) and for 9% outcome was poor (VA<6/60, Table 5). With pinhole correction this increased to 84% good outcome, 8% borderline and 8% poor. Of the 72 eyes with poor/borderline outcome, the leading causes of poor or borderline outcome were concomitant eye disease (67%) and lack of spectacle correction (24%).

For people with cataract causing VA<6/60 in either eye, we asked the reason why they had not attended for surgery. Among the 18 people with bilateral VA<6/60 who reported barriers, responses were evenly distributed (25% each) between being unaware treatment was possible, unaware how to get surgery, no need for surgery felt and fear.

Demographic and socioeconomic factors and vision loss

There was a positive association between risk of vision loss and increasing age, although this trend was driven by the significantly increased risk among people aged >80 compared to people aged 50–59 years (Odds Ratio (OR) 5.1, 95% CI 3.5–7.6, Table 6). Being female was also associated with increased risk of vision loss (OR 1.4, 95% CI 1.1–1.9). People in the poorest (OR 4.5 95% CI 1.3–3.9) and medium (OR 3.0 95% CI 1.3–3.9) SES tertiles were much more likely to have vision loss compared to those in the wealthiest tertile (p-for-trend<0.001). There was an inverse association between prevalence of vision loss and increasing level of education (p-for-trend<0.001). The association between vision loss and age, SES and education remained significant with multivariate adjustment.

Cataract surgical coverage also varied by SES level. Assuming people have cataract surgery at bilateral VA<6/60, coverage was 100% for those in the wealthiest tertile, 93% for the medium tertile and 68% for the poorest SES tertile (figure 1).

Table 4. Cataract surgical coverage* by persons and eyes.

	Persons	Eyes
Blind (VA<3/60)		
Male	96%	82%
Female	96%	83%
Total	96%	83%
Severe Visual Impairment (VA<6/60)		
Male	94%	79%
Female	93%	79%
Total	93%	79%
Visual Impairment (VA<6/18)		
Male	81%	68%
Female	80%	64%
Total	80%	65%

VA, Visual Acuity.
*Cataract surgical coverage is the proportion of persons (or eyes) with 'operable' cataract who have received cataract surgery.

Table 5. Visual acuity outcome after cataract surgery (eyes) with available correction.

	Non-IOL eyes		IOL eyes		Total	
Outcome	**n**	**%**	**n**	**%**	**n**	**%**
Available Correction						
Good[a]	1	17%	271	80%	272	80%
Borderline[a]	2	33%	39	12%	41	11%
Poor[a]	3	50%	28	8%	31	9%
Best correction						
Good[a]	2	33%	287	85%	289	84%
Borderline[a]	1	17%	25	7%	26	8%
Poor[a]	3	50%	26	8%	29	8%

[a]WHO classification of visual outcome after cataract surgery. Good: VA>6/18; borderline: VA 6/18–6/60; poor: VA<6/60.

Discussion

The prevalence of blindness (1.4%), severe visual impairment (0.9%) and visual impairment (4.9%) in people aged ≥50 years Cape Town was considerably lower than the 2002 WHO estimates, a finding which is consistent with other recent surveys conducted in the region [4,5,6,7,8,9]. This difference may be due in part to improvements in blindness prevention activities (e.g. increases in cataract surgery coverage) but may also reflect the limited data that were available when the WHO estimates were derived. The prevalence estimates in Cape Town were similar to that in urban Cameroon [8] but lower than that in rural areas in SSA [4,5,6,7,9]. A lower prevalence in urban settings may be expected as ophthalmic services are likely to be more available and accessible [32]. Surprisingly, the blindness prevalence was similar to that of a survey in rural Northern Transvaal (current day Limpopo Province) conducted more than 20 years ago [10]. This may be due to methodological differences: the authors of the survey in 'Northern Transvaal' acknowledge that the estimates should be considered 'minimum estimates' because they might have missed cases of blindness [10]. It may also reflect an older population in Cape Town and a higher contribution of posterior segment diseases, which are more difficult to treat.

Posterior segment diseases were responsible for nearly two-thirds of blindness. This is considerably higher than other surveys in the region [4,5,6,7,8,9] and is likely to be due in part to the high CSC and consequent low prevalence of cataract blindness in this setting. It may also reflect an older population and possibly higher burden of diabetes and consequent DR. The finding that posterior segment disease is an important cause of vision loss has implications for planning of eye services in Cape Town. Management of DR, glaucoma and ARMD require significantly more resources than cataract, presenting a significant challenge to blindness prevention programs. Treatment for DR and glaucoma is effective, but requires early detection (community based screening), lifelong monitoring and a high level of adherence with therapy to prevent visual loss. For age related macular degeneration there is the added challenge of minimal (in the case of atrophic disease) or limited (for exudative disease) effective treatment. The urgency of this challenge is likely to increase in this setting and throughout Africa as cataract and other avoidable causes of blindness become more under control.

Cataract accounted for 27% of bilateral blindness which is lower than that previously found in South Africa (50–54% in >40 years group [12] [13]) and elsewhere in SSA (42–65% in >50 year group) [4,5,6,7,9] but similar to that in urban Cameroon [8]. This corresponds with the higher observed CSC in Cape Town. For example, the CSC (for persons <3/60) was found to be 96% in this survey compared to 37% in the Transvaal. However, cataract still remains an important cause of vision loss in this setting and continued efforts are required if the target of eliminating avoidable blindness by 2020 is to be achieved. Encouragingly cataract surgical outcomes met the WHO recommend target of a good outcome (VA>6/18) for ≥80% of eyes with uncorrected vision. Refractive error was the leading cause of visual impairment which suggests the need for increased optical services in this setting.

There was clear variation in the prevalence of vision loss between different socio-economic groups, with the highest prevalence among people with lowest household SES and those lacking in formal education. This could be due to a higher incidence of blinding conditions in these groups. However, there was also evidence of disparity in utilisation of ophthalmic services which may explain this variation: among people needing cataract surgery at VA<6/60, only 67% of the poorest tertile had received surgery compared to 100% of the wealthiest tertile. Our findings support those in Pakistan [21], India [20] and America [33] which show poverty to be a predictor of a higher prevalence of blindness and poorer access to ophthalmic services. Vision loss may also contribute to poverty – a multicentre study showed that after sight

Table 6. The relationship between demographic and socio-economic characteristics and vision loss (bilateral VA<6/18 with available correction).

		VA<6/18		Unadjusted	Multivariate adjusted
	Total	**n**	**%**	**OR (95% CI)**	**OR (95% CI)[a]**
Age (years)					
50–59	1240	71	5.7%	Reference	Reference
60–69	817	40	4.9%	0.8 (0.6–1.3)	0.9 (0.6–1.4)
70–79	468	33	7.1%	1.3 (0.8–1.9)	1.3 (0.8–2.1)
80+	223	53	23.8%	5.1 (3.5–7.6)	6.9 (4.6–10.6)
p-for trend				<0.001	<0.001
Gender					
Male	1034	59	5.7%	Reference	Reference
Female	1712	138	8.1%	1.4 (1.1–1.9)	1.2 (0.9–1.6)
SES[b] tertile					
Poorest	890	107	12.0%	4.5 (1.3–3.9)	3.9 (2.2–6.7)
Medium	984	58	6.5%	3.0 (1.3–3.9)	1.8 (1.0–3.3)
Wealthiest	852	25	2.9%	Reference	Reference
p-for trend				<0.001	<0.001
Education					
None	172	26	15.1%	11.8 (4.0–34.4)	5.4 (1.7–16.6)
Primary	1473	116	7.9%	5.6 (2.2–14.4)	3.3 (1.3–8.6)
Secondary	42	42	5.6%	3.9 (1.5–10.3)	2.9 (1.2–7.4)
Higher	268	4	1.5%	Reference	Reference
p-for trend				<0.001	0.008

VA, Visual Acuity.
[a]Odds ratios from multivariate logistic regression analysis including all listed variables.
[b]Socio-economic status.

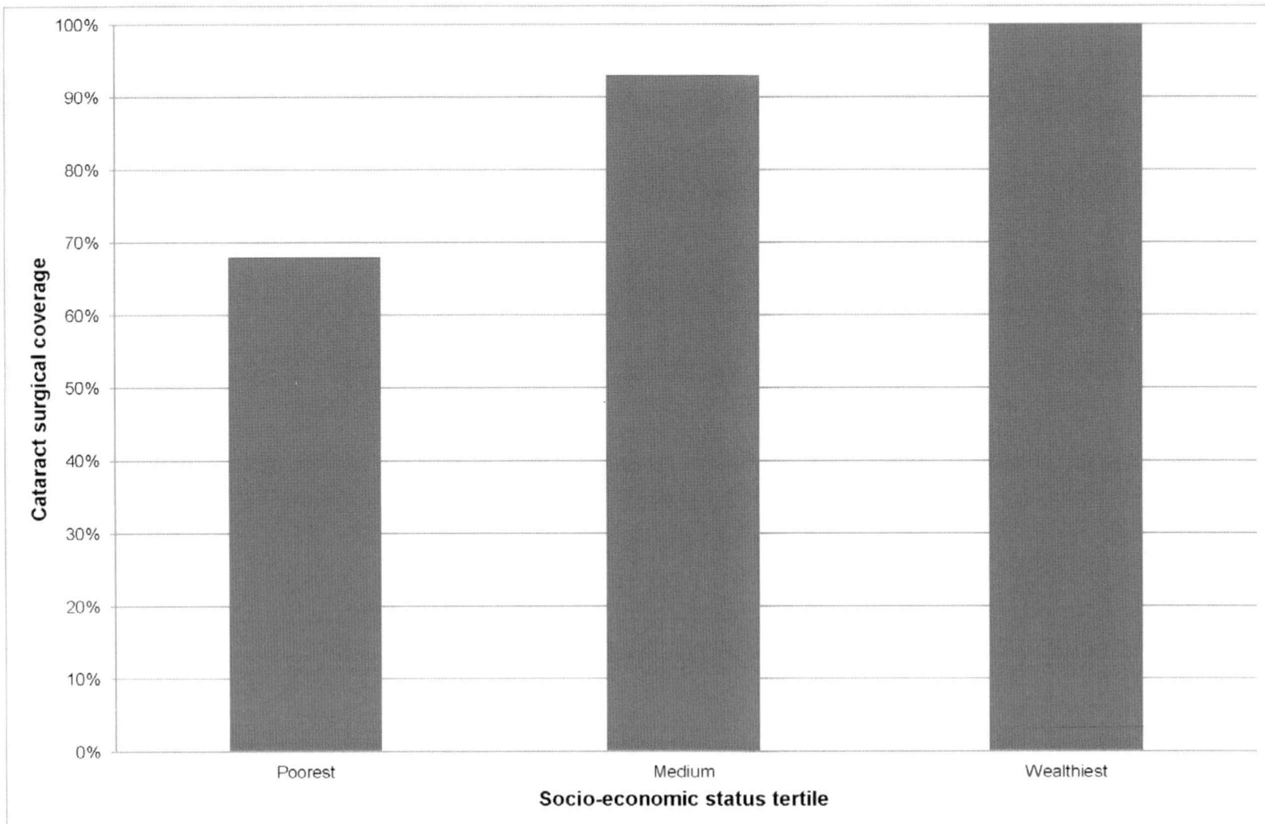

Figure 1. Cataract surgical coverage by socio-economic status. Cataract surgical coverage was defined as the proportion of people needing cataract surgery at VA<6/60 who had received it.

restoring cataract surgery, people were more likely to engage in productive activities and household expenditure increased compared to before surgery [18,19]. Lack of formal education remained a significant predictor of vision loss even after multivariate adjustment suggesting some effect of this variable independent of SES. The association between vision loss and lack of education has been noted elsewhere [34]. Our findings concur with previous studies in South Africa which have shown disparities in health status [35,36,37] and access to health services [22,23,38] among different socio-economic groups.

Interestingly, just over a third of people in the poorest tertile reported attending private health facilities for their cataract surgery. The reasons for this are unclear but may be due in part to high participation in medical insurance schemes (which all cover cataract surgery) among people in any kind of formal employment and the fact that in the public services cataract surgery is only undertaken for people with VA<6/18 in the better eye.

The trend of higher risk of vision loss among women observed in this study has been noted elsewhere [39]. This may be due to longer life expectancy among women as many eye diseases are age related, increased susceptibility to certain ophthalmic conditions or gender disparities in access to and utilisation of health services. In our study the association was no longer significant after adjustment for other socio-economic factors.

There were limitations in this study. Due to the simplified examination protocols used in RAAB it is not always possible to classify posterior segment diseases into different aetiologies. We therefore grouped posterior segment diseases together for discussion purposes. The refusal rate (5.5%) was significantly higher in Cape Town compared to other SSA studies [4,5,7,9]. This may reflect the middle income profile of Cape Town with participants placing less value on a "free eye test". Due to safety concerns, we had to reselect two clusters. We cannot rule this out as a source of bias, although the replacement clusters were from neighbouring areas with similar socio-economic characteristics. We used cluster sampling because simple random sampling is not feasible in such large populations given time and resource constraints and the lack of lists of all individuals in the population. Cluster sampling may introduce a higher sampling error, however our sample size calculation was inflated to adjust for the expected design effect from this sampling approach. Finally, this survey may underestimate the actual demand for cataract services in the public sector because patients from the surrounding districts and provinces commonly travel to Cape Town for cataract surgery.

There were also strengths. Additional efforts were made to revisit clusters at the weekend to in order to examine people who were working or away during the week days. The resulting response rate was high which reduces selection bias. We used standardised approaches to collect ophthalmic and socio-economic data. To the best of our knowledge this is the first survey in the region to examine the relationship between vision loss and socio-economic factors.

Conclusions

The prevalence of blindness in people ≥50 years in Cape Town was lower than expected probably because of high cataract surgery coverage. The contribution of posterior segment diseases as a cause of blindness is higher than previously reported in South Africa and SSA. There were socio economic disparities in prevalence of vision loss and cataract surgical coverage. These inequalities need to be addressed in order for Vision 2020 targets to be achieved in Cape Town.

Acknowledgments

We would like to thank all the people who kindly participated in the survey, the community based eye workers from the Jonga Trust, Niki Van Vuuren for data entry and Reno Morar for input on the manuscript.

Author Contributions

Conceived and designed the experiments: SP NC DS CC. Performed the experiments: NC DS KL FJ GR CC SP. Analyzed the data: NC SP. Contributed reagents/materials/analysis tools: NC DS KL FJ GR CC SP. Wrote the paper: NC SP. Revised and critically reviewed the article for important intellectual content and gave final approval for the manuscript: DS FJ KL GR CC.

References

1. Resnikoff S, Pascolini D, Etya'ale D, Kocur I, Pararajasegaram R, et al. (2004) Global data on visual impairment in the year 2002. Bull World Health Organ 82: 844–851.
2. Resnikoff S, Pascolini D, Mariotti SP, Pokharel GP (2008) Global magnitude of visual impairment caused by uncorrected refractive errors in 2004. Bull World Health Organ 86: 63–70.
3. Foster A, Resnikoff S (2005) The impact of Vision 2020 on global blindness. Eye (Lond) 19: 1133–1135.
4. Habiyakire C, Kabona G, Courtright P, Lewallen S (2010) Rapid assessment of avoidable blindness and cataract surgical services in kilimanjaro region, Tanzania. Ophthalmic Epidemiol 17: 90–94.
5. Kalua K, Lindfield R, Mtupanyama M, Mtumodzi D, Msiska V (2011) Findings from a rapid assessment of avoidable blindness (RAAB) in Southern Malawi. PLoS One 6: e19226.
6. Mathenge W, Kuper H, Limburg H, Polack S, Onyango O, et al. (2007) Rapid assessment of avoidable blindness in Nakuru district, Kenya. Ophthalmology 114: 599–605.
7. Mathenge W, Nkurikiye J, Limburg H, Kuper H (2007) Rapid assessment of avoidable blindness in Western Rwanda: blindness in a postconflict setting. PLoS Med 4: e217.
8. Oye JE, Kuper H (2007) Prevalence and causes of blindness and visual impairment in Limbe urban area, South West Province, Cameroon. Br J Ophthalmol 91: 1435–1439.
9. Oye JE, Kuper H, Dineen B, Befidi-Mengue R, Foster A (2006) Prevalence and causes of blindness and visual impairment in Muyuka: a rural health district in South West Province, Cameroon. Br J Ophthalmol 90: 538–542.
10. Bucher PJ, Ijsselmuiden CB (1988) Prevalence and causes of blindness in the northern Transvaal. Br J Ophthalmol 72: 721–726.
11. Cook CD, Knight SE, Crofton-Briggs I (1993) Prevalence and causes of low vision and blindness in northern KwaZulu. S Afr Med J 83: 590–593.
12. Rotchford AP, Johnson GJ (2002) Glaucoma in Zulus: a population-based cross-sectional survey in a rural district in South Africa. Arch Ophthalmol 120: 471–478.
13. Salmon JF, Mermoud A, Ivey A, Swanevelder SA, Hoffman M (1993) The prevalence of primary angle closure glaucoma and open angle glaucoma in Mamre, western Cape, South Africa. Arch Ophthalmol 111: 1263–1269.
14. Joubert J, Bradshaw D (2006) Population aging and health challenges. In: Steyn K, Fourie J, Temple N, eds. Chronic Diseases of Lifestyle in South Africa: 1995–2005 Technical report. Cape Town: South African Medical Research Council. 206 p.
15. Levitt NS, Katzenellenbogen JM, Bradshaw D, Hoffman MN, Bonnici F (1993) The prevalence and identification of risk factors for NIDDM in urban Africans in Cape Town, South Africa. Diabetes Care 16: 601–607.
16. Braithwaite J, Mont D (2008) Disability and poverty: a survey of World Bank poverty assessments and implications. Washington DC: World Bank.
17. Kuper H, Foster A (2005) What do we know about global blindness? Current Medical Literature Ophthalmology 15: 81–86.
18. Kuper H, Polack S, Mathenge W, Eusebio C, Wadud Z, et al. (2010) Does cataract surgery alleviate poverty? Evidence from a multi-centre intervention study conducted in Kenya, the Philippines and Bangladesh. PLoS One 5: e15431.
19. Polack S, Eusebio C, Mathenge W, Wadud Z, Mamun R, et al. (2010) The Impact of Cataract Surgery on Activities and Time-Use: Results from a Longitudinal Study In Kenya, Bangladesh and The Philippines PLoS ONE 5: e10913.
20. Dandona L, Dandona R, Srinivas M, Giridhar P, Vilas K, et al. (2001) Blindness in the Indian state of Andhra Pradesh. Invest Ophthalmol Vis Sci 42: 908–916.
21. Gilbert CE, Shah SP, Jadoon MZ, Bourne R, Dineen B, et al. (2008) Poverty and blindness in Pakistan: results from the Pakistan national blindness and visual impairment survey. BMJ 336: 29–32.
22. Harris B, Goudge J, Ataguba JE, McIntyre D, Nxumalo N, et al. (2011) Inequities in access to health care in South Africa. J Public Health Policy 32 Suppl 1: S102–123.
23. Lalloo R, Myburgh NG, Smith MJ, Solanki GC (2004) Access to health care in South Africa–the influence of race and class. S Afr Med J 94: 639–642.
24. Myburgh NG, Solanki GC, Smith MJ, Lalloo R (2005) Patient satisfaction with health care providers in South Africa: the influences of race and socioeconomic status. Int J Qual Health Care 17: 473–477.
25. Small K 2010 population estimates.City of Cape Town - Strategic Development Information and GIS Department. City of Cape Town.
26. Statistics South Africa (2011) General Household Survey 2010. Statistics South Africa, Private Bag X44, Pretoria 0001. pp 28.
27. Kuper H, Polack S, Limburg H (2006) Rapid assessment of avoidable blindness. Community Eye Health 19: 68–69.
28. Turner AG, Magnani RJ, Shuaib M (1996) A not quite as quick but much cleaner alternative to the Expanded Programme on Immunization (EPI) Cluster Survey design. Int J Epidemiol 25: 198–203.
29. Programme for the Prevention of Blindness and Deafness (1988) Coding instructions for the WHO/PBL eye examination record (version iii). Geneva: WHO 1988: 1–17. Available: http://whqlibdoc.who.int/hq/1988/PBL_88.1.pdf. Accessed 18 Dec 2011.
30. Lam D, Ardington C, Branson N, Case A, et al. (2008) The Cape Area Panel Study: A Very Short Introduction to the Integrated Waves 1-2-3-4 Data. The University of Cape Town, October 2008.
31. Filmer D, Pritchett L (2001) Estimating wealth effects without expenditure data - or tears. An application to educational enrollment in states of India. Demography 38: 115–132.
32. Lecuona K, Cook C (2011) South Africa's cataract surgery rates: why are we not meeting our targets? S Afr Med J 101: 510–512.
33. Tielsch JM, Sommer A, Witt K, Katz J, Royall RM (1990) Blindness and visual impairment in an American urban population. The Baltimore Eye Survey. Arch Ophthalmol 108: 286–290.
34. Dandona R, Dandona L (2001) Socioeconomic status and blindness. Br J Ophthalmol 85: 1484–1488.
35. Harling G, Ehrlich R, Myer L (2008) The social epidemiology of tuberculosis in South Africa: a multilevel analysis. Soc Sci Med 66: 492–505.
36. Groenewald P, Bradshaw D, Daniels J, Zinyakatira N, Matzopoulos R, et al. (2010) Local-level mortality surveillance in resource-limited settings: a case study of Cape Town highlights disparities in health. Bull World Health Organ 88: 444–451.
37. Nkonki LL, Chopra M, Doherty TM, Jackson D, Robberstad B (2011) Explaining household socio-economic related child health inequalities using multiple methods in three diverse settings in South Africa. Int J Equity Health 10: 13.
38. Kon ZR, Lackan N (2008) Ethnic disparities in access to care in post-apartheid South Africa. Am J Public Health 98: 2272–2277.
39. Abou-Gareeb I, Lewallen S, Bassett K, Courtright P (2001) Gender and blindness: a meta-analysis of population-based prevalence surveys. Ophthalmic Epidemiol 8: 39–56.

5

Population Based Outcomes of Cataract Surgery in Three Tribal Areas of Andhra Pradesh, India: Risk Factors for Poor Outcomes

Rohit C. Khanna[1,2]*, Srinivasa Reddy Pallerla[3], Shiva Shankar Eeda[3], Bala Krishna Gudapati[3], Sandra D. Cassard[4], Padmaja Kumari Rani[1,2], Ghanshyam Palamaner Subash Shantha[5], Subhabrata Chakrabarti[1], Oliver D. Schein[4,5]

1 Brien Holden Eye Research Centre, L.V. Prasad Eye Institute, Banjara Hills, Hyderabad, India, **2** Allen Foster Research Centre for Community Eye Health, International Centre for Advancement of Rural Eyecare, L.V. Prasad Eye Institute, Hyderabad, India, **3** Andhra Pradesh Right to Sight Society, Hyderabad, India, **4** Wilmer Eye Institute, Johns Hopkins University, Baltimore, Maryland, United States of America, **5** Johns Hopkins Bloomberg School of Public Health, Baltimore, Maryland, United States of America

Abstract

Purpose: To report visual outcomes and risk factors for poor outcomes of cataract surgery in three Integrated Tribal Development Agency (ITDA) areas of Andhra Pradesh, India.

Methods and Results: Using validated Rapid Assessment of Avoidable Blindness (RAAB) methodology, a population based cross-sectional study, was conducted in three ITDA areas. A two-stage sampling procedure was used to select 7281 participants aged 50 years and above. Vision assessment using a tumbling E chart and standard ocular examinations were completed. Visual outcomes and risk factors for poor outcomes were assessed among subjects undergoing cataract surgery (1548 eyes of 1124 subjects). Mean age at surgery was 67±8 years; Among the operated eyes, presenting visual acuity (PVA) and best corrected visual acuity (BCVA) worse than 6/18 was seen in 492 (31.8%; 95% CI, 29.5–34.2%) and 298 eyes (19.3%; 95% CI, 17.3–21.3%), respectively. Similarly, PVA and BCVA worse than 6/60 was seen in 219 (14.1%; 95% CI, 12.4–16%) and 147 eyes (9.5%; 95% CI, 8.1–11.1%), respectively. When either eye was taken into consideration, the PVA and BCVA worse than 6/18 was seen in 323 (20.1%; 95% CI, 18.9–23%) and 144 subjects (9.3%; 95% CI, 7.9–10.9%), respectively. PVA and BCVA worse than 6/60 was seen in 74 (4.8%; 95% CI, 3.8–6%) and 49 subjects (3.2%; 95% CI, 2.4–4.2%), respectively. Posterior capsular opacification was seen in 51 of 1316 pseudophakic eyes (3.9%; 95% CI, 2.9–5.1%). In multivariable analysis among pseudophakic subjects with PVA worse than 6/18, increasing age ($p = 0.002$) and undergoing free surgery ($p = 0.05$) were independent risk factors. Undergoing surgery before 2005 ($p = 0.05$) and being illiterate ($p = 0.05$) were independent risk factors for BCVA worse than 6/18.

Conclusions: There are changing trends with improved outcomes in cataract surgery among these tribal populations of India. However, post-operative refractive error correction remains an issue, especially for those undergoing free surgeries.

Editor: Andreas Wedrich, Medical University Graz, Austria

Funding: Funding for conducting the study was received from Department for International Development (DFID) UK. The funders had no role in study design, data collection and analysis, decision to publish, or preparation of the manuscript.

Competing Interests: The authors have declared that no competing interests exist.

* E-mail: rohit@lvpei.org

Introduction

Population based surveys in India in the past have identified cataract as the leading cause of blindness and visual impairment (VI) [1,2]. The Government of India launched a World Bank-aided project in 1994 to eliminate cataract blindness in 7 states of the country with the highest prevalence of cataract related blindness and VI [2,3]. As a result of this program, 15.3 million cataract surgeries were performed compared to a projected 11 million [3]. However, there were several concerns with respect to the quality of cataract surgeries performed under this program. Cataract surgery outcomes across different parts of the country varied significantly, with poor visual outcomes ranging between 11.8%–44.1% [4,5,6,7,8,9,10].

India has one of the largest tribal population in the world. The Government of India defined a tribal region based on certain characteristics [11], which include (and are not limited to) economically backward communities living in a primitive condition, having a distinct culture and usually living in isolation away from the mainstream. To the best of our knowledge, there are no reports on eye care and its implications from the tribal regions of India. This could be attributed to the poor accessibility of their regions of habitat [11]. The government has established the Integrated Tribal Development Agency (ITDA) to bring an overall development in these under-served areas. In the state of Andhra

Pradesh (AP) in Southern India, the government received ~1.5 million USD for Tribal Eye Care Project from the Department for International Development (DFID), UK, for a period of 3 years.

As there was no prior evidence on avoidable blindness from any tribal population in India, we conducted a Rapid Assessment of Avoidable Blindness (RAAB) survey in 3 tribal-inhabited areas of Andhra Pradesh (AP) to assess the prevalence of visual impairment and blindness in these regions. The objective of this paper is to report the visual outcomes of cataract surgery and also assess the risk factors contributing to poor outcome in these 3 ITDA areas.

Methods

Geographical distribution

The 3 ITDA selected for this study in Andhra Pradesh were Bhadrachalam in the Khammam district and Eturunagaram in the Warangal district (Area 1), Kota Rama Chandrapuram (K R Puram) in the West Godavari district and Rampa Chodavaram (R C Varam) in the East Godavari district (Area 2) and Srisailam, which is spread over 6 districts of Mahabubnagar, Nalagonda, Ranga Reddy, Kurnool, Guntur and Prakasam (Area 3). As per the 2001 census, the population of area 1 was 897,611, area 2 was 421,000 and area 3 was 554,439 [12].

Sample selection

A population based cross-sectional survey was conducted using validated RAAB methodology among subjects aged 50 years or older [13]. A two-stage sampling strategy involved Probability Proportionate to Size Sampling (PPSS) strategy for the selection of clusters (villages) followed by Compact Segment Sampling (CSS) for selection of households within the clusters [14,15]. The population sizes in these villages were obtained from 2001 census data and an annual growth rate of 1.3% was added to obtain an estimate for 2009. For sample size calculations, the prevalence of blindness in each area was estimated to be 6%. It was estimated that 13% of the population would be 50 years or older [12]. Allowing for a 95% confidence interval, a precision of 20% (lower bound of 4.8%), design effect of 1.5 for cluster of 50 subjects and 10% non-response rate, the sample size required in each area was 2500.

Study definitions

Blindness was defined as VA worse than 6/60 in the better eye with available correction and VI was defined as VA worse than 6/18 but not worse than 6/60 in the better eye with available correction [16].

Definitions of ocular pathologies

Refractive error was defined as VA <6/18 improving ≥6/18 with pin hole. Cataract was defined as visible opacity in pupillary area impairing vision and partly or complete obscuration of red reflex on distant direct ophthalmoscopy. Glaucoma was defined as any 2 of the following 4 signs i) Neuroretinal rim reduced to <=0.1 of cup disc (C:D) size ii) C:D ratio >=0.8 iii) asymmetry of the cups >=0.2 iv) any surgical/laser procedure performed for glaucoma and any fundus pathology other than glaucoma was characterized as posterior segment pathology.

The standard RAAB survey form was used (Annexure S1). Additional information was collected on the type of population residing in these areas (tribal or non-tribal) and literacy. Illiteracy was defined as not able to read or write simple text and numbers [17]. The study was approved by the Institutional Review Board of L V Prasad Eye Institute and conformed to the tenets of the Declaration of Helsinki. All subject aged 50 years and above in the population, in the research area, residing in the village at least for the previous 6 months from the initiation of the study and willing to give informed consent were enrolled. A written informed consent was obtained from all the subjects having a minimum level of literacy. However, subjects who did not have a formal education provided their consent based on a thumb impression in the consent form. All the study procedures was explained in detail to

Table 1. Comparison of characteristics of 1548 eyes based on their lens status.

Parameters	Aphakia–n (%)	Pseudophakia– n (%)	P value	Total – n (%)
Total eyes	232 (15)	1316 (85)		1548 (100)
Area 1	111 (47.8)	489 (37.2)		600 (38.8)
Area 2	33 (14.2)	283 (21.5)	0.018	316 (20.4)
Area 3	88 (37.9)	544 (41.3)		632 (40.8)
Proportion in tribals	46 (19.8)	306 (23.3)	0.34	352 (22.7)
Proportion in literate	8 (3.5)	125 (9.5)	0.004	133 (8.6)
Time of surgery				
≤1998	70 (30.2)	27 (2.1)		97 (6.3)
1999–2004	127 (54.7)	339 (25.8)	<0.001	466 (30.1)
2005–2009	35 (15.1)	950 (72.7)		985 (63.6)
Government sector operated	124 (53.4)	592 (45)	0.03	716 (46.3)
Proportion operated free	157 (67.7)	1099 (83.5)	<0.001	1256 (81.1)
V/A<6/60 (PVA)	116 (50)	103 (7.8)	<0.001	219 (14.2)
V/A<6/18 (PVA)	166 (71.6)	326 (24.8)	<0.001	492 (31.8)
V/A <6/60 (BVA)	74 (31.9)	73 (5.6)	<0.001	147 (9.5)
V/A <6/18 (BVA)	128 (55.2)	128 (55.2)	<0.001	298 (19.3)

Abbreviations: PVA: Presenting visual acuity; BVA: Best corrected visual acuity.

each subject by the study investigator, in presence of two to three community heads of the village.

Training

Training for all the team members was given at L V Prasad Eye Institute, Hyderabad and an Inter Observer Variation Test (IOVT) was performed for each of these teams for the measurement of visual acuity (VA) and lens examination and to ensure acceptable agreement (Kappa value ≥0.6). Additionally, causes of blindness and VI were assessed by qualified ophthalmologists based on clinical examinations. For quality control measures, the clinical findings of all subjects with presenting visual acuity (PVA) <6/18 in either eye, those with previous cataract surgery and 10% of normal subjects in 6 preselected clusters (2 in each area), were further assessed by a second ophthalmic assistant and an ophthalmologist. Prior to undertaking the main study, a pilot study was conducted to ensure the standardization of all protocols.

Table 2. Proportion of eyes with pseudophakia and aphakia having presenting and best corrected visual acuity <6/18.

Parameters	Pseudophakic eyes		Aphakic eye	
	(n = 1316)		(n = 232)	
	PVA<6/18	BCVA <6/18	PVA <6/18	BCVA <6/18
	n (%)	n (%)	n (%)	n (%)
Total	326 (24.8)	170 (12.9)	166 (71.6)	128 (55.2)
50–59 years	30 (14.6)	16 (7.8)	14 (66.7)	13 (61.9)
60–69 years	154 (25.9)	80 (13.5)	58 (73.4)	46 (58.2)
≥70 years	142 (27.5)	74 (14.3)	94 (71.2)	69 (52.3)
Male	134 (23.2)	71 (12.3)	62 (72.1)	51 (59.3)
Female	192 (26.0)	99 (13.4)	104 (71.2)	77 (52.7)
Tribal	83 (27.1)	41 (13.4)	31 (67.4)	26 (56.5)
Non tribal	243 (24.1)	129 (12.8)	135 (72.6)	102 (54.8)
Literate	19 (15.2)	8 (6.4)	4 (50)	4 (50)
Illiterate	307 (25.8)	162 (13.6)	162 (72.3)	124 (55.4)
Glasses				
Yes	60 (20.9)		78 (57.4)	
No	266 (25.9)		88 (91.7)	
2005–2009	221 (23.3)	108 (11.4)	25 (71.4)	20 (57.1)
1999–2004	99 (29.2)	57 (16.8)	92 (72.4)	75 (59.1)
<1999	6 (22.2)	5 (18.5)	49 (70)	33 (47.1)
Paid	37 (17.1)	19 (8.8)	48 (64)	33 (44)
Free	289 (26.3)	151 (13.7)	118 (75.2)	95 (60.5)
NGO/Private	156 (21.6)	84 (11.6)	72 (66.7)	53 (49.1)
Government	170 (28.7)	86 (14.5)	94 (75.8)	75 (60.5)
Area 1	112 (22.9)	52 (10.6)	73 (65.8)	51 (46)
Area 2	72 (25.4)	46 (16.3)	26 (78.8)	21 (63.6)
Area 3	142 (26.1)	72 (13.2)	67 (76.1)	56 (63.6)

PVA: Presenting Visual Acuity; BCVA: Best Corrected Visual Acuity; NGO: Non-governmental Organization.

Data collection procedures

The epidemiological data were collected from the last week of July to September 2009. A local health worker in each cluster helped with enumeration as well as verification of age and the examination procedure was explained to the subjects. Visual acuity was measured in daylight conditions using the tumbled 'E' charts optotype 6/60 on one side and 6/18 on other side. If the subject's VA was worse than 6/18, a pinhole test was performed. For aphakic subjects, a+10D lens or their available correction was used along with a pinhole correction. Pinhole measured visual acuity was used as a surrogate for best corrected visual acuity (BCVA). If the subject's VA did not improve with pinhole correction, the subject was examined by an ophthalmologist using a portable uni-ocular slit lamp for the anterior segment. For assessment of lens status, torch and distant direct ophthalmoscope were used in a shaded or semi-dark environment without pupillary dilatation. Then 1% Tropicamide drops were instilled and a fundus examination was done to check for any posterior segment pathology. The principal cause of blindness or VI was recorded by the ophthalmologist and if there was more than one cause, the most treatable cause was recorded. If the subject required any treatment, he was referred to the nearest secondary or tertiary eye care facility with a referral slip.

Subjects who had undergone cataract surgery were asked about the date and place of their surgery and whether they paid for the services or if it was free. If the subject was absent, two revisits were made, before classifying the subject as unavailable.

Data were collected and entered on the same day, independently by two data entry operators (Annexure S1). Both the databases were checked for consistency using the RAAB software.

Data Analysis

Data analysis was performed with Stata software (version 11.0) [18]. Continuous variables were compared using Student's t test or one-way analysis of variance (ANOVA), while categorical variables were analyzed using chi-square test. Risk factors for VA worse than 6/18 were analysed by multiple logistic regression with generalized estimating equation (GEE) along with robust variance estimation to account for the correlation between both the eyes in an individual [19,20]. Multi-collinearity between variables was assessed looking at the variance inflation factor and fitness of the model was assessed using Hosmer Lemeshow test for goodness of fit [21]. Since the two surgical procedures for aphakia

Table 3. Cause of Visual impairment and blindness stratified by category of visual impairment and blindness.

Causes	<6/18–6/60	<6/60	Total
	n (%)	n (%)	
Refractive error	174 (63.7)	17 (7.8)	191 (38.8)
Aphakia (uncorrected)	10 (3.7)	64 (29.2)	74 (15)
Surgical complications	31 (11.4)	47 (21.5)	78 (15.9)
Other corneal scars	2 (0.7)	*9 (4.1)	11 (2.2)
Glaucoma	4 (1.5)	13 (5.9)	17 (3.5)
Other posterior segment	52 (19.1)	69 (31.5)	121 (24.6)
Overall n (%)	273 (100)	219 (100)	492 (100)

*Include one eye with phthisis.

Table 4. Logistic regression showing risk factor for blindness and visual impairment for presenting visual acuity (PVA) and best corrected visual acuity (BCVA) in pseudophakic eyes.

	For PVA <6/18 in pseudophakic eyes				For BCVA <6/18 in pseudophakic eyes			
	n = 1316 eyes				n = 1316 eyes			
	*OR	P value	#OR	P value	*OR	P value	#OR	P value
Age								
50–59	Ref							
60–69	2.05	0.001	1.98	0.002	1.85	0.03	1.64	0.1
≥70	2.23	<0.001	2.19	0.001	1.99	0.02	1.80	0.05
Overall		0.001		0.002		0.05		0.14
Gender								
Male	Ref							
Female	1.17	0.27	1.16	0.31	1.11	0.57	1.08	0.7
Tribal								
Yes	Ref							
No	0.85	0.32	0.89	0.53	0.95	0.79	1.13	0.57
Literacy								
Literate	Ref							
Illiterate	1.94	0.01	1.63	0.09	2.30	0.03	2.16	0.05
Glasses								
Yes	Ref							
No	1.32	0.12	1.26	0.19				
Time								
2005–09	Ref							
1999–04	1.36	0.04	1.31	0.08	1.58	0.01	1.35	0.03
<1999	0.94	0.9	1.03	0.95	1.77	0.27	2.09	0.16
Overall		0.11		0.21		0.03		0.05
Paying								
Paid	Ref							
Free	1.74	0.005	1.52	0.05	1.66	0.046	1.57	0.12
Place								
NGO/PVT	Ref							
GVT.	1.47	0.004	1.31	0.09	1.29	0.13	1.23	0.33
Area								
Area 1	Ref							
Area 2	1.15	0.46	1.12	0.58	1.63	0.04	1.77	0.03
Area 3	1.19	0.43	1.20	0.27	1.28	0.22	1.34	0.16
Overall		0.52		0.53		0.11		0.08

PVA: Presenting Visual Acuity; BCVA: Best Corrected Visual Acuity; OR: Odds Ratio; CI: Confidence Interval; NGO: Non-governmental Organization; H-L: Hosmer-Lemeshow goodness of fit; GVT: government; NGO: non-governmental organization; PVT: private sector; *: indicates odds ratios of uni-variate analysis, #: indicates odds ratios of multi-variate analysis.

and pseudophakia are quite different, a separate logistic regression was performed for each of them.

Results

During the study period, 7500 subjects were enumerated in three tribal zones and 7281 (97.1%) were examined. 1124 subjects had undergone cataract surgery, yielding an overall prevalence of 15.4% (95% CI, 14.6–16.3%). Of them, 424 subjects (37.7%) had undergone bilateral surgery. A higher proportion of surgeries were performed in the non-tribal population compared to the tribal population (19.6% versus 9%; p<0.001) and among illiterates as compared to literates (16% versus 11%; p<0.001).

Overall, the mean ages of the subjects who underwent cataract surgery was 67±8 years (median: 65 years and range: 50–90 years). The mean age of the female subjects (n = 642) was lower than males at the time of surgery (p = 0.001). Only 25.4% of the operated subjects were using glasses. Of the unilaterally operated eyes, 59 had aphakia and 641 had pseudophakia, while among the bilaterally operated subjects, 52 had aphakia in both eyes and 303 had pseudophakia in both the eyes. The remaining 69 subjects had aphakia in one eye and pseudophakia in the other eye. Thus, despite 232 (15%) eyes being aphakic, 90.1% subjects had pseudophakia in at least one eye.

The mean time since surgery was 4.4±4.5 years (median = 3 - years). Among the different settings that were availed for surgery, 708 (45.7%) eyes were operated in a government hospital, 569 (36.8%) eyes in the non-governmental organizations, 263 (17%) eyes in the private sector and the remaining 8 (0.5%) in eye camps. Since the 8 eyes operated in camps were performed in the government sector, they were grouped with those operated in the government sector for further analysis. For comparisons across different studies, those operated in the private sector were grouped to those operated in the non-governmental organizations. A total of 1256 (81.1%) eyes were operated for free.

Table 1 provides a comparison of different characteristics of the 1548 eyes based on their lens status (aphakia and pseudophakia). As seen in this table, most of the aphakia surgeries were done before 2005 ($p<0.001$) and a relatively higher proportion of these were operated in the government sector ($p = 0.03$) and among the illiterate population ($p = 0.004$).

Visual impairment and blindness

As seen in table 1, PVA worse than 6/60 and worse than 6/18 was found in 219 (14.2%; 95% CI, 12.4–16%) and 492 eyes (31.8%; 95% CI, 29.5–34.2%), respectively. The BCVA worse than 6/60 and worse than 6/18 was found in 147 (9.5%; 95% CI, 8.1–11.1%) and 298 eyes (19.3%; 95% CI, 17.3–21.3%), respectively. When either eye was taken into consideration, the PVA and BCVA worse than 6/18 was seen in 323 (20.1%; 95% CI, 18.9–23%) and 144 subjects (9.3%; 95% CI, 7.9–10.9%), respectively. PVA and BCVA worse than 6/60 was seen in 74 (4.8%; 95% CI, 3.8–6%) and 49 subjects (3.2%; 95% CI, 2.4–4.2%), respectively. PVA and BCVA worse than 6/18 and worse than 6/60 was significantly more prevalent among the aphakic compared to pseudophakic eyes ($p<0.001$). Table 2 shows the proportion of eyes with pseudophakia and aphakia having PVA and BCVA worse than 6/18 stratified by various risk factors. There was no difference in the proportion of visual impairment ($p = 0.7$) or blindness ($p = 0.24$) in the 3 areas.

Causes of visual impairment and blindness

Overall, refractive error, uncorrected aphakia, surgical complications and posterior segment disorders were the major causes of VI and blindness (Table 3). Among the subjects with VA worse than 6/60, uncorrected aphakia, surgical complications and posterior segment disorders were relatively more common, while for those with VA worse than 6/18 but better than 6/60, uncorrected refractive error was the common cause of VI and blindness. Posterior capsular opacification was seen in 51 of 1316 pseudophakic eyes (3.9%; 95% CI, 2.9–5.1%)

Risk factors for blindness and VI

Table 4 and Table S1 exhibits the risk factor for blindness and VI for PVA and BCVA in pseudophakic eyes, wherein, for PVA, increasing age ($p = 0.002$) and availing free surgery ($p = 0.05$) were an independent risk factors, illiteracy ($p = 0.09$) and surgeries performed at the government sector ($p = 0.09$) were not the major risk factors. Similarly, for BCVA, illiteracy ($p = 0.05$) and a history of cataract surgery before year 2005 ($p = 0.05$) were marginal risk factors for blindness and VI. Among the aphakic subjects, abstaining from the use of glasses was the only independent risk factor ($p<0.001$) for PVA (data not shown). It may be noted here that the power to detect significant risk factors in aphakic subjects were limited due to vagaries of small sample size.

Discussion

The overall prevalence of cataract surgery was much higher than that reported from India a decade ago and is relatively higher compared to neighboring and some developed countries [5,6,7,8,22,23,24,25,26,27,28]. Our estimates are similar to the prevalence seen in the urban cohort (15.7%) but lower than the rural cohort (21.9%) of Chennai Glaucoma Study (CGS) and also lower than that reported from Navsari in Gujarat (17.6%) [9,10].

Among the 1548 eyes, 15% were aphakics, which was much lower than that reported a decade ago [5,6,7,8]. The overall prevalence of aphakia was comparable to reports from Navsari in Gujarat (15.9%)[10], but was lower than the urban and rural cohorts of CGS (27.2% and 44.5%, respectively) [9,10]. The proportion of intraocular lens implantation was much higher that reported a decade earlier from India [5,6,7,8]. These temporal trends suggest that most of the surgeons have passed the transition phase of conversion from non-IOL surgery to IOL surgery.

PVA and BCVA > = 6/18 were seen in 68.2% and 80.7% of the eyes, respectively and there was no significant difference in the 3 tribal areas. This was much higher than that reported from a recent study from Navsari in Gujarat (PVA and BCVA ≥6/18 seen in 50.7% and 74.5%, respectively)[10], CGS (PVA and BCVA ≥6/18 seen in 54.2% and 78.4% respectively)[9] and Bharatpur in Rajasthan (PVA and BCVA ≥6/18 seen in 31.5% and 58.8% respectively) [7]. Though the PVA was better than Tirunelveli and Sivaganga (PVA ≥6/18 seen in 64% and 60.3% respectively), the BCVA was comparable to both the areas (BCVA ≥6/18 seen in 83% and 84.5% respectively) [6,8]. It was also comparable to Lumbini zone and Chitwan district of Nepal [24], but better than Satkhira district in Bangladesh [28]. The difference in PVA and BCVA reported from other parts of India and neighboring countries could be due to the difference in proportion of pseudophakics in these populations as well as the use of IOL with appropriate power.

Based on PVA, only 14.2% eyes were blind and the proportion was significantly higher for aphakics than pseudophakics. This was lower to that observed at Navsari in Gujarat (18%) [10], and the urban and rural cohorts of CGS (17.2% and 26.8%, respectively) [9]. This was also comparable to Tirunelveli and Sivaganga (11.8% and 13.8% respectively) [6,8]; and much lower than Bharatpur in Rajasthan (44.1%) [7] and the urban and rural cohorts in the previously conducted Andhra Pradesh Eye Disease Study (APEDS) (21.4% and 24.5% respectively) [4,5]. Similar variation in proportions of blindness were reported from the neighboring regions of Lumbini zone and Chitwan district in Nepal (13.8%) [24], Ratuhat district in Nepal (20%) [27], Satkhira district in Bangladesh (23.5%) [28], Liwan in China (15.6%) [23] and Hong Kong (11.2%) [25]. It may be noted that the proportion of blindness in the population was highly influenced by the blindness in aphakics in the present study. Thus, the proportion of aphakics in other populations may also explain the differences in the prevalences of blindness among them.

Based on PVA, the proportion of blindness in pseudophakic population was only 7.8%, which is similar to that reported from Bharatpur in Rajasthan (14%) [7], CGS(11.7%) [9], Tirunelveli (5.1%) [8], Sivaganga (4.2%) [6] and APEDS (5.6%) [5]. It was also comparable to the neighboring regions of Lumbini zone and Chitwan district of Nepal (7.9%) [24], Ratuhat district in Nepal (10%) [27], Satkhira district in Bangladesh (6%) [28] and Hong Kong (7.8%) [25]. It may be stated here that as the prevalence of aphakia in a population decreases, the proportion of post-cataract surgery blindness also reduces simultaneously.

The differences in PVA and BCVA underscores the importance of adequate post-operative refraction and use of spectacles. The use of spectacles was only 25.4%, which was much lower than Navsari in Gujarat (54.2%) [10], Tirunelveli (35%) [8], Bharatpur in Rajasthan (56%) [7] and Sivaganga (48.6%) [6]. As stated earlier, this could be due to the increased proportion of pseudophakics in this population. In the pseudophakic population of Tirunelveli and Sivaganga the use of spectacles was only ranging from 10–20% [6,8]. The possible reason for low use of spectacles in the pseudophakic population could be that these subjects may not feel the need for use of spectacles as they are able to carry on their daily activities without them. Another possible reason could be due to the issues related to accessibility and affordability of refractive error services. The use of spectacles in pseudophakics was also much lower than the developed regions of Hong Kong (40%) [25] and Latinos in Los Angeles (70%) [22].

The major cause of VI was uncorrected refractive error and for blindness was uncorrected aphakia, surgical complications and posterior segment disorders. This was similar to the other studies from India [4,5,6,7,8,9,10]. This underscores the importance of rigorous pre-operative comprehensive examination to rule out any pre-existing pathology and adequate training to manage surgical complications. Posterior capsular opacification (PCO) was seen in only 3.9% of pseudophakic subjects and was comparable to Tiruneveli (5.3%) [8] and Sivaganga (2.7%) [6] and higher than reportd in Nepal (0.5%) [27]. However, it was lower than Navsari in Gujarat (16.5%) [10] and CGS (12.5%) [9]. It was also lower than Lumbini zone and Chitwan district of Nepal (8%) [24].

Analysis of risk factors for VA<6/18 in pseudophakic eyes for PVA and BCVA suggest that there are issues related to refractive error services, especially for those who were operated for free. As the use of glasses did not differ between those operated for free and the paid subjects (21.2% versus 24.9%; $p = 0.23$), this could be attributed to an incorrect prescription in these subjects. As far as the National Program for Control for Blindness (NPCB) policy is concerned, there is only one time funding provided for prescribing spectacles to the post-operative subjects. As a usual practice, most of these refractions are done still in camp settings in the rural areas where mass refractions are done in a single day. It is possible that there might be more errors in refractions done in these make shift units. Apart from this, the refractive error status of pseudophakic subjects change over a period of time. However, due to issues related to affordability and accessibility of refractive error services, these subjects are very unlikely to go for repeat refraction or for purchase of a new pair of glasses. Poor outcome for BCVA in subjects with an early surgical intervention could be due to other ocular co-morbidity in them. Illiteracy was used as proxy for socio-economic status and it is possible that various other factors associated with illiteracy or poverty might be responsible for poor outcomes in these subjects.

Despite our best efforts, there were some limitations in this study. As visual fields were not performed on these subjects, we might have missed some VI or blindness due to visual field defects. We also did not assess the type of cataract surgery performed on these subjects as well as the details of surgical complications.

In summary, compared to previous studies done a decade earlier, there was an overall changing trend related to cataract surgery outcomes seen in this population. Though we did not have a baseline data before the launch of the Tribal Eye Care project, it is possible that these results might reflect the success of the Tribal Eye Care Project launched by the government in these remote areas Andhra Pradesh. This study has also shown that there were some issues related to the use of spectacles and visual outcomes in those operated free. Proper post-operative refractions, adequate follow-up and provision of glasses might help to comprehensively address this issue.

Acknowledgments

We wish to thank Prof James Tonascia, Johns Hopkins Bloomberg School of Public Health, for his critical review of the data and providing statistical advice. We would also like to thank Prof David Friedman, Wilmer Eye Institute and Bloomberg School of Public Health, who participated in initial discussions during the analysis phase and provided valuable advice. Finally, we would also like to acknowledge all the subjects who volunteered to be a part of this study.

Author Contributions

Conceived and designed the experiments: RCK SRP SSE BKG PKR. Performed the experiments: RCK SRP SSE BKG PKR. Analyzed the data: RCK SDC GPSS SC ODS. Contributed reagents/materials/analysis tools: RCK SDC GPSS ODS. Wrote the paper: RCK SDC GPSS SC ODS. Data management: RCK SRP SSE BKG.

References

1. Angra SK, Murthy GV, Gupta SK, Angra V (1997) Cataract related blindness in India & its social implications. Indian J Med Res 106: 312–324.
2. Jose R, Bachani D (1995) World Bank-assisted Cataract Blindness Control Project. Indian J Ophthalmol 43: 35–43.
3. Dua AS (2005) National Programme for Control of Blindness. National Commission on Macroeconomics and Health Background Papers – Burden of Disease in India. NCMH Background Papers-Burden of Disease in India: Ministry of Health & Family Welfare; New Delhi. pp 299–304.
4. Dandona L, Dandona R, Anand R, Srinivas M, Rajashekar V (2003) Outcome and number of cataract surgeries in India: policy issues for blindness control. Clin Experiment Ophthalmol 31: 23–31.
5. Dandona L, Dandona R, Naduvilath TJ, McCarty CA, Mandal P, et al. (1999) Population-based assessment of the outcome of cataract surgery in an urban population in southern India. Am J Ophthalmol 127: 650–658.
6. Thulasiraj RD, Reddy A, Selvaraj S, Munoz SR, Ellwein LB (2002) The Sivaganga eye survey: II. Outcomes of cataract surgery. Ophthalmic Epidemiol 9: 313–324.
7. Murthy GV, Ellwein LB, Gupta S, Tanikachalam K, Ray M, et al. (2001) A population-based eye survey of older adults in a rural district of Rajasthan: II. Outcomes of cataract surgery. Ophthalmology 108: 686–692.
8. Nirmalan PK, Thulasiraj RD, Maneksha V, Rahmathullah R, Ramakrishnan R, et al. (2002) A population based eye survey of older adults in Tirunelveli district of south India: blindness, cataract surgery, and visual outcomes. Br J Ophthalmol 86: 505–512.
9. Vijaya L, George R, Rashima A, Raju P, Arvind H, et al. (2010) Outcomes of cataract surgery in a rural and urban south Indian population. Indian J Ophthalmol 58: 223–228.
10. Murthy GV, Vashist P, John N, Pokharel G, Ellwein LB (2009) Prevalence and vision-related outcomes of cataract surgery in Gujarat, India. Ophthalmic Epidemiol 16: 400–409.
11. Government of India, Ministry of Tribal Affairs website. Available: www.tribal.nic.in. Accessed 6 May 2011.
12. Census of India website. Available: www.censusindia.gov.in. Accessed 6 May 2011.
13. RAAB manual website: Available: www.cehjournal.org/files/raab/RAABManualVFPV4.02.pdf. Accessed 6 May 2011.
14. Kuper H, Polack S, Limburg H (2006) Rapid assessment of avoidable blindness. Community Eye Health 19: 68–69.

15. Turner AG, Magnani RJ, Shuaib M (1996) A not quite as quick but much cleaner alternative to the Expanded Programme on Immunization (EPI) Cluster Survey design. Int J Epidemiol 25: 198–203.
16. Office of The Chief Commissioner for Person with Disabilities, Ministry of Social Justice and Empowerment, Government of India website. Available: www.ccdisabilities.nic.in. Accessed 6 May 2011.
17. Park K, ed (2007) Text Book of Preventive and Social Medicine. 2007 ed: M/S Banarsidas Bhanot, Jabalpur, India.
18. StataCorp (2009) Stata Statistical Software: Release 11. College Station, TX: StataCorp LP.
19. Glynn RJ, Rosner B (1992) Accounting for the correlation between fellow eyes in regression analysis. Arch Ophthalmol 110: 381–387.
20. Zeger SL, Liang KY (1986) Longitudinal data analysis for discrete and continuous outcomes. Biometrics 42: 121–130.
21. Hosmer D, Lemeshow S (2000) Applied Logistic Regression Analysis John Wiley & Sons.
22. Baranano AE, Wu J, Mazhar K, Azen SP, Varma R (2008) Visual acuity outcomes after cataract extraction in adult latinos. The Los Angeles Latino Eye Study. Ophthalmology 115: 815–821.
23. Huang W, Huang G, Wang D, Yin Q, Foster PJ, et al. (2011) Outcomes of cataract surgery in urban southern China: the Liwan Eye Study. Invest Ophthalmol Vis Sci 52: 16–20.
24. Kandel RP, Sapkota YD, Sherchan A, Sharma MK, Aghajanian J, et al. (2010) Cataract surgical outcome and predictors of outcome in Lumbini Zone and Chitwan District of Nepal. Ophthalmic Epidemiol 17: 276–281.
25. Lau J, Michon JJ, Chan WS, Ellwein LB (2002) Visual acuity and quality of life outcomes in cataract surgery patients in Hong Kong. Br J Ophthalmol 86: 12–17.
26. Lavanya R, Wong TY, Aung T, Tan DT, Saw SM, et al. (2009) Prevalence of cataract surgery and post-surgical visual outcomes in an urban Asian population: the Singapore Malay Eye Study. Br J Ophthalmol 93: 299–304.
27. Sapkota YD, Sunuwar M, Naito T, Akura J, Adhikari HK (2010) The prevalence of blindness and cataract surgery in rautahat district, Nepal. Ophthalmic Epidemiol 17: 82–89.
28. Wadud Z, Kuper H, Polack S, Lindfield R, Akm MR, et al. (2006) Rapid assessment of avoidable blindness and needs assessment of cataract surgical services in Satkhira District, Bangladesh. Br J Ophthalmol 90: 1225–1229.

6

Non-Invasive Bleaching of the Human Lens by Femtosecond Laser Photolysis

Line Kessel[1]*, Lars Eskildsen[1,2], Mike van der Poel[2], Michael Larsen[1]

1 Department of Ophthalmology, Glostrup Hospital, University of Copenhagen, Glostrup, Denmark, 2 Department of Photonics Engineering, Technical University of Denmark, Kgs. Lyngby, Denmark

Abstract

Background: Globally, cataract is the leading cause of blindness and impaired vision. Cataract surgery is an attractive treatment option but it remains unavailable in sufficient quantity for the vast majority of the world population living in areas without access to specialized health care. Reducing blindness from cataract requires solutions that can be applied outside operating theatres. Cataract is a protein conformational disease characterized by accumulation of light absorbing, fluorescent and scattering protein aggregates. The aim of the study was to investigate whether these compounds were susceptible to photobleaching by a non-invasive procedure and whether this would lead to optical rejuvenation of the lens.

Methodology/Principal Findings: Nine human donor lenses were treated with an 800 nm infra-red femtosecond pulsed laser in a treatment zone measuring $1 \times 1 \times 0.52$ mm. After laser treatment the age-induced yellow discoloration of the lens was markedly reduced and the transmission of light was increased corresponding to an optical rejuvenation of 3 to 7 years.

Conclusions/Significance: The results demonstrate that the age-induced yellowing of the human lens can be bleached by a non-invasive procedure based on femtosecond laser photolysis. Cataract is a disease associated with old age. At the current technological stage, lens aging is delayed but with a treatment covering the entire lens volume complete optical rejuvenation is expected. Thus, femtosecond photolysis has the potential clinical value of replacing invasive cataract surgery by a non-invasive treatment modality that can be placed in mobile units, thus breaking down many of the barriers impeding access to treatment in remote and poor regions of the world.

Editor: Anna Mitraki, University of Crete, Greece

Funding: The study received financial support from the Danish Medical Research Council (grant # 721-06-0664) and the Danish National Advanced Technology Foundation (Hoejteknologifonden). The funders had no role in the study design, data collection and analysis, decision to publish, or preparation of the manuscript.

Competing Interests: The authors have declared that no competing interests exist.

* E-mail: line.kessel@dadlnet.dk

Introduction

Cataract is the world-leading cause of blindness and visual impairment accountable for almost 20 million cases of bilateral blindness [1]. Blindness from cataract could be prevented if only high quality and high volume cataract surgery was available all over the globe [2]. This is unfortunately not the case and the barriers impeding access to treatment includes lack of skilled and well-trained surgeons, lack of sterile operating facilities, lack of the high-tech equipment required for the surgical procedure, and the high cost of the procedure rendering the surgery inaccessible to a vast majority of world population. At present there is no known ways of preventing cataract formation or any non-surgical treatment modalities.

Cataract is a protein conformational disease caused by posttranslational modifications of the structural lens proteins [3]. The human lens is a highly specialized avascular tissue with little or no turn-over of its constituent structural proteins [4]. The orderly arrangement of these proteins is essential for the transparency of the lens [5–8] and for quality of vision. With time the structural lens proteins are subjected to posttranslational modifications by non-enzymatic glycation [9] and other biochemical and biophysical pathways [3] leading to an accumulation of chromophores that absorb visible light preferentially in the blue end of the spectrum [10], giving the aged human lens its characteristic yellow-brown color. Additional processes of optical degradation of the aging and cataractous lens include protein aggregation leading to increased scattering of light [11]. The end result is the milky white appearance that prompted the ancient Greeks to name the condition after their word for waterfall "katarrhaktes".

Photoactive molecules, such as chromophores, will eventually degrade upon the interaction with light. Chromophore bleaching is a phenomenon of fundamental importance for multiple life functions such as vision that is based on the photobleaching of photopigments, opsins, in the retina [12]. The fluorescent chromophores of the human lens can be bleached in vitro by broad-band ultraviolet radiation [13,14] demonstrating that lenses can be optically rejuvenated by chromophore bleaching. Ultraviolet treatment of the lens is, however, not possible in a clinical setting because of retinal phototoxicity [15,16].

Instead, we chose to explore a multiphoton approach where ultraviolet-like effects are obtained in confined space using infra-red light that is less harmful to the retina [17].

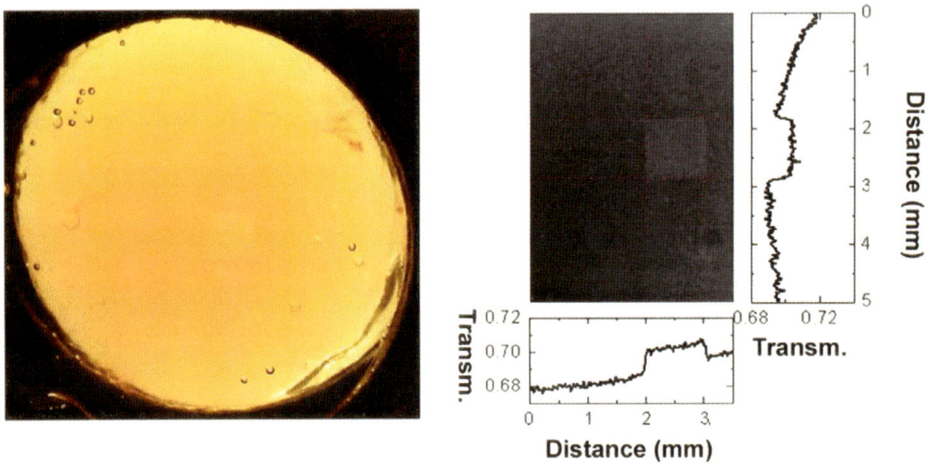

Figure 1. Photographic documentation of the laser photobleaching. To the right is shown a color photograph of a 58 year old donor lens after treatment and to the left is shown a black-and-white excerpt of the same photograph with an image analysis of the light intensity in the photograph. The treated area is seen as a lighter square and it is marked by red dotted lines on the black and white photograph. The relative transmission was calculated by using the black plastic spacer surrounding the lens as a reference for 0% transmission and the vacant space between the lens and the plastic spacer as a reference for 100% transmission.

Multiphoton effects occur when two or more photons hit a target molecule simultaneously. In practice, this requires a very high photon density that can only be obtained by using ultra-short pulsed lasers. The chosen methodology is analogue to the bleaching of artificial fluorescent dyes known by researchers in the field of multiphoton microscopy [18]. We demonstrate that a clinically relevant level of photobleaching can be obtained in a manner that is predicted to be safe for the rest of the eye.

Results

Nine human organ donor lenses aged 58 to 75 years of age were exposed to infra-red 800 nm radiation from a femtosecond pulsed Ti:Sapphire laser using pulse energies ranging from 0.10 to 0.55 μJ. The laser beam was scanned across the lens in a line-by-line raster pattern covering a volume of 1mm in height ×1 mm in width ×0.52 mm in depth. Photobleaching was visible to the unaided observer in the treated area with no signs of damage to

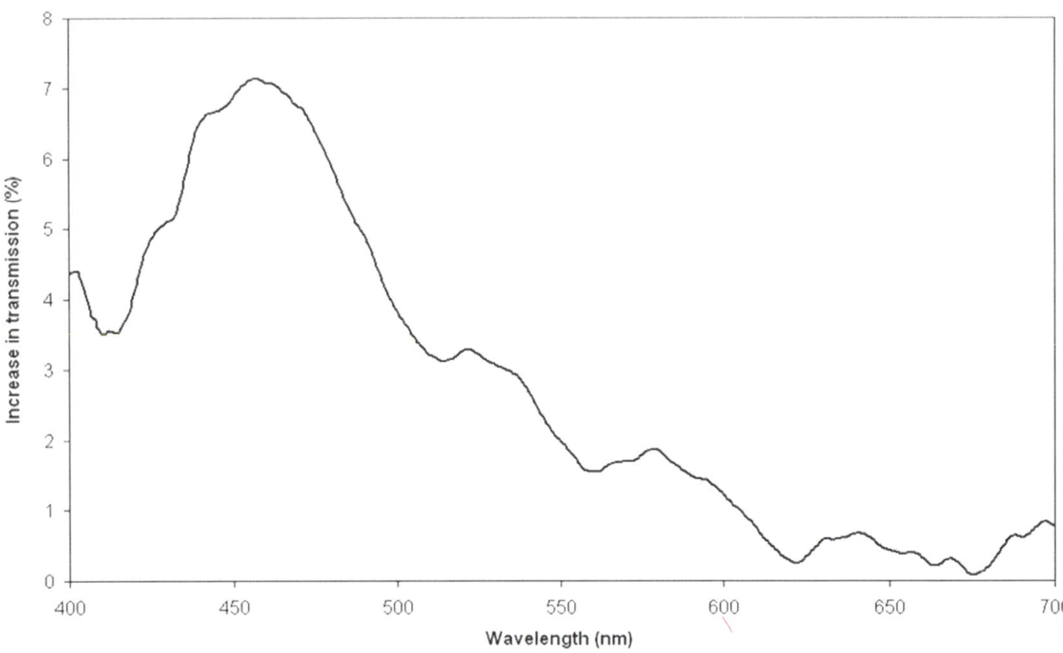

Figure 2. Changes in the transmission properties after treatment. The graph shows the spectral distribution of the increase in light transmission through a human lens (donor lens # 7 in Table 1) after femtosecond laser photolysis. On the y-axis is shown the increase in transmission after treatment. The transmission before treatment was set to 0 for all wavelengths, i.e. 0% indicates that no changes in transmission properties were observed after treatment.

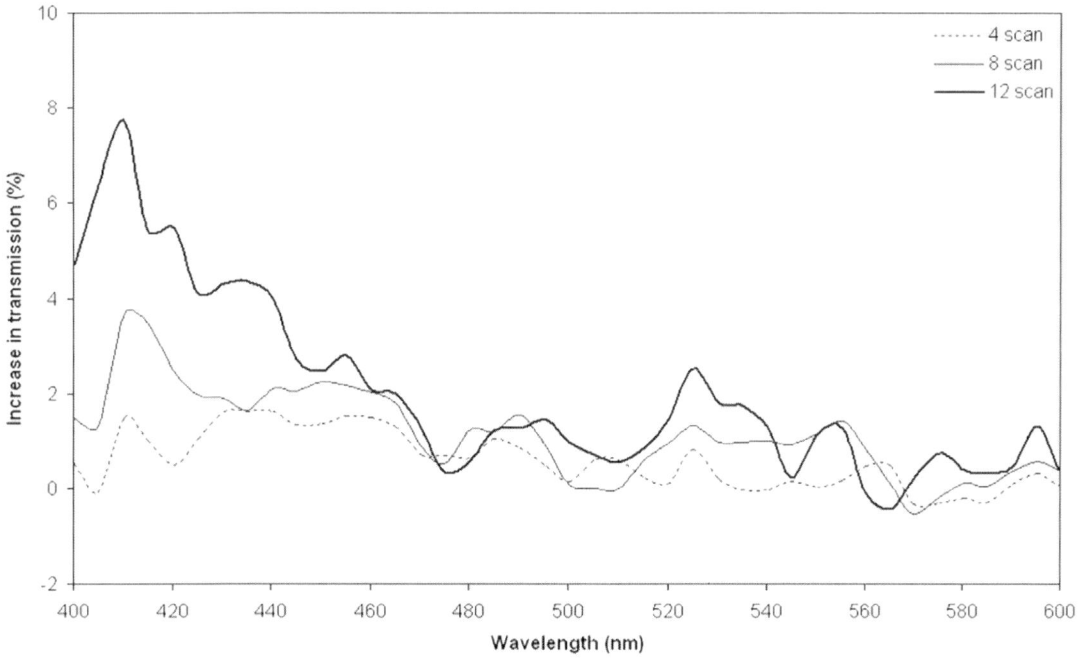

Figure 3. The treatment response depends on the laser dosage. Dose-response curve shows an increasing improvement in the transmission of light with increasing number of scans applied to the same area for a 61 year old human donor lens (donor lens # 6 in Table 1). The increase in transmission is shown in percentage on the y-axis as a function of wavelength (in nm on the x-axis). 0% indicates that no changes were observed after the laser treatment.

the untreated parts of the lens (Fig. 1). Using a slit-lamp biomicroscope it was seen that photobleaching was confined to the subvolume inside the lens targeted by the scanning procedure. The effect of the laser treatment remained visible 1 to 2 weeks after the treatment. Continued observation was not possible due to the gradual optical deterioration of the donor lenses post mortem.

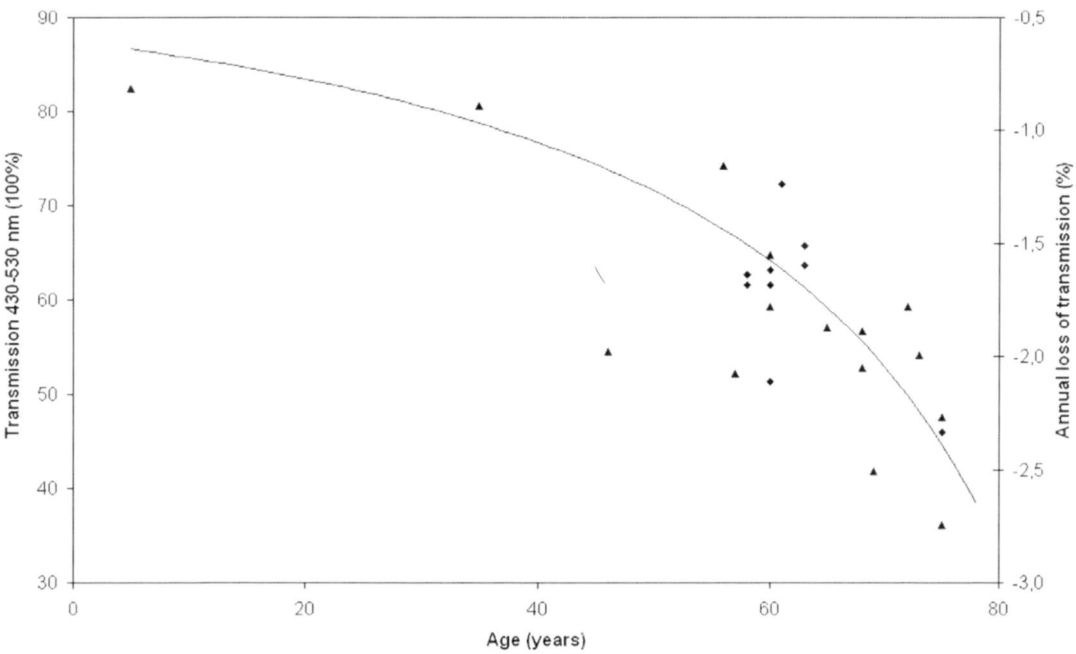

Figure 4. Age-dependent decline in the transmission of blue light. The graph shows the transmission of blue-green light (430–530 nm) measured in vitro in healthy human donor lenses in vitro as a function of age. Diamond markers indicate lenses that were also used in bleaching experiments whereas the triangular marks indicate lenses that were used for transmission measurement only. The left vertical axis shows the transmission from 430 to 530 nm in percent and the right vertical axis show the annual loss of transmission in percent. The curve was drawn based on Eq. 1.

Table 1. Increase in transmission of human lenses after femtosecond laser photolysis.

Lens no.	Donor age (years)	Transmission increase 430–530 nm (%)	Rejuvenation (years)
1	58	5.4	6.6
2	58	3.5	4.9
3	60	5.9	7.0
4	60	6.0	7.1
5	60	2.1	3.7
6	61	1.3	3.0
7	63	3.1	4.6
8	63	1.6	3.2
9	75	6.2	7.3

Rejuvenation was calculated as the difference in age of the donor lens before treatment and the age equivalent to the lens after treatment. Lenses #3 and #4 were from the same donor.

After laser treatment the transmission of light through the lens was increased over the entire visible spectrum and most prominently in the blue-green part (Fig. 2), where the age-related loss of transmission is also most pronounced. The effect of the laser treatment showed a clear dose response with the number of scans applied to the lens (Fig. 3).

To estimate the clinical relevance of the laser-induced improvement in lens transmission the age-induced changes in lens transmission was assessed in a separate experiment using twenty-five human donor lenses (Fig. 4). We found that the age-related changes in transmission properties of blue-green light from 430 to 530 nm could be approximated by Eq. 1, where *Age* is age in years, $p<0.0001$, $R^2=0.63$:

$$T_{430-530nm} = \log(2.43113 - 0.01313 * Age) \tag{1}$$

Using Eq. 1 to calculate the apparent lens age after laser treatment, the improvement in lens transmission after treatment was found to correspond to a reduction in lens age of 5.2 years (range 3.0 to 7.3 years, Table 1). Notably, the treatment effects presented in Table 1 was the result of treating a subvolume of the lens of 0.52 mm in thickness, corresponding to 1/10 of the axial thickness of a typical lens (Fig. 5).

During 800 nm femtosecond laser irradiation the lenses emitted a strong blue autofluorescence signal indicating that two-photon absorption took place (Fig. 6). The rate of two-photon absorption (R_{TPA})depends on the density (ρ) of the molecules that can be excited by two-photon absorption, the two-photon absorption cross section for the molecule (β), laser power/area (I^n, with n being the number of photons involved in the process, i.e. $n=2$ for a two-photon process), and the energy of the impinging photons ($\hbar\omega$). Assuming that the medium is optically thin, the rate of TPA of a laser beam impinging on a cylindrical volume with a cross sectional area A and length L will follow Eq. 2:

$$R_{TPA} = \frac{\rho\beta ALI^2}{(\hbar\omega)^2} \tag{2}$$

If not only the fluorescence but also the photobleaching was the result of two-photon absorption it follows from Eq. 2 that the rate of photobleaching will be faster in more densely coloured lenses and when more laser power is applied to the lens. In other words, older and more densely coloured lenses will, predictably, benefit more from the laser treatment than younger and less coloured lenses.

We found that, indeed, the photobleaching was significantly ($p=0.01$, $R^2=0.78$) greater for more densely coloured lenses combined with the square of the laser power, Eq. 3:

$$T_{increase} = 9.5 + 345.0 * I^2 - 13.0 * T_{pre} \tag{3}$$

Where $T_{increase}$ denominates the increase (in percent) in transmission after laser treatment, T_{pre} denominates the transmission before laser treatment, and I is the mean laser power (in Watt). All other variables from Eq. 2 were kept constant between experiments, i.e. the energy of the impinging photons, the area of laser spot size, and the two-photon absorption cross section. The transmission measurements before treatment was used as a surrogate measure of the density of the two-photon absorbing molecules in the lens.

Discussion

We have shown that the age-induced yellow discolouration of human donor lenses can be bleached by a non-invasive procedure

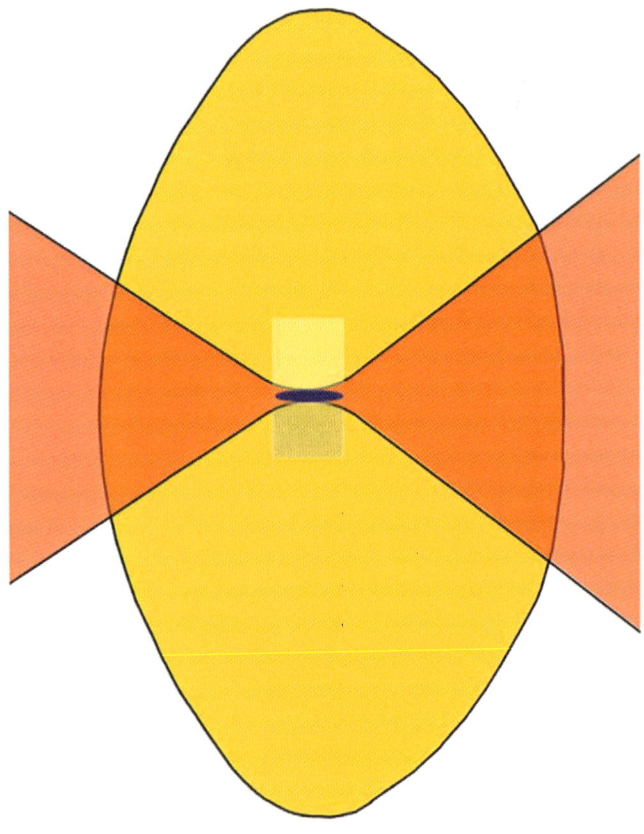

Figure 5. Schematic presentation of the laser treatment shown on a cross section of a lens in the sagittal plane. An infra-red laser (here shown in red) is focused inside a human donor lens. Emission of blue autofluorescence is seen in the focal region as a sign of two-photon absorption. The laser is scanned over the lens in a line-by-line raster pattern. The technical set-up only allowed for 2 directional scanning restricting the depth of the treatment plane to the Rayleigh length of focal region of the laser. Thus, a subvolume measuring 1.0 mm in height by 1.0 mm in width by 0.52 mm in depth was treated. The treated area is shown as a lighter area above the laser focal region and the area awaiting treatment is shown in a grey shade below the laser focal region.

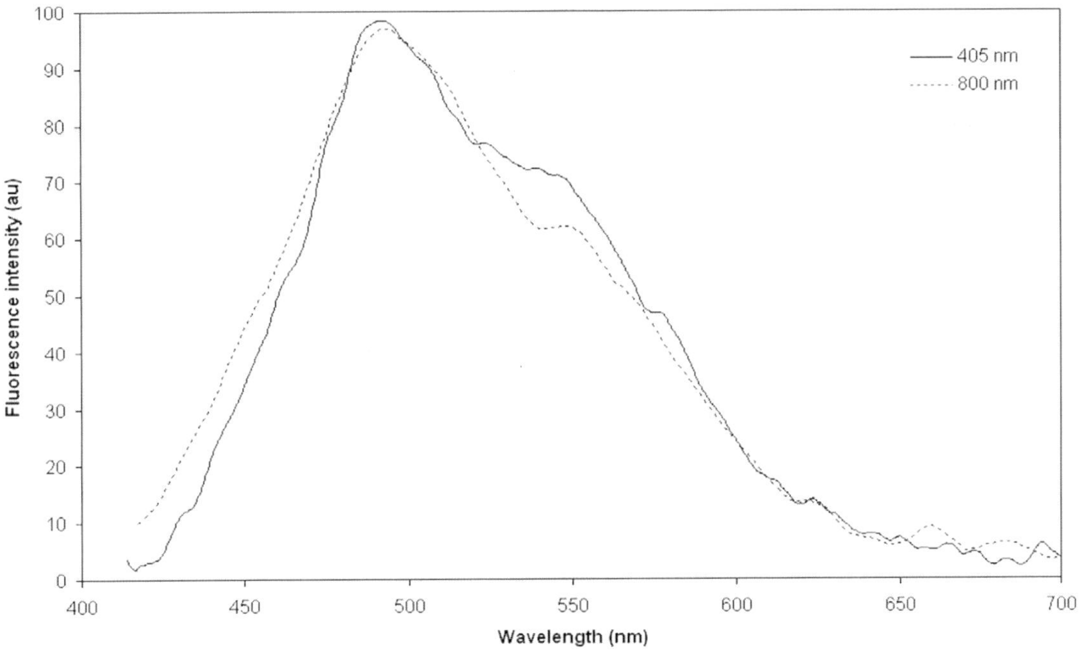

Figure 6. Fluorescence intensity profiles. Spectral characteristics of fluorescence from the human lens excited by 405 nm continuous-wave laser radiation (thin) and 800 nm femtosecond laser radiation (thick). Fluorescence was recorded at a 90 degree angle relative to the excitation laser beam and the differences in fluorescence emission spectrum for λ_{ex} at 405nm and λ_{ex} at 800 nm at the lower wavelengths are related to the 800 nm laser being focused at a greater distance from the detection source, i.e. a greater absorption of preferentially shorter wavelengths took place before the fluorescence emission reached the detector.

using femtosecond pulsed infra-red laser light. Even with the current primitive set-up clinically relevant effects corresponding to a lens rejuvenation of 3 to 7 years was obtained. Cataract is a disease associated with old age and by postponing the need for surgery by 5 years the number of surgeries performed can be reduced by 35% [19]. Treating the entire lens volume is expected to eliminate the effect of several decades of optical aging.

The observation of blue autofluorescence indicates that the photobleaching was mediated by two-photon absorption of the infra-red laser light leading to ultraviolet equivalent effects in the focal region. Multiphoton effects have a step-like progression with increasing laser intensities from no effects over photobleaching to material ablation and tissue disruption [20]. We used laser intensities well below the level required for mechanical effects [21] because we were interested in the more subtle photochemical effects. The exact photochemical reactions involved in the treatment are not known but ultraviolet irradiation has been shown to degrade one of the advanced glycation end products (AGEs) found in the aging lens [22]. Protein denaturation by advanced glycation is of major importance for the age-induced optical changes seen in human lenses [9] and photodegradation of AGEs could be a likely mechanism of action for the observed photobleaching of the aged human donor lenses.

Despite the widespread use of femtosecond laser in the treatment of medical conditions, most prominently in the LASIK procedure for refractive surgery [23], the ocular safety of multiple femtosecond pulses have only been the subject of a single study so far [24]. Comparing our procedure with this study is not simple because femtosecond retinal safety threshold depends on many different factors, such as retinal spot size [25], pulse duration [26–28], and the wavelength of the laser [29]. Nevertheless, based on the existing data our procedure is predicted to within retinal safety limits but further safety evaluation by animal studies should be performed before the treatment can be tested in clinical studies.

Our results are noteworthy because cataract is the most prominent cause of vision loss in the world today. It is responsible for an estimated number of 20 million cases of blindness and an even greater, but unknown, number of cases of impaired visual acuity [1]. Patients are not blinded or visually impaired because of a lack of treatment but because of a lack of access to treatment. A number of economic and logistic challenges are responsible for the lack of access to cataract surgery in underprivileged populations. Changing from an invasive, surgical treatment towards a non-invasive solution will break down some of the barriers impeding access to treatment. If the treatment could be placed in mobile units allowing transportation of the treatment facilities into remote and rural areas, the road is paved for an easy access to a cure for cataract world-wide. Our method has both potentials though many questions must be answered and many issues solved before the treatment can be used clinically, such as the effect of the treatment on the scattering properties of the lens and long term effects of the treatment on the lens as well as the rest of the eye.

In conclusion, our results show that the aged human donor lenses can regain the colour of younger lenses by being treated with subtle low-energy infrared femtosecond laser pulses that evoke two-photon events in a target volume inside the intact lens nucleus. This opens an entirely new prospect of developing clinically applicable non-invasive techniques for the treatment of cataract.

Materials and Methods

Human donor lenses

Human lenses were provided by the Cornea Bank NORI (Amsterdam, the Netherlands). Nine lenses from 8 individuals

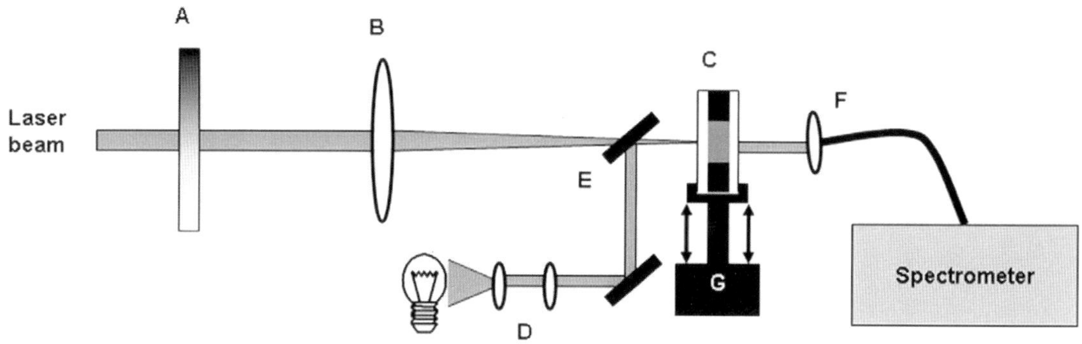

Figure 7. Experimental set-up. Diagram showing the set-up for the experimental laser exposure and transmission study of human lens. Laser intensity was adjusted using a graded neutral density filter (A) and focused using an f = 85 mm focusing lens (B) onto the lens sample (C). Spectral transmission of the lens was measured using an incandescent light source, a set of collimating lenses (D), a flip-in mirror (E), and a spectrometer. The lens sample was moved relative to the laser beam using motorized translation stages (G).

(aged 58–75 years) were used for laser irradiation experiments and these lenses plus 16 additional lenses were included in the study of lens transmission in relation to age (5–73 years). The lenses were maintained at 5°C in minimal essential medium supplemented with phenol red until use. All lenses were of normal yellow color for their age and showed no localized opacities upon microscopy. The quality of the lenses was assessed using slit lamp biomicroscopy and only lenses of good optical quality were used for the experiments. Before the experiments the lenses were removed from the MEM and surgically decapsulated. Then the lenses were sandwiched between two glass microscope mounting plates held apart by an adjustable spacing system. Under these conditions, the lenses maintained their hydration status, transparency and color for up to two weeks post mortem.

Femtosecond laser system

Experimental photolytic treatment of the lens in vitro was performed using a mode-locked Ti:Sapphire laser (Mira 900, Coherent) and a regenerative amplifier (RegA, Coherent). The system delivered a train of pulses with a Gaussian beam profile, the wavelength was centered at 800 nm with maximum pulse energy of 2 μJ and a full-width-at-half-maximum pulse duration of 200 to 300 femtoseconds (10^{-15} s). Repetition rate could be varied from 31 to 275 kHz. Pulse duration and average beam power was measured using an autocorrelator and a thermopile detector, respectively. The laser power delivered to the eye lens was controlled using a graded neutral density attenuation filter. The laser beam was focused using an 85 mm focal length lens yielding a theoretical minimum $1/e^2$ beam intensity diameter of 14 μm and a Rayleigh length of 0.26 mm. This is calculated for the conditions in the lens tissue where the index of refraction is 1.4 [30]. The thickness of the treatment plane is taken to be two times the Rayleigh length, i.e. 0.52 mm. The lens sample was scanned relative to the laser beam using computer-controlled motorized translation stages from Thorlabs (Thorlabs, Sweden). The lens was scanned in a raster pattern in the transverse plane only, meaning that the depth of the treated plane was defined theoretically by the Rayleigh length of the focused laser beam (Fig. 5). The experimental set-up is shown in Fig. 7.

Transmission measurements

Bleaching was documented by measuring the transmission of white light from an incandescent light bulb source that was collected by a spectrometer (AvaSpec-2048-2 spectrometer (Avantes, the Netherlands). To ensure that transmission was measured at the exact site of exposure, the transmission measurements were aligned with the laser exposure beam using a 100 μm (diameter) aperture. To correct for minor differences in intensity of the white light source, all transmission measurements shown have been calibrated to the transmission of near-infrared light (750–800 nm).Though measurements of scattering of light was not directly included in the study, indirect information on scattering properties can be derived from the transmission measurements since an increase in scattering (especially backward scattering, i.e. in the direction backwards to the incandescent light source) would reduce the recorded transmission.

Slit lamp biomicroscopy

The lenses were inspected visually before and after treatment using a slit lamp (BQ900, Haag-Streit, Germany). The slit lamp is a modified microscope where the object of interest can be viewed at 6.3 to 40× magnification using a height and width adjustable slit of light that illuminates the object of interest at a chosen angle, thus providing the possibility three-dimensional optical sectioning.

Photographic documentation

The lenses were photographed using a digital Canon 30D EOS camera equipped with a macrolens.

Acknowledgments

The authors are grateful for the kind and excellent service provided by Dr. Liesbeth Pels and associates at the Corneabank NORI of Amsterdam, the Netherlands in providing the human donor lenses.

Author Contributions

Conceived and designed the experiments: LK LE MvdP ML. Performed the experiments: LK LE. Analyzed the data: LK MvdP. Contributed reagents/materials/analysis tools: LK. Wrote the paper: LK MvdP ML.

References

1. Resnikoff S, Pascolini D, Etya'ale D, Kocur I, Pararajasegaram R, et al. (2004) Global data on visual impairment in the year 2002. Bulletin of the World Health Organization 82: 844–851.
2. World Health Organization (2007) Vision 2020. The right to sight. Gobal initiative for the elimination of avoidable blindness. Action plan for 2006–2011. pp 1–97.

3. Bloemendal H, de Jong W, Jaenicke R, Lubsen NH, Slingsby C, et al. (2004) Ageing and vision: structure, stability and function of lens crystallins. Progress in Biophysics & Molecular Biology 86: 407–485.
4. Lynnerup N, Kjeldsen H, Heegaard S, Jacobsen C, Heinemeier J (2008) Radiocarbon Dating of the Human Eye Lens Crystallines Reveal Proteins without Carbon Turnover throughout Life. PLoS ONE 3: e1529.
5. Benedek GB (1971) Theory of transparency of the eye. Applied Optics 10: 459–473.
6. Delaye M, Tardieu A (1983) Short-range order of crystallin proteins accounts for eye lens transparency. Nature 302: 415–417.
7. Stradner A, Foffi G, Dorsaz N, Thurston G, Schurtenberger P (2007) New insight into cataract formation: Enhanced stability through mutual attraction. Physical Review Letters 99.
8. Ponce A, Sorensen C, Takemoto L (2006) Role of short-range protein interactions in lens opacifications. Molecular Vision 12: 879–884.
9. Monnier VM, Cerami A (1981) Nonenzymatic browning in vivo: possible process for aging of long-lived proteins. Science 211: 491–493.
10. Kessel L, Lundeman JH, Herbst K, Andersen TV, Larsen M (2010) Age-related changes in the transmission properties of the human lens and their relevance to circadian entrainment. Journal of Cataract & Refractive Surgery 36: 308–312.
11. Takemoto L, Sorensen CM (2008) Protein-protein interactions and lens transparency. Exp Eye Res 87: 496–501.
12. Saari JC (2000) Biochemistry of visual pigment regeneration: the Friedenwald lecture. Invest Ophthalmol Vis Sci 41: 337–348.
13. Kessel L, Kalinin S, Soroka V, Larsen M, Johansson LBA (2005) Impact of UVR-A on whole human lenses, supernatants of buffered human lens homogenates, and purified argpyrimidine and 3-OH-kynurenine. Acta Ophthalmologica Scandinavica 83: 221–227.
14. Ortwerth BJ, Chemoganskiy V, Olesen PR (2002) Studies on Singlet Oxygen Formation and UVA Light-mediated Photobleaching of the Yellow Chromophores in Human Lenses. Exp Eye Res 74: 217–229.
15. Gorgels TG, van ND (1995) Ultraviolet and green light cause different types of damage in rat retina. Invest Ophthalmol Vis Sci 36: 851–863.
16. Ham WT, Jr., Mueller HA, Sliney DH (1976) Retinal sensitivity to damage from short wavelength light. Nature 260: 153–155.
17. Ham WT, Mueller HA, Ruffolo JJ, Clarke AM (1979) Sensitivity of the Retina to Radiation-Damage As A Function of Wavelength. Photochemistry and Photobiology 29: 735–743.
18. Denk W, Strickler JH, Webb WW (1990) Two-photon laser scanning fluorescence microscopy. Science 248: 73–76.
19. Kessel L (2010) Can we meet the future demands for cataract surgery? Acta Ophthalmol, AOS1839 [pii];10.1111/j.1755-3768.2009.01839.x [doi].
20. Heisterkamp A, Maxwell IZ, Mazur E, Underwood JM, Nickerson JA, et al. (2005) Pulse energy dependence of subcellular dissection by femtosecond laser pulses. Opt Express 13: 3690–3696.
21. Vogel A, Venugopalan V (2003) Mechanisms of pulsed laser ablation of biological tissues. Chem Rev 103: 577–644.
22. Argirov OK, Lin B, Ortwerth BJ (2005) Phototransformations of advanced glycation end products in the human eye lens due to ultraviolet A light irradiation. Maillard Reaction: Chemistry at the Interface of Nutrition, Aging, and Disease 1043: 166–173.
23. Friedlaender MH (2006) LASIK surgery using the IntraLase femtosecond laser. Int Ophthalmol Clin 46: 145–153.
24. Cain CP, Toth CA, Noojin GD, Stolarski DJ, Thomas RJ, et al. (2002) Thresholds for retinal injury from multiple near-infrared ultrashort laser pulses. Health Phys 82: 855–862.
25. Cain CP, Toth CA, Noojin GD, Stolarski DJ, Thomas RJ, et al. (2001) Visible lesion threshold dependence on retinal spot size for femtosecond laser pulses. Journal of Laser Applications 13: 125–131.
26. Cain CP, Toth CA, DiCarlo CD, Stein CD, Noojin GD, et al. (1995) Visible retinal lesions from ultrashort laser pulses in the primate eye. Invest Ophthalmol Vis Sci 36: 879–888.
27. Toth CA, Cain CP, Stein CD, Noojin GD, Stolarski DJ, et al. (1995) Retinal Effects of Ultrashort Laser-Pulses in the Rabbit Eye. Investigative Ophthalmology & Visual Science 36: 1910–1917.
28. Rockwell BA, Hammer DX, Hopkins RA, Payne DJ, Toth CA, et al. (1999) Ultrashort laser pulse bioeffects and safety. Journal of Laser Applications 11: 42–44.
29. Cain CP, Toth CA, Noojin GD, Carothers V, Stolarski DJ, et al. (1999) Thresholds for visible lesions in the primate eye produced by ultrashort near-infrared laser pulses. Investigative Ophthalmology & Visual Science 40: 2343–2349.
30. Hermans EA, Dubbelman M, Van der HR, Heethaar RM (2008) Equivalent refractive index of the human lens upon accommodative response. Optom Vis Sci 85: 1179–1184.

7

The Impact of Successful Cataract Surgery on Quality of Life, Household Income and Social Status in South India

Robert P. Finger[1,2*¶], **David G. Kupitz**[1¶], **Eva Fenwick**[2], **Bharath Balasubramaniam**[3], **Ramanathan V. Ramani**[3], **Frank G. Holz**[1], **Clare E. Gilbert**[4]

1 Department of Ophthalmology, University of Bonn, Bonn, Germany, **2** Centre for Eye Research Australia, Royal Victorian Eye and Ear Hospital, University of Melbourne, Melbourne, Australia, **3** Sankara Eye Care Institutions, Coimbatore, India, **4** International Centre for Eye Health, London School for Hygiene and Tropical Medicine, London, United Kingdom

Abstract

Background: To explore the hypothesis that sight restoring cataract surgery provided to impoverished rural communities will improve not only visual acuity and vision-related quality of life (VRQoL) but also poverty and social status.

Methods: Participants were recruited at outreach camps in Tamil Nadu, South India, and underwent free routine manual small incision cataract surgery (SICS) with intra-ocular lens (IOL) implantation, and were followed up one year later. Poverty was measured as monthly household income, being engaged in income generating activities and number of working household members. Social status was measured as rates of re-marriage amongst widowed participants. VRQoL was measured using the IND-VFQ-33. Associations were explored using logistic regression (SPSS 19).

Results: Of the 294 participants, mean age ± standard deviation (SD) 60±8 years, 54% men, only 11% remained vision impaired at follow up (67% at baseline; $p<0.001$). At one year, more participants were engaged in income generating activities (44.7% to 77.7%; $p<0.001$) and the proportion of households with a monthly income <1000 Rps. decreased from 50.5% to 20.5% ($p<0.05$). Overall VRQoL improved ($p<0.001$). Participants who had successful cataract surgery were less likely to remain in the lower categories of monthly household income (OR 0.05–0.22; $p<0.02$) and more likely to be engaged in income earning activities one year after surgery (OR 3.28; $p=0.006$). Participants widowed at baseline who had successful cataract surgery were less likely to remain widowed at one year (OR 0.02; $p=0.008$).

Conclusion: These findings indicate the broad positive impact of sight restoring cataract surgery on the recipients' as well as their families' lives. Providing free high quality cataract surgery to marginalized rural communities will not only alleviate avoidable blindness but also - to some extent - poverty in the long run.

Editor: John E Mendelson, California Pacific Medical Center Research Institute, United States of America

Funding: The project was supported by the German Ophthalmological Society (DOG), the German Research Foundation (DFG) and the Indian Academy of Science. The funders had no role in study design, data collection and analysis, decision to publish, or preparation of the manuscript.

Competing Interests: The authors have declared that no competing interests exist.

* E-mail: robertfinger@gmx.net

¶ These authors contributed equally to this work.

Introduction

Globally, cataract is the main cause of blindness with the vast majority of cataract blind living in low income countries (LIC) [1] and approximately eight million of those blind from cataract live in India. [2,3] Blindness and poverty are closely linked in a cyclic relationship, as poverty can lead to blindness from conditions such as cataract or trachoma, and blindness can worsen poverty through reduced economic productivity. [4,5,6,7,8] Furthermore visual impairment leads to reduced quality of life (QoL) [9,10], poorer general health [11], lower social status and increased mortality. [12,13] Cataract surgery is a highly cost effective intervention [14] and cataract surgical rates have increased considerably over the past decade in many LICs, including India. However, the quality of provided cataract surgery is not always optimal, with a considerable proportion of patients still blind or vision impaired after cataract surgery in a LIC setting. [15,16] Restoration of vision, for example through cataract surgery, has been demonstrated to enhance quality of life and participation in daily living and, more recently, to improve household economic status. [4].

The Millennium Development Goals (MDGs) are eight international development goals which the United Nations (UN) and all its member states aim to achieve by the year 2015. They include eradicating extreme poverty, gender equality, and developing a global partnership for development. [17] With its high success rates and cost-effectiveness, it is likely that the provision of cataract surgery may contribute towards reducing poverty as part of the MDGs.

Against this background, we assessed the impact of successful first eye cataract surgery on poverty, social status and vision-related QoL (VRQoL) in South India. We hypothesized that successful cataract surgery would reduce poverty, and improve VRQoL and social status. This information is important for the MDGs to achieve their goals and it may also help in allocating resources to ascertain high quality cataract surgical outcomes.

Methods

Ethics Statement

Ethical approval was obtained from the ethics committees of Sankara Eye Care Services and the University of Bonn. The study adhered to the tenets of the declaration of Helsinki. Every participant gave informed, written (signature or thumb imprint) consent.

This prospective study, took place from March 2009 until July 2010 in Tamil Nadu, India. Tamil Nadu is an industrialized and populous state (population 62 million in 2001) with the largest urban conglomeration in India. [18] However, there are still poor, rural areas, which are underserviced as providers tend to be concentrated in cities. The cataract surgical rate in Tamil Nadu is above the Indian average, being approximately 4000 cataract operations per million population per year. [19] This study was embedded within routine services provided by one community eyecare provider, Sankara Eye Care Services, Coimbatore. The cataract outreach program operated by Sankara has been described in detail elsewhere. [20].

Recruitment and Follow Up

Participants who were visually impaired from cataract and had not undergone prior cataract surgery in any eye were eligible. Persons who were classified as poor, aged 40 years or more, and eligible for first eye cataract surgery were recruited. Visual impairment was defined as less than 6/60 (logarithm of minimum angel of resolution (LogMAR) 1.0) in the eye assigned for surgery.

Recruitment took place at the base hospital after participants had been assessed at outreach eye clinics, which are regularly conducted. Those who agreed to participate were interviewed and underwent a full eye examination before undergoing cataract surgery. Patients' transport, surgery, and inpatient hospital stays were provided free by the hospital as patients all fell under the poverty threshold (defined below). After cataract surgery, patients were given eye drops, transported back to the outreach site and told to attend the next outreach clinic (usually a month later) for a follow up assessment of the cataract surgery. If they failed to attend they were sent a reminder by mail. Follow-up data collection for the study occurred at the patients' homes at 1 year follow up by community eye health workers local to the area who are employed full-time by Sankara.

Ocular Assessment and Cataract Surgery

Preoperative assessment included distance visual acuity (DVA) measurement using a LogMAR numbers or tumbling E chart at six meters without correction or with habitual correction and with pinhole. Participants underwent a basic eye examination by an ophthalmologist to determine the cause of visual loss and underwent a more detailed eye examination, including pupil dilation, if the cause of visual loss could not be determined. Only participants for whom cataract was the main cause of visual impairment were included. At follow up, DVA was tested using the same chart at six meters with habitual correction or uncorrected and with pinhole.

Manual small incision cataract surgery (SICS) with implantation of an intraocular lens (IOL) (rigid, single piece PMMA implant) under parabulbar anaesthesia was performed on all participants. IOL power was determined for each individual using manual keratometry (Bausch and Lomb) and an ocular ultrasound A scan (Echorule 2, Biomedix Optotechnik & Devices, India).

Measures of Poverty

Participatory approaches in ranking wealth have been found to yield useful data and valid information on household wealth. [21,22] The economic part of the baseline questionnaires was extensively discussed with key informants and patients in focus groups prior to the current study in order to reflect meaningful and culturally appropriate measures of poverty. Household income is commonly considered a gold standard measure of current socioeconomic position. [22] The most commonly used definition of global poverty is the absolute poverty line set by the World Bank, based on income and/or consumption (poverty $2 and extreme poverty $1 a day or less). [23] The Indian government defined poverty as less than Indian Rupees (Rs). 560 per month in urban areas and Rs. 368 in rural areas in 2006 [24] although definitions used by state governments may vary. In this study, poverty was defined as access to less than Rs. 1200 a month, either as personal (sole earner) or household income. This threshold is in agreement with Tamil Nadu state policy where governmental ration cards are issued when the monthly household income is less than Rs. 1200 (approx. US$25).

In the current study poverty was measured through self-reported monthly household income, employment status, occupation and number of working household members. As asset ownership was unlikely to change over the 1-year follow up period and could thus not reflect the impact of successful first eye cataract surgery, it was not assessed in this study. [5] During the baseline interview, participants were encouraged to discuss monthly household income with accompanying household members and include all sources of income, monetary and non-monetary into the final estimate. As blind persons have been found to be more likely to be unemployed and, if employed, to work more often in low wage jobs [13], we recorded employment status and occupation of all participants at baseline and follow up. In addition, the number of working household members was recorded, as households with disabled members generally have less members involved in income generating activities of any kind. [13] Working was defined as being involved in activities which directly or indirectly generate income.

Measures of Social Status

Disability, including blindness, leads to social exclusion and stigmatization which in turn impedes access to social networks and formal services or social institutions. [13] Widowers and even more so widows are particularly affected by this societal response in India, and have little resources at their disposal to cope with disability. [13] More disabled women than men are unmarried or do not remarry once widowed in India. [25] As social status or stigmatization is difficult to measure [26], we assessed whether participants who were widowed at baseline remarried following cataract surgery as a proxy of decreasing stigma and increasing societal esteem as well as an improved financial outlook of the individual or household.

Vision-related Quality of Life

VRQoL was measured using the IND-VFQ-33, a structured questionnaire which contains 33 questions (items) related to the degree of difficulty in performing vision-dependent activities (e.g., reading, climbing stairs), psychosocial impact (e.g. fear, anxiety) and visual symptoms (e.g. glare, pain). [27,28] The original IND-VFQ-33 questionnaire was developed and extensively validated in the same Indian state (Tamil Nadu), thus no cultural or linguistic adaptation was necessary. [27] In the current study, we performed Rasch analysis to assess the measurement properties of the IND-VFQ-33 in our sample population over time.

Sample Size Calculation

As no data were available to estimate the effect of cataract surgery on household income or the rate of re-marriage, we based the sample size calculations on reported changes in per capita expenditure (PCE) following cataract surgery. [5] The observed change was of a similar magnitude in all cases regardless of whether patients were blind, severely or moderately visually impaired at baseline. Assuming an odds ratio of 1.6 for an improvement in categories of household income, with a power of 0.8 at a significance level of $p = 0.05$, we would need 293 participants (G*Power 3 [29]). Accounting for a loss of 10% to follow up, we aimed to recruit 330 participants.

Psychometric Evaluation of the IND-VFQ-33

We have reported the process of psychometric evaluation of the IND-VFQ-33 using Rasch analysis in more detail elsewhere. [10] In brief, Rasch analysis is a modern psychometric method that mathematically describes the interaction between respondents and test items. We performed Rasch analysis using Winsteps software (version 3.68), Chicago, Illinois, USA. [30] It was important to establish that differences between the IND-VFQ scores at baseline and follow-up are valid indicators of changes over time. [31] Consequently, the baseline and follow-up data were stacked and the absence of differential item functioning (DIF) was used to establish invariance over time. Any change in VRQoL scores on an individual level was considered clinically meaningful if it was larger than approximately half the standard deviation of the overall mean. This is generally considered to be a useful estimate of a clinically meaningful difference [32,33], and has repeatedly been used to rate the meaningfulness of change in parameters such as VRQoL or vision-specific functioning. [10].

Statistical Analysis

The SPSS statistical software (Version 19.0, SPSS Science, Chicago, IL) was used to analyze the data. Participants lost to follow up were excluded from all analyses. Descriptive statistical analyses were performed to characterize the participants' socio-demographic, clinical and IND-VFQ-33 data. Logistic regression (binary and multinomial) models were conducted to determine the independent factors associated with measures of poverty, social status and VRQoL.

Visual acuity was converted into LogMAR for analysis. Successful cataract surgery was defined as a VA improvement equal or better than 20/63 (LogMAR 0.5). In order to demonstrate the impact of cataract surgery, analyses were based on successful cataract surgery, rather than the presence or absence of vision impairment at follow-up, as these two variables contain the same information. In 80% of cases the operated eye was the better eye at follow up.

Results

Socio-demographics and Clinical Characteristics of the Participants

A total of 313 individuals were recruited at baseline. 19 (6%) patients were lost to follow up and a further 21 (7%) participants who underwent second eye cataract surgery during follow up were excluded from all but the descriptive analyses. Baseline characteristics of patients lost to follow up were not significantly different ($p > 0.05$) with regards to age, gender, better eye VA, household size or income. The final study sample at baseline thus comprised 294 participants with a mean ± SD age of 60±8 years. Just under half of the participants were women (46%, **Table 1**). Vision significantly improved after cataract surgery (better eye LogMAR 0.7 (baseline) to 0.3 (follow up), $p < 0.001$), and only 11% of patients remained vision impaired compared to 67% at baseline, $p < 0.001$.

Measures of Poverty

Monthly household income increased to at least the next better category in 122 persons (45.5%) with most participants reporting to be in the Rs 1001–3000 category at follow up (**Table 1**, $p < 0.001$). The mean number of working household members significantly increased at follow up (0.97 to 1.49, $p < 0.001$, **Table 1**). Similarly, the number of participants engaged in income generating activities increased from 128 (44%) at baseline to 225 (77%, $p < 0.001$) at follow up, with the largest increase seen in the unskilled, daily wage category (**Table 1**). The number of participants reported to not work due to vision problems decreased from 76 at baseline to 4 at follow up.

Participants who had successful cataract surgery were significantly more likely to report a higher monthly household income 1 year after cataract surgery. Compared to the highest income category (>3000 Rs./month), participants were about five times (OR 0.22, 95%CI 0.08–0.62; $p = 0.004$) less likely to report a monthly household income of 0–1000 Rs. and about twenty times less likely to report an income of >1000–3000 Rs. (OR 0.05; 95%CI <0.01–0.64; $p = 0.021$, **Table 2**). Participants who had successful cataract surgery were more likely to be engaged in income earning activities one year after surgery (OR 3.28; 95% CI 1.40–7.82; $p = 0.006$, **Table 2**).

Social Status

Participants who had successful cataract surgery were less likely to remain widowed at one year (OR 0.02; 95% CI <0.01–0.35; $p = 0.008$, **Table 3**). At baseline, 208 (71%) participants were married, and 80 (27%) widowed or single (**Table 1**). Over the course of the year, 28 participants remarried, while 47 participants remained widowed (5 lost to follow up, **Table 3**). Stratifying this by gender, nine out of 13 widowers (69%) and 19 out of 62 widows (31%) remarried over the course of the study.

Vision-related Quality of Life

The psychometric properties of the IND-VFQ-33 are summarized in **table S1**. The IND-VFQ-33 was split into four subscales, mobility, activity limitations, psychosocial impact and visual symptoms. All subscales fit the Rasch model (table S1). However, the visual symptoms subscale was left out of all further analyses as it was not felt to add any essential information. All other subscales demonstrated an improvement in VRQoL after cataract surgery (all $p \leq 0.001$, **Table 1**). Having had successful cataract surgery was independently associated with higher reported mobility, less activity limitations and better psychosocial impact (all $p < 0.05$; **Table 4**). Marital or work status was not associated with any of the subscale scores. Participants reported better emotional well-being with an improvement of monthly household income at one year (OR 31, $p = 0.034$, **Table 4**).

Discussion

Persons who underwent successful cataract surgery reported better visual acuity and increased VRQoL in South India. Successful cataract surgery also increased the likelihood to be engaged in an income earning activity, report a higher monthly

Table 1. Characteristics of the sample at baseline and 1 year follow up.

		Baseline	1 year Follow up	p-value
		n = 294	n = 294	BL-1 yr
Age in yrs		60.07±8.29		
Gender	Female	134(45.6%)		
Education	No schooling	125(42.5%)		
	Up to 5 yrs	100(34.0%)		
	More than 5 yrs	54(18.4%)		
Mean ± standard deviation				
Visual acuity in the better eye		0.74±0.44	0.27±0.20	<0.001
VA of operated eye+		1.29±0.65	0.34±0.29	<0.001
VRQoL – subscales of the IND-VFQ 33, logits				
• Activity Limitation		65±24	80±9	<0.001
• Mobility		51±23	70±7	<0.001
• Psychosocial Impact		59±21	79±13	<0.001
No. of household members		3.87±2.17	4.00±1.99	.100
Working household members		0.97±0.75	1.49±0.70	<0.001
Proportion n(%)				
Marital status	Married	208(70.7%)	232(78.9%)	<0.001
	Widowed or Single	80(27.2%)	49(16.7%)	
Visual Impairment		196 (66.7%)	32 (10.9%)	<0.001
Working		128(43.5%)	225(76.5%)	<0.001
Occupation$	Unskilled labour (daily wage)	86(43.8%)	177(78.7%)	.061
	Land owner	16(12.5%)	32(14.2%)	
	Skilled labour	26(20.3%)	16(7.1%)	
Reason for not working#	Vision problem	76(45.8%)	4(5.8%)	.061
	Too old or retired	32(19.3%)	33(47.8%)	
	Other health problem	29(17.5%)	19(27.5%)	
	Doesn't need to work	21(12.7%)	7(10.1%)	
Household's monthly income	Rs 0–1000	143(48.7%)	59(20.1%)	<0.001
	Rs 1001–3000	92(31.3%)	207(70.4%)	
	>Rs 3000	28(9.5%)	20(6.8%)	

BL = baseline, VA = visual acuity, measured in LogMAR, VRQoL = vision-related quality of life, RS = Indian Rupees;
+Operated eye VA at baseline was taken before cataract surgery;
$question applicable to working participants only;
#question applicable to the non working participants only; p-values derived from paired sample t-tests for continuous and Wilcoxon signed rank test for categorical variables.

household income and report a higher number of working household members one year on. In addition, widowed or single participants who had successful cataract surgery were more likely to have remarried over the one year follow up period. These findings emphasize the need for high quality cataract surgery services, as unsuccessful cataract surgery may not only lead to no improvements in vision and VRQoL, but may also deprive patients of a possible future reduction of poverty at the household level and their chance to re-marry in case of widowhood.

Overall, our findings are in line with other studies, where blindness, in particular from cataract, and poverty have been found to be intricately linked. [4,6,7,34] However, there is a dearth of literature regarding the non-ocular impact of cataract surgery in low income countries. [5] Previous studies have reported that cataract surgery may lead to an improvement in VRQoL [35], per capita expenditure [5] and an increase in time spent on productive activities. [36] These non-ocular outcomes of cataract surgery are reflected by our findings of an increase in VRQoL, monthly household income, the number of working household members and the likelihood to be engaged in income generating activities one year after cataract surgery.

Several studies have found poverty to be a barrier to accessing cataract surgery services in India and elsewhere. [37,38,39] In addition, poor surgery outcomes are very likely to discourage acceptance of available cataract surgery services. [7,20] Given the important positive outcomes of cataract surgery found in this study, increased efforts are needed to encourage greater acceptance of offered cataract surgery services. Such services should ideally be of high quality and provided regularly by the same provider in the same vicinity, and tailored to the needs of impoverished communities. [20].

Table 2. Impact of successful cataract surgery on marital status and measures of poverty at follow up.

		OR	95% CI	p
Marital (social) status	Widowed	1	reference	
	Married	3.28	1.31; 8.23	**0.012**
Working/Occupation	No	1	reference	
	Yes	3.31	1.40; 7.82	**0.006**
No. of working household members		1.24	0.55; 2.81	0.603
Monthly household income	> Rs 3000	1	reference	
	>1000–3000	0.05	<0.01; 0.64	**0.021**
	0–1000	0.22	0.08; 0.62	**0.004**

OR = odds ratio, CI = confidence interval; controlling for age, gender, education and household size (no. of members) in logistic regression.

The authors are unaware of any other study which has accessed the impact of a vision-restoring intervention on social status in blind persons in South Asia. In our study, successful cataract surgery, i.e. sight restoration to levels above vision impairment, was associated with an increased likelihood of being remarried a year later if widowed at baseline. Based on published studies, one can assume a rate of remarriage after being widowed of 6–20% for women and 60–65% for men of all ages over their remaining life span in South India. [40] Unfortunately, no reports of how an existing disability affects rates of remarriage in India are available. Thus, reported rates only reflect rates of remarriage in the general population. In our sample, these high rates of re-marriage were observed in an older population during a one-year follow-up, which increases the probability of the observed rates being higher than in the general population. Whether the positive economic impact of successful cataract surgery highlighted above increases the likelihood of remarriage, or whether it is reduced stigma due to sight restoration, or a combination of these, is difficult to assess. In either case, our results suggest that successful cataract surgery may increase the likelihood of widowed persons remarrying. However, as our observations are based on a small sample and a limited follow-up with no control group, they have to be interpreted with caution. Nevertheless, this finding has a range of positive implications, as widowhood is associated with adverse health impacts, loss of opportunities to engage in income generating activities and loss of societal esteem. [41].

Strengths of our study include the provision of uniform cataract surgery of high quality with IOL implantation, with good surgical outcomes, detailed visual acuity data, little attrition to follow up and culturally appropriate and well validated questionnaires. Moreover, being embedded into routine service provision of Sankara Eye Care Services in Coimbatore, our sample is representative of the communities served by this service provider in Tamil Nadu, South India. Economic data were collected at the individual and household level, rather than inferred from district

Table 3. Characteristics of participants who re-married and participants who were still widowed/single at 1 year (5 participants lost to follow up).

		Univariate analysis			Logistic regression		
		Remarried n = 28	**Still widowed n = 47**	**p**	**OR**	**95% CI**	**p**
Age		59.93±6.95	59.04±8.24	0.635	0.98	0.90; 1.07	0.696
Gender	Male	9(32.1%)	4(8.5%)	**0.009**	0.10	0.01; 1.17	0.066
	Female	19(67.9%)	43(91.5%)		1	(reference)	
Education	No schooling	16(57.1%)	37(78.7%)	**0.035**	25.51	0.89; 728.45	0.058
	Up to 5 yrs	7(25.0%)	8(17.0%)		15.92	0.57; 444.82	0.103
	More than 5 yrs	4(14.3%)	1(2.1%)		1	(reference)	
VRQoL:							
• Mobility		71±7	70±8	0.779	Not included		
• Activity Limitation		80±9	80±9	0.567	Not included		
• Psychosocial Impact		82±13	79±12	0.322	Not included		
VI at BL		18(64.3%)	32(68.1%)	0.737	Not included		
VI at 1 year		2(7.1%)	10(21.3%)	0.109	Not included		
Successful cataract surgery at 1 year		25(89.3%)	32(68.1%)	**0.039**	0.02	<0.01; 0.35	**0.008**
Working at 1 yr		23(82.1%)	33(70.2%)	0.254	0.95	0.17; 5.19	0.952
Monthly household income at 1 yr	Rs 0–1000	8(28.6%)	15(31.9%)	0.670	0.11	<0.01; 8.14	0.310
	Rs 1001–3000	19(67.9%)	30(63.8%)		0.53	0.01; 22.99	0.743
	>Rs 3000	1(3.6%)	1(2.1%)		1	(reference)	
No. of household members at 1 yr		3.79±1.79	3.68±2.17	0.830	1.07	0.67; 1.71	0.782
No. of working household members at 1 yr		1.44±75	1.36±.74	0.626	0.59	0.14; 2.41	0.459

Data reported as mean ± standard deviation (SD) or n(%); p-values for univariate tests derived from independent samples t-tests for continuous and Mann-Whitney U test for categorical variables; OR = odds ratio; CI = confidence interval.

Table 4. Factors associated with patient-reported quality of life at 1 year in generalized linear models, adjusted for age, gender and education.

		Mobility			Activity Limitation			Psychosocial Impact		
		OR	95% CI	p	OR	95% CI	p	OR	95% CI	p
Successful cataract surgery	No (ref)	1			1			1		
	Yes	1375.50	127.17; 14877.60	**<0.001**	30.43	1.51; 611.92	**0.026**	5033.27	62.86; 403027.84	**<0.001**
Working	No(ref)	1			1			1		
	Yes	1.19	0.12; 11.99	0.884	4.15	0.22; 76.49	0.339	1.44	0.02;101.99	0.866
Marital status	Widowed/Single (ref)	1			1			1		
	Married	0.16	0.01; 2.32	0.179	0.34	0.01; 9.91	0.533	0.20	<0.01;27.78	0.526
Monthly household income	No improvement (ref)	1			1			1		
	Improvement	1.34	0.24; 7.52	0.740	1.76	0.20; 15.49	0.611	31.32	1.31;751.00	**0.034**

OR = odds ratio, CI = confidence interval, ref = reference category.

or other regional approximations such as postcodes or census data which increases accuracy. [6,42] During the one year follow-up, no new government or NGO funded programs increasing options to be engaged in income generating activities were implemented in the area. To the authors' knowledge, no new factory was opened or other large employer moved into the area, either. The use of Rasch analysis, an important step in modern scale validation, to assess the measurement properties of the IND-VFQ-33 is another strength of this study. [10] Moreover, as the IND-VFQ-33 was developed using input primarily from cataract patients in Tamil Nadu, [28] the item content is likely to be very appropriate for this sample.

Conversely, our study is limited by a relatively small sample size, and a relatively short follow up to assess the long term impact of cataract surgery on VRQoL, poverty and social status. The lack of a non-operated control group makes it difficult to generalize results. However, other case-control studies have demonstrated the overall impact of cataract surgery compared to no surgery. [4] Also, our measures of poverty differ from other studies assessing the association of blindness and poverty, which limits comparability of our findings. Assessing the impact of successful cataract surgery on rates of re-marriage is inherently difficult and our results have to be interpreted with caution. However, overall, our results compare well to other studies as well as studies assessing rates of re-marriage based on Indian census data. [40].

In conclusion, successful cataract surgery restores not only vision and improves VRQoL, but enables previously visually impaired persons to restart work, leads to a higher monthly household income, and more members of the household being engaged in income earning activities. In addition, it makes re-marriage amongst widowed elderly persons more likely. Thus, it is a public health imperative to provide high quality cataract surgery to impoverished communities in developing countries as part of achieving the MDGs.

Acknowledgments

The investigators thank both the staff at the Sankara Eye Centre in Coimbatore, who conducted the field work and translated and transcribed the data, and all participants for their time and invaluable contribution.

Author Contributions

Conceived and designed the experiments: RPF DGK BB RVR. Performed the experiments: RPF DGK BB RVR. Analyzed the data: RPF DGK EF. Contributed reagents/materials/analysis tools: RPF DGK EF BB RVR FGH CG. Wrote the paper: RPF DGK EF BB RVR FGH CG.

References

1. Pascolini D, Mariotti SP (2012) Global estimates of visual impairment: 2010. British J Ophthalmol 96: 614–618.
2. Murthy G, Gupta SK, John N, Vashist P (2008) Current status of cataract blindness and Vision 2020: the right to sight initiative in India. Indian J Ophthalmol 56: 489–494.
3. Finger RP (2007) Cataracts in India: current situation, access, and barriers to services over time. Ophthalmic Epidemiol 14: 112–118.
4. Kuper H, Polack S, Eusebio C, Mathenge W, Wadud Z, et al. (2008) A case-control study to assess the relationship between poverty and visual impairment from cataract in Kenya, the Philippines, and Bangladesh. PLoS Med 5: e244.
5. Kuper H, Polack S, Mathenge W, Eusebio C, Wadud Z, et al. (2010) Does cataract surgery alleviate poverty? Evidence from a multi-centre intervention study conducted in Kenya, the Philippines and Bangladesh. PLoS One 5: e15431.
6. Gilbert CE, Shah SP, Jadoon MZ, Bourne R, Dineen B, et al. (2008) Poverty and blindness in Pakistan: results from the Pakistan national blindness and visual impairment survey. BMJ 336: 29–32.
7. Dandona L, Dandona R, Srinivas M, Giridhar P, Vilas K, et al. (2001) Blindness in the Indian state of Andhra Pradesh. Investigative Ophthalmology and Visual Science 42: 908–916.
8. Zimmer Z (2008) Poverty, wealth inequality and health among older adults in rural Cambodia. Soc Sci Med 66: 57–71.
9. Polack S, Eusebio C, Fletcher A, Foster A, Kuper H (2010) Visual impairment from cataract and health related quality of life: results from a case-control study in the Philippines. Ophthalmic Epidemiol 17: 152–159.
10. Finger RP, Kupitz DG, Holz FG, Balasubramaniam B, Ramani RV, et al. (2011) The impact of the severity of vision loss on vision-related quality of life in India: an evaluation of the IND-VFQ-33. Investigative Ophthalmology and Visual Science 52: 6081–6088.

11. Taylor HR, Katala S, Munoz B, Turner V (1991) Increase in mortality associated with blindness in rural Africa. Bull World Health Organ 69: 335–338.
12. Sengupta M, Agree EM (2002) Gender and Disability Among Older Adults in North and South India: Differences Associated with Coresidence and Marriage. Journal of Cross-Cultural Gerontology 17: 313–336.
13. Foley D, Chowdhury J (2007) Poverty, Social Exclusion and the Politics of Disability: Care as a Social Good and the Expenditure of Social Capital in Chuadanga, Bangladesh. Social Policy & Administration 41: 372–385.
14. Baltussen R, Sylla M, Mariotti SP (2004) Cost-effectiveness analysis of cataract surgery: a global and regional analysis. Bull World Health Organ 82: 338–345.
15. Dandona L (2001) Cataract surgery in very elderly patients. Outcome of cataract surgery is poor in developing countries. BMJ 323: 455.
16. Dandona L, Dandona R, Anand R, Srinivas M, Rajashekar V (2003) Outcome and number of cataract surgeries in India: policy issues for blindness control. Clinical and Experimental Ophthalmology 31: 23–31.
17. United Nations (2012) United Nations Millenium development Goals. New York: United Nations.
18. Office of the Registrar General and Census Commissioner (2001) Census of India. Census data 2001: India at a glace. Government of India.
19. World Health Organization (2004) Cataract Surgical Rate Southeast Asia Region 2004. Geneva: World Health Organization.
20. Finger RP, Kupitz DG, Holz FG, Chandrasekhar S, Balasubramaniam B, et al. (2011) Regular provision of outreach increases acceptance of cataract surgery in South India. Tropical Medicine & International Health.
21. Adams AM, Evans TG, Mohammed R, Farnsworth J (1997) Socioeconomic stratification by wealth ranking: Is it valid? World Dev 25: 1165–1172.
22. Hargreaves JR, Morison LA, Gear JS, Kim JC, Makhubele MB, et al. (2007) Assessing household wealth in health studies in developing countries: a comparison of participatory wealth ranking and survey techniques from rural South Africa. Emerg Themes Epidemiol 4: 4.
23. World Bank (1990) World Development Report: Poverty. Washington: World Bank.
24. Department of Planning (2006) Survey for below the poverty line families. Government of Punjab.
25. Gooding K (2006) Poverty and Blindness: A survey of the literature. Haywards Heath: Sightsavers International Programme Development Unit. http://www.vision2020uk.org.uk/library.asp?section = 000100050005.
26. Krieger N, Williams DR, Moss NE (1997) Measuring social class in US public health research: concepts, methodologies, and guidelines. Annu Rev Public Health 18: 341–378.
27. Gupta SK, Viswanath K, Thulasiraj RD, Murthy GV, Lamping DL, et al. (2005) The development of the Indian vision function questionnaire: field testing and psychometric evaluation. Br J Ophthalmol 89: 621–627.
28. Murthy GV, Gupta SK, Thulasiraj RD, Viswanath K, Donoghue EM, et al. (2005) The development of the Indian vision function questionnaire: questionnaire content. Br J Ophthalmol 89: 498–503.
29. Faul F, Erdfelder E, Lang AG, Buchner A (2007) G*Power 3: a flexible statistical power analysis program for the social, behavioral, and biomedical sciences. Behavior Research Methods 39: 175–191.
30. Linacre JM (2008) WINSTEPS Rasch measurement computer program. Chicago, IL: Winsteps.com.
31. Wolfe EW, Chiu CW (1999) Measuring pretest-posttest change with a Rasch Rating Scale Model. J Outcome Meas 3: 134–161.
32. Sloan J (2005) Assessing the minimally clinically significant difference: scientific considerations, challenges and solutions. COPD 2: 57–62.
33. Norman G, Sloan J, Wyrwich K (2003) Interpreation of changes in health-related quality of life: the remarkable universality of half a standard deviation. Med Care 41: 582–592.
34. Lewallen S (2008) Poverty and cataract–a deeper look at a complex issue. PLoS Med 5: e245.
35. Polack S, Eusebio C, Mathenge W, Wadud Z, Mamunur AK, et al. (2010) The impact of cataract surgery on health related quality of life in Kenya, the Philippines, and Bangladesh. Ophthalmic Epidemiol 17: 387–399.
36. Polack S, Eusebio C, Mathenge W, Wadud Z, Rashid M, et al. (2010) The impact of cataract surgery on activities and time-use: results from a longitudinal study in Kenya, Bangladesh and the Philippines. PLoS One 5: e10913.
37. Nirmalan PK, Katz J, Robin AL, Krishnadas R, Ramakrishnan R, et al. (2004) Utilization of eye care services in rural south India: the Aravind Comprehensive Eye Survey. British J Ophthalmol 88: 1237–1241.
38. Kessy JP, Lewallen S (2007) Poverty as a barrier to accessing cataract surgery: a study from Tanzania. Br J Ophthalmol 91: 1114–1116.
39. Finger RP, Ali M, Earnest J, Nirmalan PK (2007) Cataract surgery in Andhra Pradesh state, India: an investigation into uptake following outreach screening camps. Ophthalmic Epidemiol 14: 327–332.
40. Bhat M, Kanbargi R (1984) Estimating the incidence of widow and widower re-marriages in India from census data. Population Studies 38: 89–103.
41. Chen M, Dreze J (1992) Widows and health in rural north India. Economic and Political weekly 27: 24–31.
42. Fraser S, Bunce C, Wormald R, Brunner E (2001) Deprivation and late presentation of glaucoma: case-control study. BMJ 322: 639–643.

8

Comparison of Blue Light-Filtering IOLs and UV Light-Filtering IOLs for Cataract Surgery

Xiao-feng Zhu[1], Hai-dong Zou[1]*, Yong-fu Yu[2], Qian Sun[1], Nai-qing Zhao[2]

1 Department of Ophthalmology, Shanghai First People's Hospital Affiliated Shanghai Jiao Tong University, Shanghai, China, **2** Department of Biostatistics, School of Public Health, Fudan University, Shanghai, China

Abstract

Background: A number of published randomized controlled trials have been conducted to evaluate visual performance of blue light-filtering intraocular lenses (IOL) and UV light-filtering intraocular lenses (IOL) after cataract phacoemulsification surgery. However, results have not always been consistent. Therefore, we carried out a meta-analysis to compare the effectiveness of blue light-filtering IOLs versus UV light-filtering IOLs in cataract surgery.

Methods and Findings: Comprehensive searches of PubMed, Embase, Cochrane Library and the Chinese BioMedical literature databases were performed using web-based search engines. Fifteen trials (1690 eyes) were included for systematic review, and 11 of 15 studies were included in this meta-analysis. The results showed that there were no significant differences in postoperative mean best corrected visual acuity, contrast sensitivity, overall color vision, or in the blue light spectrum under photopic light conditions between blue light-filtering IOLs and UV light-filtering IOLs [WMD = −0.01, 95%CI (−0.03, 0.01), P = 0.46; WMD = 0.07, 95%CI (−0.04, 0.19), P = 0.20; SMD = 0.14, 95%CI (−0.33, 0.60), P = 0.566; SMD = 0.20, 95%CI (−0.04, 0.43), P = 0.099]. However, color vision with blue light-filtering IOLs was significantly reduced in the blue light spectrum under mesopic light conditions [SMD = 0.74, 95%CI (0.29, 1.18), P = 0.001].

Conclusion: This meta-analysis demonstrates that postoperative visual performance with blue light-filtering IOLs is approximately equal to that of UV light-filtering IOLs after cataract surgery, but color vision with blue light-filtering IOLs demonstrated some compromise in the blue light spectrum under mesopic light conditions.

Editor: Robert S. Phillips, University of York, United Kingdom

Funding: No current external funding sources for this study.

Competing Interests: The authors have declared that no competing interests exist.

* E-mail: zouhaidong@hotmail.com

Introduction

Globally, cataract is one of the most serious blinding diseases [1]. Modern cataract surgery is routinely combined with the implantation of an intraocular lens (IOL). UV light-filtering lenses have been the dominant IOLs used in modern cataract surgery since the mid-1980 s because of the growing evidence that ultraviolet light caused photic retinopathy and cystoid macular edema [2]. Recently there has been support for increasing the absorption spectrum of IOLs. The rationale is that UV light-filtering IOLs do not protect the retina from phototoxic damage by high-energy, short-wavelength blue light (approximately 400–480 nm) which is thought to contribute to the pathogenesis of age-related macular degeneration (AMD) [3,4]. The healthy human crystalline lens gradually becomes yellow as part of the normal ageing process. This yellowing reduces the transmission of blue light, thereby blocking an amount of blue light from reaching the retina [5]. After cataract extraction, the possibility of retinal exposure to blue light may accelerate AMD [6]. To address this potential damage, several blue light-filtering IOLs have been introduced in recent years. Their yellow tint more closely replicates the spectral transmission properties of the aged human crystalline lens than do the UV light-filtering IOLs [7].

Despite the benefits of blue light filtering, concerns were raised that this could negatively affect visual performance after cataract surgery [8]. Specifically, controversy remains as to ultimate best corrected visual acuity (BCVA), contrast sensitivity, color vision and glare. In recent years, several studies were performed to test visual function with blue light-filtering IOLs. Some described a better [9–11] and others, a worse [8,12,13], outcomes. However, we find that the majority of the literature did not describe any statistically significant differences in comparisons with UV light-filtering IOLs [14–17], or, if present, these differences were most likely small.

In this paper, we conduct a systematic review and meta-analysis of published randomized controlled trials to assess the visual performance of blue light-filtering IOLs and UV light-filtering IOLs after cataract surgery.

Materials and Methods

1. Search strategy

Two independent investigators (Zhu and Yu) searched publications from 2000 to June 30th, 2011 in PubMed, Embase, Cochrane Library, and the Chinese BioMedical Literature (CBM) databases by using the combination of MeSH terms "cataract extraction" or "phacoemulsification" or "lens" or "intraocular" or "implantation" or "blue light filtering" or "blue blocking" or "AcrySof Natural" or "SN60AT" or "yellow intraocular lens" or "YA60BB". In addition, the reference lists of potentially relevant manuscripts were scanned backwards to obtain extra eligible studies. No language restrictions were applied.

2. Inclusion criteria

2.1. Type of study: For inclusion, studies had to be randomized controlled trials (RCTs) comparing postoperative visual performance of blue light-filtering IOLs and UV light-filtering IOLs. Simulation experiments with blue light-filtering IOLs and UV light-filtering IOLs and clinical trials containing aspherical or multifocal IOLs were excluded.

2.2. Object of study: Patients with age-related cataract had phacoemulsification and IOL implantation. Otherwise, patients with ocular disease, such as glaucoma or age-related macular degeneration, preexisting systemic disease such as diabetes, or history of intraocular surgery that could affect the postoperative visual outcome were excluded.

2.3. Interventions: In addition to the different types of intraocular lens (blue light-filtering IOL or UV light-filtering IOL) implanted in the two groups, the interventions were the same.

2.4. Outcome measures: Main outcome measures included postoperative best corrected visual acuity, contrast sensitivity and color vision. Secondary outcome measures included postoperative visual quality assessment and adverse visual events.

3. Data extraction

Two independent investigators (Zhu and Yu) were involved in data extraction. The third investigator (Zou) examined the results, and a consensus was reached. The outcome in patients at the end of follow-up after phacoemulsification and IOL implantation was reviewed. We extracted the following data from the eligible studies: (1) general characteristics (title, first author, journal and year of publication); (2) methodology (type of study, country of origin, sequence generation, allocation concealment, masking or blinding, incomplete outcome data, selective reporting and other sources of bias); (3) subjects (recruitment site, enrollment periods, inclusion criteria, exclusion criteria, general patient characteristics); (4) Interventions and control groups (model of IOLs); (5) outcomes (measurement, follow-up time and loss of follow-up); (6) analysis (statistical methods); (7) results (quantitative results, qualitative results, postoperative visual quality assessment and adverse visual events). If original data were unavailable in articles, a request for original data was sent to the corresponding author.

4. Assessment of methodology quality

Two independent investigators (Zhu and Yu) evaluated the quality of each study using the Jadad scale [18]. The third investigator (Zou) examined the results, and a consensus was reached. The Jadad score is obtained from a possible 5-point scale, high scores indicating high quality, by yes/no answers to two questions for randomization and masking, and one question evaluating the reporting of patient withdrawals and dropouts. One point is given for each of the following: if the study is described as randomized, if the study is described as double-blind and if there is a description of withdrawals or dropouts. Two additional points are given if the method of randomization and the method of double blinding are appropriately described.

5. Statistical analysis

The meta-analysis was performed with the Stata version 11.0 (Stata Corp). For continuous data, the weighted mean difference (WMD) and 95%CI were recommended when all trials used the same scale to report their outcomes, while standardized mean difference (SMD) and 95%CI were more appropriate when trials used different scales to report their outcomes, or the means of their outcomes differed greatly. For dichotomous data, rate ratio or relative risk (RR) was strongly recommended for effect statistics for meta-analysis of randomized trials.

Statistical heterogeneity was tested by Q-test (x^2) [19] for each outcome, with a significance set at a P value<0.10. Insignificance indicates that the results of the different trials were similar ($P\geq0.1$, $I^2\leq50\%$). We evaluated the pooled summary effect by using a fixed-effect model to reduce the effects of heterogeneity between trials. Otherwise, data were combined using the random-effect model ($P<0.1$, $I^2>50\%$). If $I^2>75\%$, subgroup analysis was used to analysis the sources of heterogeneity. Sensitivity analysis calculated within subgroups of studies decided a priori were performed to assess the robustness of the main conclusions and explain heterogeneity. To determine whether the results of the meta-analysis were unduly influenced by any outcome measures in any one study, we recomputed the meta-analysis statistic after deleting each outcome measure one at a time.

Individual and pooled results were illustrated by point estimates and 95% confidence intervals (CIs). Results where the 95% CI did not include zero (for mean difference) or one (for odds ratio) were considered statistically significant. Where data could not be combined, we conducted a descriptive analysis.

Results

1. Literature search

A total of 107 abstracts from the multiple databases were retrieved, 68 of which were based on their titles and abstracts. Only 15 randomized controlled trials (RCTs) [14,17,20–32] recruiting 1690 eyes were included in our analysis. The trials selection process is shown in Figure 1.

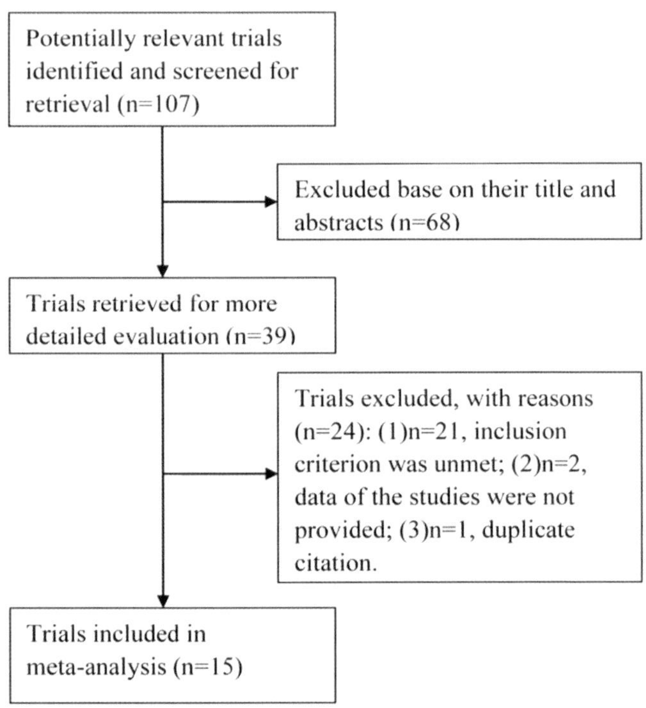

Figure 1. Process of study selection of RCTs.

2. Characteristics of eligible studies

Characteristics of RCTs included in the current meta-analysis are presented in Table 1 and Table 2. More than half of the studies [20,21,17,23,24,26,28,29,31] (60%, 9/15) were performed in Europe followed by 4 studies [14,22,30,32] in Asia; one study [25] from Australia and one study [27] from Brazil. The mean age of patients in most of the studies ranged from 50 to 88 years. The mean percentage of female patients ranged from 48.51% to 75%, as shown in Table 1. The mean follow-up time ranged from 2 months to 2 years (Table 2).

3. Quality assessment

3.1. Sequence generation: In 6 of all the RCTs included in the systematic review, the investigators described a random component in the sequence generation process such as: referring to a random number table [14] or using a computer random number generator [30] or shuffling envelopes [25,26,31]. The remainder did not describe the specific methods of random sequence generation.

3.2. Masking: Of 13 studies that described their masking or binding, 1 used triple-blinding [30], 8 used double-blinding [14,20,22–24,26,31,32] and 4 used single-blinding [17,21,25,29].

3.3. Withdrawals: All studies described the data of missing patients. Among these, 8 studies had missing cases: 6 of 80 (7.5%) [14]; 86 of 297 (28.96%) [17]; 3 of 31 (9.68%) [23]; 8 of 47 (17.02%) [24]; 10 of 80 (12.5%) [27]; 6 of 50 (12%) [28]; 7 of 80 (8.75%) [30]; and 4 of 80(5%) [31].

3.4. Other sources of bias: Only 2 studies used the following or an equivalent method to achieve allocation concealment: sealed envelopes [26] or sequential numbering [14].

Eight studies [14,17,20–22,24,25,32] described the patients' subjective satisfaction of visual quality between the blue light-filtering IOL and UV light-filtering IOL after surgery, and the other studies did not. Therefore, we do not know the existence of other potential factors.

The quality assessment of included studies is shown in Table 3.

4. Efficacy analysis

4.1. Postoperative best corrected visual acuity (BCVA): All studies described postoperative BCVA; the results of 8 studies [23,24,26–30,32] (596 eyes) were LogMAR transformation, including mean (m), standard deviation (SD) and sample size (n). Also, these studies had heterogeneity of effect size ($P = 0.0001$, $I^2 = 78.3\%$), so the random effect model was used for meta-analysis. The results are shown in Figure 2. No significant difference between the two groups [WMD = −0.01, 95%CI (−0.03, 0.01), P = 0.46], indicated that blue light-filtering IOL groups and UV light-filtering IOL groups were not significantly different in postoperative BCVA.

Subgroup analysis was conducted at the same time, according to the different IOL types. The studies were divided into four subgroups: blue light-filtering AcrySof Natural SN60AT IOL vs. UV light-filtering Sensar AR40e IOL (Subgroup 1) [27–29]; blue light-filtering Hoya YA60BB vs. UV light-filtering VA60BB (Subgroup 2) [23,24]; blue light-filtering AcrySof Natural SN60AT IOL vs. UV light-filtering AcrySof SA60AT IOL (Subgroup 3) [26,30]; and blue light-filtering Hoya YA60BB vs. UV light-filtering MC61131 (Subgroup 4) [32]. The results are shown in Figure 3.

All four subgroups were used to produce the random effect model for BCVA, and the results obtained from any subgroup show no significant differences. The results are as follows: Subgroup 1 (SN60AT vs. AR40e IOL, three studies [27–29], recruiting 258 eyes) [WMD = 0.00, 95%CI (−0.01, 0.02), P = 0.763]; Subgroup 2 (YA60BB vs. VA60BB, two studies [23,24], recruiting 134 eyes) [WMD = −0.01, 95%CI (−0.04, 0.01), P = 0.294]; Subgroup 3 (SN60AT vs. SA60AT, two studies [26,30], recruiting 125 eyes) [WMD = −0.02, 95%CI (−0.06, 0.02), P = 0.27]; Subgroup 4 (YA60BB vs. MC611, one study [32], recruiting 79 eyes) [WMD = 0.01, 95%CI (−0.01, 0.03), P = 0.42]. All the results indicated that blue light-filtering IOL groups and

Table 1. Characteristics of RCTS (n = 15) included in the meta-analysis.

First author (date)	Site	No. patients	No. eyes	Age (years) (test group/control group)	Sex(%) male: female (test group/control group)	Intervention
Hayashi 2006 [14]	Japan	80	160	71.1±6.7/70.7±6.2	12:26/12:24	YA-60BB/VA-60BB
Wirtitsch 2009 [20]	Austria	24	48	74±8	6:18	YA-60BB/VA-60BB
Barisić 2007 [21]	Croatia	60	120	68±4.5/67±4.2	9:21/9:21	Acrysof Natural IOL/AcrySof MA60BM IOL
Marshall 2005 [17]	England	297	594	≥60 (0.3/1.0)	29.3:70.7/39.5:60.5	SN60AT/SA60AT
Bhattacharjee 2006 [22]	India	13	26	62.15±6.68	6:7/6:7	SN60AT/SA60AT
Schmidinger 2008 [23]	Austria	31	62	73.40±7.64	NA	YA-60BB/VA-60BB
Mester 2008 [24]	Germany	47	94	Range 50–80	NA	YA-60BB/VA-60BB
Leibovitch 2006 [25]	Australia	19	19	74±6/74±6	3:6/6:4	SN60AT/SA60AT
Vuori 2006 [26]	Finland	37	52	72±8/73±7	NA	SN60AT/SA60AT
Rocha 2007 [27]	Brazil	40	80	71.0/69.2	2:3	SN60AT/Sensar AR40
Caporossi 2009 [28]	Italy	50	100	70.2±4.1/68.4±5.1	NA	SN60AT/Sensar AR40
Caporossi 2007 [29]	Italy	50	100	70.2±4.1/68.4±5.1	NA	SN60AT/Sensar AR40
Pandita 2007 [30]	India	80	80	61±2.7/59±3	51:49/52:48	SN60AT/SA60AT
Neumaier-Ammerer 2010 [31]	Austria	80	80	NA	NA	YA-60BB/VA-60BB & SN60AT/SA60AT
Wang 2010 [32]	China	79	79	67±8	NA	YA-60BB/MC611

NA, not available.

Table 2. Characteristics of RCTS (n = 15) included in the meta-analysis.

First author (date)	Measurement			Follow-up	Loss
	Visual acuity	Contrast sensitivity	Color Vision		
Hayashi 2006 [14]	*	* CAT-2000	NA	3 m	6 of 80 (7.5%)
Wirtitsch 2009 [20]	*	* Holladay	* Lanthony D-15	90±10 d	No
Barisić 2007 [21]	*	NA	NA	6 m	No
Marshall 2005 [17]	*	* CSV-1000E	* FM??? D-15	1 y	86 of 297 (28.96%)
Bhattacharjee 2006 [22]	*	* Pelli-Robson	* FM 100-hue	18 m	No
Schmidinger 2008 [23]	*	* Moorfields	NA	12 w	3 of 31 (9.68%)
Mester 2008 [24]	*	* ETDRS???+FACT???	* FM 100-hue	12 m	8 of 47 (17.02%)
Leibovitch 2006 [25]	*	* Pelli-Robson	* FM D-15	6 m	No
Vuori 2006 [26]	*	NA	* FM 100-hue	6 m	No
Rocha 2007 [27]	*	NA	NA	90 d	10 of 80 (12.5%)
Caporossi 2009 [28]	*	* Optec 6500	NA	2 y	6 of 50 (12%)
Caporossi 2007 [29]	*	* Optec 6500	NA	2 m	No
Pandita 2007 [30]	*	* CSV-1000E	NA	3 m	7 of 80 (8.75%)
Neumaier-Ammerer 2010 [31]	*	* CSV-1000E + Pelli-Robson	* Roth 28-hue	2 m	4 of 80 (5%)
Wang 2010 [32]	*	* ETDRS + Optec 6500	* FM 100-hue	3 m	No

*, yes; d = days; m = months; y = years; NA, not available.
① ETDRS, Early Treatment Diabetic Retinopathy Study contrast charts;
② FACT, Functional acuity contrast test;
③ FM, Farnsworth-Munsell.

UV light-filtering IOL groups were not significantly different in postoperative BCVA.

4.2. Postoperative contrast sensitivity: Twelve studies [14,17,20,22–25,28–32] compared the contrast sensitivity of blue light-filtering IOLs and UV light-filtering IOLs after implantation. The methods of assessing contrast sensitivity were described in Table 2. However, most of the literature using several different methods reported only the contrast sensitivity graph or P value, but no detailed data. On the other hand, for part of the data in reports, means and standard deviations cannot be calculated, and there was failure to pool analysis. Although we tried to contact the author, results of the corresponding data were not obtained. Thus, these could cause measurement bias. Thereafter, we conducted a descriptive analysis with results shown in Table 4.

Only two studies [22,25] recruiting 45 eyes used the same measurement method (Pelli-Robson contrast sensitivity chart), and

Table 3. Evaluation of the quality of RCTs included in the meta-analysis.

Study	Sequence generation	Double-blind	Withdrawals	Jadad score(0–5)
Hayashi 2006 [14]	Adequate	Adequate	DS	5
Wirtitsch 2009 [20]	Adequate	Adequate	DS	5
Barisić 2007 [21]	UA	SB	DS	2
Marshall 2005 [17]	UA	SB	DS	2
Bhattacharjee 2006 [22]	UA	Adequate	DS	4
Schmidinger 2008 [23]	UA	Adequate	DS	4
Mester 2008 [24]	UA	Adequate	DS	4
Leibovitch 2006 [25]	Adequate	SB	DS	3
Vuori 2006 [26]	Adequate	Adequate	DS	5
Rocha 2007 [27]	UA	NA	DS	2
Caporossi 2009 [28]	UA	NA	DS	2
Caporossi 2007 [29]	UA	SB	DS	2
Pandita 2007 [30]	Adequate	Adequate	DS	5
Neumaier-Ammerer 2010 [31]	Adequate	NA	DS	4
Wang 2010 [32]	UA	Adequate	DS	4

UA, Unclear; SB, Single blinding; DB, Double blinding; TB, Triple blinding; DS, Described; NA, not available.

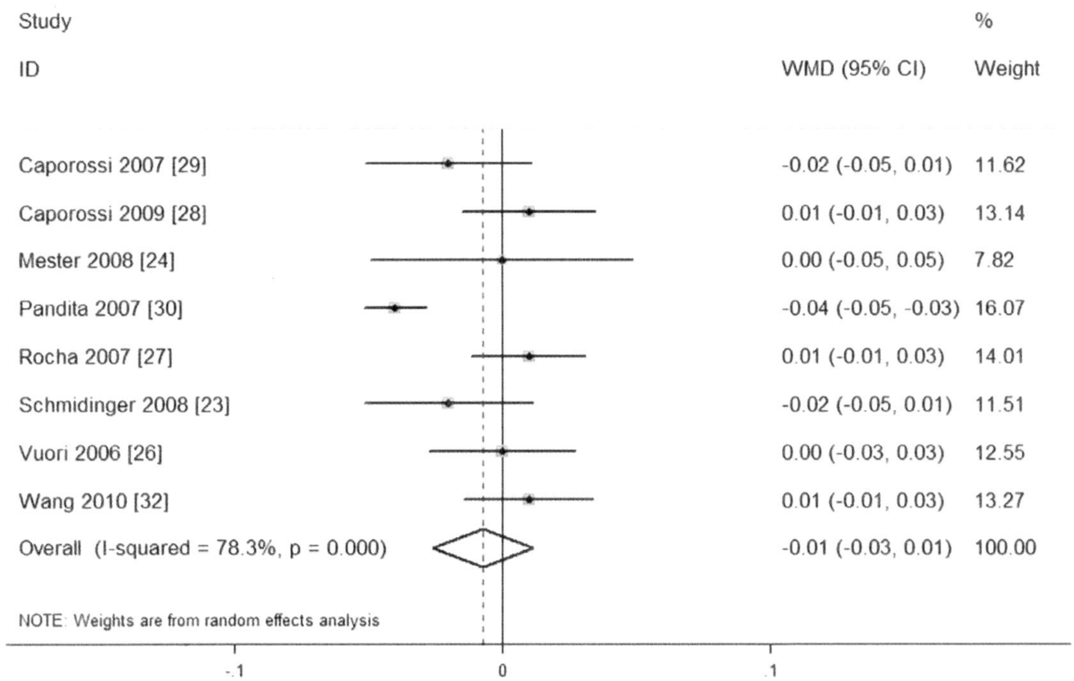

Figure 2. Meta-analysis of postoperative best corrected visual acuity (BCVA).

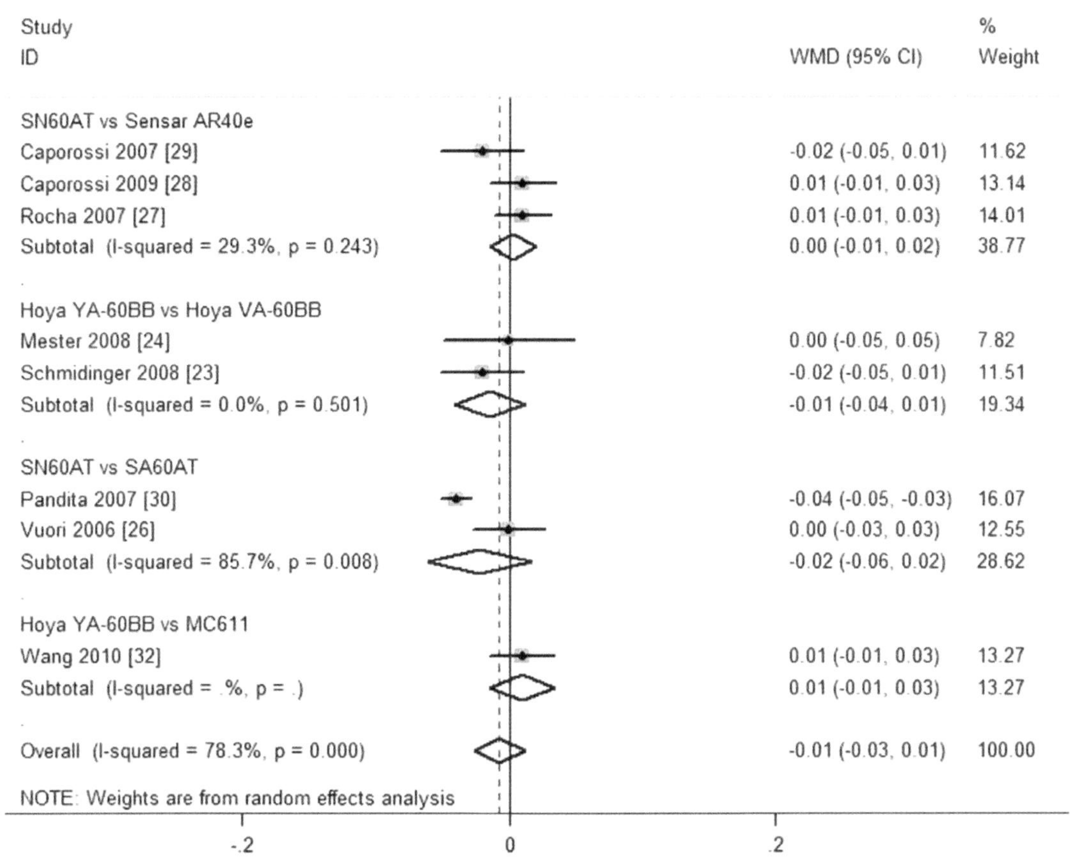

Figure 3. Subgroup analysis of postoperative best corrected distance visual acuity (BCVA).

Table 4. Comparison of postoperative contrast sensitivity in two groups.

		Photopic Conditions		Mesopic Conditions	
Model of IOLs	**Study**	**With Glare**	**Without Glare**	**With Glare**	**Without Glare**
SN60AT/SA60AT	Marshall 2005 [17]	NA	*	NA	*
	Pandita 2007 [30]	NA	*	*	*
	Neumaier-Ammerer 2010 [31]	*	*	*	*
SN60AT/Sensar AR40	Caporossi 2009 [28]	NA	*	NA	*
	Caporossi 2009 [29]	NA	*	NA	*
	Hayashi 2006 [14]	*	*	*	*
	Wirtitsch 2009 [20]	The blue light-filtering IOLs had worse contrast sensitibity compared with the UV-filtering IOL.			
YA-60BB/VA-60BB	Schmidinger 2008 [23]	NA	*	NA	NA
	Mester 2008 [24]	NA	*	*	*
	Neumaier-Ammerer 2010 [31]	*	*	*	*
YA-60BB/MC611	Wang 2010 [32]	*	*	*	*

*, No statistically significant difference; NA, not available.

reported complete data. They had no heterogeneity of effect size ($P = 0.609$, $I^2 = 0\%$), so the fixed effect model was used for meta-analysis. No significant difference between the two groups was seen [WMD = 0.07, 95%CI (−0.04, 0.19), P = 0.20], indicating that blue light-filtering IOL groups and UV light-filtering IOL groups were not significantly different in postoperative contrast sensitivity. The results are shown in Figure 4.

4.3. Postoperative color vision: Eight studies [17,20,22,24–26,31,32] compared the color vision of blue light-filtering IOLs and UV light-filtering IOLs after implantation. The methods of assessing color vision were described in Table 2. Five of them [24–26,31,32] reported complete data, and one [24] reported that color vision for blue with the blue light-filtering IOL was significantly reduced under photopic and mesopic conditions; another study [32] reported that the UV light-filtering IOL had significantly better color vision than the blue light-filtering IOL under mesopic conditions. The remaining studies showed no statistically significant difference.

Two studies [25,26] recruiting 71 eyes used different scales to report their outcomes in overall color vision, so that standardized mean differences (SMD) were more appropriate. They also had no heterogeneity of effect size ($P = 0.59$, $I^2 = 0\%$), so the fixed effect model was used for meta-analysis. No significant difference between the two groups was seen [SMD = 0.14, 95%CI (−0.33, 0.60), P = 0.566], indicating that blue light-filtering IOL groups and UV light-filtering IOL groups were not significantly different in postoperative color vision. The results are shown in Figure 5.

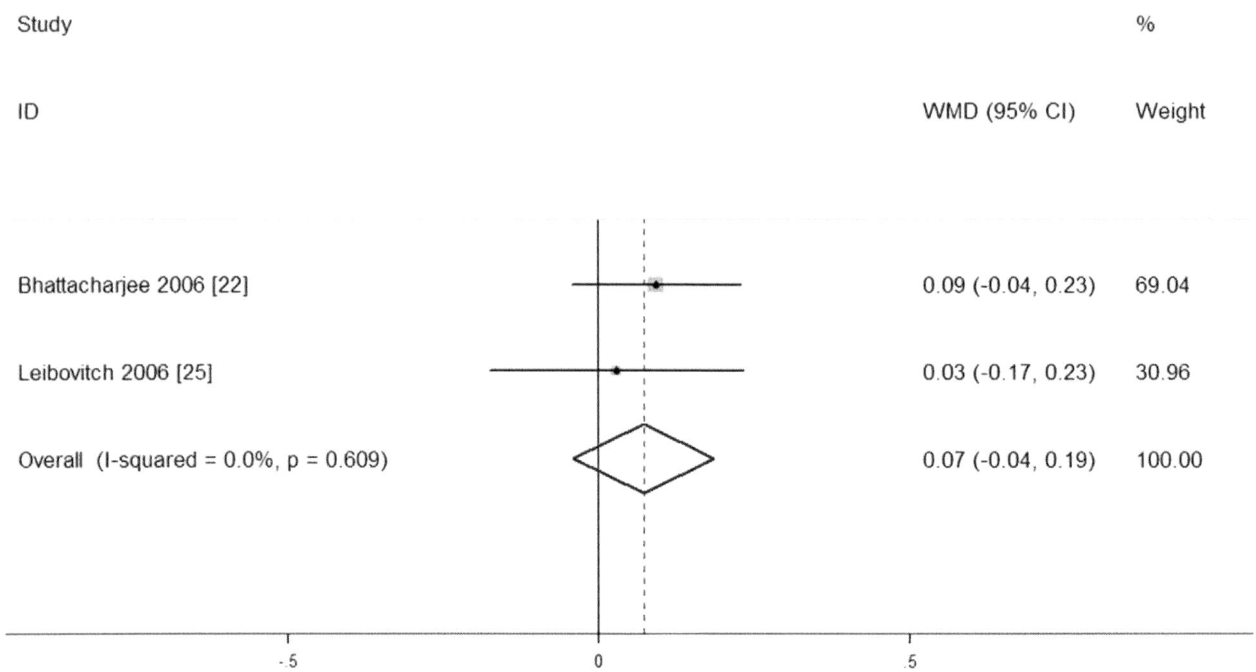

Figure 4. Meta-analysis of postoperative contrast sensitivity.

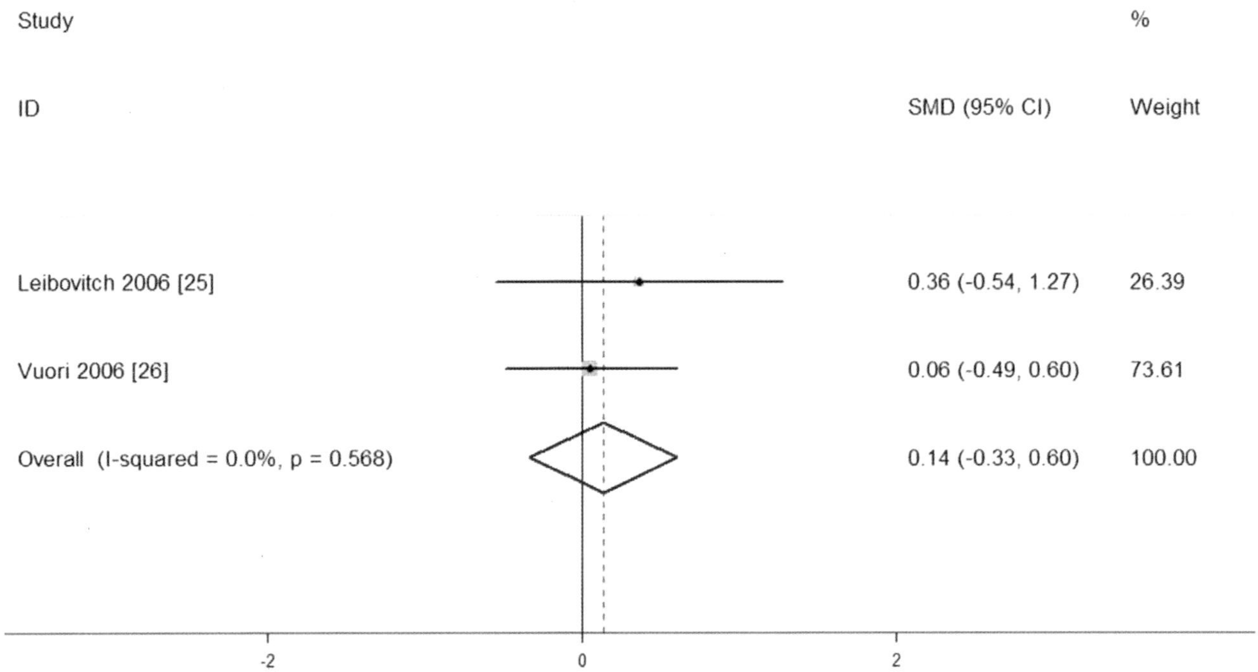

Figure 5. Meta-analysis of postoperative overall color vision.

Four studies [24,26,31,32] recruiting 281 eyes tested postoperative color vision in the blue light spectrum under photopic light conditions. They used different scales to report their outcomes, so standardized mean differences (SMD) were more appropriate. Also, they had no heterogeneity of effect size ($P = 0.806$, $I^2 = 0\%$), so the fixed effect model was used for meta-analysis. No significant differences were seen between the two groups [$SMD = 0.20$, 95%CI (-0.04, 0.43), $P = 0.099$], indicating that blue light-filtering IOL groups and UV light-filtering IOL groups were not significantly different in postoperative color vision in the blue light spectrum under photopic light conditions. The results are shown in Figure 6.

In addition, a sensitivity analysis suggested that the result was stable after deleting anyone's particular outcome. The results are shown in Figure 7.

Three studies [24,31,32] recruiting 229 eyes tested postoperative color vision in the blue light spectrum under mesopic light conditions. They used different scales to report their outcomes, so standardized mean differences (SMD) were more appropriate. Also, they had no heterogeneity of effect size ($P = 0.05$, $I^2 = 61.7\%$), so the

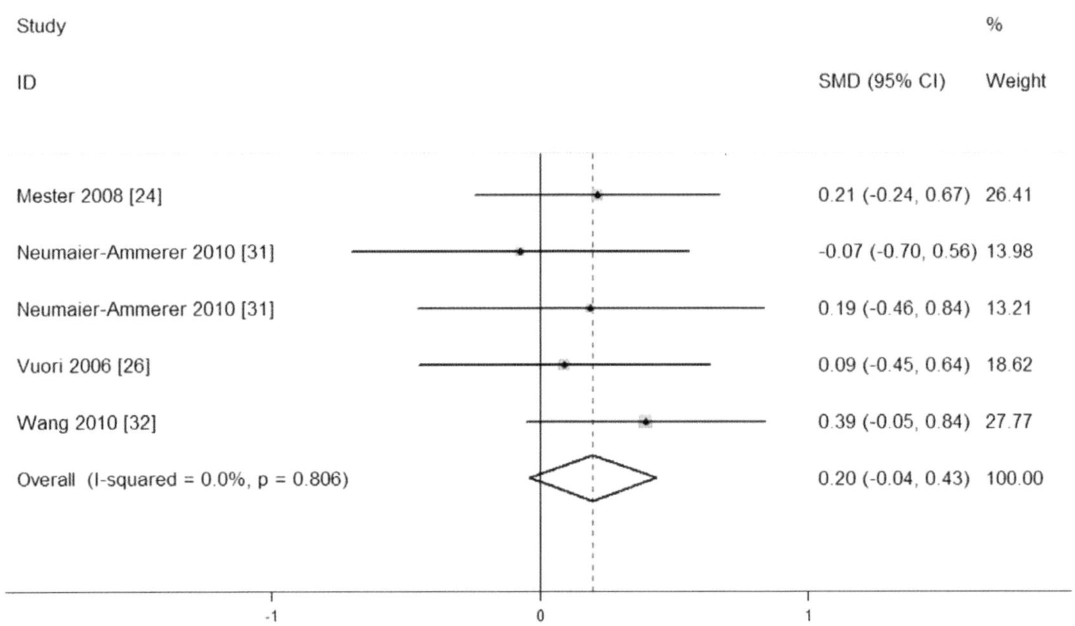

Figure 6. Meta-analysis of postoperative color vision in the blue light spectrum under photopic light condition.

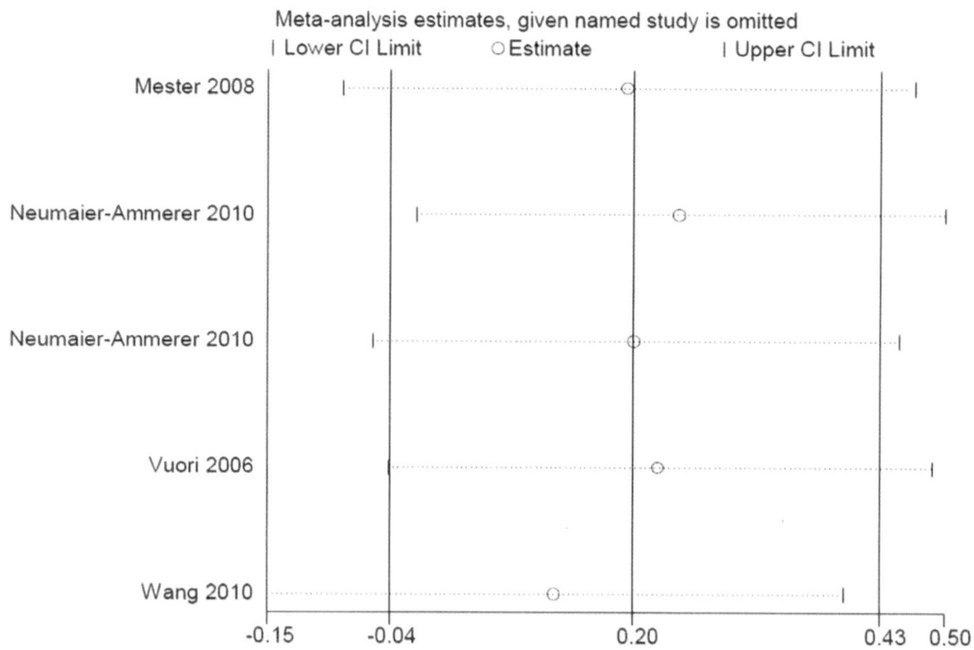

Figure 7. Sensitivity analysis of postoperative color vision in the blue light spectrum under photopic light condition.

random effect model was used for meta-analysis. There was a significant difference between the two groups [SMD = 0.74, 95%CI (0.29, 1.18), P = 0.001], indicating that color vision for blue with blue light-filtering IOLs was significantly reduced under mesopic conditions. The results are shown in Figure 8.

Additionally, the sensitivity analysis revealed that color vision with blue light-filtering IOLs was significantly reduced under mesopic conditions in the blue light spectrum. The results are shown in Figure 9.

4.4. Postoperative subjective satisfaction of visual quality and adverse visual events: Four studies [14,20,21,23] reported that different patients' subjective satisfaction of visual quality between the blue light-filtering IOL and UV light-filtering IOL after surgery. In the two studies [14,20] that

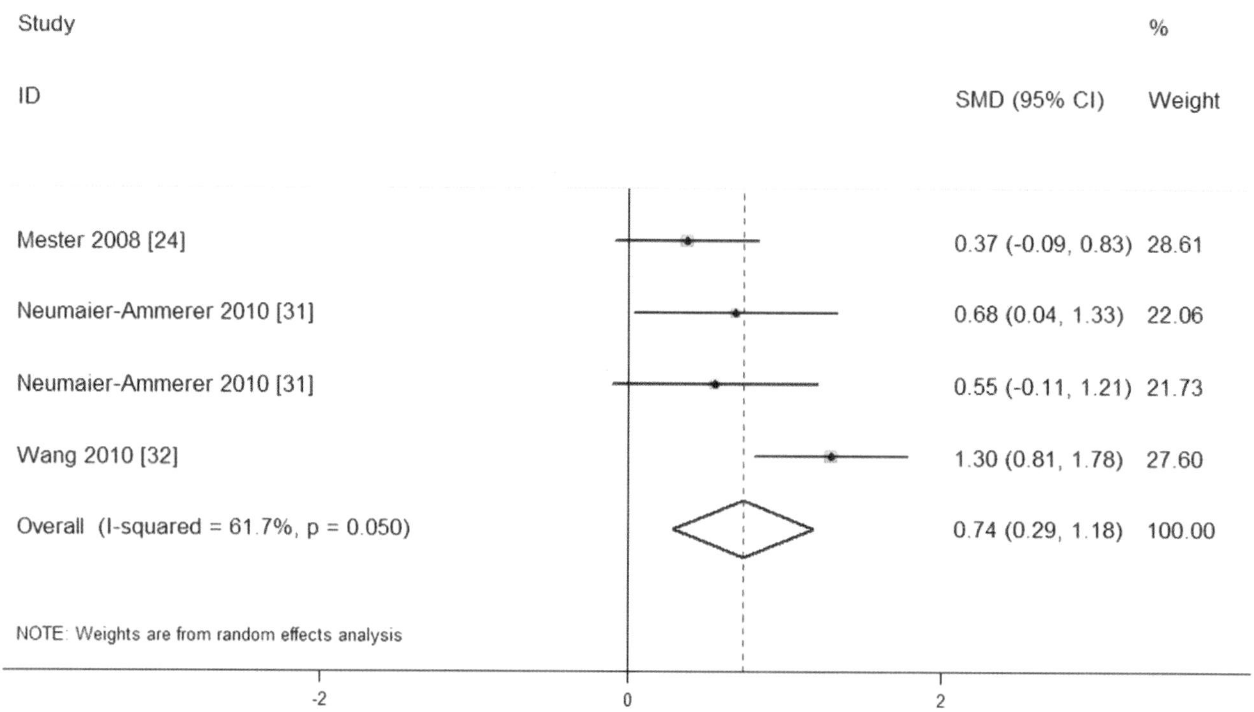

Figure 8. Meta-analysis of postoperative color vision in the blue light spectrum under mesopic light condition.

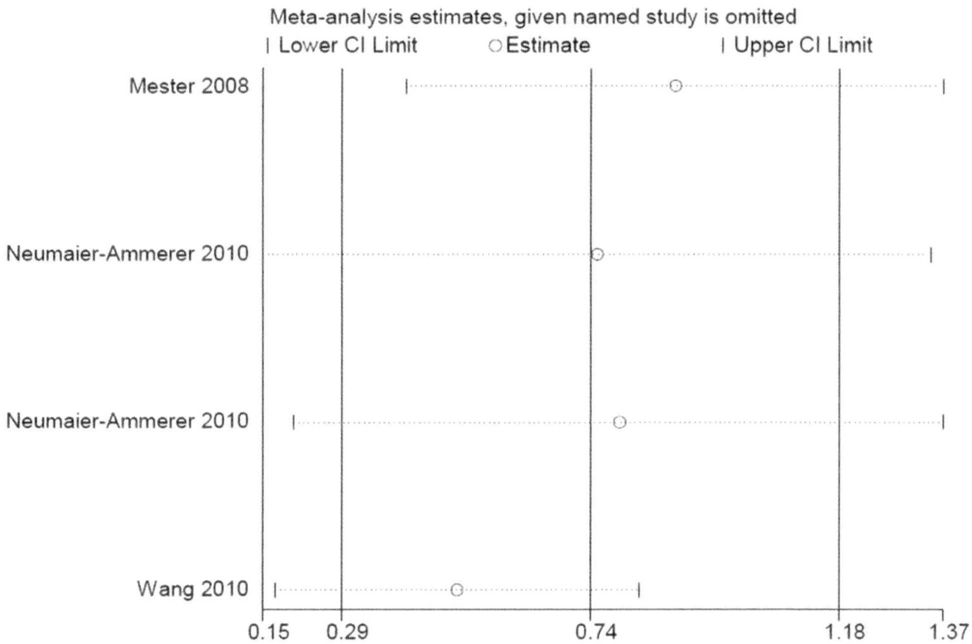

Figure 9. Sensitivity analysis of postoperative color vision in the blue light spectrum under mesopic light condition.

used questionnaires for evaluation, Wirtitsch and associates [20] using a questionnaire regarding color vision or contrast vision or vision under poor light conditions, they reported that 3 of 24 patients noticed a difference and all could correctly identify the eye implanted with the blue light-filtering IOL. However, all 3 patients said that they were not disturbed in binocular vision. In the report by Hayashi and associates [14], where patients were given a standardized questionnaire regarding glare symptoms and cyanopsia, the authors found that the incidence of patients who noticed cyanopsia was significantly less in the blue light-filtering IOL group than in the UV light-filtering IOL group at 2 weeks after surgery ($p = 0.0234$), but no patients reported cyanopsia at 3 months. In addition, another two studies [21,23] reported different patients' subjective satisfaction and subjective color vision in the left eye and right eye. Barisić and associates [21] described high satisfaction in patients who were implanted with a blue light-filtering IOL. Schmidinger and associates [23] found that 2 patients independently reported subjective changes in color vision in the eye with the blue light-filtering IOL; the changes probably resulted from the difference in color brightness because yellow IOLs reduce color brightness in the blue range of visible light. Furthermore, four studies [17,24,25,32] found no significant differences in subjective satisfaction of visual quality or lens-related adverse events in either group after surgery, which only Wang and associates [32] used the standardized questionnaire regarding subjective evaluation of glare, halo, and color vision perception. The remaining studies reported no relevant results in this regard.

Discussion

This systematic review compared the postoperative visual performance of RCTs between blue light-filtering IOLs and UV light-filtering IOLs, with the results showing that no statistically significant differences were found in comparing postoperative best corrected visual acuity, contrast sensitivity, and overall color vision. However, blue light-filtering IOLs demonstrated some compromise in the blue light spectrum under mesopic light conditions.

Large-scale epidemiological and animal studies have demonstrated that exposure to short wavelength visible light may be associated with a potential risk for accelerating the pathology of age-related macular degeneration (AMD) and retinal damage [2,3,33–35]. The natural aging crystalline lens can absorb amounts of UV and visible light, due to natural yellowing and opacification, going against the phototoxicity-AMD hypothesis [5]. Evidence suggests that blue light can damage the macula in patients who have undergone cataract surgery or clear lens extraction [6]. Therefore, an ideal IOL should be similar to that of the adult crystalline lens. Blue light-filtering IOLs show transmittance curves similar to that of a 53-year-old person's natural crystalline lens to help reduce the potential damage from blue light reaching the retina [7].

The implantation of blue light-filtering IOLs caused debate over their potential negative effects on postoperative visual performance, such as BCVA, contrast sensitivity and color vision, especially in dark conditions. We found that most of the literature overwhelmingly demonstrated that there were no detrimental effects of blue light-filtering IOLs on clinical visual recovery, which was consistent with our results. However, Mester and associates [24], in one of the included studies, mentioned that color vision in the blue light spectrum with the blue light-filtering IOLs (HOYA YA60BB) was significantly reduced under mesopic and photopic conditions: the impairment did not exceed the normal range or induce subjective disturbance of color vision. Furthermore, Barisić and associates [21] indicated that the blue light-filtering IOLs (HOYA YA60BB) had inferior contrast acuity and foveal threshold compared with the UV light-filtering IOLs. Unfortunately, we could not obtain complete data for a pooled analysis. Wang and associates [32] reported that blue light-filtering IOLs gave poor contrast sensitivity and color vision under mesopic conditions, which was in agreement with the conclusions of Neumaier-Ammerer and associates [31]. In fact, blue light-filtering IOLs have been shown to reduce the incidence of photophobia and cyanopsia in the early postoperative period [11,36].

Meta-analysis is the pooling of data from a number of different studies and objectively reanalyzing the resulting data set to provide a more precise result to assist in making clinical decisions. A possible limitation includes inappropriate pooling of data and publication bias. In our analysis, to avoid acknowledged and unintended duplication of data, we included only the most recent series of patient groups and randomized controlled trials, which are the optimal choice for meta-analyses. To minimize the publication bias, we conducted an electronic search and a manual search of the references of relevant studies to identify all the potential articles. This systematic review included 15 studies, all of which met the strict inclusion criteria; therefore, the intervention groups and control groups were comparable. However, the overall quality of the studies was not high. Only six studies had adequate sequence generation, two studies used adequate methods to achieve allocation concealment, and 2 studies made no mention of masking. In addition, different follow-up times and less reporting of postoperative visual adverse events could cause selection bias. Several studies lacked sufficient data for analysis, or involved different measurement methods, or used different units of measurement, or not used a standard questionnaire to assess: all of these could cause measurement bias. All the information in this systematic review came from the published literature, with special reports or unpublished data not being included, as they could cause publication bias. Therefore, to improve the quality of RCTs in the future, further verification of the postoperative visual performance and safety of blue light-filtering IOLs is needed. The format of reports should comply with the rules of CONSORT, providing detailed and transparent information in order to judge the authenticity of the outcomes.

In conclusion, our systematic review, as well as other clinical reports, suggests that the blue light-filtering IOLs had postoperative visual performance comparable to the UV light-filtering IOLs, but conclusions regarding color vision are still inconsistent.

Author Contributions

Conceived and designed the experiments: HZ XZ. Performed the experiments: XZ HZ QS YY. Analyzed the data: HZ XZ YY NZ. Contributed reagents/materials/analysis tools: HZ XZ YZ. Wrote the paper: XZ HZ.

References

1. Resnikoff S, Pascolini D, Etya'ale D, Kocur I, Pararajasegaram R, et al. (2004) Global data on visual impairment in the year 2002. Bull WHO 82: 844–851.
2. Ham WT, Jr., Mueller HA, Sliney DH (1976) Retinal sensitivity to damage from short wavelength light. Nature 260: 153–155.
3. Tomany SC, Cruickshanks KJ, Klein R, Klein BE, Knudtson MD (2004) Sunlight and the 10-year incidence of age-related maculopathy: the Beaver Dam Eye Study. Arch Ophthalmol 122: 750–757.
4. Taylor HR, West S, Muñoz B, Rosenthal FS, Bressler SB, et al. (1992) The long-term effects of visible light on the eye. Arch Ophthalmol 110: 99–104.
5. van Norren D, van de Kraats J (2007) Spectral transmission of intraocular lenses expressed as a virtual age. Br J Ophthalmol 91: 1374–1375.
6. Cugati S, Mitchell P, Rochtchina E, Tan AG, Smith W, et al. (2006) Cataract surgery and the 10-year incidence of age-related maculopathy. Ophthalmology 113: 2020–2025.
7. Brockmann C, Schulz M, Laube T (2008) Transmittance characteristics of ultraviolet and blue-light-filtering intraocular lenses. J Cataract Refract Surg 34: 1161–1166.
8. Mainster MA, Sparrow JR (2003) How much blue-light should an IOL transmit? Br J Ophthalmol 87: 1523–1529.
9. Niwa K, Yoshino Y, Okuyama F (1996) Effects of tinted intraocular lens on contrast sensitivity. Ophthalmic Physiol Opt 16: 297–302.
10. Rodríguez-Galietero A, Montés-Micó R, Muñoz G, Albarrán-Diego C (2005) Blue-light filtering intraocular lens in patients with diabetes: contrast sensitivity and chromatic discrimination. J Cataract Refract Surg 31: 2088–2092.
11. Yuan Z, Reinach P, Yuan J (2004) Contrast sensitivity and color vision with a yellow intraocular lens. Am J Ophthalmol 138: 138–140.
12. Schwiegerling J (2006) Blue-light-absorbing lenses and their effect in scotopic vision. J Cataract Refract Surg 32: 141–144.
13. Pierre A, Wittich W, Faubert J, Overbury O (2007) Luminance contrast with clear and yellow-tinted intraocular lenses. J Cataract Refract Surg 33: 1248–1252.
14. Hayashi K, Hayashi H (2006) Visual function in patients with yellow tinted intraocular lenses compared with vision in patients with non-tinted intraocular lenses. Br J Ophthalmol 90: 1019–1023.
15. Rodriguez-Galietero A, Montes-Mico R, Munoz G, Albarrán-Diego C (2005) Comparison of contrast sensitivity and color discrimination after clear and yellow intraocular lens implantation. J Cataract Refract Surg 31: 1736–1740.
16. Cionni RJ, Tsai JH (2006) Color perception with AcrySof Natural and AcrySof single-piece intraocular lenses under photopic and mesopic conditions. J Cataract Refract Surg 32: 236–242.
17. Marshall J, Cionni RJ, Davison J, Ernest P, Lehmann R, et al. (2005) Clinical results of the blue-light filtering AcrySof Natural foldable acrylic intraocular lens. J Cataract Refract Surg 31: 2319–2323.
18. Jadad AR, Moore RA, Carroll D, Jenkinson C, Reynolds DJ, et al. (1996) Assessing the quality of reports of randomized clinical trials: is blinding necessary? Control Clin Trials 17: 1–12.
19. Higgins JP, Thompson SG (2002) Quantifying heterogeneity in a meta-analysis. Stat Med 21: 1539–1558.
20. Wirtitsch MG, Schmidinger G, Prskavec M, Rubey M, Skorpik F, et al. (2009) Influence of blue-light-filtering intraocular lenses on color perception and contrast acuity. Ophthalmology 116: 39–45.
21. Barisić A, Dekaris I, Gabrić N, Bosnar D, Lazić R, et al. (2007) Blue light filtering intraocular lenses in phacoemulsification cataract surgery. Coll. Antropol 31(suppl): 57–60.
22. Bhattacharjee H, Bhattacharjee K, Medhi J (2006) Visual performance: Comparison of foldable intraocular lenses. J Cataract Refract Surg 32: 451–455.
23. Schmidinger G, Menapace R, Pieh S (2008) Intraindividual comparison of color contrast sensitivity in patients with clear and blue-light-filtering intraocular lenses. J Cataract Refract Surg 34: 769–773.
24. Mester U, Holz F, Kohnen T, Lohmann C, Tetz M (2008) Intraindividual comparison of ablue-light filter on visual function: AF-1 (UY) versus AF-1 (UV) intraocularlens. J Cataract Refract Surg 34: 608–615.
25. Leibovitch I, Lai T, Porter N, Pietris G, Newland H, et al. (2006) Visual outcomes with the yellow intraocular lens. Acta Ophthalmol Scand 84: 95–99.
26. Vuori ML, Mäntyjärvi M (2006) Colour vision and retinal nerve fibre layer photography in patients with an Acrysof Natural intraocular lens. Acta Ophthalmol Scand 84: 92–94.
27. Rocha KM, Soriano ES, Chamon W, Chalita MR, Nosé W (2007) Spherical aberration and depth of focus in eyes implanted with aspheric and spherical intraocular lenses: a prospective randomized study. Ophthalmology 114: 2050–2054.
28. Caporossi A, Casprini F, Martone G, Balestrazzi A, Tosi GM, et al. (2009) Contrast sensitivity evaluation of aspheric and spherical intraocular lenses 2 years after implantation. J Refract Surg 25: 578–590.
29. Caporossi A, Martone G, Casprini F, Rapisarda L (2007) Prospective randomized study of clinical performance of 3 aspheric and 2 spherical intraocular lenses in 250 eyes. J Refract Surg 23: 639–648.
30. Pandita D, Raj SM, Vasavada VA, Vasavada VA, Kazi NS, et al. (2007) Contrastsensitivity and glare disability after implantation of AcrySof IQ Natural aspherical intraocular lens: prospective randomized masked clinical trial. J Cataract Refract Surg 33: 603–610.
31. Neumaier-Ammerer B, Felke S, Hagen S, Haas P, Zeiler F, et al. (2010) Comparison of visual performance with blue light-filtering and ultraviolet light-filtering intraocular lenses. J Cataract Refract Surg 36: 2073–2079.
32. Wang H, Wang J, Fan W, Wang W (2010) Comparison of photochromic, yellow, and clear intraocular lenses in human eyes under photopic and mesopic lighting conditions. J Cataract Refract Surg 36: 2080–2086.
33. Cruickshanks KJ, Klein R, Klein BE, Nondahl DM (2001) Sunlight and the 5-year incidence of early age-related maculopathy: the Beaver Dam Eye Study. Arch Ophthalmol 119: 246–250.
34. Grimm C, Wenzel A, Williams T, Rol P, Hafezi F, et al. (2001) Rhodopsin-mediated blue-light damage to the rat retina: effect of photoreversal of bleaching. Invest Ophthalmol Vis Sci 42: 497–505.
35. Hafezi F, Marti A, Munz K, Remé CE (1997) Light-induced apoptosis: differential timing in the retina and pigment epithelium. Exp Eye Res 64: 963–970.
36. Yap M (1984) The effect of a yellow filter on contrast sensitivity. Ophthalmic Physiol Opt 4: 227–232.

9

Effect of the Gas6 c.834+7G>A Polymorphism and the Interaction of Known Risk Factors on AMD Pathogenesis in Hungarian Patients

Gergely Losonczy[1]*, Attila Vajas[1], Lili Takács[1], Erika Dzsudzsák[2], Ágnes Fekete[3], Éva Márhoffer[1], László Kardos[4], Éva Ajzner[5], Begoña Hurtado[6], Pablo Garcia de Frutos[6], András Berta[1]⁹, István Balogh[2]⁹

1 Department of Ophthalmology, University of Debrecen, Debrecen, Hungary, 2 Department of Laboratory Medicine, University of Debrecen, Debrecen, Hungary, 3 Department of Anesthesiology and Intensive Care, University of Debrecen, Debrecen, Hungary, 4 Hygiene and Infection Control Services, Kenézy Gyula County Hospital, Debrecen, Hungary, 5 Central Laboratory, Jósa András Teaching Hospital, Nyíregyháza, Hungary, 6 Department of Cell Death and Proliferation, Institute of Biomedical Research of Barcelona (IIBB-CSIC, IDIBAPS), Barcelona, Spain

Abstract

Age-related macular degeneration (AMD) is the leading cause of blindness in the elderly in the developed world. Numerous genetic factors contribute to the development of the multifactorial disease. We performed a case-control study to assess the risk conferred by known and candidate genetic polymorphisms on the development of AMD. We searched for genetic interactions and for differences in dry and wet AMD etiology. We enrolled 213 patients with exudative, 67 patients with dry AMD and 106 age and ethnically matched controls. Altogether 12 polymorphisms in Apolipoprotein E, complement factor H, complement factor I, complement component 3, blood coagulation factor XIII, HTRA1, LOC387715, Gas6 and MerTK genes were tested. No association was found between either the exudative or the dry form and the polymorphisms in the Apolipoprotein E, complement factor I, FXIII and MerTK genes. Gas6 c.834+7G>A polymorphism was found to be significantly protective irrespective of other genotypes, reducing the odds of wet type AMD by a half (OR = 0.50, 95%CI: 0.26–0.97, p = 0.04). Multiple regression models revealed an interesting genetic interaction in the dry AMD subgroup. In the absence of C3 risk allele, mutant genotypes of both CFH and HTRA1 behaved as strongly significant risk factors (OR = 7.96, 95%CI: 2.39 = 26.50, p = 0.0007, and OR = 36.02, 95%CI: 3.30–393.02, p = 0.0033, respectively), but reduced to neutrality otherwise. The risk allele of C3 was observed to carry a significant risk in the simultaneous absence of homozygous CFH and HTRA1 polymorphisms only, in which case it was associated with a near-five-fold relative increase in the odds of dry type AMD (OR = 4.93, 95%CI: 1.98–12.25, p = 0.0006). Our results suggest a protective role of Gas6 c.834+7G>A polymorphism in exudative AMD development. In addition, novel genetic interactions were revealed between CFH, HTRA1 and C3 polymorphisms that might contribute to the pathogenesis of dry AMD.

Editor: Katriina Aalto-Setala, University of Tampere, Finland

Funding: This study was supported by by the Hungarian Research Fund OTKA K68616 (to A.B.) and by the Social Renewal Operational Programme TAMOP 4.2.1./B-091/1/KONV-2010-0007 project (to A.B. and I.B.). The funders had no role in study design, data collection and analysis, decision to publish, or preparation of the manuscript.

Competing Interests: The authors have declared that no competing interests exist.

* E-mail: losigeri@gmail.com

⁹ These authors contributed equally to this work.

Introduction

Age-related macular degeneration (AMD) is the leading cause of visual impairment in the elderly in developed countries, most prominently in white populations [1,2]. The prevalence of the disease increases with age reaching as much as 15% above the age of 80 [3]. AMD is a multifactorial disease characterized by progressive degeneration of the central retina leading to visual deterioration. Early stages of AMD are characterized by retinal pigment abnormalities and accumulation of small deposits called drusen under the macular area of the retina. Two advanced forms of the disease are distinguished: extensive pigment epithelium atrophy also referred to as geographic atrophy (GA) leading to irreversible and untreatable visual deterioration or subretinal neovascular membrane (SRNVM) formation characterized by intra- or subretinal invasion of new vessels arising from the choroid. Multiple methods have been developed to determine the severity of the disease and to estimate the risk of progression from early to late stages. The neovascular form is referred to as exudative or wet type, while AMD without any neovascular component is considered non-exudative or dry type AMD [4]. Although the etiology of the disease is still largely unclear, several risk factors have been unequivocally linked to AMD, including advanced age, European origin and smoking. Other factors including high cholesterol level, sunlight exposure, blue iris, oxidative damage, hypertension, obesity and inflammation have also been linked to AMD development, however, with inconsistent results [5,6]. Cataract surgery has been shown to increase risk exclusively of dry late AMD, however carriers of two complement factor H (CFH) risk alleles are prone to develop all types of AMD [7].

In recent years a growing number of evidence has supported the role of genetic risk factors in AMD pathogenesis. The most widely studied and strongest genetic risk factors map to genes of the alternative complement pathway and its regulators, and are most likely responsible for an imbalance in the complement activation. Additionally, there is a wide range of chromosome regions and genes with different functions implicated in AMD pathogenesis. Because in most studies sharp clinical difference between cases and controls is ascertained by recruiting cases with unequivocally advanced phenotype, little is known about the genetic background of intermediate dry AMD. It is still an open question what makes the difference in the genetic etiology of exudative and non-exudative AMD [8].

After the initial reports [9,10,11], numerous case-control studies have provided supportive evidence for a strong association between AMD and the p.Tyr402His (rs1061170) polymorphism of the CFH gene in different populations. According to a very recent meta-analysis of 24 case-control studies the p.Tyr402His variant confers a 2-fold higher risk of late-AMD per copy in individuals of European descent [12].

Other components of the complement system have also been implicated in AMD pathogenesis. The initial report demonstrated that the p.Arg102Gly (rs2230199) polymorphism in the Complement factor 3 (C3) gene confers statistically significant risk to AMD with an odds ratio of 1.7 for heterozygotes and 2.6 for homozygotes in comparison to wild type subjects [13]. Later similar odds ratios were reported equally contributing to early and late AMD. The risk was independent of CFH p.Tyr402His and LOC387715 p.Ala69Ser polymorphisms [14,15].

The rs10033900 polymorphism of Complement factor I (CFI), a proteolytic regulatory enzyme inactivating C3b has been shown to be associated with AMD [16,17], however a recent paper failed to confirm this association [18].

Strong association has been confirmed between AMD and the p.Ala69Ser (rs10490924) polymorphism in LOC387715 coding a protein of unknown function [19,20] or a promoter SNP of the HTRA serine peptidase 1 (HTRA1) gene (rs11200638) [21,22,23,24]. These two polymorphisms are located in close vicinity and it is still a subject of debate which of the two plays a role in the pathomechanism of the disease.

Although lipids are major components of drusen, proteins involved in lipid transportation have been linked to AMD pathogenesis only recently [25]. Apolipoprotein E (ApoE), a polymorphic gene with three common allelic variants (E2, E3 and E4) has also been connected to the pathogenesis of AMD. E3 is the major allele among whites. E4 allele has been reported to decrease AMD risk, or at least delay the occurrence of the disease. In contrast, the presence of the E2 allele is associated with increased risk and younger age at diagnosis [26,27,28]. ApoE E4 proved to be protective with an odds ratio of 0.5 (95%CI: 0.29–0.86) in a study comprising of 3137 individuals [29]. Another study demonstrated a protective effect of the E4 allele only in the neovascular AMD patient group with an OR of 0.61 (95%CI: 0.38–0.97) [30]. In contrast with these findings, a Spanish study reported an increased risk for AMD due to the ApoE E4 allele, with an OR of 5.6 [31]. Previously we could not demonstrate statistically significant association between ApoE alleles and AMD in a Hungarian population. However, the potential risk factor E2 allele was less frequent in patients than in controls (0.066 and 0.1, respectively) while the E4 allele was more frequent in the patient group than in controls (0.108 versus 0.084, respectively), interestingly [32]. The somewhat inconsistent findings on the association of AMD and ApoE called for a recently published pooled analysis (n = 21.160) demonstrating that the E2 allele in homozygous form confers risk (OR = 1.83, 95%CI: 1.04–3.23) and the E4 allele is protective (OR = 0.72 per haplotype; 95%CI: 0.65–0.74) in late AMD [33]. A recent well powered case-control study (including 2187 cases and 2187 age and ethnically matched controls) demonstrated disease risk of the E2 allele compared to the E3/E3 genotype (OR = 1.32, 95%CI: 1.11–1.58). However, the E2 allele only conferred risk to early AMD in the never smoker and previously smoker group, while the E4 allele was protective against early AMD exclusively in the current smoker population [34].

The growth arrest–specific gene 6 (Gas6) product is a vitamin K dependent protein secreted by leukocytes and endothelial cells in response to injury. Gas6 has a high structural homology with the natural anticoagulant protein S. It has not been implicated in AMD pathogenesis so far, however there are certain functions of the protein that make it a possible candidate for AMD. It has growth factor-like properties through its interaction with receptor tyrosine kinases of the TAM family; Tyro3, Axl and MerTK, this way it contributes to the regulation of angiogenesis, cell survival, proliferation, migration and adhesion, making it a relevant participant of biological processes like atherogenesis and thrombosis [35,36,37,38]. Recently, we found that Gas6 is present in the human circulation [39]. A Gas6 polymorphism (c.834+7AA genotype) was identified as a common SNP in the general population and gave the strongest association with stroke [40]. Others found similar association with acute coronary syndrome, and type 2 diabetes [36,40,41]. TAM receptor tyrosine kinases and their ligands Gas6 and Protein S are essential for the phagocytosis of apoptotic cells and membranes in the immune, nervous, and reproductive systems [42]. Moreover, MerTK receptor is the key player involved in photoreceptor outer segment phagocytosis by RPE cells. MerTK knock-out mice develop almost total degeneration of the retinal photoreceptor layer by 10 weeks of age [43,44,45]. MerTK SNPs were selected because of their tagging properties after Haploview analysis of the genotypes downloaded from the HapMap database for CEU population (Rel20/phase II Jan06, on NCBI B35 assembly, dbSNP b125). Haplotype (defined as a group of closely linked polymorphic alleles in a chromosomal region) tagging SNPs were selected according to the following parameters: MAF>0.05 in Caucasians, $r2>0.8$ between each pair of tagged and tagging SNPs in pairwise tagging and haplotypes coverage down to 5% of their frequency in the HapMap CEU population for each analysed gene. The 4 tagSNPs selected belong to a haplotype block and were sufficient to cover the whole gene [46].

The aim of our present case-control study was to refine the association of the known polymorphisms and AMD subtypes in the Hungarian population and to explore the interplay of different polymorphisms. We considered MerTK and its ligand Gas6 as candidate genes to play a role in AMD pathogenesis and searched for association between their polymorphisms and the disease.

Patients and Methods

Ethics Statement

The study was approved by the Institutional Ethics Committee of the University of Debrecen and the procedures strictly adhered to the tenets of the declaration of Helsinki.

Patients

In total, 386 subjects were enrolled in the case-control study: 213 patients with exudative AMD, 67 patients with dry AMD and 106 unrelated ethnically matched healthy controls were ascertained in Eastern-Hungary at the Department of Ophthalmology,

University of Debrecen between 2005 and 2011. The control group consisted of individuals attending to the Outpatient Clinic because of refractive disorders, or post-cataract follow-up visits. To maximize the reliability of our study, we deliberately selected controls to be somewhat older than patients. Written informed consent was obtained from all participants. Detailed patient history was recorded with the use of a questionnaire focusing on known or suspected non-genetic risk factors of AMD such as cigarette smoking, exposure to blue light, medical history of acute myocardial infarction, ischemic heart disease and deep venous thrombosis. Cigarette smoking was determined in packyears. Smoking of one pack of cigarettes daily for a period of one year was considered one packyear. Body mass index (BMI) was calculated on the actual body height and weight values when ascertained that no considerable change in body weight occurred in the past 10 years. An average BMI was calculated in patients with significant loss or increase of body weight based on body weight values of the previous 10 years period. Color fundus photographs were taken of patients and controls. Fluorescein angiography was used to investigate patients with exudative AMD. Grading of the severity of the disease was based on the clinical age-related maculopathy staging system (CARMS) [4]. There were 5,3,18,6 and 35 patients in the dry AMD group characterized as CARMS grade 2b, 2c, 3a, 3b and 4, respectively.

For statistical analysis, patients were classified according to the more severely affected eye into two groups corresponding to either dry or wet AMD. No signs of AMD, such as abnormal pigmentation or drusen were observed in controls. Color fundus photographs and fluorescein angiograms were evaluated by two experienced ophthalmologist (T.L. and L.G.). Patients or controls with other ocular diseases interfering with reliable evaluation of AMD were not included in the study.

Molecular genetic methods

Molecular genetic methods for the detection of the common ApoE alleles, CFH p.Tyr402His polymorphism, LOC387715 rs10490924 (p.A69S) and HTRA1 rs11200638 polymorphisms were used as described earlier [32]. Factor XIII Val34Leu polymorphism was detected using fluorescent PCR and hybridization probes [47]. Similar methodology was used for the genotyping of Gas6 rs8191974 (c.834+7G>A) polymorphism and for the MerTK rs86016 (g.2920G>A) polymorphism, as described earlier [46]. Complement C3 rs2230199 (p.Arg102Gly) polymorphism was tested using a PCR-RFLP method. Amplification was performed using the primers: C3R102F: 5′- CAG GGA GTT CAA GTC AGA AAA GG -3′ and C3R102R: TCT TGT CTG TCT GGA TGA AGA GG -3′. The 131 bp PCR product was then subjected to the digestion with *Cfo*I restriction endonuclease. The sole restriction site of the enzyme in the PCR product is lost when the mutation is present. The candidate, most likely a tag SNP, that has been shown to be associated with AMD, rs10033900 in the complement factor I (CFI) gene was tested using TaqMan SNP Genotyping assay. TaqMan assays were also used for the detection of the MerTK I1b rs17835605 (g.4916C>T), MerTK I1c rs10496440 (g.8809A>C) and MerTK I4 rs7573344 (g.60127A>G), as described earlier [46]. Over 98% of controls and 96% of patients were genotyped in each test. For the verification of all in-house mutation detection methods described above, randomly selected samples were sequenced with the same primers that were used for PCR amplification. No discrepancy was found in any of the tested samples.

Statistical methods

Biallelic polymorphisms were tested using the chi-square test for the deviation of Hardy-Weinberg equilibrium in the control group. Continuous and categorical variables were described in terms of mean (SD) and frequency (%), respectively, in AMD subtype groups and in controls. Unadjusted between-group comparisons were made using ANOVA or Kruskal–Wallis tests subject to normality and homoscedasticity assumptions (continuous variables), and Fisher's exact test (categorical variables). Unadjusted effects of explanatory variables were estimated using simple logistic regression and expressed as odds ratios and 95% confidence intervals (CI). Continuous variables were transformed with the formula providing the best achievable fit. Categorical variables were regrouped by pooling groups with close to identical effects if applicable. Models were fitted for the total sample and for subsamples formed by restricting cases to dry or wet AMD variants. Adjusted effects were estimated using multiple logistic regression. The significance criterion was set at $\alpha = 0.05$ for all tests, i.e. with no formal adjustment for multiple testing. Categorical variables were regrouped by pooling groups with close to identical effects if applicable. Age and cataract surgery were included as a priori adjustment covariates without effect interpretations, due to their association with study group inherent in the control recruitment methods used. Further variable selection was based on an iterative procedure where models were started by including all explanatory variables with significant unadjusted effects, adding each of the rest one by one and keeping if meaningful, and were made parsimonious by eliminating those of neutral behavior. Possible interactions between explanatory variables of models thus developed were systematically evaluated and kept if found significant. For comparability between dry and wet AMD variant models, genetic interactions included in any subtype model were also used in the other. Model fit was checked using Hosmer–Lemeshow tests for all three final models. As HTRA1 rs11200638 and LOC rs10490924 are in linkage disequilibrium, for the analysis HTRA1 rs11200638 was selected.

Results

Characteristics of the study population

In total, 280 patients and 106 controls were enrolled in the present study. Basic characteristics of the study population are summarized in Table 1. Patients were divided into two subgroups according to disease phenotype involving 213 patients in the wet and 67 patients in the dry AMD subgroups. There was a slight female predominance among wet AMD patients which is in line with European data on gender distribution in neovascular AMD [48].

There was no significant difference between the ages of the dry and wet subgroups of patients, however, controls were significantly older than patients as a result of intentionally older control selection. Cataract surgery was also more common in the control group because of controls selection methods and probably because the older age of the controls. There was no statistically significant difference between patients and controls in terms of frequency of hypertension, deep venous thrombosis, myocardial infarct, smoking and body mass index. Interestingly, outdoor profession was significantly more frequent among controls than patients.

Genotype distribution and unadjusted odds ratios of the analyzed polymorphisms

The genotype distributions in controls and patients are shown in Table S1. Actual sample number is provided for each test. Small differences are due to the shortage of DNA sample quantity

Table 1. Characteristics of the study population.

Attributions	Dry AMD	Wet AMD	Controls	p
	N = 67	N = 213	N = 106	
Female N (%)	34 (50.7)	125 (58.7)	53 (50.0)	0.26
Male N (%)	33 (49.3)	88 (41.3)	53 (50.0)	0.26
Age (year, mean±SD)	75.4 (11.5)	76.0 (7.3)	79.1 (6.1)	0.005
Smoking (packyear, mean± SD)	12.0 (20.1)	11.2 (19.8)	11.4 (21.9)	0.76
BMI (mean±SD)	27.3 (4.5)	27.3 (4.4)	27.6 (4.7)	0.83
Hypertension N (%)	45 (67.2)	159 (75.0)	81 (79.4)	0.21
DVT N (%)	7 (10.4)	15 (7.1)	15 (14.9)	0.09
AMI N (%)	6 (9.0)	19 (9.0)	7 (7.4)	0.90
Outdoor profession N (%)	22 (32.8)	39 (18.5)	38 (38.4)	0.0004
Cataract surgery N (%)	21 (31.3)	48 (22.6)	73 (70.2)	<0.0001

BMI: body mass index, DVT: deep vein thrombosis, AMI: acute myocardial infarction.

available. The control group showed no statistical difference from Hardy-Weinberg equilibrium in the case of the tested polymorphisms. Minor alleles of genes unequivocally linked to AMD were more frequent in patients than in controls. Except IIa, MerTK receptor polymorphisms showed a very low minor allele frequency and no notable difference between cases and controls. In case of ApoE the most common E3 allele was slightly more frequent in patients than in controls while the potential risk factor E2 allele was less frequent in patients than in controls. The ApoE E4 allele had similar frequency in all the three groups. Unadjusted odds ratios, and corresponding p values for each genotype comparison are shown in Table 2.

Multiple regression models

The model of pooled dry and wet AMD variants revealed strongly significant adjusted risks in case of the presence of homozygous polymorphisms in the CFH and HTRA1 genes, increasing the odds of AMD by more than five and nearly ten times (OR = 5.3, 95%CI: 2.5–11.5, p<0.0001, and OR = 9.8, 95%CI: 3.3–29.5, p<0.0001), respectively. No significant interactions were found between any pairs of these variables.

Factors showing significant adjusted associations with dry type AMD are shown in Table 3. and Figure 1. These are genes C3, CFH, and HTRA1, with interactions between both C3 and CFH (p = 0.020) and C3 and HTRA1 (p = 0.024). The heterozygous/homozygous genotype of C3 carried a significant risk over wild type genotype in the simultaneous absence of homozygous CFH and HTRA1 polymorphisms only. In this case it was associated with a near-five-fold relative increase in the odds of dry type AMD. The stratum of subjects with homozygous mutated HTRA1 and CFH genes contained an insufficient number and distribution of observations for C3 effect estimation. In the case of wild type C3 genotype, mutated alleles of both CFH and HTRA1 behaved as strongly significant risk factors, but reduced to neutrality otherwise.

Factors found to have remarkable associations with wet type AMD included the genes Gas6, CFH, and HTRA1 (Table 4, Figure 1). Gas6 was protective irrespective of other genotypes (p = 0.04), reducing the odds of wet type AMD by a half. There was no evidence for the effect of C3 (left in the model for comparability with the dry variant), and although C3's odds ratios specific for different combinations of CFH and HTRA1 genotypes showed a fairly varied pattern, the interaction was technically not significant, unlike in the case of the dry AMD. However, there was some indication that the effect of HTRA1 (homozygous vs. wild type or heterozygous genotype) was modified by the C3 genotype, with estimated odds ratios of 45.04 (p = 0.0005) and 4.34 (p = 0.04) in C3 wild type and hetero/homozygous mutated genotypes, respectively. Homozygous CFH polymorphism was observed to be a highly significant risk factor for wet type AMD, with odds ratios slightly varying around 7.5 depending on whether mutations in C3 were present or not. All models had a sufficient goodness-of-fit by Hosmer–Lemeshow tests.

Discussion

Our understanding about the genetic causes and therefore pathological pathways involved in the development of AMD has increased substantially in the last few years. The p.Tyr402His polymorphisms of the CFH gene, the rs11200638 polymorphism of the serine peptidase HTRA1 and the p.Ala69Ser polymorphism of the LOC387715 gene are unequivocally associated to AMD in different populations with robust risks. Our results further support these observations and demonstrate robust and highly significant adjusted risk conferred by these polymorphisms as shown by the analysis of the pooled AMD population. After dividing the patient group to exudative (wet) and non-exudative (dry) subgroups, other associations and an interesting genetic interplay was revealed. The rs2230199 polymorphism of the C3 gene contributed significant disease risk to non-exudative AMD in the simultaneous absence of homozygous CFH and HTRA1 polymorphisms. Alternative complement activation is the major biological process linked to AMD development so far. C3 plays a central role in the alternative pathway and its role in AMD pathogenesis is supported by epidemiological and experimental observations. The C3 polymorphism had no significant effect on the development of wet AMD in our study population.

Epidemiological reports on the p.Arg102Gly C3 polymorphism are usually limited to advanced cases including neovascular AMD and geographic atrophy. This approach, however, falls short of detecting any difference between the etiology of dry and wet AMD. Despite the fact that CFH and C3 are members of the same biological pathway, no evidence of a genetic interplay between these two has been demonstrated so far [49]. Carriers of two risk alleles of the rs2230199 polymorphism of the C3 gene are at

Table 2. Unadjusted ORs of the examined polymorphisms.

Polymorphism	Genotypes compared	Dry AMD		Wet AMD	
		OR	p value	OR	p value
CFH rs1061170	TC+CC vs. TT	1.30	0.43	3.27	<0.0001
CFH rs1061170	TC vs. TT	0.86	0.67	2.09	0.0104
CFH rs1061170	CC vs. TC	3.86	0.003	4.17	0.0001
CFH rs1061170	CC vs. TT	3.32	0.01	8.73	<0.0001
CFH rs1061170	CC vs. TT+TC	3.60	0.002	5.45	<0.0001
LOC387715 rs10490924	GT+TT vs. GG	1.50	0.20	3.29	<0.0001
LOC387715 rs10490924	GT vs. GG	1.22	0.56	2.07	0.01
LOC387715 rs10490924	TT vs. GT	3.55	0.03	7.47	<0.0001
LOC387715 rs10490924	TT vs. GG	4.31	0.01	15.5	<0.0001
LOC387715 rs10490924	TT vs. GG+GT	3.89	0.01	10.0	<0.0001
HTRA1 rs11200638	TC+CC vs.TT	1.52	0.19	3.21	<0.0001
HTRA1 rs11200638	TC vs. CC	1.24	0.52	2.00	0.01
HTRA1 rs11200638	CC vs. TC	4.03	0.03	9.18	<0.0001
HTRA1 rs11200638	CC vs. TT	5.00	0.01	18.4	<0.0001
HTRA1 rs11200638	CC vs. TT+TC	4.46	0.01	12.2	<0.0001
Gas6 rs8191974	AA vs. GA	1.51	0.39	1.00	0.99
Gas6 rs8191974	AA vs. GG	1.03	0.96	0.61	0.21
Gas6 rs8191974	AA vs. GG+GA	1.27	0.60	0.79	0.54
Gas6 rs8191974	GA vs. GG	0.68	0.26	0.61	0.05
Gas6 rs8191974	GA+AA vs. GG	0.75	0.37	0.61	0.04
C3 rs2230199	CG+GG vs. CC	1.55	0.17	1.27	0.3237
C3 rs2230199	CG vs. CC	1.47	0.24	1.22	0.4198
C3 rs2230199	GG vs. CG	1.76	0.48	1.52	0.5409
C3 rs2230199	GG vs. CC	2.59	0.23	1.86	0.3568
C3 rs2230199	GG vs. CC+GC	2.22	0.31	1.73	0.41
CFI rs10033900	CC vs. TC	1.47	0.34	1.21	0.55
CFI rs10033900	CC vs. TT	1.54	0.34	1.31	0.44
CFI rs10033900	TC vs. TT	1.04	0.91	1.09	0.76
FXIII rs5985	GT+TT vs. GG	0.59	0.10	0.66	0.08
FXIII rs5985	GT vs. GG	0.65	0.20	0.64	0.08
FXIII rs5985	TT vs. GT	0.51	0.34	1.15	0.73
FXIII rs5985	TT vs. GG	0.34	0.11	0.74	0.46
FXIII rs5985	TT vs. GG+GT	0.40	0.18	0.90	0.78
Apo-E	3/4+4 vs. 2+2/3	1.67	0.3897	1.51	0.3512
Apo-E	3/4+4 vs. 3/3	1.00	0.9929	1.02	0.9543
Apo-E	2+2/3 vs. 3/3	0.60	0.2879	0.68	0.2632
Mertk I1a	AA vs. GA	0.96	0.9251	1.08	0.8171
Mertk I1a	AA vs. GG	0.83	0.7086	1.00	0.9910
Mertk I1a	GA vs. GG	0.87	0.6891	0.93	0.7714
Mertk I1b	CT vs. CC	0.58	0.1329	0.76	0.2919
Mertk I1b	TT vs. CC	2.50	0.0989	1.16	0.7664
Mertk I1b	TT vs. CT	4.33	0.0144	1.52	0.4218
Mertk I1c	AC vs. AA	0.54	0.2623	1.13	0.7328
Mertk I4	AG vs. AA	0.88	0.7186	0.79	0.3602
Mertk I4	GG vs. AA	*	*	0.62	0.5352
Mertk I4	GG vs. AG	*	*	0.79	0.7615

*Missing data are due to insufficient minor allele frequency.

moderate risk to develop AMD compared to wild type subjects (OR: 1.88, 95%CI: 1.59–2.23) according to a recent meta-analysis [15]. Besides that, it is well known that, drusen, the hallmark of dry AMD contains complement factors 3a and 5a among other inflammatory proteins, which therefore could play a role in drusen formation and might even have an effect on neovascularisation [50,51,52,53,54]. Experimental evidence showed that suppression of the complement cascade in the retina delayed and reversed the onset of AMD in a monkey model of dry AMD [55]. The effect of CFH and C3 polymorphisms are mutually exclusive on the risk of dry AMD in our study population. On the other hand, CFH has a robust effect on neovascular AMD independent of the C3 status. Since the two proteins are located in the same biological pathway, our results can be explained with the stronger effect overriding the other. Interestingly, the interaction between C3 and HTRA1 is very similar, which indicates that C3 and HTRA1 are also competing in dry AMD development. This finding underscores previous reports on the role of HTRA1 in complement regulation [56]. Taken together our findings indicate a central role of C3 in dry AMD formation, however, CFH and HTRA1 genotype have an influence on the effect of the C3 p.Arg102Gly polymorphism most likely explained by their complement regulatory activity. CFI has been associated to AMD development with conflicting results. Fagerness et al. reported an OR of 0.7 for the lower risk C allele ($p = 6.46 \times 10^{-8}$) of the rs10033900 polymorphism within the CFI gene in a large population of European descent [16]. Chen et al found a statistically significant association of the rs2285714 risk allele and AMD with a moderate OR of 1.31 (95%CI: 1.18–1.45, $p = 3.4 \times 10^{-7}$) [57]. Seddon et al. demonstrated that the protective effect of the hepatic lipase (LIPC) rs10468017 polymorphism on AMD pathogenesis was stronger in the presence of double wild type rs10033900 compared to the homozygous polymorphism [58]. The findings of the original article by Fagerness were reflected in three case-controls studies. A report on a Japanese population demonstrated an OR of 0.28 (95%CI: 0.11–0.69, $p = 0.0035$) for the rare homozygous CC genotype [59]. The work of Ennis et al. supports the involvement of the CFI gene in AMD development by demonstrating four SNP's in the CFI gene associating to AMD, however the effect of the rs10033900 polymorphism, which had the strongest association signal in the original work of Fagerness, was not statistically significant in their cohort ($p = 0.135$). Interestingly, the haplotype including rs10033900 polymorphism and another non-significant polymorphism together conferred statistically significant disease risk ($OR = 2.15$, $p = 0.02$) [17]. A very well powered case-control study based on independent samples from England and Scotland failed to detect any statistically significant effect of the rs10033900 polymorphism on AMD ($OR = 0.95$, 95%CI: 0.83–1.09, $p = 0.47$) [18]. Similarly to that, in the present study we could not provide any additional support for the association of the rs10033900 polymorphism and AMD. Although our sample size is not as large as some of the cited works, it is large enough to detect strong or even weak but significant associations with other well established

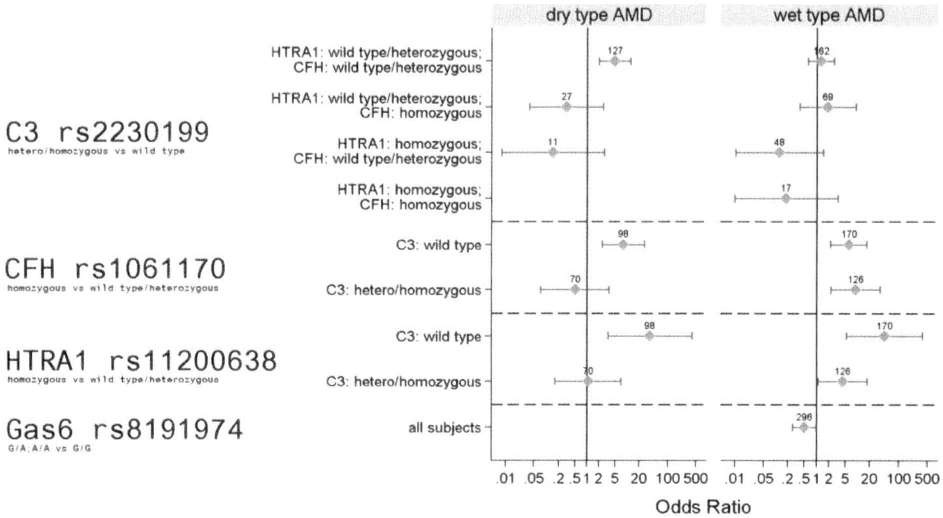

Figure 1. The effect of GAS6 c.834+7G>A polymorphism and genetic interactions on the risk of AMD. Polymorphisms with the compared genotypes are shown on the left side. Stratum of subjects involved in the corresponding analysis are on the vertical axis. Figures above markers indicate number of observations for the given stratum Adjusted odds ratios and 95% confidence intervals are represented by dots and lines, respectively. In the dry AMD group the effect of C3 polymorphism in case of double CFH/HTRA1 homozygousity could not be estimated due to low observation number. GAS6 was not included as an explanatory variable in the model for dry AMD.

risk factors of AMD as demonstrated by our findings on the CFH, LOC387715, HTRA1 and C3 polymorphisms. Our results are in line with studies showing no effect of the rs10033900 polymorphism. Although one cannot exclude such an association based on a single negative result, there are a growing number of publications falling short of detecting any effect of the polymorphism which clearly indicates that the association is not unequivocal and calls for further epidemiological and functional analysis to clarify the link between CFI and AMD.

No evidence of association with AMD could be demonstrated in the case of ApoE alleles. We neither could confirm previous reports on the protective effect of the E4 allele, nor could we show any risk related to the E2 allele. Two recent very-well powered epidemiological studies [33,34] concluded on the disease causing effect of the E2 allele and the protective role of the E4 allele. Albeit these convincing studies, our results still do not fit in the line. Interestingly, we could not observe any statistically significant disease association with any of the ApoE alleles, moreover the frequency of the E2 risk allele was higher in controls than in patients, while the protective E4 allele showed similar frequencies in the wet AMD and the control group. These data indicate that ApoE is not a key player in AMD pathogenesis in the Hungarian population. This can either be explained by a geographical difference, or by other different environmental factors, probably the different smoking habits of the Hungarian population.

Candidate gene approach is widely used to identify biological pathways and genes involved in pathological processes. Based on their biological functions, we directly tested for disease association of common polymorphisms in the FXIII, Gas6 and in one of the Gas6 receptor genes, MerTK. Blood coagulation factor XIII is a plasma transglutaminase that cross links adjacent fibrin chains in the final step of the coagulation cascade. In addition, FXIII is known to participate in wound healing, tissue remodeling and embryo implantation at least partially through its proangiogenic effect [60]. The cardioprotective p.Val34Leu polymorphism of the blood coagulation factor XIII has been associated with accelerated thrombin activation, recurrent subconjunctival haemorrhage, intracerebral haemorrhage, and a decreased immune reaction in humans [61,62,63]. Most importantly, since angiogenesis plays a crucial role in neovascular AMD, we found it reasonable to investigate if the polymorphism had any effect on AMD formation. However, we failed to detect any association of AMD and the polymorphism in our present study, indicating a neutral polymorphism in relation to both dry and wet AMD development.

Gas6, a Protein S structural homologue, has important functions in the regulation of angiogenesis, cell migration and proliferation. Its common polymorphism Gas6 c.834+7G>A is

Table 3. Polymorphisms showing significant association with dry AMD using multiple logistic regression.

Polymorphism	Genotypes compared	Stratum of subjects	OR	95% CI	p value
C3 rs2230199	CG+GG vs. CC	**HTRA1**: TT+TC **CFH**: TT+TC	4.93	1.98–12.25	0.0006
CFH rs1061170	CC vs. TT+TC	**C3**: CC	7.96	2.39–26.50	0.0007
HTRA1 rs11200638	TC+CC vs.TT	**C3**: CC	36.02	3.30–393.02	0.0033

Stratum represents genotype of subjects involved in the analysis.

Table 4. Polymorphisms showing significant association with wet AMD using multiple logistic regression.

Polymorphism	Genotypes compared	Stratum of subjects	OR	95% CI	p value
CFH rs1061170	CC vs. TT+TC	**C3**: CC	6.08	2.17–17.04	0.0006
CFH rs1061170	CC vs. TT+TC	**C3**: CT+TT	8.96	2.24–35.79	0.002
HTRA1 rs11200638	TC+CC vs.TT	**C3**: CC	45.04	5.30–382.83	0.0005
HTRA1 rs11200638	TC vs. CC	**C3**: CT+TT	4.34	1.09–17.28	0.04
Gas6 rs8191974	GA+AA vs. GG	n.a.	0.5	0.26–0.97	0.04

Stratum represents genotype of subjects involved in the analysis.

associated with decreased risk of cardiovascular diseases. Its receptors (TAM) play a crucial role in phagocytosis of apoptotic cells in the immune, nervous, and reproductive systems. These functions make Gas6 and its receptors a potential candidate involved in both dry and wet AMD development. In the pooled early and late AMD population the Gas6 polymorphism showed no statistically significant association to AMD. When analyzing dry and wet subgroups separately, no association with the dry AMD could be demonstrated; however a protective effect was detected in the wet AMD subgroup ($p = 0.04$). As formation of new vessels is a hallmark of wet AMD, it is likely that it is this function of Gas6 that is important in the context of the disease. Gas6 is able to inhibit VEGF-A signaling through Axl activation of SHP-2 phosphatases [38]. Recently, a similar inhibitory effect has been shown in metastasis induced angiogenesis [64]. This finding suggests a role of Gas6 in controlling pathological angiogenesis, and that c.834+7G>A polymorphism of the GAS6 gene, which has been linked to disease repeatedly [36,40,41], could have a direct effect on the function of the gene through an unknown mechanism. Future epidemiological and functional studies are required to further evaluate the effect of the GAS6 polymorphism on AMD development. It is to be noted, that no formal correction for multiple testing was applied in the multiple logistic regression analysis, however, this does not invalidate the conclusion that the suggested effect of the GAS6 polymorphism is worthy of further investigations.

In our case-control study we confirmed previous findings on the association of AMD and genetic polymorphisms in the CFH, LOC387715 and HTRA1 genes, however could not demonstrate any association with the CFI gene. More interestingly, we found a genetic interplay of CFH, HTRA1 and C3 genes, showing that the C3 polymorphism is a major contributor of dry AMD in the absence of the other polymorphisms, while has no effect on wet AMD development in our population. This result indicates that C3 plays a critical role in dry AMD rather than wet AMD pathogenesis, and its effect can be overdriven by other known genetic risk factors in the CFH and HTRA1 genes. We detected a protective effect of a common Gas6 c.834+7G>A polymorphism on wet AMD formation. Our results suggest a possible new player and novel genetic interactions in AMD pathogenesis, however our data should be confirmed in other populations, especially in the case of the Gas6 polymorphism.

Author Contributions

Conceived and designed the experiments: GL LT IB AB EM EA AF. Performed the experiments: GL AV EM AF ED IB LT BH PGdF LK. Analyzed the data: GL LK IB EA AB. Contributed reagents/materials/analysis tools: GL AB IB ED LK EA BH PGdF. Wrote the paper: GL LK IB AB.

References

1. Klein R, Peto T, Bird A, Vannewkirk MR (2004) The epidemiology of age-related macular degeneration. Am J Ophthalmol 137: 486–495.
2. Friedman DS, Katz J, Bressler NM, Rahmani B, Tielsch JM (1999) Racial differences in the prevalence of age-related macular degeneration: the Baltimore Eye Survey. Ophthalmology 106: 1049–1055.
3. Friedman DS, O'Colmain BJ, Munoz B, Tomany SC, McCarty C, et al. (2004) Prevalence of age-related macular degeneration in the United States. Arch Ophthalmol 122: 564–572.
4. Seddon JM, Sharma S, Adelman RA (2006) Evaluation of the clinical age-related maculopathy staging system. Ophthalmology 113: 260–266.
5. Coleman HR, Chan CC, Ferris FL 3rd, Chew EY (2008) Age-related macular degeneration. Lancet 372: 1835–1845.
6. Chakravarthy U, Wong TY, Fletcher A, Piault E, Evans C, et al. (2010) Clinical risk factors for age-related macular degeneration: a systematic review and meta-analysis. BMC Ophthalmol 10: 31.
7. Ho L, Boekhoorn SS, Liana, van Duijn CM, Uitterlinden AG, et al. (2008) Cataract surgery and the risk of aging macula disorder: the rotterdam study. Invest Ophthalmol Vis Sci 49: 4795–4800.
8. Francis PJ, Klein ML (2011) Update on the role of genetics in the onset of age-related macular degeneration. Clin Ophthalmol 5: 1127–1133.
9. Klein RJ, Zeiss C, Chew EY, Tsai JY, Sackler RS, et al. (2005) Complement factor H polymorphism in age-related macular degeneration. Science 308: 385–389.
10. Edwards AO, Ritter R 3rd, Abel KJ, Manning A, Panhuysen C, et al. (2005) Complement factor H polymorphism and age-related macular degeneration. Science 308: 421–424.
11. Haines JL, Hauser MA, Schmidt S, Scott WK, Olson LM, et al. (2005) Complement factor H variant increases the risk of age-related macular degeneration. Science 308: 419–421.
12. Sofat R, Casas JP, Webster AR, Bird AC, Mann SS, et al. (2012) Complement factor H genetic variant and age-related macular degeneration: effect size, modifiers and relationship to disease subtype. Int J Epidemiol 41: 250–262.
13. Yates JR, Sepp T, Matharu BK, Khan JC, Thurlby DA, et al. (2007) Complement C3 variant and the risk of age-related macular degeneration. N Engl J Med 357: 553–561.
14. Despriet DD, van Duijn CM, Oostra BA, Uitterlinden AG, Hofman A, et al. (2009) Complement component C3 and risk of age-related macular degeneration. Ophthalmology 116: 474–480 e472.
15. Thakkinstian A, McKay GJ, McEvoy M, Chakravarthy U, Chakrabarti S, et al. (2011) Systematic review and meta-analysis of the association between complement component 3 and age-related macular degeneration: a HuGE review and meta-analysis. Am J Epidemiol 173: 1365–1379.
16. Fagerness JA, Maller JB, Neale BM, Reynolds RC, Daly MJ, et al. (2009) Variation near complement factor I is associated with risk of advanced AMD. Eur J Hum Genet 17: 100–104.
17. Ennis S, Gibson J, Cree AJ, Collins A, Lotery AJ (2010) Support for the involvement of complement factor I in age-related macular degeneration. Eur J Hum Genet 18: 15–16.

18. Cipriani V, Matharu BK, Khan JC, Shahid H, Hayward C, et al. (2012) No evidence of association between complement factor I genetic variant rs10033900 and age-related macular degeneration. Eur J Hum Genet 20: 1–2; author reply 3.
19. Jakobsdottir J, Conley YP, Weeks DE, Mah TS, Ferrell RE, et al. (2005) Susceptibility genes for age-related maculopathy on chromosome 10q26. Am J Hum Genet 77: 389–407.
20. Rivera A, Fisher SA, Fritsche LG, Keilhauer CN, Lichtner P, et al. (2005) Hypothetical LOC387715 is a second major susceptibility gene for age-related macular degeneration, contributing independently of complement factor H to disease risk. Hum Mol Genet 14: 3227–3236.
21. Yang Z, Camp NJ, Sun H, Tong Z, Gibbs D, et al. (2006) A variant of the HTRA1 gene increases susceptibility to age-related macular degeneration. Science 314: 992–993.
22. Dewan A, Liu M, Hartman S, Zhang SS, Liu DT, et al. (2006) HTRA1 promoter polymorphism in wet age-related macular degeneration. Science 314: 989–992.
23. Yoshida T, DeWan A, Zhang H, Sakamoto R, Okamoto H, et al. (2007) HTRA1 promoter polymorphism predisposes Japanese to age-related macular degeneration. Mol Vis 13: 545–548.
24. Cameron DJ, Yang Z, Gibbs D, Chen H, Kaminoh Y, et al. (2007) HTRA1 variant confers similar risks to geographic atrophy and neovascular age-related macular degeneration. Cell Cycle 6: 1122–1125.
25. Wang L, Clark ME, Crossman DK, Kojima K, Messinger JD, et al. (2010) Abundant lipid and protein components of drusen. PLoS One 5: e10329.
26. Souied EH, Benlian P, Amouyel P, Feingold J, Lagarde JP, et al. (1998) The epsilon4 allele of the apolipoprotein E gene as a potential protective factor for exudative age-related macular degeneration. Am J Ophthalmol 125: 353–359.
27. Baird PN, Guida E, Chu DT, Vu HT, Guymer RH (2004) The epsilon2 and epsilon4 alleles of the apolipoprotein gene are associated with age-related macular degeneration. Invest Ophthalmol Vis Sci 45: 1311–1315.
28. Baird PN, Richardson AJ, Robman LD, Dimitrov PN, Tikellis G, et al. (2006) Apolipoprotein (APOE) gene is associated with progression of age-related macular degeneration (AMD). Hum Mutat 27: 337–342.
29. Francis PJ, Hamon SC, Ott J, Weleber RG, Klein ML (2009) Polymorphisms in C2, CFB and C3 are associated with progression to advanced age related macular degeneration associated with visual loss. J Med Genet 46: 300–307.
30. Yu Y, Reynolds R, Fagerness J, Rosner B, Daly MJ, et al. (2011) Association of variants in the LIPC and ABCA1 genes with intermediate and large drusen and advanced age-related macular degeneration. Invest Ophthalmol Vis Sci 52: 4663–4670.
31. Asensio-Sanchez VM, Rodriguez-Martin T, Gala-Molina I, Rodriguez-Fernandez I (2006) [Age-related macular degeneration: its association with the epsilon4 allele of the apolipoprotein E gene]. Arch Soc Esp Oftalmol 81: 9–12.
32. Losonczy G, Fekete A, Voko Z, Takacs L, Kaldi I, et al. (2011) Analysis of complement factor H Y402H, LOC387715, HTRA1 polymorphisms and ApoE alleles with susceptibility to age-related macular degeneration in Hungarian patients. Acta Ophthalmol 89: 255–262.
33. McKay GJ, Patterson CC, Chakravarthy U, Dasari S, Klaver CC, et al. (2011) Evidence of association of APOE with age-related macular degeneration: a pooled analysis of 15 studies. Hum Mutat 32: 1407–1416.
34. Adams MK, Simpson JA, Richardson AJ, English DR, Aung KZ, et al. (2012) Apolipoprotein E gene associations in age-related macular degeneration: the Melbourne Collaborative Cohort Study. Am J Epidemiol 175: 511–518.
35. Fernandez-Fernandez L, Bellido-Martin L, Garcia de Frutos P (2008) Growth arrest-specific gene 6 (GAS6). An outline of its role in haemostasis and inflammation. Thromb Haemost 100: 604–610.
36. Jiang L, Liu CY, Yang QF, Wang P, Zhang W (2009) Plasma level of growth arrest-specific 6 (GAS6) protein and genetic variations in the GAS6 gene in patients with acute coronary syndrome. Am J Clin Pathol 131: 738–743.
37. Lutgens E, Tjwa M, Garcia de Frutos P, Wijnands E, Beckers L, et al. (2008) Genetic loss of Gas6 induces plaque stability in experimental atherosclerosis. J Pathol 216: 55–63.
38. Gallicchio M, Mitola S, Valdembri D, Fantozzi R, Varnum B, et al. (2005) Inhibition of vascular endothelial growth factor receptor 2-mediated endothelial cell activation by Axl tyrosine kinase receptor. Blood 105: 1970–1976.
39. Balogh I, Hafizi S, Stenhoff J, Hansson K, Dahlback B (2005) Analysis of Gas6 in human platelets and plasma. Arterioscler Thromb Vasc Biol 25: 1280–1286.
40. Munoz X, Obach V, Hurtado B, de Frutos PG, Chamorro A, et al. (2007) Association of specific haplotypes of GAS6 gene with stroke. Thromb Haemost 98: 406–412.
41. Lee CH, Chu NF, Shieh YS, Hung YJ (2012) The growth arrest-specific 6 (Gas6) gene polymorphism c.834+7G>A is associated with type 2 diabetes. Diabetes Res Clin Pract 95: 201–206.
42. Rothlin CV, Lemke G (2010) TAM receptor signaling and autoimmune disease. Curr Opin Immunol 22: 740–746.
43. Duncan JL, LaVail MM, Yasumura D, Matthes MT, Yang H, et al. (2003) An RCS-like retinal dystrophy phenotype in mer knockout mice. Invest Ophthalmol Vis Sci 44: 826–838.
44. Hall MO, Obin MS, Heeb MJ, Burgess BL, Abrams TA (2005) Both protein S and Gas6 stimulate outer segment phagocytosis by cultured rat retinal pigment epithelial cells. Exp Eye Res 81: 581–591.
45. Chen YY, Lu QJ, Lu QX, Wang NL (2011) Gene expression profile changes caused by the dysfunction of Mer during retinal pigment epithelium phagocytosis. Chin Med J (Engl) 124: 1145–1155.
46. Hurtado B, Abasolo N, Munoz X, Garcia N, Benavente Y, et al. (2010) Association study between polymorphisms in GAS6-TAM genes and carotid atherosclerosis. Thromb Haemost 104: 592–598.
47. Shemirani AH, Muszbek L (2004) Rapid detection of the factor XIII Val34Leu (163 G→T) polymorphism by real-time PCR using fluorescence resonance energy transfer detection and melting curve analysis. Clin Chem Lab Med 42: 877–879.
48. Rudnicka AR, Jarrar Z, Wormald R, Cook DG, Fletcher A, et al. (2012) Age and gender variations in age-related macular degeneration prevalence in populations of European ancestry: a meta-analysis. Ophthalmology 119: 571–580.
49. Spencer KL, Olson LM, Anderson BM, Schnetz-Boutaud N, Scott WK, et al. (2008) C3 R102G polymorphism increases risk of age-related macular degeneration. Hum Mol Genet 17: 1821–1824.
50. Mullins RF, Russell SR, Anderson DH, Hageman GS (2000) Drusen associated with aging and age-related macular degeneration contain proteins common to extracellular deposits associated with atherosclerosis, elastosis, amyloidosis, and dense deposit disease. FASEB J 14: 835–846.
51. Johnson LV, Ozaki S, Staples MK, Erickson PA, Anderson DH (2000) A potential role for immune complex pathogenesis in drusen formation. Exp Eye Res 70: 441–449.
52. Anderson DH, Mullins RF, Hageman GS, Johnson LV (2002) A role for local inflammation in the formation of drusen in the aging eye. Am J Ophthalmol 134: 411–431.
53. Johnson LV, Leitner WP, Staples MK, Anderson DH (2001) Complement activation and inflammatory processes in Drusen formation and age related macular degeneration. Exp Eye Res 73: 887–896.
54. Nozaki M, Raisler BJ, Sakurai E, Sarma JV, Barnum SR, et al. (2006) Drusen complement components C3a and C5a promote choroidal neovascularization. Proc Natl Acad Sci U S A 103: 2328–2333.
55. Chi ZL, Yoshida T, Lambris JD, Iwata T (2010) Suppression of drusen formation by compstatin, a peptide inhibitor of complement C3 activation, on cynomolgus monkey with early-onset macular degeneration. Adv Exp Med Biol 703: 127–135.
56. An E, Sen S, Park SK, Gordish-Dressman H, Hathout Y (2010) Identification of novel substrates for the serine protease HTRA1 in the human RPE secretome. Invest Ophthalmol Vis Sci 51: 3379–3386.
57. Chen W, Stambolian D, Edwards AO, Branham KE, Othman M, et al. (2010) Genetic variants near TIMP3 and high-density lipoprotein-associated loci influence susceptibility to age-related macular degeneration. Proc Natl Acad Sci U S A 107: 7401–7406.
58. Seddon JM, Reynolds R, Rosner B (2010) Associations of smoking, body mass index, dietary lutein, and the LIPC gene variant rs10468017 with advanced age-related macular degeneration. Mol Vis 16: 2412–2424.
59. Kondo N, Bessho H, Honda S, Negi A (2010) Additional evidence to support the role of a common variant near the complement factor I gene in susceptibility to age-related macular degeneration. Eur J Hum Genet 18: 634–635.
60. Dardik R, Loscalzo J, Inbal A (2006) Factor XIII (FXIII) and angiogenesis. J Thromb Haemost 4: 19–25.
61. Kovar FM, Marsik CL, Jilma B, Mannhalter C, Joukhadar C, et al. (2009) The inflammatory response is influenced by FXIII VAL 34 LEU polymorphism in a human LPS model. Wien Klin Wochenschr 121: 515–519.
62. Balogh I, Szoke G, Karpati L, Wartiovaara U, Katona E, et al. (2000) Val34Leu polymorphism of plasma factor XIII: biochemistry and epidemiology in familial thrombophilia. Blood 96: 2479–2486.
63. Ariens RA, Philippou H, Nagaswami C, Weisel JW, Lane DA, et al. (2000) The factor XIII V34L polymorphism accelerates thrombin activation of factor XIII and affects cross-linked fibrin structure. Blood 96: 988–995.
64. Png KJ, Halberg N, Yoshida M, Tavazoie SF (2011) A microRNA regulon that mediates endothelial recruitment and metastasis by cancer cells. Nature 481: 190–194.

10

An Objective Scatter Index Based on Double-Pass Retinal Images of a Point Source to Classify Cataracts

Pablo Artal[1]*, Antonio Benito[1], Guillermo M. Pérez[1], Encarna Alcón[1], Álvaro De Casas[2], Jaume Pujol[3], José M. Marín[2]

1 Laboratorio de Óptica, Universidad de Murcia, Murcia, Spain, **2** Hospital Universitario Virgen de la Arrixaca, Murcia, Spain, **3** Centre de Desenvolupament de Sensors, Instrumentació i Sistemes (CD6), Universidad Politécnica de Cataluña, Tarrasa, Barcelona, Spain

Abstract

Purpose: To propose a new objective scatter index (OSI) based in the analysis of double-pass images of a point source to rank and classify cataract patients. This classification scheme is compared with a current subjective system.

Methods: We selected a population including a group of normal young eyes as control and patients diagnosed with cataract (grades NO2, NO3 and NO4) according to the *Lens Opacities Classification System* (LOCS III). For each eye, we recorded double-pass retinal images of a point source. In each patient, we determined an objective scatter index (OSI) as the ratio of the intensity at an eccentric location in the image and the central part. This index provides information on the relevant forward scatter affecting vision. Since the double-pass retinal images are affected by both ocular aberrations and intraocular scattering, an analysis was performed to show the ranges of contributions of aberrations to the OSI.

Results: We used the OSI values to classify each eye according to the degree of scatter. The young normal eyes of the control group had OSI values below 1, while the OSI for subjects in LOCS grade II were around 1 to 2. The use of the objective index showed some of the weakness of subjective classification schemes. In particular, several subjects initially classified independently as grade NO2 or NO3 had similar OSI values, and in some cases even higher than subjects classified as grade NO4. A new classification scheme based in OSI is proposed.

Conclusions: We introduced an objective index based in the analysis of double-pass retinal images to classify cataract patients. The method is robust and fully based in objective measurements; i.e., not depending on subjective decisions. This procedure could be used in combination with standard current methods to improve cataract patient surgery scheduling.

Editor: Amy Lo, The University of Hong Kong, Hong Kong

Funding: This work has been supported by "Ministerio de Educación y Ciencia," Spain (grant FIS2007-64765) and "Fundación Séneca," Murcia, Spain (grant 04524/GERM/06). The funders had no role in study design, data collection and analysis, decision to publish, or preparation of the manuscript.

Competing Interests: Co-authors Artal, Benito, Perez and Pujol hold a patent application on the reported approach (United States Patent Application 20100195876; Artal Pablo et al. August 5, 2010). Co-authors Artal and Pujol are minority investors in Visiometrics SL, the manufacturer of the OQAS instrument.

* E-mail: pablo@um.es

Introduction

Intraocular scattering may severely degrade the retinal image quality [1]. In eyes suffering early cataracts symptoms this can produce visual disturbances, even if visual acuity remains normal [2]. This has important practical implications; for example the optimal scheduling of a cataract surgery should be determined by the moment when the visual impairment produced by the cataract affects the normal daily activities [3]. The subjectivity implicit in this definition has stimulated the development of a variety of methods for classifying cataracts, that may permit a somehow standardized procedure. However, until today there is no consensus on the most adequate technique to predict the visual disturbances associated with a gradation of cataracts.

A first group of methods to evaluate cataract is composed by those based on the analysis of slit-lamp pictures of the patient's crystalline lens. The Lens Opacities Classification System III (LOCS III) [4] is one of the most representatives. Although the analysis considers different aspects like color, grade of opacification or cataract type, the final decision strongly depends on the subjective criterion of the clinician. In addition, the slit-lamp images only provide information related to the back-scattered light, while actually is forward scatter, the responsible of the degradation of retinal image in cataract patients [5]. On other hand, the relationship between the backward and the forward scatter produced in the crystalline lens depends on the type of cataract [6], which increases the difficulty of a direct interpretation of the slit-lamp images to evaluate the detrimental effect of the cataract on visual performance.

There are procedures based on the objective analysis of the image of the crystalline lens acquired either with a standard slit-lamp device [7], or with a Scheimpflug camera [8]. More recently, a method based on the analysis of the dynamic light scattering of the crystalline lens has been proposed [9]. All these techniques evaluate the development of the cataract process by the analysis of the image of the crystalline lens, but they do not directly consider the actual degradation of the retinal image and the associated impairment on the visual performance.

There is a second group of methods based on the evaluation of the degradation produced by the cataract on different visual functions. The evaluation of visual acuity or contrast sensitivity in the presence of a glare source [10,11] can be considered as classical examples of these methods. Other approaches are based on a more specific analysis of the contribution of the intraocular scattering. One of these systems is the C-Quant instrument (Oculus GmbH, Wetzlar-Dutenhofen, Germany) that uses the compensation-comparison method [12] to evaluate intraocular scattering [13,14]. These types of procedures capture the impact of forward scatter in vision, but since they are subjective, the active participation of the patient is required.

We propose here a new optical method to estimate the contribution of forward scattering that affects vision to characterize the severity of cataracts. The method is based on the analysis of the double-pass (DP) image of a point source projected on the retina. The DP technique has been widely used in the past to evaluate the optical quality of the retinal image [15,16] for a variety of conditions [17–19]. A different analysis of the light distribution in the DP image has been developed to quantify intraocular scattering [20,21]. The procedure has been applied in a control group and in eyes with different scatter severity to demonstrate its validity as a predictor of the effect of cataracts.

Methods

Subjects

We tested the procedure in 53 eyes: 15 corresponding to a group of normal young subjects (average age = 28±5 y/o); and the other 38 eyes (average age = 73±7 y/o) were patients with diagnosed cataracts. One eye per patient was evaluated. Every patient was informed of the subject of the study, and a written informed consent obtained, following the tenets of the Declaration of Helsinki. The study protocol was approved by the "Hospital Virgen de la Arrixaca" ethics committee. Firstly, we evaluate the subjects' visual acuity and refraction. In every subject, an ophthalmological exam was completed, including Optical Coherence Tomography (OCT) measurements to discard macular problems and the recording of images of the crystalline lens provided by a slit-lamp device, after dilating the pupil by instilling 0.2 ml of tropicamide (1%).

Inclusion criteria for the group of cataract patients was nuclear cataract with increasing lens opacity, although not all cases were purely nuclear cataracts, as some subjects also showed slight degree of capsular opacification. Every patient was classified according to the degree of nuclear opacification (NO), by using the LOCSIII chart [4], following the subjective decision of the ophthalmologists participating in the study. The 38 cataract eyes were classified as follows: 12 eyes as grade 2 (NO2), 18 eyes as grade 3 (NO3), and 8 eyes as grade 4 (NO4).

DP images acquisition and processing: Objective Scatter Index

We used a clinical double-pass instrument (OQAS II, Visiometrics S.L., Tarrasa, Spain) to acquire the DP images. This DP system is based on an unequal pupil configuration [22] with a diameter of 2-mm in the entrance pupil and a variable diameter for the exit pupil. In this study, the diameter of the exit pupil was set to 4 mm for the whole procedure. Fig. 1 shows a schematic representation of the instrument. An infrared diode laser is collimated (CL) and after passing the entrance aperture (P1) enters the eye. After reflection in the retina and double-pass through the ocular media, the light is reflected in a beam splitter and passes the exit aperture (P2) to be recorded in a digital camera. We acquired DP images of every eye at best focus, corrected internally by the instrument by an optometer which ranges from −8D to +6D. The astigmatism was also corrected by using the appropriate cylindrical lens on a holder placed in front of the eye.

We recorded series of images from every eye assuring that the peak intensity level was above 200 (as a maximum value of 255) and background images, with a light trap in place of the eye. Both, the series of DP retinal images and the background images were averaged, and a final image was obtained for each eye as the subtraction of the mean background from the mean DP image.

From each image, we defined an Objective Scatter Index (OSI) to quantify the magnitude of the intraocular scattering. It is based on the analysis of the intensity distribution in the outer parts of the DP image. The parameter OSI is defined as the ratio between the integrated light in the periphery and in the surroundings of the central peak of the DP image. The eccentricity and width of the specific areas for this calculation depends on the acquisition parameters of the DP system. In the particular case of the instrument OQAS, the central area selected was a circle of a radius of 1 minute of arc, while the peripheral zone was a ring set between 12 and 20 minutes of arc. The extension of the areas considered imposes a limit for a hypothetical eye with maximum scatter (i.e.; a uniform distribution of intensity on the image). A multiplying factor of 0.1 limits the accessible values of OSI from 0 to a maximum of 25. OSI for normal eyes would range around 1, while values over 5 would represent highly scattered systems.

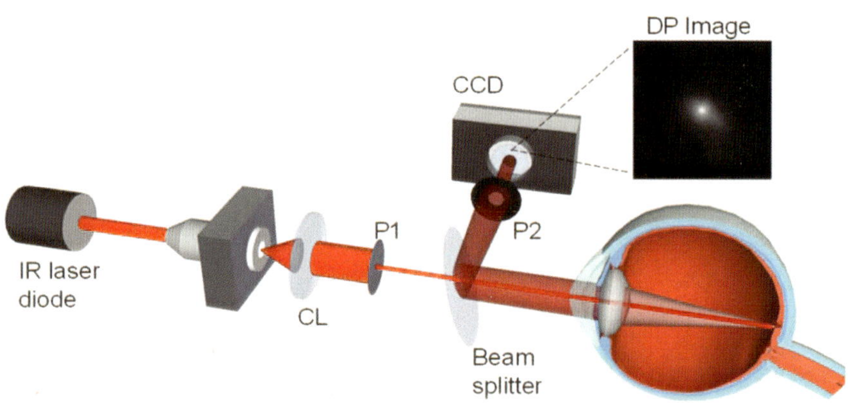

Figure 1. Schematic representation of the double-pass method. See text for further details.

Fig. 2 shows two examples on how the 2D double-pass retinal images are converted into 1D intensity profiles as radial averaged and the areas selected to integrate the intensity. A system with more scatter (example image B in figure 2) will produce an image with higher intensity in the peripheral areas and then an elevated value of OSI.

Impact of aberrations in the Objective Scatter Index

The retinal image is affected by both ocular aberrations and intraocular scattering [23,24]. These two factors influence the light distribution on the retina. While the ocular aberrations influence the light distribution at the central region of the image, the intraocular scattering cause an increment of the intensity further away from the central maximum of the retinal image, leading to a wide angle halo. The effect of the combination of both factors on the visual quality is not a simple summation of the degrading effects since, as it has been recently discovered, the addition of spherical aberrations improved contrast in the presence of scatter [25].

The interpretation of the OSI as a parameter related to the intraocular scattering requires an evaluation of the contribution of ocular aberrations on this index. It may be possible that the presence of aberrations could contribute to the outer areas of the DP images affecting the OSI values. There is a trade-off between the area registered within the DP and the amount of aberrations that would affect the parameter. We addressed this issue by comparing experimental DP images with simulated ones, calculated from actual data of the aberrations measured in the same eye using a Hartmann-Shack (HS) wave sensor [26].

Fig. 3 shows a schematic representation of the procedure to compute a synthetic DP image by using exclusively the information provided by the HS images (related only to aberrations). The DP image is the convolution of the point-spread function (PSF) corresponding with the first and the second passes [15]. From the HS images recorded for every analyzed eye, we obtained the wave aberrations and the PSF of the incoming pass (PSF1) and the PSF of the outgoing pass (PSF2) were calculated. Finally, the synthetic DP image is the result of the convolution between these two PSFs. The synthetic DP image can be compared with the experimental DP for the same eye. They should be very similar in eyes with small amount of scatter (the optical quality dominated by aberrations) and different in eyes severely affected by scatter. Fig. 4 shows an example of both, the measured DP and the calculated from the aberrations, together with a radial averaged section for each case. The results if this figure justifies the selected area (12–20 minutes of arc) that affect scatter to calculate the OSI parameter.

From a practical perspective, in addition to high order aberrations, the OSI parameter could also be largely affected by uncorrected refractive errors (defocus and astigmatism). To define the acceptable range of uncorrected defocus, we recorded a series of DP images in a young eye for different amounts of induced defocus from 0 to 2.0 D. The calculated OSI as a function of defocus is shown in Fig. 5. For uncorrected values over 1.0 D, significantly large OSI values (more than 1) are obtained. To avoid this type of artifact in the OSI determination, the DP images need to be recorded with both, defocus and astigmatism, corrected at least with a precision better than 1.0 D of spherical equivalent.

Results

The OSI parameter was estimated from the DP images obtained for the 53 eyes included in the study. Figure 6 shows, as an example, DP and slit-lamp images in four representative eyes from each group: control and NO2-NO4. DP images are clearly deteriorated for increasing levels of scatter. We calculated the average values of OSI in the patients following the LOCSIII classification. Figure 7 shows the average values of OSI for each group: 0.7±0.3 for the control group; 3.0±1.0 for the NO2 group, 6.0±2.0 for the NO3 group, and 9.0±3.0 for the NO4 group. Although the OSI values clearly increased following the subjective classification, there was a significant dispersion especially in groups NO3 and NO4.

Figure 8 shows the individual values of OSI in all tested eyes. While the normal young eyes (left) showed small and similar OSI values (typically below 1), in the case of the cataract eyes, in some individuals we found OSI values either lower or higher than the average value for the corresponding group. For example, an eye classified as NO4 (the last sample right in the panel) had an OSI value similar to other eyes that were classified as NO2.

By using the measured OSI values, we are able to establish a new classification of the eyes with different degrees of intraocular scattering (Figure 9). Following this scale, the patients could be separated out in different groups: the first range (white bars) with an OSI below 1 corresponds to eyes with low amounts of scatter that can be considered as normal eyes. The next range (light grey bars) included eyes with an OSI between 1 and 3, corresponding to older eyes with associated scatter of an early cataract. The third

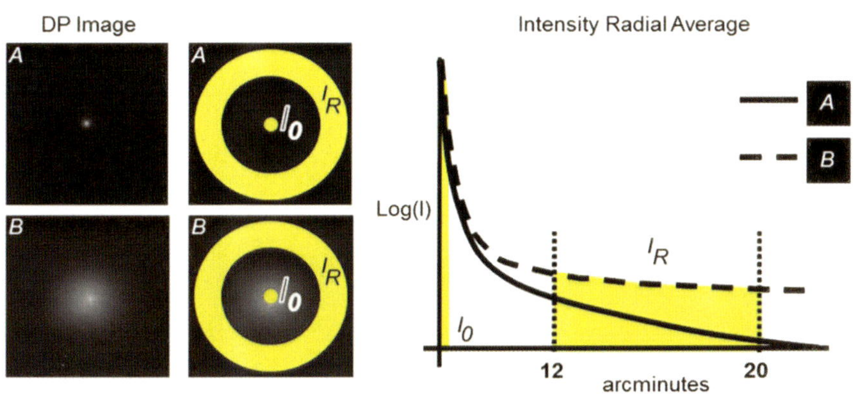

Figure 2. Example of the selection of the zone in the double-pass image used to define the objective scatter index (OSI). We compute the relation between the intensity in the peak of the image, the central area within 1 minute, with that in a ring comprised between 12 and 20 minutes. Two DP images with different levels of scatter (A less scatter, B more scatter) are represented to illustrate the procedure.

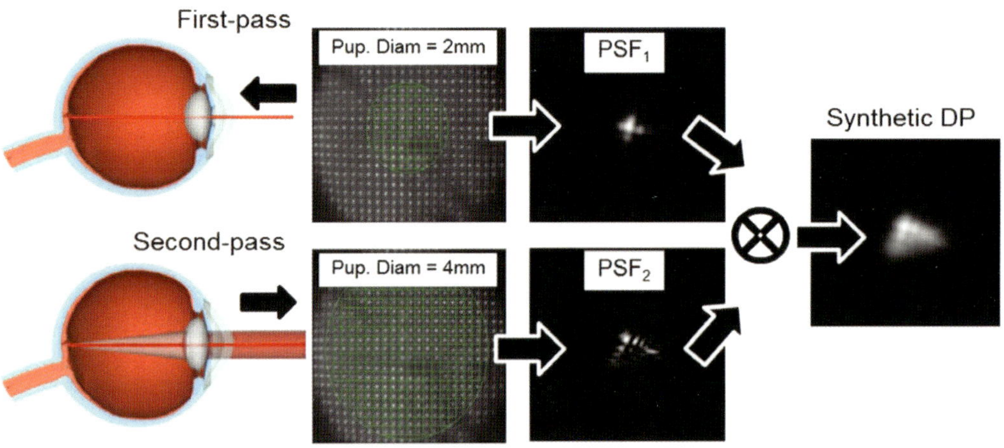

Figure 3. Schematic representation of the procedure to compute the synthetic DP image from wavefront aberration data. We computed the PSF for a 2-mm (first-pass) and 4 mm (second-pass) pupil diameter. Convolution of both PSFs renders the synthetic DP image.

range with OSI values between 3 and 7, corresponds to developed cataracts that should undergo surgery. Finally, eyes with severe cataracts and large amount of associated intraocular scattering (dark grey bars) presented values of OSI higher than 7. Figure 10 shows as an example DP images representative of the four ranges with the actual OSI value for each case.

Discussion

Westheimer and Liang [27] proposed to analyze the intensity distribution of the DP images to extract information about the combined contribution of the ocular aberrations and the intraocular scattering on the retinal image. In a later work, they combined the information of the DP images with subjective measurements to separate out the influence of the intraocular scattering on the visual performance [28]. However, they did not evaluate the contribution of the ocular aberrations on the DP images. In addition, in those studies the procedure was not applied in eyes where scatter was the main degrading effect.

We have further refined this approach to evaluate the contribution of scatter separated from refractive errors and higher order aberrations, with the main intention to classify the degree of cataracts. The main consequence of the definition of the scale of values of OSI is that we can establish a comparison between the particular positions of any of the analyzed eyes in this classification and the position of the same eye in the gradation made by the LOCSIII system. This analysis would give a percentage of agreement regarding to the number of eyes classified in equivalent levels by the two scales.

It should be noted the significant advantages of the combined use of both approaches. OSI gradation directly relates with the visual degradation (forward scatter), while the information in the slit-lamp images is useful to understand the nature and type of the cataract, although it is not always simple to predict the actual

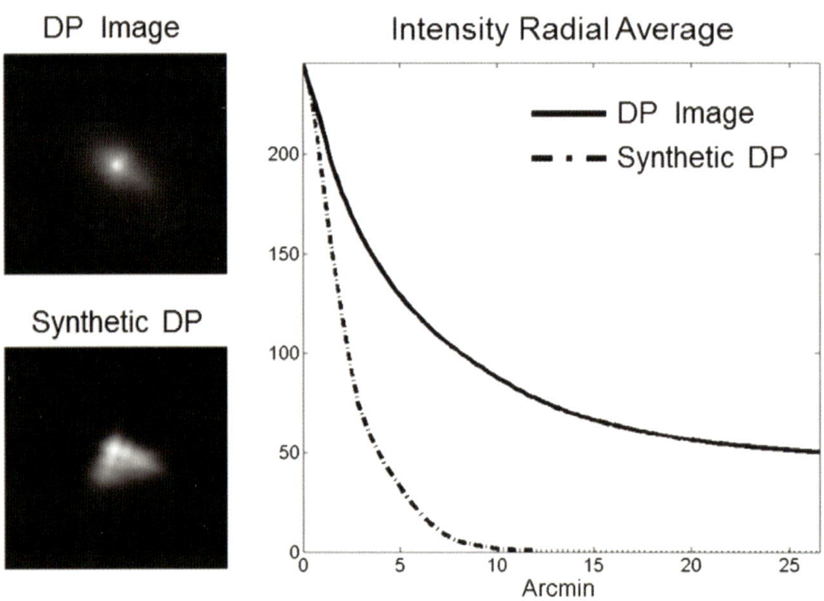

Figure 4. Example of comparison of actual and synthetic DP images. The 1D section shows the range where scatter is significant and used to calculate the OSI parameter.

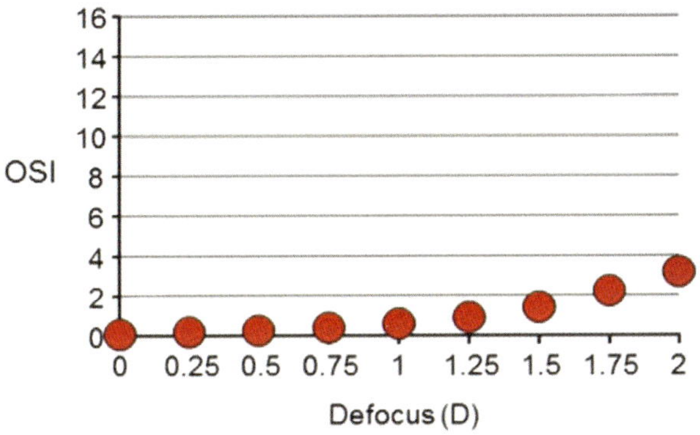

Figure 5. Estimated value of OSI as a function of induced defocus. Uncorrected refractive errors over 1 diopter induce artifacts ion the determination of OSI over the value of 1 (standard value in normal eyes). This indicates that refractive errors need to be well corrected during the DP data collection to provide accurate values of OSI. The y-axis is kept scaled to16 as in the figures where OSI is represented. This will permit a direct comparison on the impact of uncorrected defocus on OSI.

visual impact. The DP image is affected by both the forward and the backward scattering, produced in the first and the second pass of the light through the crystalline lens; the analysis of the energy distribution on this image reveals the contribution of the light scattering which really impairs visual performance.

We found an agreement of 75% by considering the complete population between the two schemes (OSI versus LOCSIII). This means that 40 of the 53 eyes were sorted as equivalent by using both methods. Although this percentage is relevant, in the daily clinical practice the capability of detecting an early cataract is especially useful and therefore, it would be very interesting to show the agreement between the eyes ranked in one of the two first levels in both scales. The percentage of agreement between the eyes classified in one of the two first levels in both scales was 84%. This means that 21 of the 25 eyes, which were ranked by the values of OSI on the first and second levels, were classified accordingly to the LOCSIII chart. This further emphasizes that a value of OSI lower than 1 characterizes a non-cataract eye,

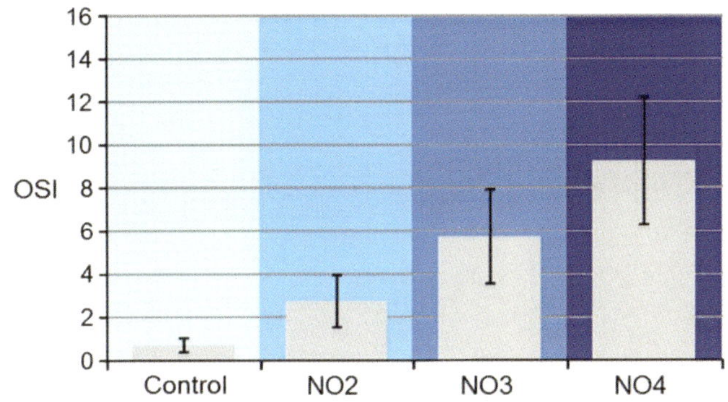

Figure 7. Average OSI for the four groups analyzed: control group (left), and groups of eyes with opacification according to the LOCSIII chart classification (groups NO2, NO3 and NO4). The error bar represents standard deviation.

whereas a value of OSI around 2 would correspond with an early cataract eye, corresponding to NO2 in the LOCSIII chart. With regard to the eyes classified in the third and fourth level of the OSI scale, they were all mature cataracts. In this case, the disagreement between LOCSIII and the OSI rankings was not quite relevant since, from a practical point of view, it does not affect the diagnosis capability of early cataract process.

The correspondence between the classification made by clinicians, by the LOCSIII chart, and the gradation established from the values of OSI, supports the applicability of this objective method to make a sound decision on the proper timing for a cataract surgery. Moreover the quantification provided by an objective gradation as OSI, can be also very useful to complete the available data from anamnesis, or reduced visual acuity in the diagnosis of an early cataract process.

In addition, it would be important to evaluate the values of OSI in other types of lens opacification, as well as to refine the possible ranges for classifying these cataracts depending on the intraocular scattering measured by OQAS. Having new data about intraocular scattering in cataracts may also be helpful to understand the developing process on cataracts, as well as to better understand the way the crystalline lens evolves from being

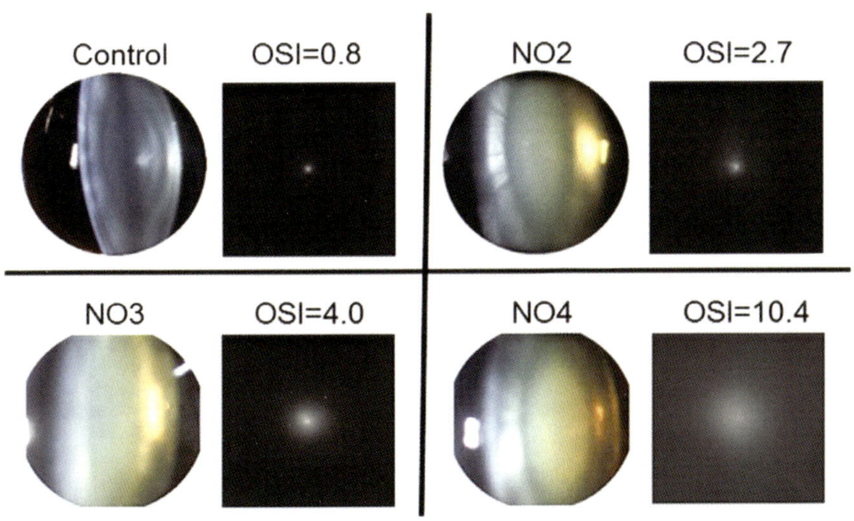

Figure 6. Example of DP and slit-laps images in four eyes as example of the four groups. The actual OSI value in each eye is noted.

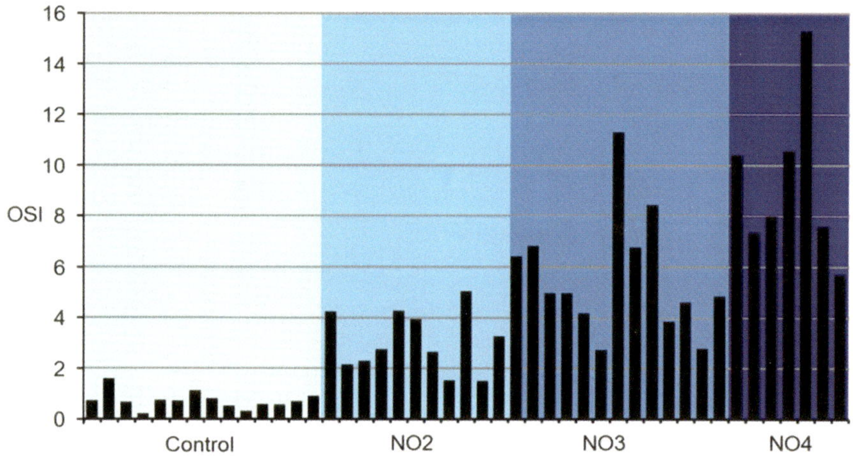

Figure 8. Individual OSI values for every tested eye. Normal young eyes (Control; left) showed small values of OSI. The eyes in groups NO2, NO3 and NO4 showed increasing OSI values, although with clear individual variability.

transparent to increased dispersion as well as other morphological and optical changes, as could be the increased aberrations with age [29].

Patients mainly affected by nuclear cataract were primarily selected among a large number of potential candidates by using slit-lamp images. However, some concomitancy between nuclear with cortical or capsular cataracts is not possible to avoid. Different types of cataracts may have a different contribution on the ocular scattering. The impossibility for estimating whether there was or not some contribution of other type of cataract together with the predominant nuclear type, could be considered as one of the factors to explain the differences between the gradation made by the LOCS and the objective classification based on OSI.

The DP image, and therefore the scatter index, is affected by the complete eye. It would be possible in some particular cases to measure an elevated OSI due to corneal haze, which is not related to cataract. In the DP instrument, the laser beam in the first pass has a small diameter (1.5 mm diameter) and reaches the eye within the pupil center area. With a localized cataract the actual impact location of the beam could affect directly the image in the retina. In the second pass, after retinal reflection, the situation is different since the light fills the whole area of the pupil, and hence, the entire crystalline lens (within the area of the pupil) is considered. DP image actually contains information from the whole pupil area. However, some minor variability in the results could be observed due to the impact of the first pass. In an instrument with a large beam also in the first pass, this problem could be avoided. We should emphasize that the reported method provides average information within the complete pupil area; i.e, it is not spatially resolved. This technique, although useful, should be combined with complementary techniques routinely. The DP images were recorded using near infrared light. This is an advantage for the patient's comfort during image acquisition. However, the magnitude of scatter in infrared light can be different than in visible light. The impact of retinal scatter could be also larger in infrared since light penetrates deeper in the retina. This is a limitation for the absolute characterization of scatter, but not very relevant for the relative gradation of cataract of this study.

The changes in the cornea and the vitreous as a function of age may also increase the overall amount of ocular scattering. However, in non pathological cases, the magnitude of these effects would be smaller than that of the lens in early cataract.

In conclusion, a new objective optical method has been developed to quantify the degree of cataract. It is based on the

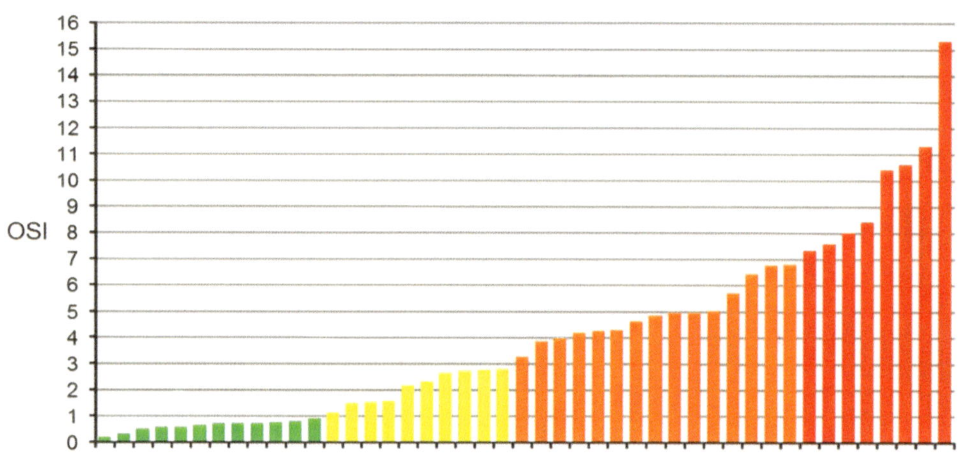

Figure 9. Subjects classified according to obtained OSI values. Increasing grey scale represents the gradation proposed by the quantification of cataracts, according to this objective parameter.

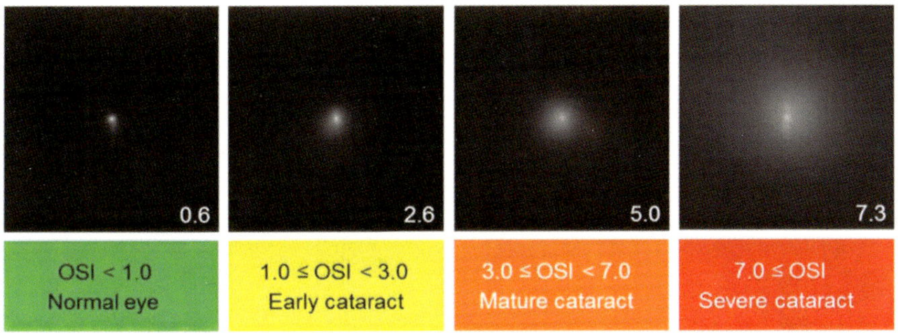

Figure 10. Example of DP images for the different range following the OSI classification scheme. Double-pass (DP) images from four eyes and corresponding OSI values. Below, proposed classification ranges of eyes according to the measured OSI values.

recording and processing of double pass retinal images of a point source. We demonstrated the potential of the technique in a group of cataract patients. The correlation of the cataract gradation between this approach and a standard subjective method (LOCSIII) is significant.

However the higher sensitivity and the intrinsic nature of this approach to detect forward scattering renders our method more powerful specially in the detection of earlier stages of cataract and to relate cataract symptoms with visual complaints. The method is robust and fully based on objective measurements; i.e., not depending on subjective decisions. This procedure could be used in combination with standard current methods to improve cataract surgery patients scheduling.

Acknowledgments

The authors thank Sergio Luque and Fernando Diaz for their help with the software development, Salome Abenza for help in the clinic and all the patients participating in the study.

Author Contributions

Conceived and designed the experiments: PA. Performed the experiments: AB GP EA ADC. Analyzed the data: PA AB GP EA ADC JP JMM. Contributed reagents/materials/analysis tools: JP JMM. Wrote the paper: PA.

References

1. Allen MJ, Vos JJ (1967) Ocular scattered light and visual performance as a function of age. Am J Optom Arch Am Acad Optom 44: 717–727.
2. de Wit GC, Franssen L, Coppens JE, van den Berg TJ (2006) Simulating the straylight effects of cataracts," J Cataract Refract Surg 32: 294–300.
3. Steinberg EP, Bass EB, Luthra R, Schein OD, Sharkey P, et al. (1995) Variation in ophthalmic testing before cataract surgery. Results of a national survey of ophthalmologists. Arch Ophthalmol 112: 896–902.
4. Chylack LT, Wolfe JK, Singer DM, Leske MC, Bullimore MA, et al. (1993) The Lens Opacities Classification System III. The Longitudinal Study of Cataract Study Group. Arch Ophthalmol 111: 831–836.
5. Paulsson LE, Sjöstrand J (1980) Contrast sensitivity in the presence of glare light. Theoretical concepts and preliminary clinical studies. Invest Ophthalmol Vis Sci 19: 401–406.
6. de Waard PW, IJspeert JK, van den Berg TJ, de Jong PT (1992) Intraocular light scattering in age-related cataracts. Invest Ophthalmol Vis Sci 33: 618–625.
7. Duncan DD, Shukla OB, West SK, Schein OD (1997) New objective classification system for nuclear opacification. J Opt Soc Am A 14: 1197–1204.
8. Vivino MA, Chintalagiri S, Trus B, Datiles M (1993) Development of a Scheimpflug slit lamp camera system for quantitative densitometric analysis. Eye 7: 791–798.
9. Datiles MB, Ansari RR, Reed GF (2002) A clinical study of the human lens with a dynamic light scattering device. Exp Eye Res 74: 93–102.
10. Holladay JT, Prager TC, Trujillo J, Ruiz RS (1987) Brightness acuity test and outdoor visual acuity in cataract patients. J Cataract Refract Surg 13: 67–69.
11. Bailey IL, Bullimore MA (1991) A new test for the evaluation of disability glare. Optom Vis Sci 68: 911–917.
12. Franssen L, Coppens JE, van den Berg TJ (2006) Compensation comparison method for assessment of retinal straylight. Invest Ophthalmol Vis Sci 47: 768–776.
13. van den Berg TJ, van Rijn LJ, Michael R, Heine C, Coeckelbergh T, et al. (2007) Straylight effects with aging and lens extraction. Am J Ophthalmol 144: 358–363.
14. van den Berg TJ, IJspeert, JK (1992) Clinical Assessment of Intraocular Stray Light. App Opt 31: 3694–3696.
15. Santamaria J, Artal P, Bescós J (1987) Determination of the point-spread function of human eyes using a hybrid optical-digital method, J Opt Soc Am A 4: 1109–1114.
16. Artal P (1990) Calculations of two-dimensional foveal retinal images in real eyes. J Opt Soc Am A 7: 1374–1381.
17. Artal P, Ferro M, Miranda I, Navarro R (1993) Effects of aging in retinal image quality. J Opt Soc Am A 10: 1656–1662.
18. Guirao A, González C, Redondo M, Geraghty E, Norrby S, et al. (1999) Average optical performance of the human eye as a function of age in a normal population. Invest Ophthalmol Vis Sci 40: 203–213.
19. Artal P, Marcos S, Navarro R, Miranda I, Ferro M (1995) Through focus image quality of eyes implanted with monofocal and multifocal intraocular lenses. Opt Eng 34: 772–779.
20. Alcon E, Benito A, Perez GM, De Casas A, Abenza S, et al. (2007) Quantifying intraocular scattering in cataract patients. ARVO Meeting Abstracts 48: 3821.
21. Benito A, Alcon E, Perez GM, Abenza S, De Casas A, et al. (2007) An Objective classification scheme for cataracts. ARVO Meeting Abstracts 48: 3822.
22. Artal P, Iglesias I, Lopez N, Green DG (1995) Double-pass measurements of the retinal image quality with unequal entrance and exit pupils sizes and the reversibility of the eye's optical system. J Opt Soc Am A 12: 2358–2366.
23. Artal P (2000) Understanding aberrations by using double-pass techniques. J Refract Surg 16: 560–562.
24. Díaz-Doutón F, Benito A, Pujol J, Arjona M, Güell J, et al. (2006) Comparison of the retinal image quality with a Hartmann-Shack wavefront sensor and a double-pass instrument. Inv Ophthalmol Vis Sci 47: 1710–1716.
25. Perez GM, Manzanera S, Artal P (2009) Impact of scattering and spherical aberration in contrast sensitivity. J Vis 9: 1–10.
26. Prieto PM, Vargas-Martín F, Goelz S, Artal P (2000) Analysis of the performance of the Hartmann-Shack sensor in the human eye. J Opt Soc Am A 17: 1388–1398.
27. Westheimer G, Liang J (1994) Evaluating diffusion of light in the eye by objective means. Invest Ophthalmol Vis Sci 35: 2652–2657.
28. Westheimer G, Liang J (1995) Influence of ocular light scatter on the eye's optical performance. J Opt Soc Am A 12: 1417–1424.
29. Artal P, Berrio E, Guirao A, Piers P (2002) Contribution of the cornea and internal surfaces to the change of ocular aberrations with age. J Opt Soc Am A 19: 137–143.

11

Ionizing Irradiation Not Only Inactivates Clonogenic Potential in Primary Normal Human Diploid Lens Epithelial Cells but Also Stimulates Cell Proliferation in a Subset of This Population

Yuki Fujimichi, Nobuyuki Hamada*

Radiation Safety Research Center, Nuclear Technology Research Laboratory, Central Research Institute of Electric Power Industry (CRIEPI), Komae, Tokyo, Japan

Abstract

Over the past century, ionizing radiation has been known to induce cataracts in the crystalline lens of the eye, but its mechanistic underpinnings remain incompletely understood. This study is the first to report the clonogenic survival of irradiated primary normal human lens epithelial cells and stimulation of its proliferation. Here we used two primary normal human cell strains: HLEC1 lens epithelial cells and WI-38 lung fibroblasts. Both strains were diploid, and a replicative lifespan was shorter in HLEC1 cells. The colony formation assay demonstrated that the clonogenic survival of both strains decreases similarly with increasing doses of X-rays. A difference in the survival between two strains was actually insignificant, although HLEC1 cells had the lower plating efficiency. This indicates that the same dose inactivates the same fraction of clonogenic cells in both strains. Intriguingly, irradiation enlarged the size of clonogenic colonies arising from HLEC1 cells in marked contrast to those from WI-38 cells. Such enhanced proliferation of clonogenic HLEC1 cells was significant at ≥2 Gy, and manifested as increments of ≤2.6 population doublings besides sham-irradiated controls. These results suggest that irradiation of HLEC1 cells not only inactivates clonogenic potential but also stimulates proliferation of surviving uniactivated clonogenic cells. Given that the lens is a closed system, the stimulated proliferation of lens epithelial cells may not be a homeostatic mechanism to compensate for their cell loss, but rather should be regarded as abnormal. This is because these findings are consistent with the early *in vivo* evidence documenting that irradiation induces excessive proliferation of rabbit lens epithelial cells and that suppression of lens epithelial cell divisions inhibits radiation cataractogenesis in frogs and rats. Thus, our *in vitro* model will be useful to evaluate the excessive proliferation of primary normal human lens epithelial cells that may underlie radiation cataractogenesis, warranting further investigations.

Editor: Melinda Duncan, University of Delaware, United States of America

Funding: The authors have no support or funding to report.

Competing Interests: The authors have declared that no competing interests exist.

* E-mail: hamada-n@criepi.denken.or.jp

Introduction

The ocular lens is a transparent, avascular tissue that refracts incoming light onto the retina and grows throughout life without developing tumors [1]. The lens capsule, lens epithelium, lens cortex and lens nucleus compose the lens, and the boundary between its anterior and posterior surfaces is called an equator. The lens epithelium comprises a single layer of cuboidal epithelial cells located in the anterior subcapsular region. Lens epithelial cells in the germinative zone around the equator divide, migrate posteriorly, and terminally differentiate into fiber cells that possess no organelles [2]. Newly formed fibers wrap around existing cortical fibers, and become more internalized and tightly packed mature nuclear fibers. The lens capsule encases the entire lens, so that all cells stay inside the lens throughout life.

A cataract is a clouding of the lens. Posterior subcapsular (PSC) cataracts are one of the three major types of cataracts, and most common in ionizing radiation-induced cataracts. Such radiogenic cataracts have been described for over a century [3] and regarded as typical late effects of radiation. The International Commission on Radiological Protection (ICRP) considers that the lens is among the most radiosensitive tissues [4]. ICRP has recommended dose limits for the lens to prevent vision-impairing cataracts since 1954 [5], because cataracts limit occupational performance and interfere with daily life activities even if surgically curable and not life threatening. In 2011, ICRP recommended reducing occupational dose limit for the lens by a factor of 7.5 [6], which was revised 21 years after the previous revision [7]. Such lowering may affect some medical or nuclear workers (and perhaps even some patients as well), thereby creating a surge of interest in cataracts [8]. From a therapeutic viewpoint, 10 Gy and 18 Gy are considered as tolerance dose that causes cataracts requiring surgical intervention in 5% and 50% of patients within 5 years post therapy, respectively [9] (c.f., ICRP considers 0.5 Gy as a threshold dose that causes vision-impairing cataracts in 1% of exposed individuals with >20 years follow-up [6]), and treatment planning is made to minimize the lens dose. Nonetheless, children with retinoblastoma are often treated with radiation due to its radiosensitive nature, and this leads to cataracts for which pediatric surgery is a challenge [10]. Manned space missions also raise a concern for cataracts [11]. Despite such a long history documenting radiogenic cataracts, the underlying mechanisms remain unclear, and mitigators are yet to be established [6].

A colony formation assay has been the most extensively used technique in the field of radiation biology since its establishment in 1956 [12]. This assay evaluates the radiosensitivity in terms of the clonogenic survival, where a cell that retains the ability to form a colony containing ≥50 cells (referred hereinafter to as a clonogenic colony) typically in two weeks (a period that varies with cell type) is regarded as a surviving cell. In these experiments, fibroblasts have been most widely used among various types of primary normal human diploid cells. Conversely, there has been no information available hitherto as to the clonogenic survival of lens epithelial cells (i.e., the only possible clonogenic population within the lens structures), which was evaluated here in parallel with fibroblasts for comparison.

Materials and Methods

Cell Cultures

The ScienCell Research Laboratories (Carlsbad, CA) sells several lots of primary normal human lens epithelial cells derived from different donors under the same name (HLEpiC) and catalog number (6550). Of these, the lot 5971 (cytokeratin 18-positive HLEpiC harvested from a 24-week gestation female fetus and subsequently passaged once during which time 5 population doublings occurred *in vitro* before shipping) was purchased, and renamed HLEC1 to avoid possible confusion that our future use of different lots of HLEpiC may cause. All flasks and dishes used for HLEC1 cells were precoated with poly-*L*-lysine (PLL), and HLEC1 cells were routinely subcultured in EpiCM [epithelial cell culture medium containing 2% fetal bovine serum (FBS), 1% growth supplement (components not disclosed by the manufacturer), 19 U/ml penicillin and 19 μg/ml streptomycin, pH of 7.4 with an atmosphere of 95% air/5% CO_2] in 75-cm^2 tissue culture (T75) flasks, following the manufacturer's instruction. HLEC1, PLL and EpiCM were purchased from ScienCell. WI-38 primary normal human diploid lung fibroblasts were established by Hayflick as his 38th fibroblast strain at the Wistar Institute of Anatomy and Biology (Philadelphia, PA) in 1962, and derived from a surgically aborted three-month gestation Caucasian female fetus [13,14]. WI-38 cells that underwent 19 population doublings *in vitro* were purchased from American Type Culture Collection (CCL-75, Manassas, VA), and passaged in T75 flasks in Dulbecco's modified Eagle's medium (DMEM, D8437, Sigma, St Louis, MO) supplemented with 10% heat-inactivated FBS (171012, Nichirei Bioscience, Tokyo, Japan). All cell cultures were maintained at 37°C in a humidified atmosphere of 5% CO_2 in air, except where otherwise specified.

Primary normal human cells have a finite replicative lifespan *in vitro* as firstly proposed by Hayflick and Moorhead in 1961 [15]. To evaluate this, cells were serially passaged. The population doubling number (PDN) was calculated as $\log_2(N_H/N_P)$, where N_P and N_H are cell numbers plated and those harvested, respectively. The cumulative population doubling (CPD) level was calculated as the initial PDN (i.e., 5 for HLEC1 and 19 for WI-38) plus the PDN increased by additional passages. The end of the replicative lifespan was defined by failure of the population to increase after a minimum of three weeks in culture with weekly refeedings. The population doubling time was calculated as the reciprocal of q, when growth curves were fitted against the data points in the exponential growth phase to $y = qx+s$ where y, x, q and s are CPD, time (h), slope and intercept, respectively.

Preparation of Metaphase Chromosome Spreads

Exponentially growing cells were treated with 25 ng/ml colcemid (Gibco, Grand Island, NY). After mild trypsinization and mitotic shake off, cells were hypotonized with 75 mM KCl, fixed in 3:1 methanol:acetic acid, dropped onto cleaned slides, and stained with 6% Giemsa (Wako, Osaka, Japan). Chromosome numbers in each metaphase were counted under an Olympus BX51 microscope.

Irradiation and Colony Formation

At one day prior to irradiation, 1.8×10^5 cells were seeded onto each T25 flask. Cells were exposed to single, graded doses of X-rays at room temperature from an X-ray generator (MBR-1505R2, Hitachi Medico, Tokyo, Japan) operated at 150 kV and 5 mA with a 1-mm aluminum plus 0.2-mm copper filter, followed by incubation at 37°C in 95% air/5% CO_2. Only one T25 flask was placed at a time in a single exposure in the central 15.8-cm-diameter circle at the distance from the radiation source to the cell surface of 250 mm, and irradiated at a dose rate of 0.43±0.005 Gy/min for HLEC1 and 0.43±0.008 Gy/min for WI-38. The dose uniformity within the T25 flask was ±4.9%, and the half value layer of X-rays used was 5.5 mm. Control cells were sham-irradiated and manipulated in parallel with the test cells. Within 1 h postirradiation, cells were rinsed, trypsinized, and suspended in EpiCM (for HLEC1) or DMEM with 10% FBS (for WI-38). Then, cells were counted, diluted in DMEM with 20% FBS, and reseeded into 10-cm dishes in quadruplicate, and incubated for 14 days, at which time they were fixed and stained with crystal violet. Stained cells were viewed under a Nikon SM2645 stereomicroscope, and the 8-bit RGB color JPEG images were captured with a Panasonic DMC-TZ30 digital camera. Note that the difference in cell numbers replated after irradiation for colony formation was statistically insignificant between HLEC1 and WI-38 (Table S1).

Hereafter, a colony with 2–49 cells is referred to as an abortive colony, a cell capable of producing a clonogenic colony as a clonogenic cell, and a cell incapable of producing a clonogenic colony as a nonclonogenic cell. The plating efficiency of sham-irradiated cells was calculated as the number of clonogenic colonies divided by that of plated cells. The surviving fraction of irradiated cells was calculated as the number of clonogenic colonies divided by that of plated cells with correction for the plating efficiency. Survival curves were fitted against the means of independent experiments to the exponential equation $y = \exp(-kx)$, where y, x and k are surviving fraction, the dose and slope, respectively. The dose required to reduce the surviving fraction to 0.1 (10% survival dose, D_{10}) and that to $1/e$ (mean lethal dose, D_0) was calculated as $[\ln(1/0.1)]/k$ and $1/k$, respectively.

To quantify differences among clonogenic colonies, colony size was evaluated based on the methods explained in Figures S1, S4, S5 and S6. Briefly, cell numbers in all manually countable clonogenic colonies were directly counted under the stereomicroscope, and this was the case for most colonies with <1,500 cells. The area of each clonogenic colony, and cell numbers in manually uncountable clonogenic colonies were evaluated using the captured images and the ImageJ 1.47 freeware (http://rsb.info.nih.gov/ij/).

Statistical Analysis

Data were calculated as the means and standard deviations (SD) of three repeated experiments unless otherwise described. Statistical comparisons between groups were made by Student's *t*-test, and a p value of <0.05 was considered to be significant.

Results

HLEC1 and WI-38 are Diploid, and HLEC1 has a Shorter Replicative Lifespan than WI-38

Cells need to go through a minimum of 5.64 doublings for clonogenic colony formation, but the proliferative potential of HLEC1 lens epithelial cells is uncharacterized nor is its ploidy unlike the case for WI-38 lung fibroblasts [13]. To this end, we evaluated the ploidy and proliferative potential. The karyotype analysis of metaphase chromosome spreads confirmed that both strains are diploid (Table 1 and Figure 1). Serial passages revealed that HLEC1 and WI-38 have a population doubling time of 66.6 and 32.4 h, and reach the end of their replicative lifespan at CPD 17.1 and 69.1, respectively (Figure 2). Young cells (i.e., CPD 11.0 for HLEC1 and CPD 32.0 for WI-38) were thus used for subsequent experiments.

Clonogenic Survival of HLEC1 and WI-38 Similarly Declines with Radiation Dose, Whilst HLEC1 has a Lower Plating Efficiency than WI-38

HLEC1 at CPD 11.0 and WI-38 at CPD 32.0 were reinoculated within 1 h postirradiation, followed by colony formation for 14 days. Note that CPD 11.0 was the youngest HLEC1 experimentally available to us. The colony formation assay revealed that the clonogenic survival similarly decreases with increasing dose of X-rays in both strains (Figure 3). Whereas the plating efficiency of HLEC1 was significantly lower than that of WI-38 (1.6±0.6% vs 19.5±3.6%, $p=0.0056$), the difference between these two survival curves was statistically insignificant at all five dose points tested (i.e., 0.5–6 Gy) for which p values ranged from 0.11 to 0.50. These results suggest that whilst HLEC1 has a smaller fraction (~one-twelfth) of clonogenic cells than WI-38, irradiation with the same dose inactivates the same fraction of clonogenic cells in both strains.

Irradiation Stimulates the Proliferation of Surviving Uninactivated Cells in HLEC1 but not in WI-38

Interestingly, the colony formation assay also led us to the observation that clonogenic colonies arising from irradiated HLEC1 look obviously larger than those from sham-irradiated counterparts (Figure 4). This potentially challenges the long-held tenet among users of the colony formation assay that irradiation suppresses proliferation and increases killing of cells thereby resulting in dose-dependent clonogenic inactivation [3,12]. We hence decided to quantify these differences in clonogenic colonies.

To confirm our above-described impression, the area of clonogenic colonies was first analyzed as explained in Figure S1. Figure 5A illustrates that whereas the area of clonogenic colonies derived from HLEC1 and that from WI-38 does not differ significantly at 0 Gy ($p=0.24$), the former was significantly larger than the latter at ≥0.5 Gy ($p<0.001$). Frequency of clonogenic colonies did not exhibit multimodal distributions for both strains and at all dose points (Figure S2), so that clonogenic colonies exceeding the mean plus 2SD area of sham-irradiated controls were judged as "large" colonies. As regards WI-38, the area of clonogenic colonies decreased significantly at ≥1 Gy compared with sham-irradiated controls (Figure 5A). Decreases were also observed in the fraction of large colonies among all clonogenic colonies and that among all plated cells (Figure 5B and 5C). The exponential equation fitted the latter fraction data well with a correlation coefficient square (R^2) of 0.979 (Figure 5C). Given a dose-dependent decrease in the size of clonogenic colonies, this is not surprising because the curve of this sort should reflect the clonogenic survival when colonies above the mean plus 2SD area (e.g., with several thousand cells) were judged as survivors instead of a general criterion of 50 cells. These observations obtained with WI-38 reconfirmed the rationale of the colony formation assay, such that irradiation inactivates clonogenic potential and decreases the clonogenic survival both of which occur dose dependently. With respect to HLEC1, the area of clonogenic colonies was elevated with dose, and such increases were significant at ≥2 Gy compared with sham-irradiated controls (Figure 5A). Surprisingly, large colonies accounted for as high as 33.8% and 34.6% of all clonogenic colonies at 4 and 6 Gy, respectively (Figure 5B), whereas its fraction was similar to WI-38 at 0 Gy and 0.5 Gy. When the data for the fraction of large colonies among all plated cells were fitted to the exponential equation, the curve looked much flatter than the case for WI-38 (Figure 5C), and such difference should be attributable to the increased proliferation following irradiation. Refitting of these data at 0.5–4 Gy to the linear equation yielded the line with a slope of 2.6×10^{-5}, nearly parallel to the x-axis (Figure S3). These findings suggest that irradiation not only inactivates clonogenic potential but also stimulates cellular proliferation, and imply that such cells whose proliferation is activated by irradiation exist in the population at a similar rate independent of dose.

Cell numbers in clonogenic colonies arising from HLEC1 were further evaluated as described in Figures S4, S5 and S6, because the increased colonial area may not necessarily reflect the increased proliferation. Cell numbers in clonogenic colonies significantly increased at ≥2 Gy, and ranged from 50 cells/colony

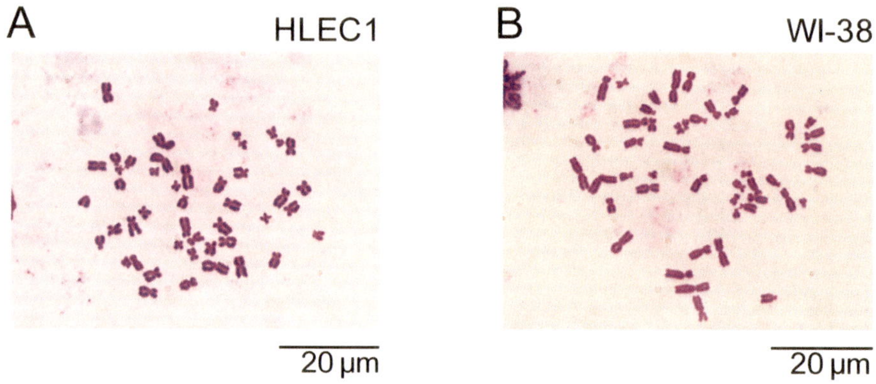

Figure 1. Representative images of metaphase chromosomes in HLEC1 at CPD 14.5 (A) and WI-38 at CPD 44.7 (B). Bars, 20 μm.

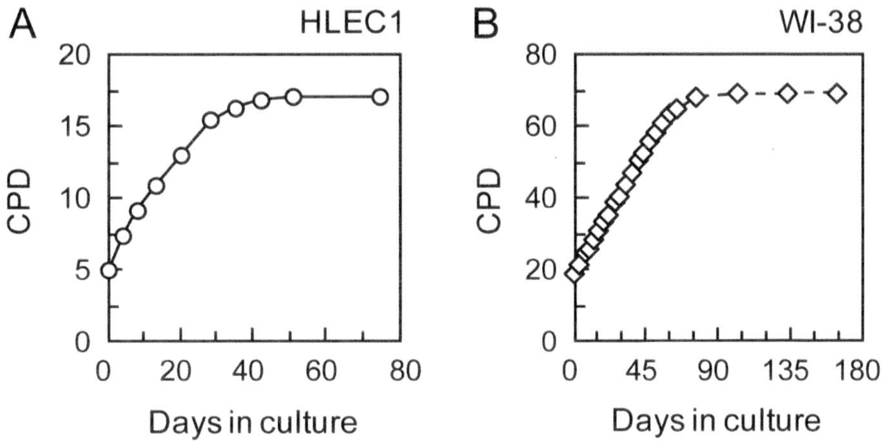

Figure 2. Growth curve of HLEC1 (A) and WI-38 (B). HLEC1 at CPD 5.0 and WI-38 at CPD 19.0 were plated and serially passaged with weekly replenishment. The population doubling times of HLEC1 and WI-38 were estimated to be 66.6 h at CPD 5.0–15.5 and 32.4 h at CPD 19.0–64.9, respectively. HLEC1 and WI-38 ceased to divide at CPD 17.1 and 69.1, respectively.

(i.e., criteria for a survivor in the colony formation assay) observed at 0, 0.5 and 1 Gy to 57,745 cells/colony observed at 6 Gy each of which corresponded to PDN 5.64 and 15.8, respectively (Figure 6A). Figure 6B clearly shows that irradiation greatly increases PDN of clonogenic cells during a period of 14 days for colony formation (e.g., PDN 12.6 at 6 Gy increased from PDN 10.0 at 0 Gy). This finding reinforces the observation that irradiation stimulates the proliferation of clonogenic cells, but the impact of irradiation on nonclonogenic cells was still unclear. To address this, the number of all cells outside clonogenic colonies (i.e., cells in abortive colonies or other nonclonogenic cells) was counted. Then, the changes in CPD of the whole population were reasonably evaluated (Figure 6C), such that CPD in sham-irradiated controls that actually increased after 14 days (>4) was not so different from that assumed given a population doubling of 66.6 h (<5). As a whole population, a replicative lifespan (~17.1 CPD) was not exceeded irrespective of dose, and irradiation reduced population doublings. The CPD for HLEC1 was less reduced at high dose due to cellular proliferation in clonogenic colonies than WI-38 cells (Figure 6C), and this led to changes in the shape of the survival curve for HLEC1 (Figure 7).

Discussion

Here we have carried out the colony formation assay of two primary normal human diploid female fetal cell strains: HLEC1 lens epithelial cells and WI-38 lung fibroblasts. HLEC1 had the lower plating efficiency than WI-38, but a difference in the clonogenic survival (colony number-based survival) between two strains was insignificant (Figure 3), indicating that the same dose inactivates the same fraction of clonogenic cells in both strains. For WI-38, the fraction and size of clonogenic colonies declined with dose to a parental cell (Figures 5A and S5), and a difference between the colony number-based survival and the cell number-based survival was insignificant (Figure 7). These findings conform to the general principle of the colony formation assay [12] and are also consistent with our previous findings obtained with AG01522D primary normal human diploid male nonfatal foreskin fibroblasts [16,17,18]. Intriguingly, however, the reverse held true for HLEC1. The area of clonogenic colonies and its cell numbers escalated significantly at ≥2 Gy (Figures 5A and 6A), and the "large" colonies explained nearly one-third of all clonogenic colonies at 4 and 6 Gy (Figure 5B). It is evident from these findings that irradiation stimulates the proliferation of surviving uninactivated clonogenic cells. Findings obtained with HLEC1 are discussed in more detail below.

The Results of Cell Numbers and PDN may be Underestimated

The colony formation assay is unable to exactly determine cell numbers, the temporal kinetics of cell divisions, and the doubling number of individual cells. This is not only because some cells are lost while cells are washed, fixed and stained after colony formation, but also because the assay does not provide the information on the timing of each event (e.g., death and proliferation) that occurs during colony formation. Cells to be lost should consist of spontaneously occurring "nonattached" cells, and radiation-induced detached/floating cells due to death, inactivation and/or mitosis of irradiated cells and their progeny cells. Of these, spontaneous cell loss should partly be reflected in

Table 1. Karyotype.

	Cell types	
	HLEC1	WI-38
CPD at the time of analysis	14.5	44.7
Number of metaphases analyzed	52	66
Number of chromomosomes/cell	46	46

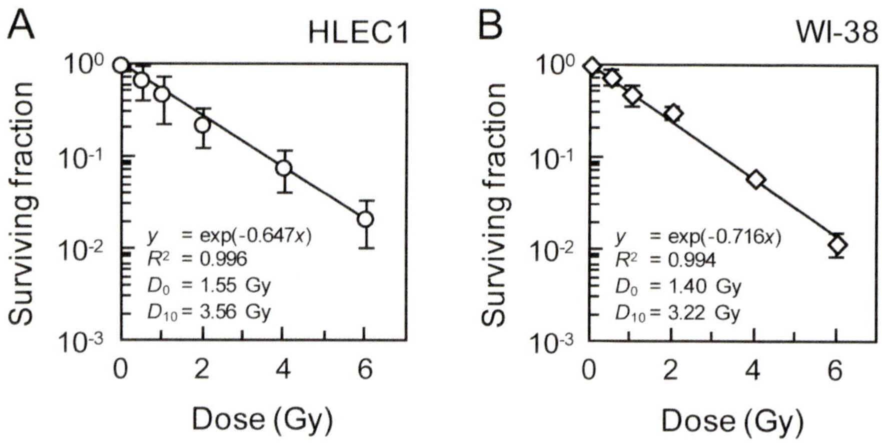

Figure 3. Clonogenic survival of HLEC1 (A) and WI-38 (B). Within 1 h after exposure to indicated dose of X-rays at a dose rate of 0.43±0.01 Gy/min, cells were reinoculated for colony formation and incubated for 14 days at which time they were fixed and stained. At the time of reinoculation, CPD of HLEC1 and WI-38 was 11.0 and 32.0, respectively (n.b., CPD 11.0 was experimentally available youngest HLEC1 in our hand). The plating efficiency of HLEC1 and WI-38 was 1.6±0.6 and 19.5±3.6%, respectively. Curves were fitted to the exponential equation $y = \exp(-kx)$, and D_0 and D_{10} were calculated as $1/k$ and $[\ln(1/0.1)]/k$, respectively. R^2, correlation coefficient square. The data are presented as means and SD of three independent experiments with quadruplicate measurements.

the plating efficiency, but radiation-induced cell loss should rise with dose. Pertinently, PDN was calculated by transformation of the relative cell numbers (e.g., cell numbers at days 0 versus 14) to the base-2 logarithm. However, the kinetics of cells with *n* divisions should not always obey the *n*-th power of 2, and should be more complicated such as by delayed reproductive death that occurs dose dependently and explained by a branching process model [16,17,18,19]. Accordingly, these should cause underestimation of cell numbers, PDN and individual cell divisions at high dose. In other words, it seems likely that compared with the present results, cells experienced more divisions and colonies contained more cells when parental cells received high dose.

The computerized video time-lapse analysis may overcome limitations of the colony formation assay such as those just discussed above, but still has difficulty in tracing the fate of all cells during the entire colony formation process (e.g., due to limited

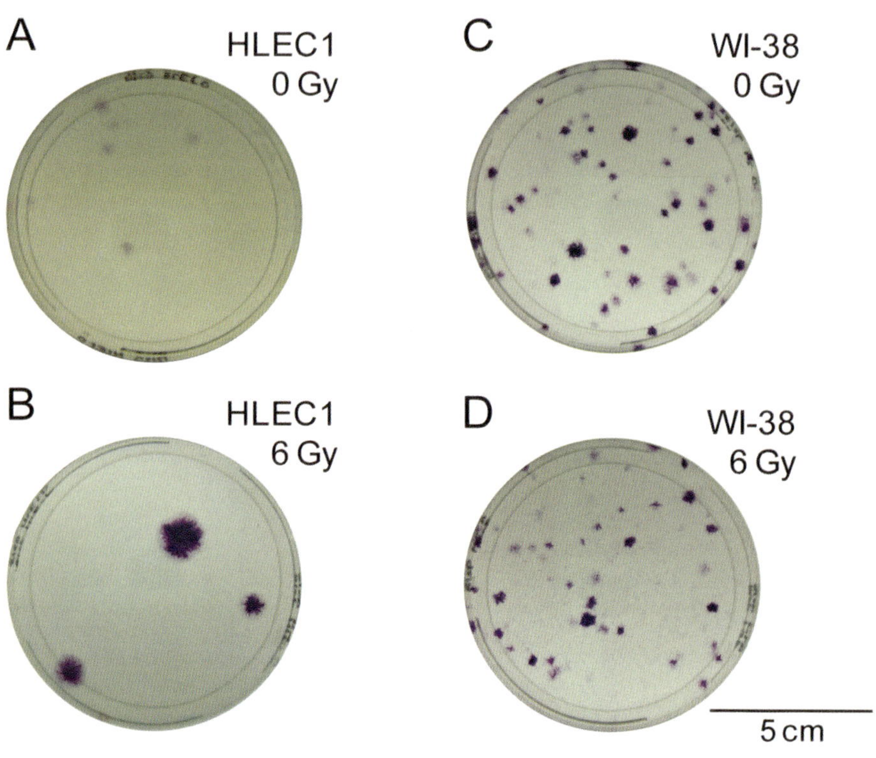

Figure 4. Representative images of colonies arising from sham-irradiated HLEC1 (A), 6 Gy-irradiated HLEC1 (B), sham-irradiated WI-38 (C), and 6 Gy-irradiated WI-38 (D). Shown are colonies that were formed during 14 days in 10-cm dishes and stained with crystal violet. Bar, 5 cm.

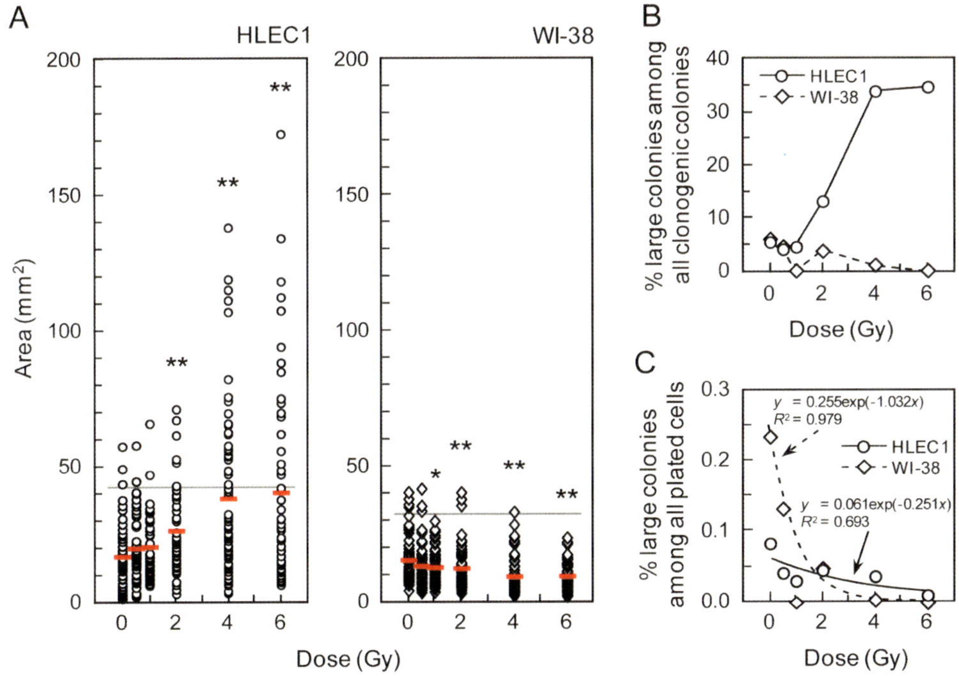

Figure 5. The area of clonogenic colonies. (A) The area distribution of clonogenic colonies arising from HLEC1 (left panel) and WI-38 (right panel) as a function of dose. The area of clonogenic colonies (45–68 colonies for HLEC1 and 54–93 colonies for WI-38 per dose point) was measured as described in Figure S1. Red bars indicate the means at each dose point. The horizontal lines indicate the mean+2SD area in sham-irradiated controls (41.7 mm^2 for HLEC1 and 31.7 mm^2 for WI-38). *$0.01 \leq p < 0.05$ and **$p < 0.01$ compared with sham-irradiated controls. See Figure S2 for the frequency distribution replotted as a function of the area. (B) The fraction of clonogenic colonies exceeding the mean+2SD area of sham-irradiated controls among all clonogenic colonies analyzed. (C) The fraction of clonogenic colonies exceeding the mean+2SD area of sham-irradiated controls among all plated cells. Curves were fitted to the exponential equation, though the data points for 1 Gy and 6 Gy for WI-38 were excluded because of zero values. R^2, correlation coefficient square. When the intercept of the exponential curve for WI-38 was changed from 0.255 to 1, its slope changed from 1.032 to 0.716, and changed from 0.979 to 0.994. For Figure 5B and 5C, circles with solid lines and diamonds with dotted lines indicate the data for HLEC1 and WI-38, respectively.

capacity and occasional cell loss from the field of view [20]). This awaits further development of a time-lapse analysis system, but the colony formation assay would serve as a feasible and easy technique to know the fate of irradiated cells and their descendants.

Stimulated Proliferation Should be Regarded as Excessive Rather than Compensatory

Irradiation increased PDN of the clonogenic cell population during 14 days (e.g., 2.6 population doublings at 6 Gy additional to 0 Gy, Figure 6B). The most pronounced clone with 15.8 doublings at 6 Gy was estimated to have a doubling time of 21.0 h given a constant growth rate during 14 days (c.f., the population doubling time of 66.6 h presented in Figure 2). As a whole, CPD of the whole cell population (nonclonogenic plus clonogenic cells) during colony formation did not exceed the replicative lifespan of ~CPD 17.1 (Figures 2 and 6C). The CPD of the irradiated population was less than the unirradiated control, but would have been even more reduced if surviving uninactivated cells had not been stimulated to divide (Figure 6C). In general, such stimulated proliferation may act as a homeostatic, preventive mechanism to compensate for cell loss, but this should not be the case for the lens. This is because the lens is a closed system inside which all live and dead cells stay throughout life. Namely, not only cells in clonogenic colonies but also all of other cells (e.g., cells in abortive colonies, and detached cells) observed in our *in vitro* system would not go outside the lens *in vivo*, though its accurate numerical data cannot be obtained as discussed above. Thus, the stimulated proliferation of the lens epithelial cells should be regarded as the abnormal, excessive proliferation.

Incidentally, the clonogenic survival of HLEC1 and WI-38 did not differ significantly, when a general criterion of 50 cells was used to define survivors (Figure 3). For WI-38, this survival was commensurate with the survival for which a criterion of the mean plus 2SD area was used (Figure 5C) as well as with the cell number-based survival (Figure 7). This is somewhat reminiscent of our previous result with AG01522D that the survival does not much vary when a criterion of 10 to 100 cells was used [18]. For HLEC1, however, these curves looked different (Figures 5C and 7) because of the stimulated proliferation, so that a general criterion of 50 cells should be used.

What is the Potential Etiological Significance of the Excessive Proliferation?

Lens epithelial cells in the germinative zone of the lens epithelium around the equator divide [2]. Rodent cataracts have been reported to occur after the equatorial region was locally irradiated [21], but not after irradiation when the germinative zone was shielded [22,23,24], indicating that cells in the germinative zone are the relevant cells at risk. To our knowledge, only a few papers [25,26,27] reported the radiation-induced excessive proliferation of lens epithelial cells, ahead of this work Dating back to the 1950s, von Sallman et al. observed that excessive proliferation of lens epithelial cells in the germinative zone within 21 days after X-irradiation of the rabbit eye occurred slightly at 125 r, became evident at 250 r and more manifested at

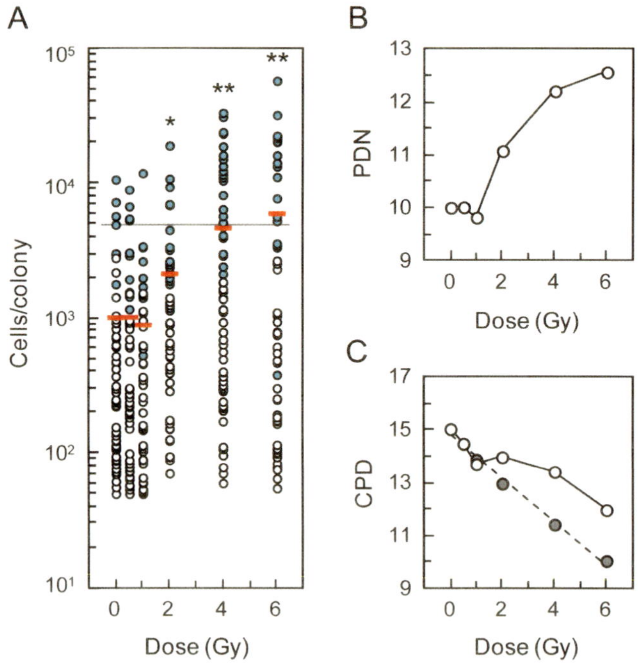

Figure 6. Changes in population doublings of HLEC1. (A) Cell numbers in individual clonogenic colonies. Cell numbers in 218 countable clonogenic colonies (open circles) were directly counted under the stereomicroscope, and those in 99 uncountable colonies (blue-filled circles) were estimated as described in Figures S4, S5 and S6. Red bars indicate the means at each dose point. A horizontal line indicates the mean+2SD value (4,944 cells) in sham-irradiated controls. $^*0.01 \leq p < 0.05$ and $^{**}p < 0.01$ compared with sham-irradiated controls. (B) PDN of clonogenic cells experienced during colony formation. To calculate PDN, cell numbers in individual clonogenic colonies (shown in Figure 6A) were summed, divided by the number of clonogenic colonies (i.e., the number of clonogenic cells plated), and then transformed to the logarithm to base 2. (C) CPD of all cells in the whole population. For calculation of the data, cell numbers in clonogenic colonies (shown in Figure 6A) were first summed. Second, the number of all cells situated outside clonogenic colonies (i.e., cells in abortive colonies or other nonclonogenic cells) was directly counted under the stereomicroscope and summed. Third, the sum of these cell numbers was divided by the number of plated cells, and transformed to the base-2 logarithm. Finally, 11.0 (CPD when plated) was added to these numbers, and shown as open circles with a solid line. Gray-filled circles with a dotted line represent CPD of all cells calculated assuming that irradiation does not alter the proliferation of clonogenic cells (i.e., PDN of irradiated clonogenic cells is the same as PDN of sham-irradiated controls regardless of dose).

higher dose (tested up to 2,000 r) [26]. Likewise, Pirie and observed overshoot of mitosis, which was maximal at 3–4 weeks and returned to a control level at 6–8 weeks after irradiation of the rabbit eye with 1400 r or 1600 r of X-rays [27]. Whereas they studied rabbit lens *in vivo*, we used HELC1 human cells *in vitro* where the microenvironment of their *in vitro* growth system for studying the HLEC1 radiation response may not necessarily mimic the normal growth signaling milieu of migrating lens epithelial cells within the capsule *in vivo*. Despite such great difference in experimental approaches, the findings obtained were surprisingly consistent especially in terms of dose range, considering that 1 Gy roughly equals 100 r. Taken together, there is evidence that inhibition of lens epithelial cell divisions prevents the occurrence of radiogenic cataracts in frogs and rats [28,29,30], showing that dividing lens epithelial cells are the target of radiation cataracts. All together, these findings suggest that excessive proliferation of lens epithelial cells in the germinative zone underlies radiation cataractogenesis, and highlight that our *in vitro* model system will be useful to evaluate the excessive proliferation of primary normal human lens epithelial cells.

Cell divisions should vary temporally with dose and among clones to produce a clonogenic colony with the same cell number (e.g., one cell grows constantly in 14 days, another cell grows fast only in the first few days, and the other cell grows fast only in the last few days), but the colony formation assay does not provide such information as discussed above. The only available pertinent information comes again from von Sallman et al. [26] who documented that following exposure to 250 or 500 r, mitotic cell counts returned to control level at day 5 and thereafter remain excessive at least up to day 21 [26].

What is the Nature of Surviving Uninactivated Radioresistant Cells of which Proliferation is Stimulated by Irradiation?

The curve for the fraction of large colonies among all plated cells looked much flatter than the case for WI-38 (Figures 5C and S3), implying that the cells whose proliferation is stimulated by irradiation exist in the population at a similar rate independent of dose. Such surviving uninactivated cells should certainly be radioresistant, but its nature and whether such cells in the irradiated population originate from clonogenic cells or from nonclonogenic cells in the sham-irradiated population are unknown. Nevertheless, if the latter is the case, it is tempting to speculate that a candidate might be slow cycling radioresistant tissue stem or progenitor cells that become rapidly cycling stem cells or give rise to other cell types upon irradiation. There is evidence for such phenomena in highly regenerative tissues like the intestine [31] and for radiation-induced proliferation of intestinal stem cells [32]. In this regard, lens stem cells remain unidentified, but its putative slow cycling stem cells have been reported to locate around the germinative zone of the lens epithelium [33]. Future studies should characterize the nature of lens stem cells and surviving uninactivated radioresistant cells.

Due to the limited number of HLEC1 available for experiments, this study employed the low plating density before irradiation, but this does not duplicate the conditions of the lens epithelium *in vivo* where cells are in close contact. Given that radiation responses depend on cell density in various cell types, it would be important to test if plating density at the time of irradiation affects the phenomena observed here.

Generally, depending on cell cycle phases at the time of irradiation, irradiation with the higher dose causes more prolonged cell cycle arrest and cell death. In contrast, for the radiogenic excessive proliferation, cell cycling may become faster at higher dose (e.g., by shortening G1 and/or G2 phases). Thus, further studies should address how radiation responses of synchronized cells and non-synchronized cells are different, and determine which cell cycle phase is most susceptible for the radiogenic excessive proliferation.

What are the Implications of the Excessive Proliferation?

Radiation cataract is a typical tissue reaction with a dose threshold below which no effect would occur [6]. This belief has prevailed since 1969 [34], but has been challenged by mounting epidemiological evidence documenting no threshold [6,8]. This necessitates the elucidation of biological mechanisms. In this respect, it would be important to consider different underlying etiologies, as Worgul et al. mentioned earlier that though the reason for the varying response of epithelial cells to different doses

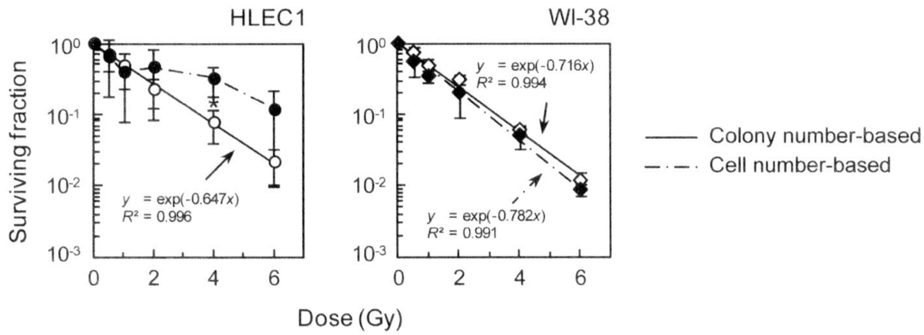

Figure 7. The impact of cell numbers in clonogenic colonies on the surviving fraction in HLEC1 (left panel) and WI-38 (right panel). The general "colony number-based" surviving fraction was calculated from the number of clonogenic colonies divided by the number of plated cells with correction for the plated efficiency. This was compared here with the "cell number-based" surviving fraction that was calculated as the sum of the integrated density of clonogenic colonies (i.e., cell numbers in clonogenic colonies given a linear relationship between the integrated density and cell numbers in each clonogenic colony) divided by the number of plated cells with correction for that at 0 Gy. Colony number-based survival curves (open symbols with solid lines) were taken from Figure 3, and the data of the integrated density of clonogenic colonies presented in Figure S5 were used to obtain cell number-based curves (closed symbols with dotted lines). The data represent means and SD of three independent experiments with quadruplicate measurements. *$0.01 \leq p < 0.05$ compared between two types of survival curves at each dose. For WI-38, the difference between the colony number-based survival curve and the cell number-based survival curve was insignificant for all 5 dose points tested ($p > 0.10$), indicating that the colony number-based survival fraction is akin to the cell number-based one. For HLEC1, the difference between two types of survival curves reached a statistical significance only at 4 Gy ($p = 0.02$), but there was clearly a tendency toward the increased surviving fraction at 2 Gy and 6 Gy.

is unknown, it is possible that the production of radiation cataract may involve more than one mechanism [35]. Human radiation cataracts are typical late effects that reportedly take a few months to decades to appear [36,37]. Common radiogenic cataracts are PSC cataracts, but cortical cataracts have also been associated with radiation exposure [38,39]. It should be pointed out that whereas a latency period of PSC cataracts greatly varies from months to decades, cortical cataracts only appear many years after exposure. For instance, it was in 2004 that the first description of cortical cataracts in atomic bomb survivors of Hiroshima and Nagasaki emerged [40]. This suggests the different mechanisms for production of early onset cataracts (e.g., PSC cataracts taking months to years to appear) and late onset cataracts (e.g., PSC and cortical cataracts taking years to decades to appear). Early onset cataracts may be accounted for, at least in part, by the excessive proliferation such that whereas complete loss of organelles during lens fiber cell terminal differentiation is responsible for lens transparency [41], excessive proliferation may cause meridional row disorganization (the known essential event associated with cataract severity) and force undifferentiated epithelioid cells to move posteriorly before organelle loss, which may eventuate in PSC opacification [2,42]. The excessive proliferation of HLEC1 cells observed here was significant at ≥2 Gy (Figures 5A and 6A), and this passably resembles the acute threshold of 0.5–2 Gy for detectable lens opacities and 2–10 Sv for vision-impairing cataracts that ICRP recommended for almost two decades before 2011 [43,44]. A threshold for early onset cataracts thus sounds biologically plausible. Considering that the lens is a closed system, cells that constitute opacities should not be limited to excessively proliferated cells and its progeny cells, and may include inactivated cells and dead cells. Figure S7 demonstrates that unlike the case for AG01522D fibroblasts where the frequency of abortive colonies rises with dose [16], the frequency of abortive colonies does not much alter at ≤2 Gy and greatly declined (colonies with 8–15 cells disappeared) at 4 and 6 Gy (n.b., due to the different radiosensitivities, the survival at 2 and 6 Gy in HLEC1 roughly corresponds to that at 4 and 8 Gy in AG01522D, respectively). This suggests that irradiated HLEC1 cells except for surviving uninactivated radioresistant cells are relatively "quiet" (dormant, quiescent or slow cycling) because of high sensitivity to radiation-induced inactivation and cell death (e.g., via premature senescence, apoptosis, necrosis and autophagy [45] for which further analysis is under way), and/or because of nonpermanent albeit very long term cell cycle arrest. Such inactivated cells may also move posteriorly (but slower than excessively proliferated cells) contributing to late onset cataract. Descendent cells arising from irradiated cells (e.g., uninactivated cells or very slowly recovered cells, including stem or progenitor cells) may contribute to late onset cataracts. If abnormal cells arising from damaged single cells form cataracts, then no threshold for cataracts may sound biologically plausible. Pertinent to this, a recent report highlights that a lens progenitor-like cell differentiated from human embryonic stem cells generates a lentoid body [46], warranting further extensive studies to test if an irradiated single lens stem cell forms a cloudy lentoid body.

The lens with progressive PSC cataract is smaller in size than that with stationary PSC cataract for the subject's age (n.b., the analysis included all kinds of etiological agents that induce PSC cataract) [47], further corroborating the key role of cell proliferation in radiation cataractogenesis. One might assume that progressive PSC cataract would have more proliferation than stationary PSC cataract, but the reverse may be true considering the data in Figure 6C where the CPD was reduced even when the excessive proliferation occurred.

There have been no established mitigators for radiogenic cataracts [6], but this situation may be improved if the mechanisms behind the radiation-induced excessive proliferation are revealed. In this light, it should be noted that although primary tumors of the human lens are not known, yet spontaneous cataractogenesis seems to involve a variety of tumor suppressor genes and DNA repair genes (e.g., p53, $p16^{Ink4a}$, $p19^{Arf}$ or $p14^{Arf}$, $p27^{Kip1}$, ATM, RAD9, BRCA1, NBS1, WRN, XRCC1 and HSF4) [1,8]. These molecules may be candidate contributors as many of them are also key players in cell cycle checkpoints and general radiation responses. Furthermore, evidence is available that p53 prevents spontaneous PSC cataract formation by suppression of cellular proliferation in mice [2]. Taken together, a recent study has documented that p53 delays while p21 drives spontaneous cataractogenesis in BubR1 progeroid mice [48]. Thus, it would be worth testing if enhancement of p53 function suppresses radiation-induced excessive proliferation *in vitro* using our system, followed by *in vivo* testing [2,8].

Conclusions

This study is the first to report the clonogenic survival of lens epithelial cells exposed to ionizing radiation, which was evaluated with the colony formation assay. The data clearly showed that irradiation not merely inactivates clonogenic potential dose dependently but even stimulates the proliferation of HLEC1 primary normal human diploid lens epithelial cells. Lines of *in vivo* evidence support the possibility that such excessive proliferation may be one of the mechanisms underpinning radiation cataractogenesis. In contrast to the case for surviving uninactivated radioresistant clonogenic cells that underwent excessive proliferation, irradiated nonclonogenic cells seemed quiet because of high radiosensitivity to inactivation and cell death, and/or because of nonpermanent yet very long term cell cycle arrest. Such on-off behavior of irradiated HLEC1 cells (i.e., to be stimulated to divide or contrarily to be inactivated) appears very unique. Though whether our present findings obtained with HLEC1 can be generalized in primary human diploid lens epithelial cells from different donors needs to be further clarified, our *in vitro* system would surely be invaluable to evaluate manifestations and mechanisms of such unique behavior of primary human diploid lens epithelial cells. A question of why cataractogenic potential of neutrons and heavy ions is very high remains fully open despite significant relevance to radiation protection, radiation therapy and space missions [3], and our *in vitro* system may help answer this fascinating question.

Supporting Information

Figure S1 Methods used to choose clonogenic colonies for the analysis and evaluate its area.

Figure S2 The frequency distribution of area of clonogenic colonies arising from HLEC1 and WI-38.

Figure S3 The fraction of clonogenic colonies exceeding the mean+2SD area of sham-irradiated controls among all plated cells.

Figure S4 Methods used to evaluate cell numbers in each clonogenic colony arising from HLEC1.

Figure S5 The integrated density of clonogenic colonies arising from HLEC1 and WI-38.

Figure S6 The relationship between the integrated density and cell numbers in all countable clonogenic colonies arising from HLEC1.

Figure S7 Alterations in the distribution of colonies in HLEC1 and AG01522D.

Table S1 Number of cells replated per 10-cm dish after irradiation for colony formation.

Acknowledgments

The authors are grateful to Dr Motohiro Yamauchi (Nagasaki Univ., Japan) for technical assistance with the chromosome analysis. Thanks are also due to Dr Toshiso Kosako (Univ. of Tokyo, Japan) for discussion.

Author Contributions

Conceived and designed the experiments: NH. Performed the experiments: NH YF. Analyzed the data: YF NH. Contributed reagents/materials/analysis tools: NH YF. Wrote the paper: NH.

References

1. Graw J (2009) Mouse models of cataract. J Genet 88: 469–486.
2. Wiley LA, Rajagopal R, Dattilo LK, Beebe DC (2011) The tumor suppressor gene *Trp53* protects the mouse lens against posterior subcapsular cataracts and the BMP receptor Acvr1 acts as a tumor suppressor in the lens. Dis Model Mech 4: 484–495.
3. Hamada N (2014) What are the intracellular targets and intratissue target cells for radiation effects? Radiat Res 181: 9–20.
4. ICRP (2007) The 2007 Recommendations of the International Commission on Radiological Protection. ICRP Publication 103. Ann ICRP 37(2–4): 1–332.
5. ICRP (1955) Recommendations of the International Commission on Radiological Protection. Br J Radiol (Suppl. 6): 1–92.
6. ICRP (2012) ICRP Statement on tissue reactions/Early and late effects of radiation in normal tissues and organs – threshold doses for tissue reactions in a radiation protection context. ICRP Publication 118. Ann ICRP 41(1/2): 1–322.
7. ICRP (1980) Statement and recommendations of the International Commission on Radiological Protection from its 1980 meeting. Br J Radiol 53: 816–818.
8. Hamada N, Fujimichi Y, Iwasaki T, Fujii N, Furuhashi M, et al. (2014) Emerging issues in radiogenic cataracts and cardiovascular disease. J Radiat Res 55: in press (doi:10.1093/jrr/rru036).
9. Emami B, Lyman J, Brown A, Coia L, Goitein M, et al. (1991) Tolerance of normal tissue to therapeutic irradiation. Int J Radiat Oncol Biol Phys 21: 109–122.
10. Osman IM, Abouzeid H, Balmer A, Gaillard MC, Othenin-Girard P, et al. (2011) Modern cataract surgery for radiation-induced cataracts in retinoblastoma. Br J Ophthalmol 95: 227–230.
11. Cucinotta FA, Schimmerling W, Wilson JW, Peterson LE, Badhwar GD, et al. (2001) Space radiation cancer risks and uncertainties for Mars missions. Radiat Res 156: 682–688.
12. Puck TT, Marcus PI (1956) Action of x-rays on mammalian cells. J Exp Med 103: 653–666.
13. Hayflick L (1965) The limited *in vitro* lifetime of human diploid cell strains. Exp Cell Res 37: 614–636.
14. Wadman M (2013) Medical research: cell division. Nature 498: 422–426.
15. Hayflick L, Moorhead PS (1961) The serial cultivation of human diploid cell strains. Exp Cell Res 25: 585–621.
16. Hamada N, Hara T, Funayama T, Sakashita T, Kobayashi Y (2008) Energetic heavy ions accelerate differentiation in the descendants of irradiated normal human diploid fibroblasts. Mutat Res 637: 190–196.
17. Sakashita T, Hamada N, Kawaguchi I, Ouchi NB, Hara T, et al. (2013) A framework for analysis of abortive colony size distributions using a model of branching processes in irradiated normal human fibroblasts. PLoS ONE 8: e70291.
18. Sakashita T, Hamada N, Kawaguchi I, Hara T, Kobayashi Y, et al. (2014) A branching process model for the analysis of abortive colony size distributions in carbon ion-irradiated normal human fibroblasts. J Radiat Res 55: in press (doi:10.1093/jrr/rrt129).
19. Hamada N, Funayama T, Wada S, Sakashita T, Kakizaki T, et al. (2006) LET-dependent survival of irradiated normal human fibroblasts and their descendents. Radiat Res 166: 24–30.
20. Endlich B, Radford IR, Forrester HB, Dewey WC (2000) Computerized video time-lapse microscopy studies of ionizing radiation-induced rapid-interphase and mitosis-related apoptosis in lymphoid cells. Radiat Res 153: 36–48.
21. Goldmann H, Liechti A (1938) Experimentelle untersuchungen über die genese des röntgenstars. Albrecht von Graefes Arch Ophthalmol 138: 722–736.
22. Alter AJ, Leinfelder PJ (1953) Roentgen-ray cataract. Effects of shielding of the lens and ciliary body. Arch Ophthalmol 49: 257–260.
23. Leinfelder PJ, Riley EF (1956) Further studies of effects of x-radiation on partially shielded lens of rabbit. Arch Ophthalmol 55: 84–86.
24. Pirie A, Flanders PH (1957) Effect of X-rays on partially shielded lens of the rabbit. Arch Ophthalmol 57: 849–854.
25. von Sallmann L, Munoz CM, Drungis A (1953) Effects of β irradiation on the rabbit lens. Arch Ophthalmol 50: 727–736.
26. von Sallmann L, Tobias CA, Anger HO, Welch C, Kimura SF, et al. (1955) Effects of high-energy particles, X-rays, and aging on lens epithelium. Arch Ophthalmol 54: 489–514.

27. Pirie A, Drance SM (1959) Modification of X-ray damage to the lens by partial shielding. Int J Radiat Biol 1: 293–304.
28. Worgul BV, Rothstein H (1975) Radiation cataract and mitosis. Ophthalmic Res 7: 21–32.
29. Hayden JH, Rothstein H, Worgul BV, Merriam GR Jr (1980) Hypophysectomy exerts a radioprotective effect on frog lens. Experientia 36: 116–118.
30. Rothstein H, Worgul BV, Medvedovsky C, Merriam GR Jr (1982) G_0/G_1 arrest of cell proliferation in the ocular lens prevents development of radiation cataract. Ophthalmic Res 14: 215–220.
31. Montgomery RK, Carlone DL, Richmond CA, Farilla L, Kranendonk ME, et al. (2011) Mouse telomerase reverse transcriptase (mTert) expression marks slowly cycling intestinal stem cells. Proc Natl Acad Sci U S A 108: 179–184.
32. Yamauchi M, Otsuka K, Kondo H, Hamada N, Tomita M, et al. (2014) A novel *in vitro* survival assay of small intestinal stem cells after exposure to ionizing radiation. J Radiat Res 55: 381–390.
33. Oka M, Toyoda C, Kaneko Y, Nakazawa Y, Aizu-Yokota E, Takehana M (2010) Characterization and localization of side population cells in the lens. Mol Vis 16: 945–953.
34. ICRP (1969) Radiosensitivity and spatial distribution of dose. ICRP Publication 14. Oxford: Pergamon Press. 118 p.
35. Worgul BV, Merriam GR, Szechter A, Srinivasan D (1976) Lens epithelium and radiation cataract. I. Preliminary studies. Arch Ophthalmol 94: 996–999.
36. Merriam GR Jr, Focht EF (1957) A clinical study of radiation cataracts and the relationship to dose. Am J Roentgenol 77: 759–785.
37. Neriishi K, Nakashima E, Akahoshi M, Hida A, Grant EJ, et al. (2012) Radiation dose and cataract surgery incidence in atomic bomb survivors, 1986–2005. Radiology 265: 167–174.
38. Nakashima E, Neriishi K, Minamoto A (2006) A reanalysis of atomic-bomb cataract data, 2000–2002: a threshold analysis. Health Phys 90: 154–160.
39. Worgul BV, Kundiyev YI, Sergiyenko NM, Chumak VV, Vitte PM, et al. (2007) Cataracts among Chernobyl clean-up workers: implications regarding permissible eye exposures. Radiat Res 167: 233–243.
40. Minamoto A, Taniguchi H, Yoshitani N, Mukai S, Yokoyama T, et al. (2004) Cataract in atomic bomb survivors. Int J Radiat Biol 80: 339–345.
41. Wride MA (2011) Lens fibre cell differentiation and organelle loss: many paths lead to clarity. Philos Trans R Soc Lond B Biol Sci 366: 1219–1233.
42. von Sallmann L (1950) Experimental studies on early lens changes after X-ray irradiation. Trans Am Ophthalmol Soc 48: 228–242.
43. ICRP (1984) Nonstochastic effects of ionizing radiation. ICRP Publication 41. Ann ICRP 14(3): 1–33.
44. Hamada N, Fujimichi Y (2014) Classification of radiation effects for dose limitation purposes: history, current situation and future prospects. J Radiat Res 55: in press (doi:10.1093/jrr/rru019).
45. Jinno-Oue A, Shimizu N, Hamada N, Wada S, Tanaka A, et al. (2010) Irradiation with carbon ion beams induces apoptosis, autophagy, and cellular senescence in a human glioma-derived cell line. Int J Radiat Oncol Biol Phys 76: 229–241.
46. Yang C, Yang Y, Brennan L, Bouhassira EE, Kantorow M, et al. (2010) Efficient generation of lens progenitor cells and lentoid bodies from human embryonic stem cells in chemically defined conditions. FASEB J 24: 3274–3283.
47. Brown N, Tripathi R (1974) The loss of the anterior sub-capsular clear zone of the lens Prognostic significance in cataract formation. Trans Ophthal Soc UK 94: 29–45.
48. Baker DJ, Weaver RL, van Deursen JM (2013) p21 both attenuates and drives senescence and aging in BubR1 progeroid mice. Cell Rep 3: 1164–1174.

12

The LEGSKO Mouse: A Mouse Model of Age-Related Nuclear Cataract Based on Genetic Suppression of Lens Glutathione Synthesis

Xingjun Fan[1]*, Xiaoqin Liu[1], Shuyu Hao[1], Benlian Wang[2], Michael L. Robinson[3], Vincent M. Monnier[1,4]*

1 Department of Pathology, Case Western Reserve University, Cleveland, Ohio, United States of America, **2** Case Center for Proteomics and Mass Spectrometry, Case Western Reserve University, Cleveland, Ohio, United States of America, **3** Department of Zoology, Miami University, Oxford, Ohio, United States of America, **4** Department of Biochemistry, Case Western Reserve University, Cleveland, Ohio, United States of America

Abstract

Age-related nuclear cataracts are associated with progressive post-synthetic modifications of crystallins from various physical chemical and metabolic insults, of which oxidative stress is a major factor. The latter is normally suppressed by high concentrations of glutathione (GSH), which however are very low in the nucleus of the old lens. Here we generated a mouse model of oxidant stress by knocking out glutathione synthesis in the mouse in the hope of recapitulating some of the changes observed in human age-related nuclear cataract (ARNC). A floxed Gclc mouse was generated and crossed with a transgenic mouse expressing Cre in the lens to generate the LEGSKO mouse in which *de novo* GSH synthesis was completely abolished in the lens. Lens GSH levels were reduced up to 60% in homozygous LEGSKO mice, and a decreasing GSH gradient was noticed from cortical to nuclear region at 4 months of age. Oxidation of crystallin methionine and sulfhydryls into sulfoxides was dramatically increased, but methylglyoxal hydroimidazolones levels that are GSH/glyoxalase dependent were surprisingly normal. Homozygous LEGSKO mice developed nuclear opacities starting at 4 months that progressed into severe nuclear cataract by 9 months. We conclude that the LEGSKO mouse lens mimics several features of human ARNC and is thus expected to be a useful model for the development of anti-cataract agents.

Editor: K. Krishna Sharma, University of Missouri-Columbia, United States of America

Funding: This work was supported by grants EY-07099 to VMM, the Vilma and Robert R. Kohn Biology of Aging Research Fund, and grant P30EY-11373 to the Visual Sciences Research Center at Case Western Reserve University. The funders had no role in study design, data collection and analysis, decision to publish, or preparation of the manuscript.

Competing Interests: The authors have declared that no competing interests exist.

* E-mail: xxf3@cwru.edu (XF); vmm3@case.edu (VMM)

Introduction

Cataract is a leading cause of blindness, accounting for 50% of blindness worldwide [1]. The cumulative incidence of cataract is strongly age-related and ranges from 2% at ages 45–54 years to 45% at ages 75–85 [1], with nuclear cataracts accounting for 30% of all age-related cataracts [2]. Surgical removal of the cataractous lens remains the only therapy, yet the National Eye Institute has estimated that a ten-year delay in the onset of cataract would result in a 50% reduction in the prevalence of cataract [3]. Both lens nuclear opacity and nuclear cataract surgery are associated with increased mortality according to the Beaver Dam Eye Study [1] and the Age-Related Eye Disease Study (AREDS) [4]. Thus, understanding the pathogenesis of age-related nuclear cataracts remains an important goal of vision research that may also provide clues on broader mechanisms of aging.

Age-related cataract is strongly related to the accumulation of damage to its long-lived proteins, the crystallins. Major age-related lens protein modifications include deamidation, deamination, racemization, accumulation of truncation products, accumulation of UV active, fluorescent, and non-UV active protein adducts and crosslinks from glycation, ascorbylation and lipoxidation reactions [5]. Collectively, these modifications contribute toward decreasing protein stability, partly by impairing the chaperone function of α-crystallins, the levels of which decrease with age due to insolubilization [6]. Overall, the aging human lens is constantly exposed to chemical and physical stresses. However, while oxidative damage is subdued during normal aging, it is a major cause or consequence of nuclear cataracts, the most common types of age-related cataracts, whereby the loss of glutathione (GSH) and formation of disulfides are considered to be the key factors in oxidative stress and nuclear cataractogenesis [7].

To protect from oxidation the lens has evolved as an anaerobic system with millimolar concentrations of both glutathione (GSH) and ascorbic acid. However, both protective systems are impaired during aging whereby GSH level significantly declines in the lens nucleus [8,9]. This is in part attributed to lowered γ-glutamyl-cysteine ligase (Gcl) activity [10] and a barrier to GSH diffusion toward the nucleus [9]. As a result ascorbic acid is increasingly oxidized throughout life leading to accelerated accumulation of crystallin-bound advanced glycation end products (AGEs) that contribute to cataractogenesis [11,12,13]. Concomitantly, increased protein residue oxidation is observed, as reflected by the formation of methionine sulfoxide, protein disulfides, kynurenine, and o-tyrosine from methionine, cysteine, tryptophan and phenylalanine, respectively [13,14,15].

In spite of considerable progress in the field, it has been extraordinarily difficult to study the relationship between the protein modifications and carbonyl stress or oxidant stress due to lack of appropriate animal models. One recent model of carbonyl stress developed by us successfully mimics the carbonyl stress component of the aging lens [12]. However, while several models illustrate the role of glutathione for sulfhydryl homeostasis, its role for lens transparency during aging has not been unequivocally established. Indeed most chemically or genetic induced models of disrupted GSH homeostasis only produced opacity in pups or very young animals, with uncertainties as to whether the observed lenticular changes were due to developmental abnormalities or chemical toxicity via pathways unrelated to oxidation itself. For this reason, we set out to genetically lower lenticular glutathione levels specifically in the lens (since the systemic knockout is lethal [16]) by disrupting the catalytic subunit of γ-glutamyl- cysteine ligase (Gclc) using a conditional Cre/LoxP approach. The predicted slow decline in glutathione levels using this approach is hypothesized to mimic the processes underlying the oxidative arm of human ARNC. Below we present the genetic, biochemical and biological phenotypes of resulting from the loss of Gclc function in the lens of the Lens Glutathione Synthesis KnockOut (LEGSKO) mouse.

Results

Conditional Deletion of Gclc Impairs Lens GSH Synthesis

In order to specifically delete Gclc from the lens, we crossed the $Gclc^{fl/fl}$ mice with MRL10-Cre mice [17] that express Cre recombinase in lens epithelia and fibers to ultimately generate mice homozygous for the conditional allele and hemizygous for MLR10 transgene. These mice $Gclc^{-/-}$/$MRL\text{-}10^{+/-}$ are deficient for Gclc specifically in the lens and are, herein named homozygous lens GSH knockout mice (HOM-LEGSKO). Similarly, the $Gclc^{fl/+}$/$MRL\text{-}10^{+/-}$ mice were named heterozygous lens GSH knockout mice (HET-LEGSKO) and should exhibit reduced Gclc levels in the lens. No lens abnormalities have been reported for mice that are hemizygous or homozygous for the MRL10-cre transgene in the absence of floxed alleles [17], and therefore phenotypes manifested in LEGSKO mice were contributed by Gclc deficiency alone. The LEGSKO mice were continuously crossbred with $Gclc^{fl/fl}$ mice (C57BL/6) to convert the genomic background towards C57BL/6. All the data provided in this paper are based on B6/FVB mixed background at third generation bred mice. The same breeding pattern and age matched control mice were used as wild type controls ($Gclc^{fl/fl}$).

LEGSKO mice exhibited reduced expression of Gclc transcripts and protein. HOM-LEGSKO lenses exhibited nearly undetectable levels of Gclc mRNA by real-time PCR, and Gclc transcripts were reduced nearly 50% in HET-LEGSKO lenses compared to wild type lenses (Fig. 1A). The levels of Gclc mRNA and protein were indistinguishable between $Gclc^{fl/fl}$ lenses (without MLR10 transgene) and lenses of wild-type mice (data not shown). The lens Gclc protein expression was completely abolished in HOM-LEGSKO lenses compared to wild type lenses based on western-blot analysis (Fig.1B). This was also confirmed by immunohistochemistry analysis using monoclonal Gclc antibody (data not shown). The deletion of Gclc gene had no impact on glutamate-cysteine ligase, modifier subunit (Gclm) protein level (Fig. 1B). Most importantly, the Gclc activity determined by monobromobimane derivatization and HPLC analysis with fluorescence detection clearly demonstrated no detectable activity in HOM-LEGSKO lenses (Fig.1C). Interestingly, however, there was only 20% reduction of Gclc activity in HET-LEGSKO lenses compared to wild type lenses. HET-LEGSKO lenses had a ~50% reduction of Gclc mRNA (Fig.1A) and 25% lower protein expression (Fig. 1B). The most intriguing finding was that HET-LEGSKO mice lenses maintained quasi-normal GSH level (reduced <10%), while HOM-LEGSKO GSH levels were more than 60% reduced compared to wild type lenses at 3months of age (Fig.1D). These results indicate that compensatory mechanisms might be involved in lens GSH homeostasis, most likely via transporter(s) systems as suggested by others [18]. Moreover, analysis of cortical and nuclear GSH content in the HOM-LEGSKO lenses at 5 months of age (Table 1) revealed a GSH gradient from cortex to nucleus, with over 75% decreased in GSH in the nuclear vs. only a 50% decrease of GSH within the cortical region.

Impact of Suppressed GSH Levels on the Lens: Elevated ROS

The GSSG/GSH ratio, an index of ROS production, was mildly and strongly increased in HET-LESGKO vs. HOM-LEGSKO mice, respectively (Fig. 1E). One of the major protein modifications associated with oxidative stress during human lens aging is methionine sulfoxide (MetSOX), which increases with age and is highly elevated in cataractous lenses, with over 50% of membrane bound protein methionine present in oxidized form [15,19]. LC/MS based methionine sulfoxide determination indicated that the HOM-LEGSKO lenses protein bound methionine oxidation was significantly increased compared to heterozygous and wild type control lenses, and it was also elevated with age as measured at 9 months compared to 3 months of age (Fig. 1F). GSH antioxidative cycle enzymes glutathione reductase (GR) and glutathione peroxidase (GPx) activity were mildly but significantly decreased (Fig. 1G&F). Surprisingly, however, we did not find elevation of protein modification by glycation in HOM-LEGSKO mice (Fig.2), such as carboxymethyl-lysine (CML), carboxyethyl-lysine (CEL), methylglyoxal hydroimidazolone-1 (MG-H1), and glyoxal hydroimidazolone-1 (G-H1), which are known to positively correlate with aging in the human lens [20,21]. An explanation for this finding is provided in the Discussion.

As the 40% reduction of GSH in the cortical region was predicted to increase oxidative stress, we investigated ROS production in living lenses ex vivo. Freshly isolated 6 months old HOM-LEGSKO and age matched control lenses were stained vitally with dihydrorhodamine 123 (DHR), a reactive oxygen species marker, and co-stained DNA with Hoechst 33342 to mark lens cell nuclei. Fluorescence (green) of DHR indicated much stronger ROS also present at cortical region of HOM-LEGSKO lens vs. age matched control lens (Fig.3).

Impact of Suppressed GSH Levels on Lens Transparency

About 20% of the homozygous mice developed nuclear opacification starting at 3 months of age based on the sensitivity of Slit-lamp detection, which progressed into severe nuclear cataract at 9 months age. In this report, we define opacity as a white area the size of at least 0.3 micrometer diameter. A typical cataract image (Fig. 4A) shows the same lens at 4 and 9 months of age, whereby the nuclear cataract was found to progress from a small opacity at 4 months to severe nuclear cataract at 9 months. The LEGSKO lenses have relative similar size and weight compared to wild type lenses. The GSH level in the lens nucleus was barely detectable and GSH level in the lens cortex dropped over 60% compared to age matched wild type lenses (Table 1).

The kinetics of the cataract formation was assessed quantitatively using Slit-lamp (Fig. 4B). 50% of HOM-LEGSKO mice had mature cataracts by 4 months compared to age matched wild type mice.

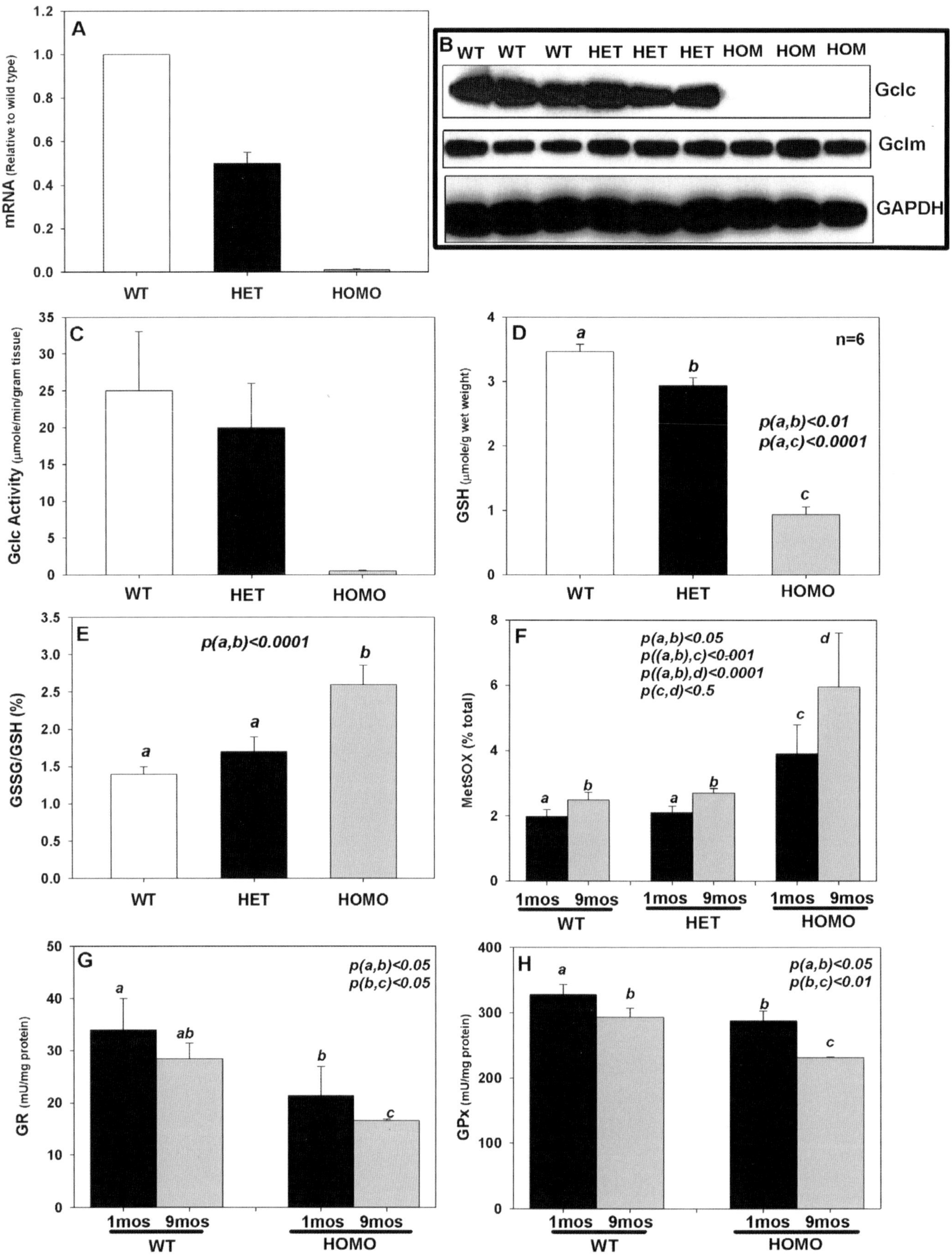
A
mRNA (Relative to wild type)
WT
HET
HOMO
B
WT WT WT HET HET HET HOM HOM HOM
Gclc
Gclm
GAPDH
C
Gclc Activity (μmole/min/gram tissue)
D
GSH (μmole/g wet weight)
n=6
p(a,b)<0.01
p(a,c)<0.0001
E
GSSG/GSH (%)
p(a,b)<0.0001
F
MetSOX (% total)
p(a,b)<0.05
p((a,b),c)<0.001
p((a,b),d)<0.0001
p(c,d)<0.5
1mos 9mos
G
GR (mU/mg protein)
p(a,b)<0.05
p(b,c)<0.05
H
GPx (mU/mg protein)
p(a,b)<0.05
p(b,c)<0.01

Figure 1. Charaterization of the GSH genotype and phenotype of LEGSKO mouse. 3mos old LEGSKO mouse lens (without cataract) total RNA was extracted and Gclc mRNA was determined by real-time PCR. The data was calculated relative to age matched wild type lenses. Gclc enzyme activity was determined by HPLC by monobromobimane fluorescent derivatization. Gclc protein expression was determined by Western-blot. (A). Gclc mRNA was reduced 50% in heterozygous mouse lenses and completely abolished in homozygous mouse lenses (n = 6). (B). Gclc protein level was reduced in heterozygous mouse lenses and abolished in homozygous lenses. Mouse liver protein extract was used as positive control. (C). Gclc activity was mildly reduced in heterozygous mouse lenses and quasi no detectable in homozygous mouse lenses (n = 6). (D). Fresh lenses (n = 6) were snap frozen, thaw at room temperature for 1 min and dissected immediately. The protein was precipitated, and the supernatant was subjected to GSH analysis by glutathione reductase (GR) and β-NADPH enzymatic recycling method. (E). the percentage of GSSG vs. GSH was significantly ($p<0.0001$) elevated in homozygous mouse lenses vs. wild type/heterozygous lenses. (F). Methionine sulfoxide was significantly ($p<0.001$) elevated in homozygous vs. wild type/heterozygous lenses, and also significantly increased with age ($P<0.05$). (G). Glutathione reductase (GR) activity, expressed as unit per milligram of protein, was mildly but significantly ($P<0.01$) reduced in homozygous lenses vs. wild type, and also significantly reduced with age. (H). Glutathione peroxidase (GPx) activity, expressed as unit per milligram of protein was mildly but significantly reduced in homozygous lens at 9 months old of age ($p<0.05$). One-Way ANOVA followed by Post-Hoc analysis was used for all comparisons (n = 10, per group, except GSSG/GSH which is 6 per group).

Discussion

This study shows that genetic suppression of lenticular glutathione synthesis generates phenotypic protein and GSH homeostatic changes that closely resemble those present in the nuclear region of the aging human lens, including cataractogenesis. Several authors have previously contributed to this paradigm by demonstrating that e.g. gamma-glutamyl transpeptidase deficient mice develop nuclear opacities at 1 week secondary to cysteine deficiency [22], or that treatment with buthionine sulfoxide (BSO) results in lowered GSH levels and cataract in newborn rats [23] and very young mice [24]· Vice-versa, oxidative stress from hyperbaric oxygen duplicates many changes observed in the aging human lens [25]. Knocking out glutathione peroxidase (GPX-1) in mice leads to cataract formation [26], whereby changes in lens epithelial cell morphology and DNA breaks were also found under oxidant stress generated by either hydrogen peroxide (H_2O_2) treatment or GPX-1 null condition [27]. Lens cells behave similarly when glutathione reductase or glutathioredoxin 2 synthesis have been knocked out [28,29]. Interestingly, in mouse lenses, free GSH detoxifies more H_2O_2 (54% to 72%) than GPX-1 (15%) or catalase (30%) [30].

In old or cataractous human lens there is a GSH gradient from the cortical to the nuclear region [8]. Truscott et al [9] proposed that a diffusion barrier forms with age, and therefore is an impediment for GSH diffusion. The data from LEGSKO mouse lenses confirm the presence of this gradient with non-detectable GSH in the nucleus of cataractous lenses. These data suggest that a barrier may also form in mouse lenses, and that impaired GSH synthesis is in part responsible for the gradient. Takemoto et al [31] discovered that crystallins were involved in inter-disulfide cross-linking with membrane, and tight binding of protein to the membrane has been proposed as a potential mechanisms of barrier formation in aged human lenses [32]. In human, lens nucleus enriched crystallins, such as gamma crystallins, have large numbers of free cysteine residues (i.e. 8 cys in human gamma C) compared to alpha crystallin, which only have two cysteine residues. These cysteine residues are maintained in either free form or as intramolecular disulfides to maintain crystallin protein stability in young and normal lenses. However, during aging, with elevated oxidation from reduced GSH level, these cysteine residues are oxidized and form intermolecular disulfide crosslinks. Such transition may impact on crystallin stability, and may cause crystallin unfolding and formation of aggregates with other proteins. Studies will be needed to elucidate the fundamental nature of the protein changes under reduced GSH levels. Because the LEGSKO mouse lenses are too young to accumulate other modifications than those resulting from oxidation, and because these mice are free of diabetes, it will be possible to selectively study the consequences of protein oxidation for protein aggregation.

It has been suggested that maintenance of a threshold of GSH concentration above 1 mM in human lens nucleus was critical for keeping the lens transparent [9,33]. This may explain the rapid cataract rate of LEGSKO mice at 9mos, since nuclear GSH is in much lower level i.e. 0.5 mM). In addition, ascorbic acid oxidation may play a key role in crystallin damage in the human lens nucleus when the GSH level drops below a certain threshold. In contrast, the mouse lens has barely detectable ascorbic acid [12]. Furthermore, we found elevated oxidation in the cortical region of LEGSKO lenses compared to wild type lenses, but we did not observe opacity in cortex at 9mos of LEGSKO mice. Thus it remains to be seen if cortical cataract will also form with age.

Another important function of GSH is the detoxification of the oxoaldehydes glyoxal and methylglyoxal, the latter being one of the most important sources of protein damage in aging and

Table 1. GSH and GSSG level (n = 6).

Genotype	Age (wks)	GSH (μmole/g wet weight)		GSSG(μmole/g wet weight)	
		Cortical	Nucleus	Cortical	Nucleus
WT	4	3.23±0.23	3.07±0.21	0.031±0.005	0.03±0.006
LEGSKO	4	1.62±0.18	1.46±0.10	0.027±0.004	0.022±0.003
WT'	36	3.08±0.33	2.65±0.39	0.03±0.007	0.032±0.003
LEGSKO	36	0.97±0.29	0.47±0.10	0.22±0.003	0.11±0.001
LEGSKO Cataract	36	0.89±0.31	N.D	0.21±0.005	N.D

N.D. : not detectable.

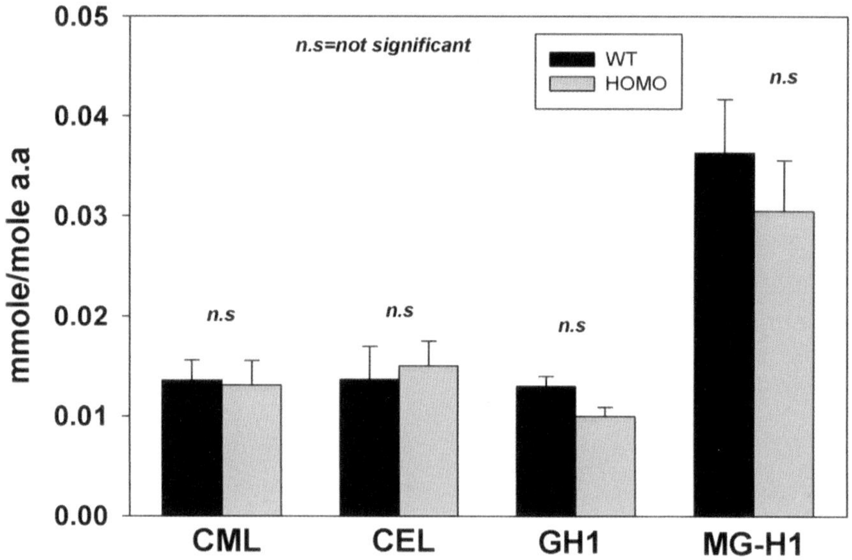

Figure 2. Quantitative comparison of mean levels ± SD for protein modification by glycation at 9 mos old of WT and Homo-LEGSKO mice lenses. Carboxymethyl-lysine (CML), carboxyethyl-lysine (CEL), methylglyoxal hydroimidazolone-1 (MG-H1), and glyoxal hydroimidazolone-1 (G-H1) were determined by LC/MS. No significant (n.s) change was observed between WT and LEGSKO lenses. Student's *t* test was used for data analysis.

cataractous lenses [12,13,34]. For this reason we expected to find increased levels of carboxymethyl-lysine (CML), carboxyethyl-lysine (CEL) and MG-H1 hydroimidazolone. At first we were surprised that none of these modifications were increased. This may mean there was enough residual glutathione as cofactor of glyoxylase I for the detoxification of these AGE precursors. However, the most likely explanation is that AGE levels are very low because vitamin C is absent in normal and LEGSKO mouse lens (both are ~100 μM), except in the hSVCT2 transgenic mouse [12]. Indeed previous data from our and other laboratories have unequivocally established ascorbic acid as a major source of these AGEs in the aging lens [12,35,36]. Breeding experiments between the LEGSKO mouse and the hSVCT2 mouse will confirm the extent to which the GSH/glyoxalase system is important for protection against ascorbic acid derived AGEs. Similarly, exposure of the hSVCT2, LEGSKO and hSVCT2xLEGSKO F1 mouse to UV/VIS light is expected to provide important in vivo information on the role of GSH for protection against photoxidative damage and formation of photosensitizers resulting from tryptophan oxidation.

In summary, lens-specific suppression of GSH synthesis in the LEGSKO mouse, while maintaining all other metabolic body functions intact, resulted in biochemical, biological and cataractous changes mimicking those of age-related human nuclear cataracts. Thus, the LEGSKO mouse is expected to be a useful tool for the development of pharmacological agents that can either restore the antioxidant reserve of the lens or block the distal effects of oxidant stress resulting from GSH deficiency.

Materials and Methods

Creation of Gclc Floxed Mouse

Gclc conditional knockout (Gclc$^{fl/fl}$) target ES cells with C57BL/6 genetic background were obtained from the European Conditional Knockout Mouse Program (EUCOMM). The Gclc$^{fl/fl}$ exon 2 is flanked by two loxP sites, and the Neo cassette is flanked by two FRT sites. Microinjection of ES cells into C57BL/6J blastocysts was done at the University of Michigan Transgenic Facility, and resulting chimeric male mice were bred with albino female mice to obtain the germ-line. F1 heterozygous Gclc$^{fl/fl}$ mice were bred with mice carrying a ubiquitously expressing Flp knockin mouse (the Jackson lab, stock No. 009086) on a C57BL/6 background to remove the Neo cassette. The resulting Gclc$^{fl/fl}$ mice were cross-bred to generate the homozygous Gclc$^{fl/fl}$ mouse line. The presence of a floxed Gclc allele was identified by PCR using tail DNA with a primer pair (forward primer, 5′-CATGAGGAA CTGAACTGAAGGATTGA-3′; reverse primer, 5′-CAAGGAGGCTCACACATCCCAGAAC-3′), which generated a 310-bp amplicon.

Creation of Lens Conditional Knockout Mouse (Gclc$^{fl/fl}$/MRL10$^{+/-}$)

In order to delete Gclc specifically from the lens epithelium and fibers, we crossed the Gclc$^{fl/fl}$ mice with MRL10-Cre mice (FVB background) that express Cre recombinase in lens epithelium and fibers [17]. F1 mice (*Gclc*$^{fl/wt}$/*MRL10*$^{+/-}$) were backcrossed to Gclc$^{fl/fl}$ mice to generate homozygous lens conditional knockout mice (*Gclc*$^{fl/fl}$/*MRL10*$^{+/-}$). All the data provide in this paper is based on B6/FVB mixed background. Mice conditionally lacking *Gclc* in lens (*Gclc*$^{fl/fl}$/*MRL10*$^{+/-}$), hereafter called LEGSKO, were identified by PCR using both conditional allele (Gclc$^{fl/fl}$) genotype primer pair and primers pair that amplifies a 190-bp fragment of Cre recombinase coding region (forward primer, 5′-AATTTGCCTGCAT-TACCGGTCGATGCAACG-3′ and reverse primer 5′-CCATTTCCGGTTATTCAACTTGCACCATGC-3′). Mice were housed under diurnal lighting conditions and allowed free access to food and water. All animals were used in accordance with the guidelines of the Association for Research in Vision and Ophthalmology for the Use of Animals in Ophthalmology and Vision Research, and experimental protocols for this study were approved by the Institutional Animal Care and Use Committee (IACUC) of Case Western Reserve University.

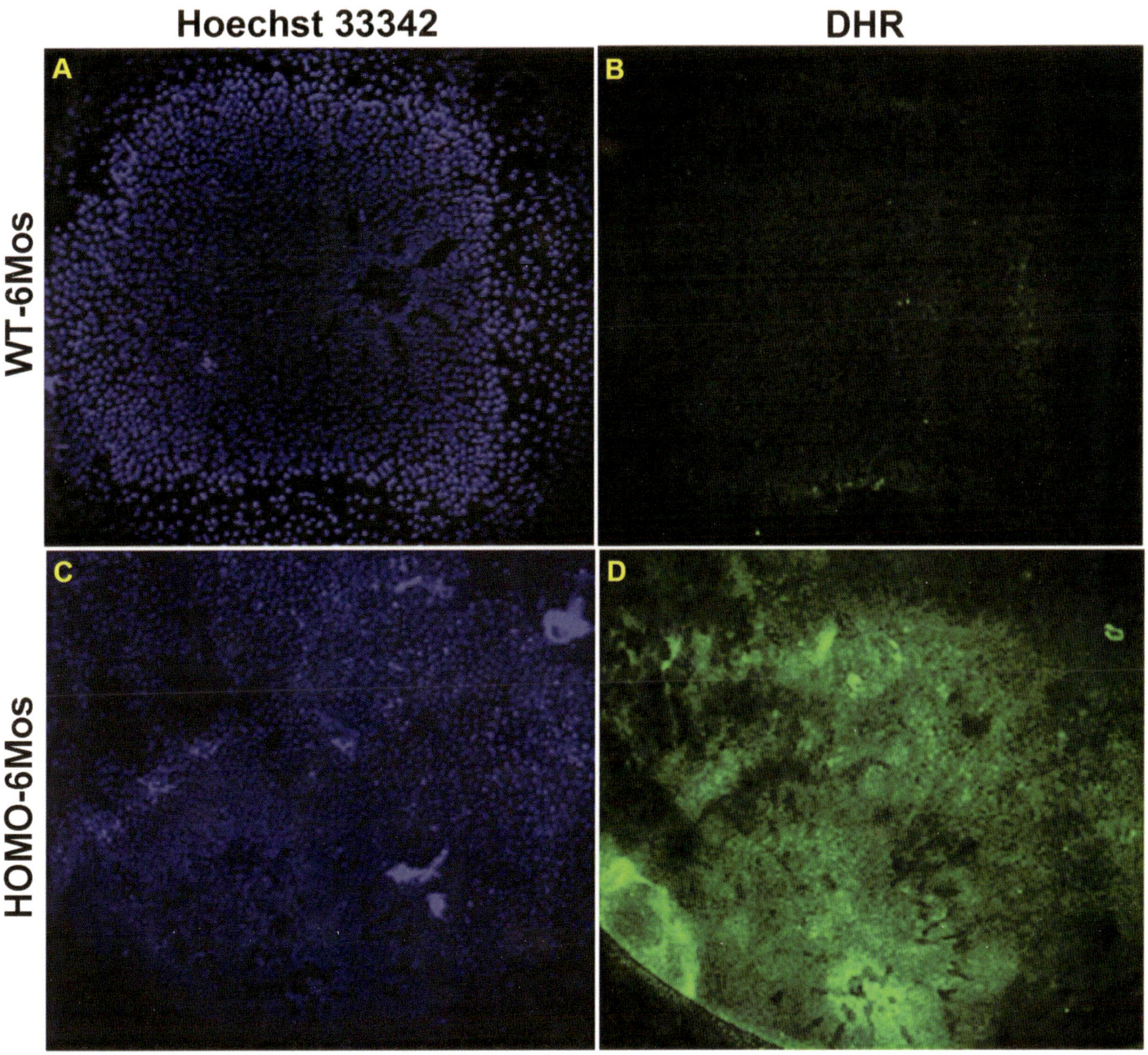

Figure 3. Comparison of lens anterior surfaces of 6 mos wild type and Homo-LEGSKO mouse lenses vitally stained for DNA and ROS. Fresh lenses were stained with both Hoechst 33342 and Dihydrorhodamine 123 (DHR). The Lens anterior was scanned using 10X objective, and 65 μm deep into the cortex and 0.8 μm layer Z-scan was performed and projection image was obtained with same method for both WT and LEGSKO lenses. (A) and (C). Comparison of DNA staining with Hoechst 33342 (blue) of the anterior surface of Wt and LEGSKO lenses. (B) and (D). Comparison of vital staining for ROS fluorescence with DHR stain (green) of the same surface areas.

Quantitative Determination of Reduced Glutathione (GSH) and Oxidized Glutathione (GSSG)

Eyes were removed immediately after sacrifice. Lenses were homogenized in 200 μl ice-cold 5% metaphosphoric acid and 0.6% sulfosalicylic acid mixture in 0.1 M potassium phosphate buffer and 5 mM EDTA buffer (pH 7.5). The supernatant was analyzed for GSH and GSSG using glutathione reductase (GR) and β-NADPH enzymatic recycle method followed by colorimetric assay after derivatization with 5,5′-dithio-bis(2-nitrobenzoic acid) (DTNB) as described [37]. Commercially available GSH (G6529, Sigma, St. Louis) and GSSG (49740, Sigma, St. Louis) were used for standard curve calibration.

Lens fibers were subdivided onto cortex and nuclear fraction by a freeze-thawing technique whereby quick freezing at −80°C was followed by thawing at room temperature for 1 min, creating a clear white opacity in nucleus. The cortical and nucleus regions can then be easy separated for GSH and GSSG determination.

γ-Glutamyl Cysteine Ligase Activity Assay

Gcl activity in lens extract was measured using monobromobimane derivatization and HPLC analysis with fluorescence detection as previously reported [38].

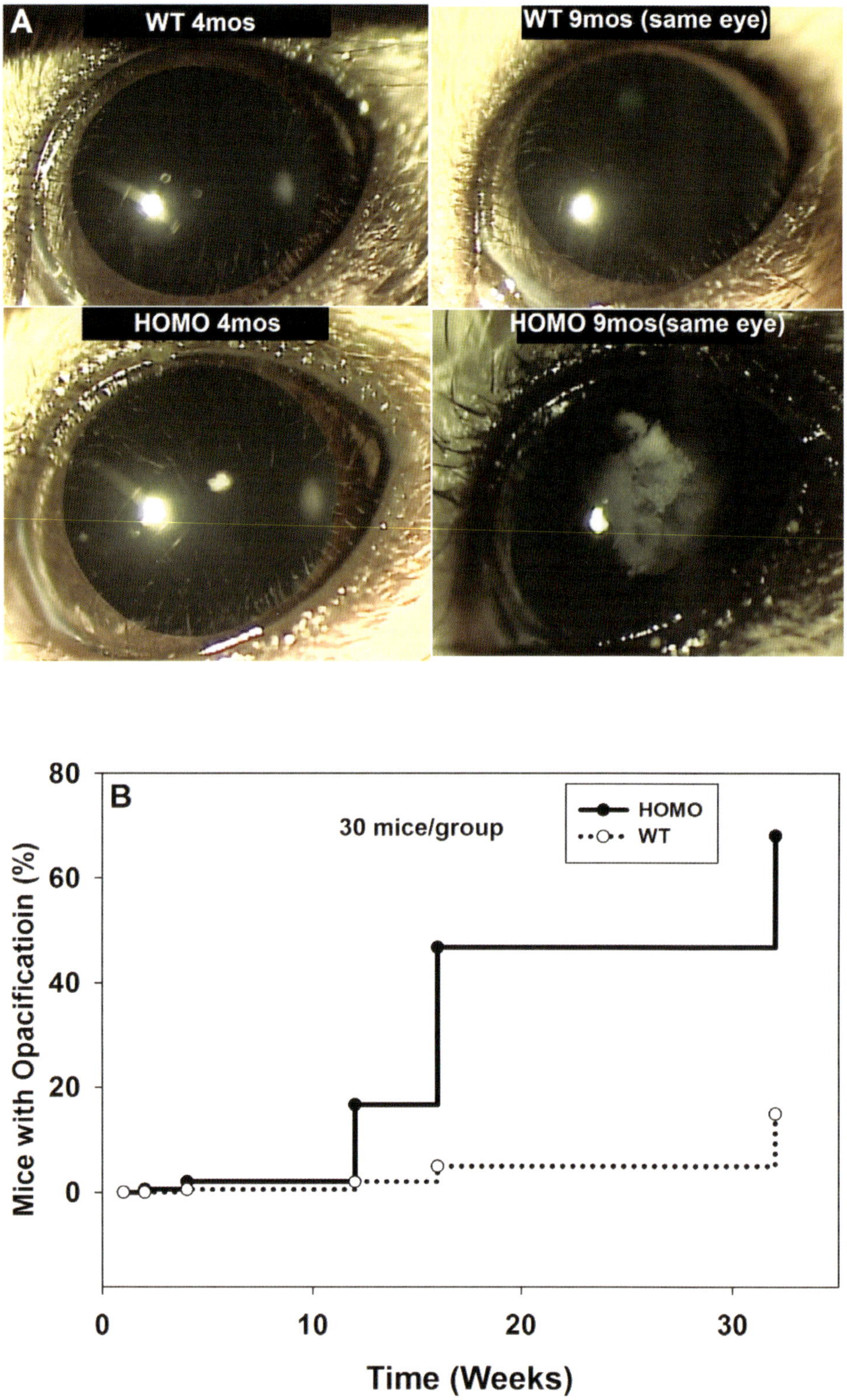

Figure 4. Slit-lamp image of LEGSKO and age matched wild type mouse lens. (A). Representative images of HOM-LEGSKO mouse lens at 4 and 9 months compared with age matched control wild type mouse lens. The same mouse was followed over a period of 9 months and lens images were taken every two months. (B). Slit-lamp images were taken periodically and lens opacity/cataract of any size were recorded for 9 months in homozygous LEGSKO mice vs. age matched wild type mice (n = 30 mice per group). LEGSKO mice developed lens opacities and cataract at much higher rate compared to wild type mice.

RNA Extraction and Quantitative mRNA Analysis of Gene Expression

Minimum Information for Publication of Quantitative Real-Time PCR Experiments (MIQE) guidelines [39] was followed for real time PCR analysis. Eyes were removed immediately after sacrifice. Lenses were collected and quickly frozen with liquid nitrogen and stored at −80°C. Total RNA was prepared from single lens using TRIzol reagent (Invitrogen, Grand Island, NY). RNA concentration was measured with a Nanodrop instrument (2000c, Thermal Sci). Only RNA samples with UV 260 nm/280 nm ratio of 1.9–2.0 and UV 260 nm/230 nm ratio >1.8 were used for subsequent experiments. For real time PCR, total RNA was deoxyribonuclease-treated (Invitrogen, Grand Island, NY) and transcribed to complementary DNA with oligo(dT) or random hexamer primer (Invitrogen, Grand Island, NY) and Moloney murine leukemia virus reverse transcriptase (New England Biolabs, Ipswich, MA). Real time PCR was performed with the SYBR Green method and an Applied Biosystems instrument (ABI StepOne Plus). Relative expression was calculated using the ΔΔCt method with normalization to constitutive genes as indicated in the figure legends. Specific primer sequences are available on request. All reactions were performed in triplicate. Data analysis was carried out using the cycle threshold values of target gene expression normalized by GAPDH as the internal control.

Western Blot

Lens fiber fractions (cortex or nucleus) were collected in 50 mM potassium phosphate buffer (pH 7.4), homogenized, and centrifuged. Whole protein extracts were further processed for immunoblot analysis and probed against Gclc using an anti-Gclc antibody (1:2000; Abnova). All data were normalized to the level of GAPDH and compared with age-matched wild type mice.

Lens Protein Enzymatic Digestion for Advanced Glycation Endproduct Analysis

For AGE analysis by LC/MS, 1 mg of lens protein extract was enzymatically digested in Chelex treated phosphate buffer with sequential additions of peptidase (Sigma P7500), protease K, pronase and aminopeptidase M (Roche, IN) as described earlier [12]. Corresponding enzyme blanks were incubated without added protein as a background control. Protein concentration was determined using the ninhydrin assay, as described earlier [12].

AGEs Determination by LC-MS/MS

Amounts of carboxymethyl-lysine (CML) and carboxyethyl-lysine (CEL), fructose-lysine (FL), methionine sulfoxide (MetSOX), glyoxal immidazolone-1 (G-H1) and methylglyoxal immidazolone-1 (MG-H1) in enzymatically digested samples were measured by electronspray positive ionization-mass spectrometric multiple reaction monitoring (ESI+MRM) with a LC-MS/MS system composed of a 2690 Separation module with a Quattro Ultima triple quadropole mass spectrometry detector (Water-Micromass, Manchester, U.K.) following the previously published procedure [40,41]. Analytes released by self-digestion of proteases in assay blanks were subtracted from analytic estimates.

Staining of Freshly Isolated Lenses with Hoechst 33342 and Dihydrorhodamine 123 (DHR)

Fresh isolated lenses were placed in chamber slides and stained with 7.5 μM dihydrorhodamine 123 (DHR) on ice for 45 min, followed by staining with 10 μM Hoechst 33342 for 15 min as described by Wolf et al [42]. The lens in M199 medium was then subjected to confocal image scanning.

Image Analysis Using Confocal Microscope

A laser scanning confocal microscope (Carl Zeiss LSM510 META) was used for whole lens analysis upon vital staining with DNA fluorochrome Hoechst 33342 and ROS marker DHR. The excitation/emission at 405 nm/450 nm was used for Hoechst 3342 and 488 nm/550 nm was used for DHR image. Lens anterior was scanned using 10X objective, and 65 μm deep into the cortex and 0.8 μm layer Z-scan was performed. The image was analyzed with LSM images analysis software from Zeiss.

Statistical Analysis

All values are expressed as means ± S.D. Statistical significance of difference in mean values was assessed by analysis of variance or Student's *t* test. Only p values <0.05 were considered statistically significant.

Acknowledgments

We thank Christopher Strauch for LC/MC analyses of advanced glycation and oxidation products.

Author Contributions

Conceived and designed the experiments: XF VMM. Performed the experiments: XF XL SH BW. Analyzed the data: XF VMM. Contributed reagents/materials/analysis tools: MLR. Wrote the paper: XF VMM.

References

1. Javitt JC, Wang F, West SK (1996) Blindness due to cataract: epidemiology and prevention. Annu Rev Public Health 17: 159–177.
2. Klein BE, Klein R, Lee KE, Gangnon RE (2008) Incidence of age-related cataract over a 15-year interval the Beaver Dam Eye Study. Ophthalmology 115: 477–482.
3. Panel C (1983) Vision Resarch : a national plan. Washington DC US DHHS:NIH publ: 83–2473.
4. Clemons TE, Kurinij N, Sperduto RD (2004) Associations of mortality with ocular disorders and an intervention of high-dose antioxidants and zinc in the Age-Related Eye Disease Study: AREDS Report No. 13. Arch Ophthalmol 122: 716–726.
5. Sharma KK, Santhoshkumar P (2009) Lens aging: Effects of crystallins. Biochim Biophys Acta 1790: 1095–1108.
6. Heys KR, Friedrich MG, Truscott RJ (2007) Presbyopia and heat: changes associated with aging of the human lens suggest a functional role for the small heat shock protein, alpha-crystallin, in maintaining lens flexibility. Aging Cell 6: 807–815.
7. Hains PG, Truscott RJ (2008) Proteomic analysis of the oxidation of cysteine residues in human age-related nuclear cataract lenses. Biochim Biophys Acta 1784: 1959–1964.
8. Bhat KS, John A, Reddy PR, Reddy PS, Reddy VN (1991) Effect of pigmentation on glutathione redox cycle antioxidant defense in whole as well as different regions of human cataractous lens. Exp Eye Res 52: 715–721.
9. Sweeney MH, Truscott RJ (1998) An impediment to glutathione diffusion in older normal human lenses: a possible precondition for nuclear cataract. Exp Eye Res 67: 587–595.
10. Rathbun WB (1984) Lenticular glutathione synthesis: rate-limiting factors in its regulation and decline. Curr Eye Res 3: 101–108.
11. Cheng R, Feng Q, Argirov OK, Ortwerth BJ (2004) Structure elucidation of a novel yellow chromophore from human lens protein. J Biol Chem 279: 45441–45449.
12. Fan X, Reneker LW, Obrenovich ME, Strauch C, Cheng R, et al. (2006) Vitamin C mediates chemical aging of lens crystallins by the Maillard reaction in a humanized mouse model. Proc Natl Acad Sci U S A 103: 16912–16917.
13. Fan X, Sell DR, Zhang J, Nemet I, Theves M, et al. (2010) Anaerobic vs aerobic pathways of carbonyl and oxidant stress in human lens and skin during aging and in diabetes: A comparative analysis. Free Radic Biol Med 49: 847–856.
14. Fu S, Dean R, Southan M, Truscott R (1998) The hydroxyl radical in lens nuclear cataractogenesis. J Biol Chem 273: 28603–28609.

15. Garner MH, Spector A (1980) Selective oxidation of cysteine and methionine in normal and senile cataractous lenses. Proc Natl Acad Sci U S A 77: 1274–1277.
16. Dalton TP, Dieter MZ, Yang Y, Shertzer HG, Nebert DW (2000) Knockout of the mouse glutamate cysteine ligase catalytic subunit (Gclc) gene: embryonic lethal when homozygous, and proposed model for moderate glutathione deficiency when heterozygous. Biochem Biophys Res Commun 279: 324–329.
17. Zhao H, Yang Y, Rizo CM, Overbeek PA, Robinson ML (2004) Insertion of a Pax6 consensus binding site into the alphaA-crystallin promoter acts as a lens epithelial cell enhancer in transgenic mice. Invest Ophthalmol Vis Sci 45: 1930–1939.
18. Kannan R, Yi JR, Zlokovic BV, Kaplowitz N (1995) Molecular characterization of a reduced glutathione transporter in the lens. Invest Ophthalmol Vis Sci 36: 1785–1792.
19. Hanson SR, Hasan A, Smith DL, Smith JB (2000) The major in vivo modifications of the human water-insoluble lens crystallins are disulfide bonds, deamidation, methionine oxidation and backbone cleavage. Exp Eye Res 71: 195–207.
20. Nagaraj RH, Monnier VM (1990) Non-tryptophan fluorescence and high molecular weight protein formation in lens crystallins of rats with chronic galactosemia: prevention by the aldose reductase inhibitor sorbinil. Exp Eye Res 51: 411–418.
21. Nagaraj RH, Sell DR, Prabhakaram M, Ortwerth BJ, Monnier VM (1991) High correlation between pentosidine protein crosslinks and pigmentation implicates ascorbate oxidation in human lens senescence and cataractogenesis. Proc Natl Acad Sci U S A 88: 10257–10261.
22. Chevez-Barrios P, Wiseman AL, Rojas E, Ou CN, Lieberman MW (2000) Cataract development in gamma-glutamyl transpeptidase-deficient mice. Exp Eye Res 71: 575–582.
23. Martensson J, Steinherz R, Jain A, Meister A (1989) Glutathione ester prevents buthionine sulfoximine-induced cataracts and lens epithelial cell damage. Proc Natl Acad Sci U S A 86: 8727–8731.
24. Calvin HI, Medvedovsky C, Worgul BV (1986) Near-total glutathione depletion and age-specific cataracts induced by buthionine sulfoximine in mice. Science 233: 553–555.
25. Gosselin ME, Kapustij CJ, Venkateswaran UD, Leverenz VR, Giblin FJ (2007) Raman spectroscopic evidence for nuclear disulfide in isolated lenses of hyperbaric oxygen-treated guinea pigs. Exp Eye Res 84: 493–499.
26. Reddy VN, Giblin FJ, Lin LR, Dang L, Unakar NJ, et al. (2001) Glutathione peroxidase-1 deficiency leads to increased nuclear light scattering, membrane damage, and cataract formation in gene-knockout mice. Invest Ophthalmol Vis Sci 42: 3247–3255.
27. Reddy VN, Lin LR, Ho YS, Magnenat JL, Ibaraki N, et al. (1997) Peroxide-induced damage in lenses of transgenic mice with deficient and elevated levels of glutathione peroxidase. Ophthalmologica 211: 192–200.
28. Giblin FJ, McCready JP, Schrimscher L, Reddy VN (1987) Peroxide-induced effects on lens cation transport following inhibition of glutathione reductase activity in vitro. Exp Eye Res 45: 77–91.
29. Wu H, Lin L, Giblin F, Ho YS, Lou MF (2011) Glutaredoxin 2 knockout increases sensitivity to oxidative stress in mouse lens epithelial cells. Free Radic Biol Med.
30. Spector A, Ma W, Wang RR, Yang Y, Ho YS (1997) The contribution of GSH peroxidase-1, catalase and GSH to the degradation of H2O2 by the mouse lens. Exp Eye Res 64: 477–485.
31. Kodama T, Takemoto L (1988) Characterization of disulfide-linked crystallins associated with human cataractous lens membranes. Invest Ophthalmol Vis Sci 29: 145–149.
32. Truscott RJ, Comte-Walters S, Ablonczy Z, Schwacke JH, Berry Y, et al. (2011) Tight binding of proteins to membranes from older human cells. Age (Dordr) 33: 543–554.
33. Giblin FJ (2000) Glutathione: a vital lens antioxidant. J Ocul Pharmacol Ther 16: 121–135.
34. Ahmed N, Thornalley PJ, Dawczynski J, Franke S, Strobel J, et al. (2003) Methylglyoxal-derived hydroimidazolone advanced glycation end-products of human lens proteins. Invest Ophthalmol Vis Sci 44: 5287–5292.
35. Dunn JA, Ahmed MU, Murtiashaw MH, Richardson JM, Walla MD, et al. (1990) Reaction of ascorbate with lysine and protein under autoxidizing conditions: formation of N epsilon-(carboxymethyl)lysine by reaction between lysine and products of autoxidation of ascorbate. Biochemistry 29: 10964–10970.
36. Ortwerth BJ, Bhattacharyya J, Shipova E (2009) Tryptophan metabolites from young human lenses and the photooxidation of ascorbic acid by UVA light. Invest Ophthalmol Vis Sci 50: 3311–3319.
37. Rahman I, Kode A, Biswas SK (2006) Assay for quantitative determination of glutathione and glutathione disulfide levels using enzymatic recycling method. Nat Protoc 1: 3159–3165.
38. Kavanagh TJ (2001) Current Protocols in Toxicology: John Wiley & Sons, Inc.
39. Bustin SA, Benes V, Garson JA, Hellemans J, Huggett J, et al. (2009) The MIQE guidelines: minimum information for publication of quantitative real-time PCR experiments. Clin Chem 55: 611–622.
40. Fan X, Zhang J, Theves M, Strauch C, Nemet I, et al. (2009) Mechanism of lysine oxidation in human lens crystallins during aging and in diabetes. J Biol Chem.
41. Ahmed N, Thornalley PJ (2003) Quantitative screening of protein biomarkers of early glycation, advanced glycation, oxidation and nitrosation in cellular and extracellular proteins by tandem mass spectrometry multiple reaction monitoring. Biochem Soc Trans 31: 1417–1422.
42. Pendergrass W, Penn P, Possin D, Wolf N (2005) Accumulation of DNA, nuclear and mitochondrial debris, and ROS at sites of age-related cortical cataract in mice. Invest Ophthalmol Vis Sci 46: 4661–4670.

13

Findings from a Rapid Assessment of Avoidable Blindness (RAAB) in Southern Malawi

Khumbo Kalua[1,2]*, Robert Lindfield[2], Maxwell Mtupanyama[3], Davie Mtumodzi[4], Vincent Msiska[5]

1 Department of Ophthalmology, College of Medicine, University of Malawi, Blantyre, Malawi, **2** International Centre for Eye Health, London School of Hygiene and Tropical Medicine, London, United Kingdom, **3** Ministry of Health, Chiradzulu District Hospital, Chiradzulu, Malawi, **4** Ministry of Health, Thyolo District Hospital, Thyolo, Malawi, **5** Ministry of Health, Mzuzu Central Hospital, Mzuzu, Malawi

Abstract

Background: Data on prevalence and causes of avoidable blindness in Malawi are not readily available. The purpose of this study was to determine the prevalence and causes of blindness in persons aged 50 and above in southern Malawi to plan eye care services for the community.

Methodology: A population-based survey was conducted in 7 districts in southern Malawi. Villages were selected by probability proportionate to size within each district. Clusters were further subdivided into segments. A predetermined number of segments were selected randomly in each cluster. The survey team moved from house to house in each segment until they had examined 50 people over the age of 50. Examination consisted of visual acuity measurement with tumbling "E" chart and ocular examination by an ophthalmologist. Participants were categorized by visual acuity. Those who were visually impaired (VA<6/18 in the better eye with available correction) were assigned a main cause of visual loss. Further information was sought from anyone who had received cataract surgery.

Results: A total number of 3,583 persons aged 50 and above were sampled; among these 3,430 (95.7%) were examined. The prevalence of blindness (presenting visual acuity <3/60 in the better eye) among persons aged 50 and above was 3.3% (95% CI 2.5–4.1). Cataract was the most common cause of blindness contributing to 48.2% of all cases, followed by glaucoma (15.8%) and cornea scarring (12.3%). The cataract surgical coverage in blind persons was 44.6%.

Conclusion: The prevalence of blindness and visual impairment in persons aged 50 and above was lower than the WHO estimate for Malawi. The majority of the causes were avoidable, with cataract accounting for approximately half of all cases of blindness. The data suggests that expansion of eye care programs to address avoidable causes of blindness is necessary in this area of southern Malawi.

Editor: Jos H. Verbeek, Finnish Institute of Occupational Health, Finland

Funding: Sight Savers funded the study. The funders had no role in study design, data collection and analysis, decision to publish, or preparation of the manuscript.

Competing Interests: The authors have declared that no competing interests exist.

* E-mail: khumbokalua@yahoo.com

Introduction

Vision 2020: The Right to Sight, is a global initiative to eliminate avoidable blindness by the year 2020 [1,2,3]. It is a collaboration between the International Agency for the Prevention of Blindness (an organization representing non-governmental bodies working in prevention of blindness) and the World Health Organization (WHO) [4,5]. Recent WHO estimates indicate that, globally, there are 45 million blind people and 153 million with visual impairment, with the highest prevalence of blindness reported in Sub-Saharan Africa [6,7]. Extrapolation from WHO data suggests that 1% of people (all ages) in Malawi are blind, and that 80% of these are aged 50 and above [7]. Findings from prevalence surveys in east Africa (Rwanda [8], Kenya [9] and Tanzania [10]) and other African countries [11] have revealed that the overall prevalence of blindness in these countries may be much lower than the WHO estimates. It is unclear whether this is the case in Malawi. A study conducted in the late 1990's in Southern Malawi suggested a reduction in the prevalence of blindness over the previous 16 years [12]. However this study only covered a small geographical area and no other surveys have been conducted to validate its findings. A reduction in the prevalence of blindness is supported by an increase in the number of cataract surgeries performed in Malawi from approximately 300 surgeries per million population in 2003 to the current estimate (2010) of 850 surgeries per million population per year.

As part of the strategy to achieve the aim of VISION 2020 in Malawi, the Government of Malawi, in collaboration with Sight Savers, recently launched a five year Comprehensive Eye Service (CES) in the South West Zone of Malawi which comprises of 7 districts. This required robust information to plan the delivery of effective services to the population.

The Rapid Assessment of Avoidable Blindness (RAAB) survey is a relatively cheap and easy means of generating population-based data on prevalence and causes of blindness in persons aged 50 and over. Many countries are now using the RAAB as a planning tool for Vision 2020 programmes.

The aim of this study was to conduct a RAAB survey in 7 districts within Southern Malawi, and generate information that will be used for planning a VISION 2020 programme in the area.

Methods

The study was conducted by Ministry of Health in Malawi, with technical support from International Centre for Eye Health, London School of Hygiene and Tropical Medicine (LSHTM). Ethical clearance for the study was obtained from the National Health Services Research Committee (NHSRC) in Lilongwe and permission was sought from the district Health Administrative Officers responsible for supervision and coordination of health activities within the districts. Following explanation of the purpose of the study, written informed consent was obtained from all subjects who participated in the study.

The study took place in 7 districts from the South West Zone of Malawi (Blantyre, Chikwawa, Nsanje, Thyolo, Chiradzulu, Mwanza and Neno) with a total population of 2,141,805 (National Statistical Office results, population and housing census, Zomba, Malawi 2008) [13].

Sample Size Calculation

A prevalence of blindness of 5% in persons aged 50 and above was used, based on experience from the trachoma surveys in that area, and other RAAB surveys in sub-Saharan Africa. Using 95% confidence interval, a precision of 20% (worst acceptable prevalence 6%), design effect (DEFF) of 1.6 and a non-response rate of 10%, a sample size of 3600 was calculated which would require 72 clusters of 50 people aged 50 and above.

Sampling Frame

Using the National Census in 2008 as the sampling frame, a list was produced of enumeration areas (called villages) and their respective population sizes of people aged 50 years and above. Villages were then selected using probability proportionate to size.

Compact segment sampling was used to select households within each village. Each village area as divided into segments containing approximately 50 people over the age of 50 and one segment was chosen at random by drawing lots. Starting at the edge of the segment, all households in the segment were included in the sample sequentially until 50 people aged 50 and above were identified. To be eligible for inclusion an individual had to reside in a household for at least six months of the previous year.

The survey was carried out by two survey teams each led by an ophthalmologist. The study took place between November 2009 and March 2010 with breaks in December and January due to heavy rain. In each cluster, the survey team visited households door-to-door, accompanied by community health workers working in the village or a local village guide (volunteer). All the examinations were conducted in the household compound.

When an eligible person was absent, the survey team left a message and returned at the end of the day to examine the individual before leaving the area. In rare circumstances where the individual was not available, information about their visual status was sought from relatives or neighbours.

Eye Examination

Information was gathered using a standardised RAAB questionnaire and a standard protocol was followed for examination. VA was measured with a tumbling illiterate Snellen "E" chart using optotype size 6/18 on one side and size 6/60 on the other. All measurements were taken in full daylight with available spectacle correction. If the VA was less than 6/18 in either eye, then pinhole vision was also measured. A simple ocular examination was performed on every participant. This included an undilated assessment of the lens using a direct ophthalmoscope. If there was any uncertainty about the diagnosis then the individual was dilated for further examination. The principal cause of blindness or visual impairment was recorded according to the standard WHO convention.

Table 1. Demography of coverage, absenteeism and refusals.

	Male		Female		Total	
	N	%	N	%	N	%
Examined	1296	95.2	2134	96	3430	95.7
Not available	58	4.3	72	3.2	130	3.6
Refused	1	0.1	4	0.2	5	0.1
Not capable	6	0.4	12	0.5	18	0.5
Total	**1361**	**100**	**2222**	**100**	**3583**	**100**
% of all examined	38		62		100	

Training

Two teams made up of an ophthalmologist and ophthalmic clinical officer, received one week of training by an experienced trainer (RL) and had another week refresher training before starting the survey. In both training sessions inter-observer agreement was measured through repeat examination of 50 patients by each of the two teams. Agreement between the teams was assessed using kappa and had to be greater than 0.7 to proceed with the survey.

Data entry and Analysis

Two data entry clerks were trained in data entry and double entered the data from the survey into the RAAB software programme which allowed assessment of data entry errors and missing data.

Results

3,583 persons aged 50 and above were included in the sample. Among these 3,430 (95.7%) were examined. 1,361(38%) were males and 2,222 (62%) were females. Coverage, absenteeism and refusals are shown in Table 1. Overall 3.6% were not available, 0.1% refused and 0.5% were not capable of completing an examination. Some participants were unaware of their date of birth. The state of emergency in Malawi during 1959 was used as

Table 2. Age and sex structure of the population of persons aged 50 and above from the entire southern region of Malawi.

Age	Male		Female		Total
	N	%	N	%	
50–59	95964	45.1	116916	54.9	212880
60–69	63697	46.0	74860	54.0	138557
70–79	39468	42.7	53071	57.3	92539
80–89	18262	38.4	29291	61.6	47553
90+	7738	34.9	14454	65.1	22192
Total	**225129**	**43.8**	**288592**	**56.2**	**513721**

Table 3. The distribution by visual acuity with available correction in the better eye.

Visual Acuity	Males (N = 1296)				Females (N = 2134)				Total (N = 3430)			
	N	%	95% CI		N	%	95% CI		N	%	95% CI	
Blind	47	3.6	2.5	4.8	67	3.1	2.2	4	114	3.3	2.5	4.1
Severe Visual Impairment	41	3.2	2.1	4.2	53	2.5	1.7	3.2	94	2.7	2.1	3.4
Visual Impairment	126	9.7	7.9	11.6	200	9.4	7.9	10.9	326	9.5	8.2	10.8
Bilateral aphakia/Pseudophakia	13	1	0.5	1.5	9	0.4	0.1	0.7	22	0.6	0.4	0.9
Unilateral aphakia/Pseudophakia	16	1.2	0.7	1.8	18	0.8	0.4	1.3	34	1	0.6	1.4

entry criteria for the study. If the individual was alive in 1959 then they were definitely older than 50 years. Table 2 shows age and sex structure of the population of persons aged 50 and above from the southern region of Malawi.

Table 3 describes the distribution of visual acuity with available correction in the better eye down into blindness (VA<3/60 in the better eye with available correction), severe visual impairment (SVI) (VA<6/60 to ≥3/60 in the better eye with available correction) and visual impairment (VI) (VA<6/18 to ≥6/60 in the better eye with available correction). The overall prevalence of blindness (unadjusted) from all causes in the examined adults aged 50 and above was 3.3% (95% CI 2.5–4.1). Twenty two (0.6%) people examined had bilateral aphakia/pseudophakia while 34(1%) had unilateral aphakia/pseudophakia.

Table 4 describes the causes of visual loss in those examined. Untreated cataract was the commonest cause of blindness, SVI and VI contributing to 48.2% of all blind persons, 57.4% of SVI and 46.3% of VI. Glaucoma was the second most common cause of blindness (15.8%) followed by other non-trachomatous corneal scarring (12.3%).

Avoidable causes of blindness accounted for 75.4% of all cases. Two of the original VISION 2020 priority diseases (trachoma & onchocerciasis) had a very low prevalence, with trachoma contributing to 4.4% of all cases of blindness and onchocerciasis being completely absent. 1.8% of blindness was attributed to cataract surgical complications.

Table 4. Causes of blindness, SVI and VI in persons examined.

Cause	Blind		SVI		VI	
	N	%	N	%	N	%
Cataract untreated	55	48.2	54	57.4	151	46.3
Glaucoma	18	15.8	13	13.8	12	3.7
Other cornea scar	14	12.3	2	2.1	7	2.1
Other post segment CNS	10	8.8	10	10.6	16	4.9
Phthisis	9	7.9	0	0.0	2	0.6
Trachoma	5	4.4	0	0.0	3	0.9
Surgical complication	2	1.8	2	2.1	1	0.3
Aphakia uncorrected	1	0.9	0	0.0	0	0.0
Refractive errors	0	0.0	13	13.8	134	41.1
Onchocerciasis	0	0.0	0	0.0	0	0.0
Diabetic retinopathy	0	0.0	0	0.0	0	0.0
Globe abnormality	0	0.0	0	0.0	0	0.0
AMD	0	0.0	0	0.0	0	0.0
		0.0		0.0		0.0
Total	**114**	100.0	**94**	100.0	**326**	100.0

Table 5 describes the cataract surgical coverage (the number of people in the survey who had cataract surgery compared to the number who required it). The cataract surgical coverage (CSC) for blind persons was 44.6% (61.5% for males and 29.5% for females), for SVI persons it was 34.5% (51% males, 22.4% females) and for those with VI it was 15.8% (24.8% males, 10.3% females). Males had a much higher CSC at all levels of visual acuity. The overall CSC for blind eyes was low (27.0%).

In terms of barriers to cataract surgery, old age ('no need felt') was reported to be the commonest barrier (23.5%) followed by 'no one to accompany' (22.1%), 'no services nearby' (13.2) and 'unaware that treatment was available' (11.8%).

Table 6 shows the visual acuity in people who had undergone cataract surgery tabulated by available correction and best correction. Presenting post-operative visual acuity was good (can see 6/18) in 40.8% of persons who had IOL surgery, and improved to 56.3% after best correction. Presenting visual acuity was poor (could not see 6/60) in 32.4% of persons and, even after best correction, 28.2% still had poor visual acuity. Among the eyes with poor outcomes and which had been operated less than 3 years ago, the causes of poor outcome were attributed to pre-operative morbidity (selection) in 40%, to surgical complications in 46.7% and long term sequel in 13.3%.

Among the persons who had non IOL surgery (N = 7), 5 (71.4%) had poor visual outcome (could not see 6/60).

The postoperative presenting visual acuity and the satisfaction levels with results of IOL surgery are shown in Table 7. 84.8% of all persons who had surgery were either very satisfied or partially

Table 5. Cataract surgical coverage in persons and eyes.

Persons	Male	Female	Total
	%	%	%
VA<3/60	61.5	29.5	44.6
VA<6/60	51	22.4	34.5
VA<6/18	24.8	10.3	15.8
Eyes			
VA<3/60	36.5	20.7	27
VA<6/60	27.8	16	20.7
VA<6/18	15.8	7.8	10.5

Table 6. Visual acuity from operated eyes obtained after cataract surgery.

Correction	Visual acuity	IOL eyes (N = 71)		No IOL (N = 7)		All (N = 78)	
		N	%	N	%	N	%
Available correction	Can see 6/18	29	40.8	1	14.3	30	38.5
	Cannot see 6/18 but can see 6/60	19	26.8	1	14.3	20	25.6
	Cannot see 6/60	23	32.4	5	71.4	28	35.9
Best correction	Can see 6/18	40	56.3	1	14.3	41	52.6
	Cannot see 6/18 but can see 6/60	11	15.5	1	14.3	12	15.4
	Cannot see 6/60	20	28.2	5	71.4	25	32.1

satisfied. Only 3% of persons were very unsatisfied with the results of surgery.

Extrapolating results to the south west zone of Malawi

Using the prevalence of blindness in persons aged 50 and above (3.3%) and the national statistical estimate (approximately 5% of the population being above the age of 50 in the south west zone) this translates to a total of 3,534 blind people of whom 1,703 (48.2%) have unoperated cataract.

Discussion

This study was conducted in order to generate information about the magnitude and causes of blindness and to use the information for planning a VISION 2020 programme in the south west zone of Malawi.

The survey found that 3.3% (95% CI 2.5–4.1) of the population over the age of 50 were blind. The main causes of blindness were cataract, glaucoma and non-trachomatous corneal scarring. It is estimated that approximately 1,703 people in the Southern Region of Malawi are blind from cataract.

There were more females (62%) than males (38%) in the sample. Table 2 shows that this is representative of the population of Southern Malawi where the census in 2008 revealed a female predominance.

The prevalence of blindness in persons aged 50 and above found in this survey is much lower than the WHO estimate (9%) [7]. This is probably a function of the limited data available at the time the WHO estimates were developed (prior to 2004), and the on-going development of prevention of blindness activities (in particular a large increase in the numbers of cataract surgeries being performed) that have become established in east and southern Africa.

The prevalence estimate in Malawi is higher than those from other RAAB surveys within the region: Rwanda (1.8%) [8];Kenya (2%) [9]; and Tanzania (2.4%) [10]; however the confidence intervals of all estimates of the prevalence of blindness overlap with the estimate from Malawi suggesting similar findings in each survey.

In this study almost 75% of blindness was avoidable. This finding mirrors the VISION 2020 estimate of avoidable blindness of 80% [5].The overall contribution of cataract as a cause of blindness (48.2%) and glaucoma (15.8) are very similar to the recent WHO estimates of causes of blindness [7]. The finding that the majority of causes of blindness are avoidable is encouraging, especially when there are new initiatives to address blindness in the area.

Even though refractive errors were not a major cause of blindness or SVI (13.8%), they were a significant cause of VI (41.1%) suggesting that a key component of any prevention of blindness programme in this area should be the correction of refractive error.

The prevalence of blindness was higher in men than women. This pattern of blindness has not been found in other RAAB surveys in east or southern Africa. The reason for the male preponderance of blindness appears to be due to many more men than women having surgery. Men were more affected by poor outcomes after surgery leaving more of them permanently blind. This finding emphasizes the importance of ensuring high quality cataract surgery as those with poor outcomes remain permanently blind.

If the cut-off for cataract surgery is taken as 6/60 (a common cut off for cataract surgery in many low income settings) then this study suggests that there are approximately 3,360 people in the survey area who might benefit from surgery in at least one eye (termed the 'backlog' of cataract).

The cataract surgical coverage (CSC) in this region was much lower (44.6%) than that reported from studies from Kenya (78%) [9] and Tanzania (68.8%) [10] but similar to findings from Rwanda (47%). It is important to note that, for many years, the

Table 7. Post operative presenting visual acuity and satisfaction with results of IOL surgery.

	Very satisfied		Partially satisfied		Indifferent		Partially unsatisfied		Very unsatisfied		Total
	N	%	N	%	N	%	N	%	N	%	
Can see 6/18	24	83	5	17.2	0		0		0		29
Cannot see 6/18 but can see 6/60	10	77	8	61.5	1	8	0		0		19
Cannot see 6/60	2	8.7	11	47.8	5	22	3	13	2	9	23
Total	**36**	**51**	**24**	**33.8**	**6**	**8**	**3**	**4**	**2**	**3**	**71**

entire region was served by one expatriate ophthalmologist based at the tertiary hospital in Blantyre who conducted infrequent cataract camps in the districts covered by this survey. The lack of frequent screening visits and access to surgical services would explain why the CSC is low and equivalent to Rwanda which also had limited services for a long time due to conflict. Malawi currently still has a very few Ophthalmologists (nine for a population of 13.6 million); and unless plans to scale up the number of individuals conducting cataract surgeries are achieved within the next few years, it is unlikely that the CSC will markedly increase.

The cataract surgical coverage was much higher in males than females, a finding that has been repeated by other researchers in many countries. It has been reported that men have a much higher chance of accessing cataract surgery services than women [14,15,16,17,18,19,20] and women are less likely to report a need for sight than men [21]. Recent evidence suggest that gender disparity in accessing eye services also occur in children, with more boys accessing eye services than girls [22]. Case finding activities for cataract should prioritise women and service providers should monitor the gender mix of surgeries to ensure that women are receiving the surgery they need.

Poor outcomes of cataract surgery as seen in this survey arise from both the service providers (medical staff) and consumers (patients). Doctors often perform surgeries under suboptimal conditions in outreach camps and may lack skills to handle cases effectively when complications arise, which can result in poor visual outcomes. It can be difficult to screen patients for pre-existing eye diseases (e.g. glaucoma) when they have a dense cataract which means that post-operatively their vision might not improve despite having perfect surgery. Frequently biometry is not available which means standard intraocular lenses are inserted which might not be appropriate for the patient. Finally post operative patients from eye camps are often left without adequate medication or follow up meaning that complications, such as uveitis, are more likely to arise and lead to permanent damage. One solution is for all cataract patients to be referred to dedicated eye centres where they can be appropriately assessed and operated on under the best possible conditions.

The strengths of this study were that there was recent population census data from 2008 to derive the sample, and that accurate village-level data was available to identify those older than 50 years (although this was compounded by many individuals lack of knowledge about their age). The survey was conducted by two experienced ophthalmologists whose diagnostic agreement was found to be robust.

Limitations of the study were the small numbers of people found to be blind in the survey meaning that extrapolations and sub-group analyses had wide confidence limits. The absence of specialised diagnostic equipment meant that cases of posterior segment disease such as glaucoma and age-related macular degeneration were identified by clinical examination only which meant that results for posterior segment causes of blindness must be interpreted with care. A final limitation of the RAAB methodology is that the patient reports (satisfaction with surgery, reasons for not having surgery) are not validated and whilst useful for service planners, should be explored further if more information is required.

In conclusion this survey found a lower than expected prevalence of blindness and visual impairment in persons age 50 and above in southern Malawi, with the majority of causes of blindness and visual impairment being avoidable. The survey provides important information for planning a VISION 2020 programme for the area and can be used as baseline information for an assessment of the impact of any programme at a later time.

Acknowledgments

Staff from Sight Savers (Malawi office) played an important role in organising the logistics for the survey and we would like to thank Country Representative and the entire team.

We would also like to thank the District Health Management Teams (DHMT) from the 7 districts comprising the South West Zone for providing staff from the environmental health departments, in particular Health Surveillance Assistants (HSA's), who provided village registers for all the selected clusters. Lastly we would like to thank the village chiefs and volunteers who assisted in identifying the boundaries of the villages.

Author Contributions

Conceived and designed the experiments: KK RL. Performed the experiments: KK MM DM VM. Analyzed the data: KK. Contributed reagents/materials/analysis tools: KK RL. Wrote the paper: KK RL.

References

1. (2008) www.VISION2020.org.
2. Foster A (2003) VISION 2020:from epidemiology to program. In: Johnson G, Minassian D, Weale R, West S, eds. The Epidemiology of Eye Disease. second ed. London: Arnold. pp 373–383.
3. Resnikoff S, Kocur I, Etya'ale DE, Ukety TO (2008) Vision 2020 - the right to sight. Ann Trop Med Parasitol 102 Suppl 1: 3–5.
4. Foster A, Resnikoff S (2005) The impact of Vision 2020 on global blindness. Eye (Lond) 19: 1133–1135.
5. Oie M, Rund BR (1999) Neuropsychological deficits in adolescent-onset schizophrenia compared with attention deficit hyperactivity disorder. Am J Psychiatry 156: 1216–1222.
6. Resnikoff S, Pascolini D, Mariotti SP, Pokharel GP (2008) Global magnitude of visual impairment caused by uncorrected refractive errors in 2004. Bull World Health Organ 86: 63–70.
7. Resnikoff S, Pascolini D, Etya'ale D, Kocur I, Pararajasegaram R, et al. (2004) Global data on visual impairment in the year 2002. Bull World Health Organ 82: 844–851.
8. Mathenge W, Nkurikiye J, Limburg H, Kuper H (2007) Rapid Assessment of Avoidable Blindness in Western Rwanda: Blindness in a Postconflict Setting. PLoS Med 4.
9. Mathenge W, Kuper H, Limburg H, Polack S, Onyango O, et al. (2007) Rapid assessment of avoidable blindness in Nakuru district, Kenya. Ophthalmology 114: 599–605.
10. Habiyakire C, Kabona G, Courtright P, Lewallen S (2010) Rapid assessment of avoidable blindness and cataract surgical services in kilimanjaro region, Tanzania. Ophthalmic Epidemiol 17: 90–94.
11. Oye JE, Kuper H, Dineen B, Befidi-Mengue R, A F (2006) Prevalence and causes of blindness and visual impairment in Muyuka: A rural health district in South West Province, Cameroon. Br J Ophthalmol 90: 538–542.
12. Courtright P, Hoechsmann A, Metcalfe N, Chirambo M, Noertjojo K, et al. (2003) Changes in blindness prevalence over 16 years in Malawi: reduced prevalence but increased numbers of blind. Br J Ophthalmol 87: 1079–1082.
13. (2008) Malawi Housing and Population 2008 census. National Statistical office, Zomba Malawi.
14. Courtright P, Lewallen S (2007) Improving gender equity in eye care: advocating for the needs of women. Community Eye Health 20: 68–69.
15. Lewallen S, Mousa A, Bassett K, Courtright P (2009) Cataract surgical coverage remains lower in women. Br J Ophthalmol 93: 295–298.
16. Courtright P, Metcalfe N, Hoechsmann A, Chirambo M, Lewallen S, et al. (2004) Cataract surgical coverage and outcome of cataract surgery in a rural district in Malawi. Can J Ophthalmol 39: 25–30.
17. Lewallen S, Courtright P (2006) Increasing uptake of eye services by women. Community Eye Health 19: 59–60.
18. Courtright P, Lewallen S (2009) Why are we addressing gender issues in vision loss? Community Eye Health 22: 17–19.
19. Lewallen S, Courtright P (2002) Gender and use of cataract surgical services in developing countries. Bull World Health Organ 80: 300–303.
20. Abou-Gareeb I, Lewallen S, Bassett K, Courtright P (2001) Gender and blindness: a meta-analysis of population-based prevalence surveys. Ophthalmic Epidemiol 8: 39–56.

21. Geneau R, Lewallen S, Bronsard A, Paul I, Courtright P (2005) The social and family dynamics behind the uptake of cataract surgery: findings from Kilimanjaro region, Tanzania. Br J Ophthalmol 89: 1399–1402.

22. Courtright P, Williams T, Gilbert C, Kishiki E, Shirima S, et al. (2008) Measuring cataract surgical services in children: an example from Tanzania. Br J Ophthalmol 92: 1031–1034.

The Impact of Cataract Surgery on Activities and Time-Use: Results from a Longitudinal Study in Kenya, Bangladesh and the Philippines

Sarah Polack[1]*, Christina Eusebio[2], Wanjiku Mathenge[3], Zazkia Wadud[4], Mamunur Rashid[5], Allen Foster[1], Hannah Kuper[1]

1 Department of Infectious and Tropical Diseases, London School of Hygiene and Tropical Medicine, Keppel Street, London, United Kingdom, **2** Cataract Foundation of the Philippines, Bacolod, Philippines, **3** Eye Unit, Rift Valley Provincial Hospital, Nakuru, Kenya, **4** Child Sight Foundation, Dhaka, Bangladesh, **5** CSS Rawm Hospital, Khulna, Bangladesh

Abstract

Background: Cataract is the leading cause of blindness in the world, and blindness from cataract is particularly common in low-income countries. The aim of this study is to explore the impact of cataract surgery on daily activities and time-use in Kenya, Bangladesh and the Philippines.

Methods/Principal Findings: A multi-centre intervention study was conducted in three countries. Time-use data were collected through interview from cases aged ≥50 years with visually impairing cataract (VA <6/24) and age- and gender-matched controls with normal vision (VA≥6/18). Cases were offered free/subsidized cataract surgery. Approximately one year later participants were re-interviewed about time-use. At baseline across the three countries there were 651 cases and 571 controls. Fifty-five percent of cases accepted surgery. Response rate at follow up was 84% (303 out of 361) for operated cases, and 80% (459 out of 571) for controls. At baseline, cases were less likely to carry out and spent less time on productive activities (paid and non-paid work) and spent more time in "inactivity" compared to controls. Approximately one year after cataract surgery, operated cases were more likely to undertake productive activities compared to baseline (Kenya from 55% to 88%; Bangladesh 60% to 95% and Philippines 81% to 94%, $p<0.001$) and mean time spent on productive activities increased by one-two hours in each setting ($p<0.001$). Time spent in "inactivity" in Kenya and Bangladesh decreased by approximately two hours ($p<0.001$). Frequency of reported assistance with activities was more than halved in each setting ($p<0.001$).

Conclusions/Significance: The empirical evidence provided by this study of increased time spent on productive activities, reduced time in inactivity and reduced assistance following cataract surgery among older adults in low-income settings has positive implications for well-being and inclusion, and supports arguments of economic benefit at the household level from cataract surgery.

Editor: Nancy Mock, Tulane University, United States of America

Funding: This study was funded by grants from CBM (http://www.cbmi.org/), SightSavers International (http://www.sightsavers.org/default.html) and ORBIS UK (http://www.orbis.org/). Representatives from these non-governmental organizations (NGO) were part of the steering committee for the study, which gave guidance towards conduct of the study but they were not involved in the study design, data collection and analysis, decision to publish, or preparation of the manuscript.

Competing Interests: Professor Allen Foster (one of the co-authors) was involved in this study in his position as Director of the International Centre for Eye Health at the London School of Hygiene & Tropical Medicine. At the time of the study Professor Foster was also the Medical Advisor to CBM, one of the international development organizations that co-funded this study. In January 2006, two years into the study, Professor Foster was appointed President of CBM. He contributed to the conception of the study question, study design and critically reviewed the draft of the article. He was not involved in the data collection, data analysis or interpretation of results.

* E-mail: sarah.polack@lshtm.ac.uk

Introduction

Cataract is the leading cause of blindness and low vision worldwide[1]. The burden of visual impairment from cataract is particularly high in the poorest countries, where it is commonly responsible for at least 50% of all blindness[2]. Visual impairment from cataract is associated with increased difficulties with activities of daily living and reduced quality of life.[3–6]

Engagement in leisure and productive activities (paid and non-paid e.g. domestic activities, home food production, child-care) is an important component of well-being in later life. [7–8] Productive activities are also likely to contribute to individual and household economy.[9] In rural low-income settings, where the prevalence of un-operated cataract is highest, all household members regardless of age commonly contribute to the basic needs of a household [10]. While direct employment opportunities may be limited in these settings, particularly in the age group most affected by cataract, the economic contribution of non-paid productive activities is well recognised. [9]

A positive effect of increased engagement in daily activities following cataract surgery is frequently asserted, yet there is a lack of empirical evidence either supporting or refuting this. Previous studies have shown using visual functioning questionnaires that people report less difficulty undertaking daily activities after cataract surgery.[11–14]. However, information is lacking on whether actual participation in and time spent on different daily activities changes following cataract surgery. No prospective studies comparing time-use patterns before and after cataract surgery could be identified. This link is likely to be complicated because cataract predominantly affects older people who may experience other co-morbidities influencing their engagement in activities.

The 'Cataract Impact Study' was undertaken to explore the impact of cataract surgery on poverty, quality of life and time-use in Kenya, Bangladesh and the Philippines among people aged ≥50 years. At baseline we found that people visually impaired from cataract (cases) were less likely to participate in and spent less time on productive activities compared to age- and gender-matched controls with normal vision.[15] Cases also spent more time in 'inactivity' and were more likely to require assistance with activities. At baseline, cases were offered cataract surgery and were followed up after one year. The aim of the current paper is to assess the impact of cataract surgery by comparing participation, time spent and assistance with different daily activities before and one year after cataract surgery in these three different low-income settings.

Methods

Ethical approval for this study was granted by ethics committees of the London School of Hygiene &Tropical Medicine, Kenya Medical Research Institute, Bangladesh Medical Research Council and the University of St. La Salle, Bacolod, The Philippines. Informed signed/thumb-printed consent was obtained from all study participants.

Study overview

The 'Cataract Impact Study' was a longitudinal intervention study conducted in Kenya (Nakuru district), Bangladesh (Satkhira district) and the Philippines (Negros Island and Antique district). At baseline cases with visual impairment from cataract and controls without visual impairment were identified and interviewed about time-use, health related quality of life and poverty. All cases were offered free or subsidized surgery. Approximately one year later cases and controls were re-traced, re-examined and re-interviewed. This paper presents the findings from the time-use data.

Study population

Sample size calculations were powered to detect a 30% increase in time spent on productive activities, with an alpha of 0.05 and 80% power. To detect this improvement required 100 operated cases in each country examined at baseline and follow-up.

Cases and controls were identified primarily through population-based surveys of blindness which included >3600 people aged ≥50 years in each setting.[16] Clusters were selected using systematic cluster sampling with probability proportionate to size and within clusters, households were selected through compact segment sampling.[17] People identified in the survey aged ≥50 years with pinhole corrected visual acuity (VA) <6/24 in the better eye due to cataract were eligible to be cases. VA was measured using a tumbling E chart and the presence of cataract was assessed through ophthalmic examination with a direct ophthalmoscope. One (or up to two in Bangladesh) age- gender and cluster matched controls without visual impairment from cataract were selected per case identified in the survey. During the survey the eligible controls in each cluster were listed by gender and age group (50–54, 55–59, 65–69 and ≥70 years). When a case was identified, one control (or up to two in Bangladesh) of the same gender and age group were selected at random for inclusion. If there were no matching controls at that time then the subsequent eligible control identified in the cluster was recruited.

Due to logistical and time constraints, additional cases were identified in each setting through community-based case detection. In Kenya and Negros (Philippines) additional clusters were selected using probability proportionate to size sampling after completion of the population based-survey. These clusters were visited in advance and asked that all people aged ≥50 years with eyesight problems come to a central point on a specified day and that people unable to attend (e.g. due to blindness or physical disability) be noted. All people attending the central point and those unable to leave their households underwent an eye examination using the procedures described above. People who met the case definition were invited to participate in the study and were interviewed in their homes. In Bangladesh and Antique (Philippines), case finding was conducted simultaneously with the survey so that age- gender matched controls were also included for these cases. In each cluster the teams asked to be taken to a community member with eye problems living within the boundaries of the cluster but outside the selected segment. The ophthalmologist conducted the ophthalmic examination at the household to identify eligible cases. In Kenya the first 50 patients (from a set date) attending the local hospital for cataract surgery and meeting the case definition were also recruited for the study.

Baseline and follow up

Baseline surveys were conducted between Jan 2005-May 2006. All cases were counselled and offered surgery at one hospital in the study district. In Kenya and Bangladesh free surgery was offered. In the Philippines a fee was requested but those who could not afford the fee were offered free surgery. Follow up surveys were undertaken approximately one year later, during the same climatic season. Interviews were conducted in respondents' own homes (except for hospital cases in Kenya) by trained interviewers who were regularly observed by supervisors. The same interviewers were involved at baseline and follow up, except in Bangladesh where two additional people were trained at follow up. Visual acuity of cases and controls at follow up was assessed using the same procedure as baseline.

Measuring time-use

Time-use data were collected using the 'stylised activity list' developed for the World Bank's Living Standards Measurement Survey.[10] Participants were asked whether they had been involved in each of a preset list of common daily activities during the last week and if yes, if they had been involved in the activity yesterday. Those who had been involved in an activity 'yesterday' were asked to estimate how much time they had spent and whether they received any assistance from another person in performing that activity. Interviewers were instructed to check that total time reported was 22–26 hours and if not, to go through the list again with the respondent. Activities were grouped as follows:

- Personal: Sleep, bathing, dressing, eating, other
- Household/family: Cooking/washing dishes, cleaning house/clothes, shopping, looking after children/elderly/sick, other
- Paid work: paid employment, commission work, self employed/own business, other

- Work for own use: Agriculture, animal rearing, fetching firewood/water, processing agricultural products/food, other
- Leisure outside home: social visits, attending ceremonies, attending meetings
- Leisure inside home: reading/listening to radio/watching TV; chatting, relaxing with friends/family; prayer (in Bangladesh), other
- No activity
- Travel

Household/family work, work for own use and paid work were all defined as productive activities.

Covariates

Data were collected on standard socio-demographic indicators and a socio-economic-status (SES) index for each household was developed using Principal Components Analysis, separately for each country.[18]

Statistical analysis

For the purposes of these analyses only controls with VA≥6/18 were included. The mean proportion of time spent on each activity group was calculated by dividing total minutes on specific activity group by the sum of minutes reported on all activities for that individual (as not all totals were exactly 24 hours). To ease interpretation, we then converted the proportion of time into hours and minutes (e.g. if the proportion of reported time on household work was 25%, this was presented as 6hours). All eligible respondents were included in this calculation whether or not they had participated in that activity. Participants were excluded from the analysis of time spent on activities if the total reported time spent on all activities was <19 hours or >30 hours.

We assessed changes in time-use following cataract surgery by comparing time-use at baseline and follow up restricted to participants who had data at both time points. McNemars test was used to compare engagement in activities during the last week (binary variable) among operated cases, un-operated cases and controls (separately). Average time spent on each activity 'yesterday' (continuous variable) was compared for each group using confidence intervals and paired t-tests. Since a substantial number of participants did not participate in household work, work for own use, paid work and leisure outside the home during the previous day, we calculated bootstrap confidence intervals for these variables and the statistical comparison of baseline and follow up time use was repeated using Wilcoxon signed rank test. Findings were essentially unchanged and therefore parametric results are presented. Case/Control comparisons were controlled for the matching variables (age and gender) and SES. Multivariate linear regression analyses were undertaken to explore socio-demographic and ocular (baseline and follow up VA) predictors of change in time spent on productive activities and 'inactivity' among operated cases. For these analyses the data for all three countries were combined. This was considered acceptable because consistent trends in change in time-use were observed between the three settings.

Results

At baseline we included 196 cases visually impaired from cataract in Kenya and 128 controls with normal vision, 217 cases and 280 controls in Bangladesh, and 238 cases and 163 controls in Philippines. All controls and the majority of cases (n = 389, 60%) were identified through the survey, rather than case finding (n = 213, 33%) or from the hospital (n = 49, 8%, Kenya only). Sixty-eight percent of cases (n = 132) identified at baseline attended for surgery in Kenya, 46% (n = 117) in Bangladesh and 47% (n = 112) in the Philippines ("operated cases").

Overall response rate at follow-up was high. In Kenya we re-examined 80% (n = 106) of the operated cases, 65% (n = 40) of un-operated cases and 75% (n = 96) of controls (table 1). Response rates were similar in Bangladesh (85%, 71%, 80%) and the Philippines (88%, 73%, 86%). The causes of non-response were death or the person not available. Refusals to participate at follow up were rare (2 participants in Kenya, 3 in Bangladesh and 3 in the Philippines). Operated cases and controls lost to follow up did not differ systematically from those included in terms of socio-demographic characteristics (data not presented). Operated cases lost to follow up were slightly more likely to participate in productive activities at baseline compared to the operated cases included at follow-up, reaching statistical significance only in the Philippines (data not presented). The final analyses included 106 operated cases and 96 controls in Kenya, 99 operated cases and 223 controls in Bangladesh and 98 operated cases and 140 controls in the Philippines. Among the operated cases at follow up, 71% in Kenya and 72% in the Philippines had presenting VA ≥6/18 in the better eye while this was higher in Bangladesh (84%).

Operated cases and controls were similar in age, gender and marital status but in Kenya and Bangladesh operated cases were less likely to have had a formal education or be in the highest SES group compared to controls (table 2). Un-operated cases were significantly older than operated cases in Kenya and the

Table 1. Loss to follow up statistics by country for operated cases, un-operated cases and controls.

Country	Participant type	Total at Baseline N	Examined at follow up N (%)	Lost to follow-up N (%)
Kenya	Operated cases	132	106 (80%)	26 (20%)
	Controls	128	96 (75%)	32 (25%)
	Un-operated cases	62	40 (65%)	22 (35%)
Bangladesh	Operated cases	117	99 (85%)	18 (15%)
	Controls	280	223 (80%)	57 (20%)
	Un-operated cases	100	71 (71%)	29 (29%)
Philippines	Operated cases	112	98 (88%)	14 (12%)
	Controls	163	140 (86%)	23 (14%)
	Un-operated cases	126	92 (73%)	34 (27%)

Table 2. Demographic and visual acuity characteristics of operated cases and controls examined at baseline and follow-up.

	Kenya			Bangladesh			The Philippines		
	Operated cases (n = 106)	Controls (n = 96)	p-value*	Operated cases (n = 99)	Controls (n = 223)	p-value*	Operated cases (n = 98)	Controls (n = 140)	p-value*
Mean age (95% CI)	74 (72–76)	73 (71–75)	0.7	70 (68–72)	68 (67–69)	0.1	71 (69–73)	70 (69–72)	0.6
Female	56%	56%	0.9	53%	57%	0.4	61%	54%	0.2
Married	52%	58%	0.4	49%	58%	0.1	44%	57%	0.04
Education	25%	45%	0.004	18%	34%	0.04	90%	92%	0.5
Highest SES±	18%	38%	0.002	16%	29%	0.01	18%	29%	0.07
Baseline VA¥									
≥6/18	0%	100%		0%	100%		0%	100%	
<6/24–6/60	39%			29%			23%		
<6/60–3/60	17%			16%			22%		
<3/60>PL	21%			12%			28%		
PL	24%			42%			28%		
Follow up VA†									
≥6/18	71%			84%			72%		
<6-18–6/60	21%			6%			20%		
<6/60	8%			10%			8%		
Surgery	57%			74%			71%		
Unilateral	43%			26%			29%		
Bilateral									

*P-value from anova (continuous variables) or chi Square (categorical variables) comparing operated cases and controls.
±Highest quartile of socio-economic status (SES).
¥Presenting visual acuity in the better eye at baseline.
†Presenting visual acuity in the better eye among operated cases at follow up classified by WHO cataract surgical outcome categories.
PL, Perception of light.

Philippines and were less likely to be married in Kenya and Bangladesh (data not presented). In Kenya un-operated cases had better vision at baseline compared to operated cases but in the other two countries the baseline VA distribution was similar between operated and un-operated cases.

Changes in time-use after cataract surgery

i) Activities carried out during previous week

At baseline in each country cases were significantly less likely than controls to undertake productive activities (Kenya, odds ratio (OR) 0.2, 95% Confidence Intervals (CI) 0.1–0.3; Bangladesh OR 0.1, 95% CI 0.1–0.2; Philippines OR 0.3 95% CI 0.2–0.6). At follow-up, the proportion of operated cases that carried out productive activities had increased significantly (table 3). Overall, nearly 25% more operated cases undertook productive work at follow-up in Kenya and Bangladesh, while for the Philippines the increase was 10% (reflecting the higher proportion engaged at baseline). In contrast, among controls, engagement in productive activities remained similar at baseline and follow up.

In each country there was an increase of at least 20% in the proportion of operated cases participating in leisure outside of the household ($p<0.005$). However this trend was also observed among controls in the Philippines and Bangladesh.

ii) Time spent on activities during previous day

The proportion of outliers excluded from these analyses was 6% in Kenya (<19 hours 4%, >29 hours 2%), 0.4% Bangladesh (<19 hours 0.2%, >29 hours 0.2%) and 12% in The Philippines (<19 hours10%, >29 hours 2%).

Productive activities. At baseline, cases spent significantly less time on productive activities in each country compared to controls (table 4). At follow-up, mean time spent on productive activities by operated cases increased compared to baseline in all three settings ($p<0.001$) (table 4). There was an average increase of 1hr 5mins (95% CI 0:21–1:47) in Kenya, 1hr 20mins (95%CI 0:40–1:59) in Bangladesh and 1hr 51mins (95%C I 0:50–2:52) in the Philippines (figure 1). In contrast among controls, time spent on productive activities either stayed the same (the Philippines) or decreased (Bangladesh and Kenya).

Leisure. At baseline, cases in Kenya spent significantly less time than controls on leisure outside of the household, while in the Philippines cases spent more time on leisure activities inside the household. At follow up, time spent on leisure outside of the household by operated cases increased in Kenya (from 21minutes (95% CI 0:12–0:31) to 1hrs 12mins (95% CI 0:48–1:30), $p<0.001$) and Bangladesh (30mins (95%CI 0:17–0:44) to 1hr13mins (95%Ci 0:59–1:28) $p<0.001$). However, a significant increase was also observed among controls in Bangladesh. In the Philippines, in contrast to the other two countries, time spent on leisure inside the home by operated cases decreased, though not significantly.

No activity. At baseline, in Kenya and Bangladesh, cases on average spent nearly two hours more in inactivity compared to controls (<0.001), while there was little difference in the Philippines. At follow-up there was a reduction of nearly two hours in average time spent on 'no activity' compared to baseline by operated cases in

Table 3. Activities carried out (during previous week) and assistance with activities (previous day) among operated cases and controls at follow up compared to baseline in Kenya, Bangladesh and the Philippines.

		Kenya			Bangladesh			Philippines		
Activity group	**Case/control**	**Baseline N (%)**	**Follow up N (%)**	**p-value***	**Baseline N (%)**	**Follow up N (%)**	**p-value***	**Baseline N (%)**	**Follow up N (%)**	**p-value***
Productive activities										
	Operated cases	53 (52%)	76 (75%)	<0.001	59 (60%)	82 (83%)	<0.001	79 (81%)	89 (91%)	0.01
	Controls	81 (88%)	75 (82%)	0.2	211 (95%)	204 (92%)	0.1	132 (94%)	131 (94%)	0.9
	p-value: cases vs controls†	<0.001	0.4		<0.001	0.02		0.001	0.2	
Leisure outside household										
	Operated cases	34 (33%)	58 (59%)	<0.001	37 (37%)	69 (70%)	<0.001	37 (38%)	56 (57%)	0.005
	Controls	56 (61%)	58 (63%)	0.8	91 (41%)	69 (70%)	<0.001	62 (44%)	103 (74%)	0.001
	p-value: cases vs controls†	<0.001	0.2		0.6	0.5		0.3	0.02	
Leisure inside household										
	Operated cases	81 (79%)	85 (83%)	0.4	98 (99%)	99 (99%)	N/A	91 (93%)	95 (97%)	0.2
	Controls	79 (86%)	82 (89%)	0.4	222 (99%)	222 (99%)	N/A	133 (95%)	138 (99%)	0.06
	p-value: cases vs controls†	0.2	0.2		0.6	0.5		0.5	0.7	
Assistance with any activity										
	Operated	26 (25%)	12 (12%)	0.01	43 (43%)	19 (19%)	<0.001	23 (23%)	1 (1%)	<0.001
	Controls	2 (2%)	6 (7%)	0.2	20 (9%)	35 (16%)	0.03	12 (9%)	7 (5%)	0.2
	p-value: cases vs controls†	<0.001	0.2		<0.001	0.4		0.02	<0.001	

*P-value from McNemars chi squared test comparing participation at baseline and follow up among i) operated cases and ii) controls.
†P-value from chi square comparing participation between operated cases and controls at i) baseline and ii) follow up.
NB Data are not presented for inactivity as nearly all (>97%) cases and controls engaged in this at baseline and follow up.

Kenya and Bangladesh ($p<0.001$, figure 1) with no change in the Philippines. Time spent on 'no activity' among controls did not change significantly from baseline and follow up.

Assistance with activities at baseline and follow up

At baseline 26% (n = 26, Kenya), 43% (n = 43, Bangladesh) and 23% (n = 23, Philippines) of cases reported receiving assistance while this was lower for controls (n = 2, 2% Kenya; n = 20, 9% Bangladesh; n = 12, 9% Philippines, $p<0.001$). At follow up the proportion of operated cases reporting assistance with any activity during the previous day reduced by at least half compared to baseline in each country (table 3), although a decrease was also observed for un-operated cases in the Philippines (from n = 14, 15% to n = 5, 5%, p = 0.03, data not presented). Among controls, the proportion reporting receiving assistance increased in Bangladesh (from n = 20, 9% to n = 35, 16%, p = 0.03), but not in the other two countries. Most reported assistance was for personal activities (sleeping, bathing, dressing and eating).

Comparison of cases and controls at follow up

After cataract surgery, time-use patterns of operated cases became more similar to controls (tables 3 and 4). The average time spent on productive activities by operated cases remained less than controls (approximately 1hour in Kenya and Bangladesh, 30mins in Philippines), although this difference was smaller than at baseline and not significant for most activity groups. In contrast, un-operated cases continued to spend between 2–3hrs less time ($p<0.04$), on productive activities and more time (1½–2hrs) doing 'no activity' compared to controls ($p<0.003$ in each country, data not presented).

Predictors of change in time-use among operated cases

We explored the predictors of change in time spent on productive activities and inactivity from baseline to follow-up among the operated cases. Increases in time spent on productive activities were significantly larger among operated cases aged 50–60 years compared to those aged ≥80 years (p = 0.04, table 5) but no associations with other socio-demographic variables were found. People who were severely visually impaired (VA<6/60–3/60), blind (VA<3/60) or had perception of light at baseline had larger increases in time on productive activities compared to those with moderate visual impairment (VA <6/24–6/60) (p-for-trend = 0.001). Increases in time on productive activities were smaller among operated cases with poor VA outcome from surgery (VA<6/60) compared to those with good outcome (VA ≥6/18, p = 0.02). Change in time spent in inactivity was not associated with the socio-demographic and ocular factors included.

Discussion

The Cataract Impact Study found that adults aged ≥50 years were more likely to undertake and spent significantly more time on productive activities after cataract surgery compared to before and this was consistent across three different low-income settings. Further, after surgery their time-use patterns become similar to those of age- gender-matched controls with normal vision. To our knowledge this is the first time the impact of cataract surgery has been explored through comparison of time-use patterns.

Time-spent on productive activities, after cataract surgery, increased by an average of one-two hours. Time spent in

Table 4. Comparison of time spent on different activity categories at baseline and follow up among operated cases and controls.

		Kenya			Bangladesh			The Philippines		
Activity category	Case/ control	Baseline Mean time* hrs:mins (95%CI)	Follow up Mean time* hrs:mins (95%CI)	P-value†	Baseline Mean time* hrs:mins (95%CI)	Follow up Mean time* hrs:mins (95%CI)	p-value†	Baseline Mean time* hrs:mins (95%CI)	Follow up Mean time* hrs:mins (95%CI)	p -value†
Productive										
	Operated cases	2:24(1:48–3:00)	3:30(2:54–4:12)	0.008	2:03(1:34–2:32)	3:26(2:47–4:05)	<0.001	3:42(2:57–4:27)	5:24(4:37–6:11)	0.001
	Controls	5:18(4:30–6:12)	4:36(3:48–5:24)	0.2	5:06(4:42–5:29)	4:29(4:04–4:54)	0.003	5:56(5:15–6:38)	6:01(5:24–6:39)	0.1
	p-value‡ case vs control	<0.001	0.1		<0.001	0.03		<0.001	0.06	
Leisure outside household										
	Operated cases	0:21(0:12–0.31)	1:12(0:48–1:30)	<0.001	0:30(0:17–0:44)	1:13(0:59–1:28)	<0.001	0:59(0:40–1:18)	1:11(0:51–1:30)	0.3
	Controls	1:12(0:42–1:42)	1:30(1:06–1:54)	0.4	0:37(0:25–0:49)	1:04(0:54–1:15)	<0.001	1:04(0:46–1:22)	1:15(0:57–1:32)	0.3
	p-value‡ case vs control	<0.001	0.3		0.7	0.3		0.6	0.7	
Leisure inside household										
	Operated cases	2:48(2:18–3:12)	3:30(3:00–4:00)	0.02	3:50(3:28–4:12)	3:56(3:34–4:17)	0.7	4:39(3:57–5:22)	3:58(3:28–4:29)	0.08
	Controls	3:06(2.36–3:30)	3:24(2:54–3:54)	0.3	3:22(3:11–3:34)	3:38(3:25–3:51)	0.04	3:07(2:42–3:32)	3:33(3:12–3:54)	0.05
	p-value‡ case vs control	0.4	0.8		0.06	0.3		<0.001	0.3	
No activity										
	Operated cases	6:36(5:54–7:24)	4:30(4:06–5:00)	<0.001	5:20(4:48–5:52)	3:26(2:57–3:56)	<0.001	4:14(3:22–5:07)	4:05(3:18–4:52)	0.5
	Controls	4:00(3:24–4:42)	3:48(3:18–4:18)	0.6	3:06(2:48–3:24)	3:07(2:48–3:26)	0.9	4:33(3:50–5:15)	4:09(3:31–4:47)	0.4
	p-value‡ case vs control	<0.001	0.04		<0.001	0.5		0.6	0.9	

*Mean time spent by participants with complete data at baseline and follow up. Participants with outlier values at either baseline or follow up were excluded.
†P-value from paired t-test comparing time-use at baseline and follow up.
‡P-value from anova comparing time-use among operated cases versus controls at a) baseline and b)follow up, controlling for age and gender.

'inactivity' reduced by nearly two hours in Kenya and Bangladesh and in the Philippines time spent on leisure inside the home decreased by nearly an hour. This corresponds with findings from baseline; in Kenya and Bangladesh at baseline, cases spent much more time "doing nothing" than controls while in the Philippines there were no differences in inactivity, but cases spent more time on leisure in the home. Reductions in both these activity groups may indicate a change towards increased engagement in more 'active' pastimes. The decreased proportion of operated cases reporting assistance at follow up, in each country, also indicates increased independence following cataract surgery.

Time use patterns can vary for a number of different reasons from one year to the next and it was to address this issue that control subjects were included in the study. The fact that increases in productive activities (engagement and time-spent) and reductions with reported assistance were consistently observed among operated cases, but not their age- gender matched controls lends important support to cataract surgery being the major causal factor in these changes among operated cases.

Many cultural and personal factors influence how people spend their time and it is neither possible nor desirable to define an 'ideal' time-use pattern. However the observed increase in productive activities supports the frequently postulated economic impact of cataract surgery. While this is most obvious for paid work, non-paid productive activities also make important economic contributions through different routes.[9] Where money for purchasing food is scarce, producing food for own use is an economic imperative. Domestic activities are essential components without which other activities contributing more directly to a household's economy cannot occur. Child-care undertaken by older adults may free up time for other household members to engage in income generating activities.[19] The reduced need for assistance with daily activities observed in this study after surgery may also contribute to this effect. Estimates from a UNDP report suggest that on a global level if "unpaid activities were treated as market transactions at the prevailing wages they would yield huge monetary valuations – a staggering $16 trillion".[9] The increased participation in different produc-

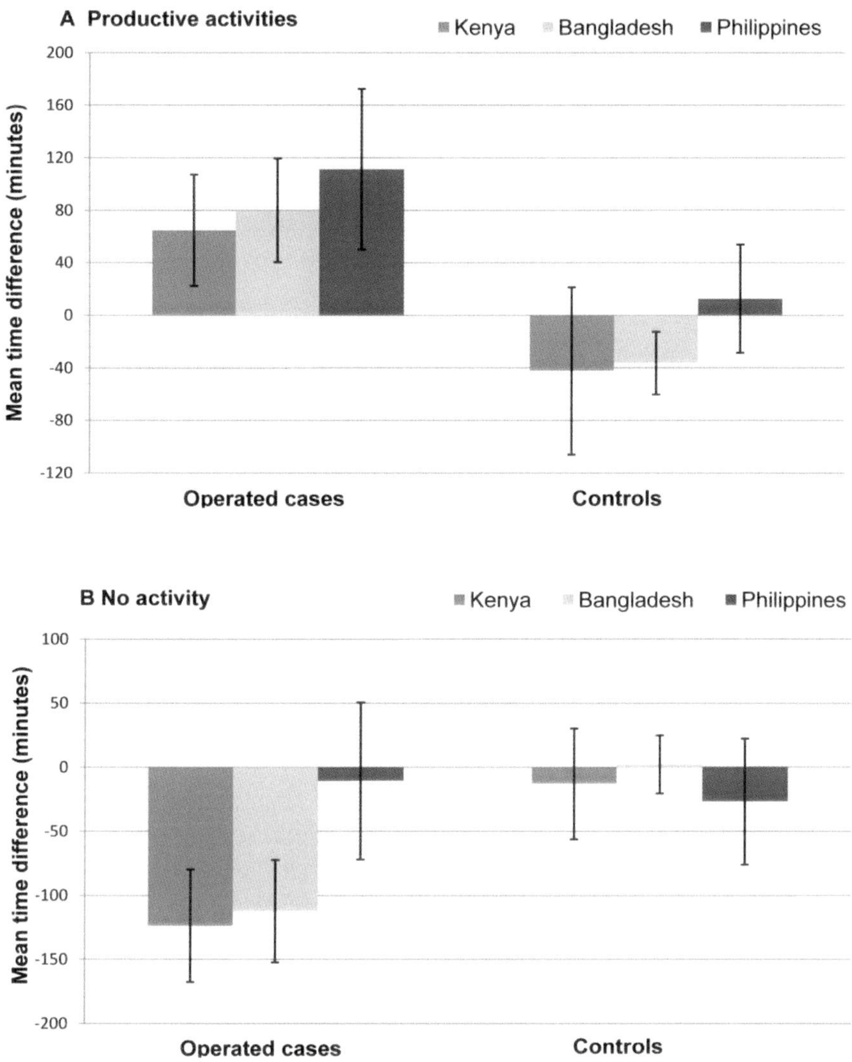

Figure 1. Change in time spent on productive activities and inactivity between baseline and follow up.

tive activities observed in this study therefore provide some evidence of a mechanism by which cataract surgery may contribute to improved economy.

Increased engagement in daily activities and reduced inactivity and need for assistance also have important implications for well-being. Previous studies have shown a positive relationship between involvement in activities and well-being, cognitive function and life satisfaction among older adults. [7–8,20] Further, these findings may indicate an increased role in family and community, supporting a human rights argument for sight restoration on the basis of improved inclusion in society.

The differences in time-use between operated cases and controls reduced compared to baseline. However, the overall time spent on productive activities by operated cases remained slightly lower at follow up, perhaps because of continued loss of functioning due to vision or other age-related conditions beside cataract or the difficulty in reversing a less active role in a household.

Limited research has been conducted in this area to allow comparison and no studies were identified that interviewed patients pre and post-operatively. Our findings support, to some extent, those of Javitt et al (1983) who found re-engagement in paid work and household activities following cataract surgery in India.[19] The reported proportion returning to paid work was much higher than in the current study (85% men, 58% women), perhaps because the study population was younger and the majority were in paid employment prior to sight loss.

The direct cost of cataract surgery to the patient in the study settings is between US$40–60 including follow up appointments and medicines. In each of these settings however, systems are in place to provide free surgery for patients who are unable to pay.

Limitations

Limitations of the time-use data collection method include the reliance on recall of time-use and the collection of time-use for a single day, which may not be a 'typical' day. [10] Follow-up interviews were not always conducted in the same month as baseline and time of year may influence time-use patterns. It was not possible to mask interviewers as to the case/control status at baseline or follow up. There was no assessment of preferences regarding different activities and changes in time-use. We acknowledge that while there is a tendency to view productive activities as positive, the burden of too much work can also be a negative phenomenon. [21]. Increased participation in leisure outside of the home was observed for controls as well as operated cases in Bangladesh and the Philippines and

Table 5. Predictors of change in time spent on productive activities from baseline to follow up among operated cases across the three countries combined.

Variable		N	Mean change in time spent minutes (95% CI)	Coefficient (95% CI)*	p-value*
Age group (years)	50–59	28	197 (113–282)	Reference	
	69–69	73	82 (26–138)	−99.2 (−196.7– −1.6)	0.05
	70–79	108	56 (13–99)	−121.7 (−215.1–28.3)	0.01
	≥80	62	70 (23–116)	−109.3(−210.0– −8.6)	0.03
	*P for trend**			0.07	
Gender	Male	122	79 (38–122)	Reference	
	Female	149	82 (47–117)	1.0 (4.8–166.1)	0.97
Baseline VA**	<6/24 - 6/60	82	8 (−38–55)	Reference	
	<6/60 - 3/60	104	104 (46–163)	85.5 (4.8–166.2)	0.04
	<3/60 >PL	88	88 (17–158)	89.5 (10.2–168.2)	0.03
	PL	130	130 (86–176)	121 (54.3–188.4)	<0.001
	*P for trend**			0.001	
Follow up VA**	>6/18	205	97 (66–126)	Reference	
	6/18–6/60	41	51 (−23–126)	−55.0 (−130–20.9)	0.16
	<6/60	25	2 (−88–92)	−106 (−72.3–55.3)	0.02
	*P for trend**			0.01	

*Coefficients, 95% Confidence Intervals and P-values are derived from the multivariate linear regression analysis.
**Presenting visual acuity in the better eye.
PL Perception of light.
There was no association between change in time spent and SES, literacy, marital status and unilateral/bilateral surgery and these data are not presented.

therefore cannot be attributed to cataract surgery. This may be explained by timing of surveys in relation to community events (end of Eid during the baseline in Bangladesh and fiestas during follow up in the Philippines).

Simplified examination techniques were used to diagnose visual impairment from cataract and therefore co-morbidities contributing to poor vision may not have been detected. However this reflects the 'real world' situation where patients with co-morbidity commonly undergo surgery even if only small increases in vision are expected and, if anything, would likely result in smaller changes in time-use following cataract surgery. A substantial proportion of the cases did not attend for surgery in each country. Few socio-demographic differences between operated and un-operated cases were observed limiting the potential affect on external validity. The exception was that un-operated cases were older than the operated cases. It is therefore possible that if more of the un-operated cases had undergone surgery and been included at the follow up, average increases in time spent on productive activities may have been slightly smaller.

Strengths

This was a large multi-country longitudinal study and similar trends in time-use change were seen across three countries. Cases and controls were population based, recruited from randomly selected clusters in the survey area (with the exception of 50 hospital cases in Kenya) and were therefore likely to be representative of the general population in the study areas. The relative stability of time-use among controls provides support to the reliability of the questionnaire and to cataract surgery being a major factor in the time-use changes observed among operated cases.

Conclusion

In conclusion, this study provides empirical evidence of increased time spent on productive activities and less time in inactivity following cataract surgery among older adults in low-income settings. As well as the positive implications for well-being and inclusion, this provides support to arguments of economic gain from sight restoring cataract surgery.

Acknowledgments

We would like to thank all the people who kindly participated in this study. We would also like to thank all the ophthalmologists, doctors, interviewers who undertook the data collection, the village guides and health workers who assisted with this study and the office managers and data entry staff.

Author Contributions

Performed the experiments: SP. Analyzed the data: SP. Wrote the paper: SP. Substantial contribution to design of study: SP, AF, HK. Substantial contribution to acquisition of data: SP, CE, WM, ZW, MR, HK. Substantial contribution to analysis and interpretation of data: SP, HK. Responsible for drafting the article: SP, HK. Approved final version to be published: SP, CE, WM, ZW, MR, AF, HK. Substantial contribution to the critical revision of the article for important intellectual content: CE, WM, ZW, MR, AF, HK. Substantial contribution to the conception of the study: AF, HK.

References

1. Resnikoff S, Pascolini D, Mariotti SP, Pokharel GP (2008) Global magnitude of visual impairment caused by uncorrected refractive errors in 2004. Bull World Health Organ 86: 63–70.
2. Resnikoff S, Pascolini D, Etya'ale D, Kocur I, Pararajasegaram R, et al. (2004) Global data on visual impairment in the year 2002. Bull World Health Organ 82: 844–851.

3. He M, Xu J, Li S, Wu K, Munoz SR, et al. (1999) Visual acuity and quality of life in patients with cataract in Doumen County, China. Ophthalmology 106: 1609–1615.
4. Nirmalan PK, Tielsch JM, Katz J, Thulasiraj RD, Krishnadas R, et al. (2005) Relationship between vision impairment and eye disease to vision-specific quality of life and function in rural India: the Aravind Comprehensive Eye Survey. Invest Ophthalmol Vis Sci 46: 2308–2312.
5. Nutheti R, Shamanna BR, Nirmalan PK, Keeffe JE, Krishnaiah S, et al. (2006) Impact of impaired vision and eye disease on quality of life in Andhra Pradesh. Invest Ophthalmol Vis Sci 47: 4742–4748.
6. Polack S, Kuper H, Wadud Z, Fletcher A, Foster A (2008) Quality of life and visual impairment from cataract in Satkhira district, Bangladesh. Br J Ophthalmol 92: 1026–1030.
7. Menec VH (2003) The relation between everyday activities and successful aging: a 6-year longitudinal study. J Gerontol B Psychol Sci Soc Sci 58: S74–82.
8. Steinkamp MW, Kelly JR (1987) Social integration, leisure activity, and life satisfaction in older adults: activity theory revisited. Int J Aging Hum Dev 25: 293–307.
9. UNDP (1995) Human Development Report. Chapter: 4 Valuing women's work. UNDP. pp 87–98.
10. Harvey AS, Taylor ME (2000) Time Use. In: Grosh M, Glewwe P, eds. Designing household survey questionnaires for developing countries Lessons from 15 years of the Living Standards Measurement Study. Washington: The World Bank. pp 249–275.
11. Applegate WB, Miller ST, Elam JT, Freeman JM, Wood TO, et al. (1987) Impact of cataract surgery with lens implantation on vision and physical function in elderly patients. Jama 257: 1064–1066.
12. Fletcher A, Vijaykumar V, Selvaraj S, Thulasiraj RD, Ellwein LB (1998) The Madurai Intraocular Lens Study. III: Visual functioning and quality of life outcomes. Am J Ophthalmol 125: 26–35.
13. Mamidipudi PR, Vasavada AR, Merchant SV, Namboodiri V, Ravilla TD (2003) Quality-of-life and visual function assessment after phacoemulsification in an urban indian population. J Cataract Refract Surg 29: 1143–1151.
14. McGwin G, Jr., Scilley K, Brown J, Owsley C (2003) Impact of cataract surgery on self-reported visual difficulties: comparison with a no-surgery reference group. J Cataract Refract Surg 29: 941–948.
15. Polack S, Kuper H, Eusebio C, Mathenge W, Wadud Z, et al. (2008) The impact of cataract on time-use: results from a population based case-control study in Kenya, the Philippines and Bangladesh. Ophthalmic Epidemiol 15: 372–382.
16. Kuper H, Polack S, Eusebio C, Mathenge W, Wadud Z, et al. (2008) A case-control study to assess the relationship between poverty and visual impairment from cataract in Kenya, the Philippines, and Bangladesh. PLoS Med 5: e244.
17. Turner AG, Magnani RJ, Shuaib M (1996) A not quite as quick but much cleaner alternative to the Expanded Programme on Immunization (EPI) Cluster Survey design. Int J Epidemiol 25: 198–203.
18. Filmer D, Pritchett L (2001) Estimating wealth effects without expenditure data - or tears. An application to educational enrollment in states of India. Demography 38: 115–132.
19. Javitt J, Venkataswamy G, Sommer A (1983) The economic and social aspect of restoring sight. In: Henkind P, ed. ACTA: 24th International Congress of Ophthalmology. New York: JP Lippincott. pp 1308–1312.
20. Hawkins BA (2005) Aging well: toward a way of life for all people. Prev Chronic Dis 2: A03.
21. Baker L, Cahalin L, Gerst K, Burr J (2005) Productive activities and subjective well-being among older adults: the influence of the number of activities and time commitment. Social Indicators Research 73: 431–458.

A Rapid Assessment of Avoidable Blindness in Southern Zambia

Robert Lindfield[1]*, Ulla Griffiths[2], Fiammetta Bozzani[2], Musonda Mumba[3], Joseph Munsanje[4]

1 International Centre for Eye Health, London School of Hygiene and Tropical Medicine (LSHTM), London, United Kingdom, **2** Department of Global Health and Development, London School of Hygiene and Tropical Medicine (LSHTM), London, United Kingdom, **3** Lusaka Eye Hospital, Lusaka, Zambia, **4** S & S Development Consultants, Lusaka, Zambia

Abstract

Introduction: A rapid assessment of avoidable blindness (RAAB) was conducted in Southern Zambia to establish the prevalence and causes of blindness in order to plan effective services and advocate for support for eye care to achieve the goals of VISION 2020: the right to sight.

Methods: Cluster randomisation was used to select villages in the survey area. These were further subdivided into segments. One segment was selected randomly and a survey team moved from house to house examining everyone over the age of 50 years. Each individual received a visual acuity assessment and simple ocular examination. Data was recorded on a standard proforma and entered into an established software programme for analysis.

Results: 2.29% of people over the age of 50 were found to be blind (VA <3/60 in the better eye with available correction). The major cause of blindness was cataract (47.2%) with posterior segment disease being the next main cause (18.8%). 113 eyes had received cataract surgery with 30.1% having a poor outcome (VA <6/60) following surgery. Cataract surgical coverage showed that men (72%) received more surgery than women (65%).

Discussion: The results from the RAAB survey in Zambia were very similar to the results from a similar survey in Malawi, where the main cause of blindness was cataract but posterior segment disease was also a significant contributor. Blindness in this part of Zambia is mainly avoidable and there is a need for comprehensive eye care services that can address both cataract and posterior segment disease in the population if the aim of VISION 2020 is to be achieved. Services should focus on quality and gender equity of cataract surgery.

Editor: Andreas Wedrich, Medical University Graz, Austria

Funding: The study was funded by Sightsavers International (www.sightsavers.org). Sightsavers paid for the field work costs (equipment, consumables, costs for field staff and transport). The funders had no role in study design, data collection and analysis, decision to publish, or preparation of the manuscript.

Competing Interests: One author is currently employed by S&S Development Consultants; however, at the time of the data collection he was employed by Sightsavers International (the funding agency) to oversee the survey. Since working for S&S Development Consultants he has commented on the draft paper.

* E-mail: Robert.lindfield@lshtm.ac.uk

Introduction

Approximately 39 million people are blind globally [1]. Over 90% of those who are blind reside in low or middle income countries. Causes of blindness can be divided into avoidable (preventable or treatable) and non-avoidable [2].

VISION 2020 is a global initiative to eliminate avoidable blindness by the year 2020 [2]. It is led by a consortium of international non-government organisations under an umbrella organisation, the International Agency for the Prevention of Blindness (IAPB) in partnership with the World Health Organization (WHO). VISION 2020 emphasises the importance of understanding both the burden and causes of blindness as a critical part of planning robust eye care programmes [3].

Several surveys have been conducted to describe the prevalence and causes of blindness in sub-Saharan Africa[4–7]. The rapid assessment of avoidable blindness (RAAB) survey technique was developed as an efficient and quick way to describe blindness at district level (populations of approximately 1–2 million people) [8]. RAAB is a cross-sectional community-based survey aimed at assessing the prevalence of avoidable eye conditions and the coverage and outcomes of cataract surgery in a population above 50 years of age. The choice of an age group with the highest expected prevalence minimizes sample size requirements and ensures RAAB surveys are rapid and relatively cheap [8].

Zambia is a country in southern Africa of approximately 13 million people. It ranks as 164 out of 187 countries in the human development index (a marker of poverty) [9].

No information is available about the prevalence or causes of blindness in Zambia. However a previous estimate based on studies in other African countries suggested the prevalence of blindness for all age groups in the region is around 1%[10–11].The Zambian Government in partnership with Sightsavers International, an international non-governmental organisation, and Seeing is Believing, a funding collaboration between Standard Chartered Bank and IAPB, established a project in southern

Zambia called The Livingstone to Lusaka Comprehensive Urban Eye Care Project that aims to reduce avoidable blindness. As part of this project a RAAB survey was conducted in the project area to establish baseline information about the prevalence and causes of blindness.

Results

3,629 people were examined (response rate of 94.9%). 60.5% were women. 148 individuals (3.9%) were unavailable, 33 (0.9%) refused and 9 (0.2%) were not capable of taking part in the survey.

The survey took place in 80 clusters in eight districts within two provinces (Southern and Lusaka) in Southern Zambia. Table 1 shows the total population by age and gender of the survey area compared to the sample. The distribution of the population sampled is broadly similar to the population of the survey area.

Prevalence of Blindness

83 (2.3% 95%CI 1.8–2.8) people were found to be blind (defined as visual acuity worse than 3/60 in the better eye with available correction). 41 (49.4%) were women. Table 2 shows the prevalence of blindness, severe visual impairment (visual acuity worse than 6/60 but equal or better to 3/60 in the better eye with available correction) and visual impairment (visual acuity worse than 6/18 but equal or better to 6/60 in the better eye with available correction) by gender. With best correction the prevalence of blindness decreased to 2.2% (80 people) (95%CI 1.6–2.8).

Causes of Blindness and Visual Impairment

Cataract was the main cause of blindness (39.8%) followed by posterior segment disease (34.9%). Overall 65.1% of blindness was avoidable. Table 3 shows the percentage of major causes by degree of visual loss. Causes such as glaucoma, age-related macular degeneration and diabetic retinopathy were grouped into posterior segment causes of visual loss because of diagnostic uncertainty. However, the survey suggested that approximately 47% of posterior segment disease was due to glaucoma.

Cataract was the leading cause of severe visual impairment and visual impairment. The second largest cause of visual impairment was refractive error (29.2%).

Cataract Surgery

86 people (113 eyes) had received cataract surgery at the time of the survey indicating a cataract surgical coverage of 46% (34% of eyes). Of all operated patients, 27 (0.7%) had received bilateral surgery.

26 (0.7%) people were bilaterally blind due to cataract, 148 (4.1%) people had one eye which was blind due to cataract. Table 4 summarises their answers when those who were bilaterally or unilaterally blind from cataract were asked why they had not had cataract surgery. 36.1% reported that they were unaware that any treatment was available for their condition.

Table 1. Age and gender distribution of the sample compared to the total population in the survey area.

Age Group	Male		Female		Total	
	Sample	Population	Sample	Population	Sample	Population
50-54	24.4%	26.8%	29.5%	30.5%	27.5%	28.5%
55-59	17.4%	19.7%	17.4%	20.9%	17.4%	20.3%
60-64	16.8%	17.3%	16.0%	19.8%	16.3%	18.5%
65-69	13.5%	14.1%	12.2%	13.5%	12.7%	13.9%
70-74	12.1%	9.8%	9.7%	8.9%	10.7%	9.4%
75-79	6.4%	6.1%	7.3%	0.5%	6.9%	3.5%
80+	9.3%	6.1%	7.9%	5.9%	8.5%	6.0%

Outcome of Cataract Surgery

Of the 113 eyes that received cataract surgery at any time in the past; all except two had an intraocular lens (IOL) inserted. Figure 1 describes the outcome of surgery. 34 (30.1%) eyes had a presenting visual acuity of worse than 6/60 (termed 'poor outcome'). The proportion decreased to 25.4% in those who had cataract surgery within 5 years of the survey date.

67 (59.2%) eyes had received cataract surgery in the five years preceding the survey. 17 (25.4%) eyes had a poor outcome and 36 (53.7%) had a good outcome, which increased to 40 (59.7%) with best correction.

The main causes of poor outcome after cataract surgery were co-morbidity (such as retinal disease or glaucoma) and complications during surgery.

When asked whether they were satisfied with the results of the surgery by eye, individuals reported they were very satisfied in 71% of surgeries and very unsatisfied in 15% of surgeries.

Gender

Cataract surgical coverage (the proportion of those who are blind compared to those who have had surgery) suggests that women (65.0% coverage, 31.7% of operated eyes) were less likely to receive surgery than men (72.1% coverage, 40.9% of operated eyes). This is despite the fact that a similar proportion of men and women were blind from cataract.

Extrapolation to the Survey Area

Assuming a prevalence of 2.29% and a population of 420,000 people over 50 in the survey area, it can be estimated that there were approximately 9600 people over 50 who were blind in the survey area at the time of the survey [12]. Approximately 4500 of these were blind due to cataract.

Based on the most recent WHO estimates, it is expected that 0.08% of the population under 15 years of age in Southern Province is blind [1]. The corresponding proportion in the age group between 15 and 49 is 0.16%[1]. Thus, approximately 13,300 people in all age groups in Southern Province were blind at the time of the survey, corresponding to an all age prevalence of 0.83%., with over 70% of cases occurring in people above 50 years of age [12].

Discussion

This population-based survey established that approximately 2.3% of people in the area running along the railway line between Livingstone and Lusaka were blind. Over 65% of blindness was avoidable with the main cause being cataract, which affected approximately 8400 people over 50. More women than men were examined in the survey but this was a reflection of the population over 50 in the survey area.

The findings were similar to those of other RAAB surveys conducted in sub-saharan Africa where the prevalence of blindness ranged from 1.8% in Rwanda [6] to 3.3% in Malawi [4], a population with similar demographics to that in Zambia. The survey in Malawi reported cataract as the leading cause of

Table 2. Prevalence of Visual Loss by Gender.

	Male (n = 1,434)		Female (n = 2,195)		Total (n = 3,629)	
Visual Acuity	**n**	**%**	**n**	**%**	**n**	**%**
Blind with best correction *	39	2.72	41	1.87	80	2.2
Blind with available correction (presenting)†	42	2.93	41	1.87	83	2.29
Severe Visual Impairment (presenting)	29	2.02	34	1.55	63	1.74
Visual Impairment (presenting)	87	6.07	166	7.56	253	6.97
Total	158	11.02	241	10.98	399	11.00

blindness (48.2%). Posterior segment disease (reported as glaucoma) was found to be the second leading cause of blindness.

The survey in Malawi reported a very low number of cataract surgeries performed on women compared to this study. This was probably due to the predominantly rural location of the Malawi survey compared to the mixed urban-rural setting in this survey. However, the present survey also revealed a gender discrepancy between the proportion of men and women receiving cataract surgery in Zambia. Despite having a similar prevalence of cataract blindness, fewer women had received surgery than men. This difference has been found in different RAAB surveys[5–7,14] in sub-Saharan Africa and remains an important issue for providers of cataract surgery who need to ensure their services reach everyone affected by disease.

This survey also found a high proportion of people who were blind from posterior segment disease (34.9%). The diagnosis was grouped in this way because it was made using a direct ophthalmoscope without any other tests, such as intraocular pressure measurement or bio-microscopy. Results from the survey suggest that the majority of posterior segment disease was due to glaucoma. This suggests that, with increasing cataract surgical services and, as a consequence, fewer people with cataract, diseases like glaucoma are becoming more prevalent causes of blindness.

The outcome of cataract surgery was suboptimal for many individuals, with over 30% of surgeries having a poor outcome despite an IOL being inserted. If surgeries are restricted to the five years before the survey, then the proportion of poor outcome decreases to 24%; however this still means that nearly one in four people do not see better than 6/60 despite having surgery. The main causes of poor outcome were co-morbidity and surgical complications. These results are similar to previous studies in sub-saharan Africa (including the survey in Malawi) and emphasise the importance of monitoring outcome and ongoing assessment of the quality of the services provided [4,7,15].

Limitations of the Study

Precise, detailed examination was not possible as all diagnosis was made with a direct ophthalmoscope. This means that any posterior segment causes of visual loss should be interpreted with care. However, it was felt that the diagnosis was robust as agreement was tested prior to the survey beginning.

Care must be taken in interpreting the responses given by individuals to the question about why they had not had cataract surgery as this was not a rigorous qualitative assessment of the barriers to surgery and must only be used as a pointer to the main reasons why people did not take up surgery.

Table 3. Degree and cause of presenting visual loss by person.

	Blind		SVI		VI		Total	
	n	**%**	**n**	**%**	**n**	**%**	**n**	**%**
Cataract	33	39.8	37	58.7	118	29.2	188	47.2
Posterior Segment*								
Glaucoma	25	30.1	8	12.7	4	1.6	37	9.3
Diabetic Retinopathy	0	0	0	0	3	1.2	3	0.75
Age-related Macular Degeneration	2	2.4	2	3.2	10	4	14	3.5
Other	2	2.4	3	4.8	16	6.3	21	5.3
Total	29	34.9	13	20.6	33	13	75	18.8
Corneal Scarring	12	14.5	7	11.1	22	8.7	41	10.3
Phthysis	5	6	0	0	0	0	5	1.3
Refractive Error	2	2.4	4	6.3	74	29.2	80	20.1
Surgical Complications	2	2.4	2	3.2	5	2	9	2.3
Total	83	100	63	100	252	100	398	100

***Note: Posterior segment is presented overall and broken into component diseases.**

Table 4. Reasons given for not having cataract surgery.

	Bilaterally blind from cataract		Unilaterally blind from cataract		Total	
	n	%	n	%	n	%
Unaware of treatment	18	42.9	87	34.9	105	36.1
Destiny/God's will	7	16.7	38	15.3	45	15.5
How to get surgery	2	4.8	33	13.3	35	12.0
No services	2	4.8	29	11.6	31	10.7
Wait for maturity	3	7.1	22	8.8	25	8.6
No-one to accompany	4	9.5	9	3.6	13	4.5
Cannot afford	2	4.8	9	3.6	11	3.8
Contra-indication	0	0	6	2.4	6	2.1
One eye not blind	0	0	5	2	5	1.7
Old age: no need	1	2.4	3	1.2	4	1.4
Fear of operation	2	4.8	2	0.8	4	1.4
Fear of losing sight	0	0	4	1.6	4	1.4
No time	1	2.4	2	0.8	3	1.0
Total	42	100	249	100	291	100

There was a marked discrepancy between the proportion of men and women examined in the survey. This reflects the population distribution of the country where there are a higher proportion of women than men over 50 years old and is similar to the situation in Malawi. However there was approximately equal representation between men and women who were blind. It is

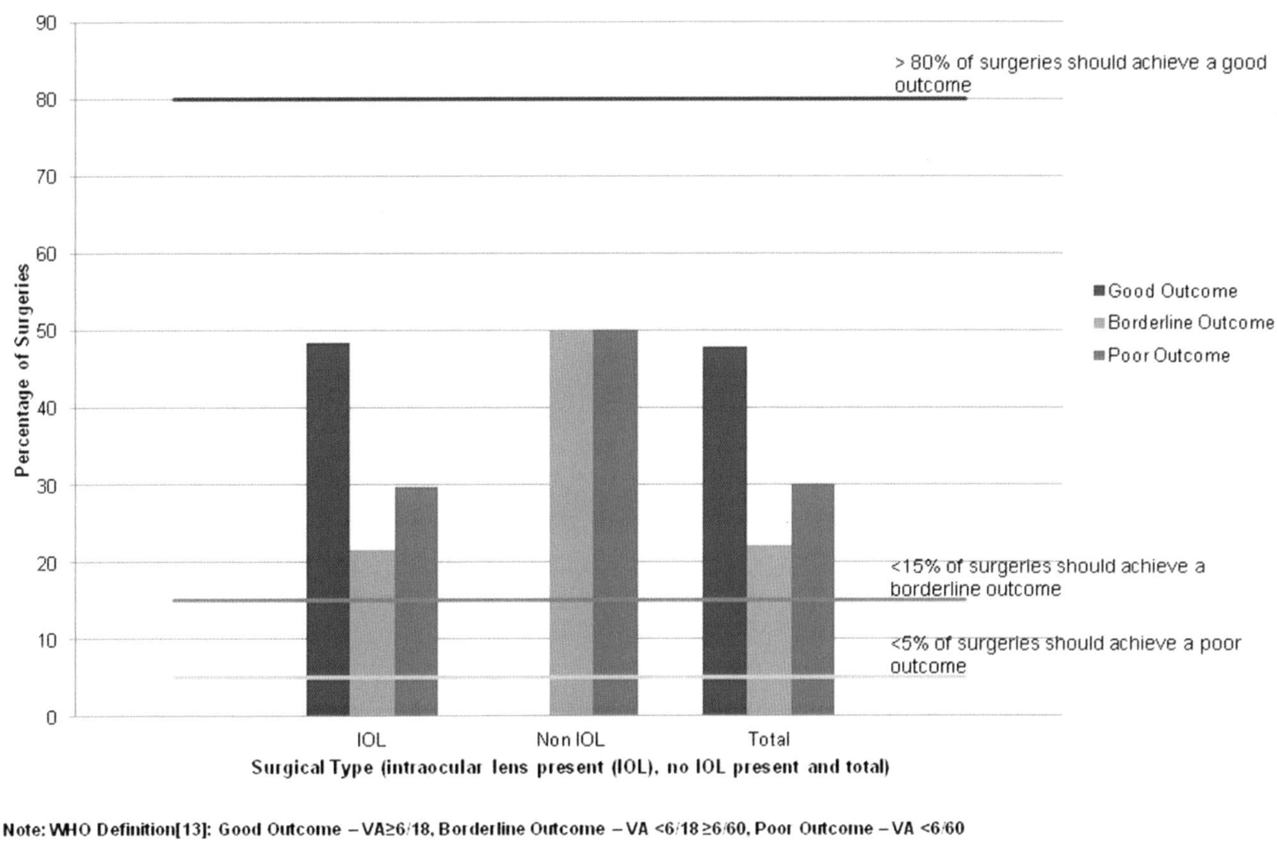

Figure 1. Percentage of poor outcomes with and without IOL insertion following cataract surgery in Southern Zambia compared to the WHO recommendations.

possible that blind men were over-represented in the sample because they remain at home whereas normal sighted men are able to leave the house and work.

Conclusion

Blindness in the survey area between Lusaka and Livingstone affects approximately 1 in 50 of the population over 50. Nearly half is due to cataract – a treatable cause of blindness. The results from the RAAB Survey in Zambia provide important information to allow service providers, government and non-governmental organisations to plan services and advocate for eye care.

Methods

Ethical Approval

Ethical approval was granted by the Medical Research Ethics Committee of the University of Zambia.

Timescale

The survey took place in June and July 2010.

Setting

The survey area runs between Livingstone and Lusaka along a railway line and covers a population of approximately 3 million people, 12% of whom are aged above 50 [12].

An up-to-date age-specific list of the population per village was established using records from Central Statistical Office of Zambia in each district. This was thought to be the most reliable source of population data and was used as the sampling frame.

Sample Size Calculation

The sample size was calculated using an estimated prevalence of 4%, with a variation of 20%, a non-compliance of 10%, a design effect of 1.5 and a 95% confidence limit. This was based on previous RAAB surveys in sub-Saharan Africa[4–6]. This gave a sample size of 3,830 people over the age of 50.

The sample size meant that 80 clusters (villages) were selected for the survey.

Teams

Four teams were trained to conduct the survey. Each team consisted of an ophthalmologist or senior ophthalmic nurse and an assistant, either an ophthalmic clinical officer or an ophthalmic nurse.

Training

Teams received one weeks training from an accredited RAAB trainer (RL) before starting the survey. Agreement between teams was assessed using a formal test where each team examined the same patient, assessing visual acuity and lens examination, and cause of any visual loss and reported their findings. Kappa was calculated and each team had to achieve at least 0.70 before the survey could commence.

Selecting the Sample

There was a two stage sample selection. The first stage involved selecting villages from the sampling frame using probability proportional to size. The second stage consisted of dividing the village into segments of approximately 50 people over the age of 50. The segment of the village to be surveyed was selected using simple random sampling.

Each team moved from house to house in the selected segment. In each house every eligible person over the age of 50 was enumerated even if they were absent from the house. Eligibility was defined as residing in the house for more than 6 months in the previous twelve months, and sleeping in the house either the preceding or following nights. 50 people over the age of 50 were examined in each segment. If fewer than 50 people over the age of 50 were resident in the segment then a second segment from the cluster was selected by random and the survey continued until 50 people were found. Data collection lasted for six weeks.

If an eligible person was absent from the house at the time the survey team visited, then every effort was made to find and examine the individual. This included returning to the house at a later time, seeking the individual in another location or asking the individual to find the team when able. If it was not possible to examine the individual, family and friends were asked whether the person was blind.

Individuals who were eligible but for some reason unable to be examined (e.g. learning disabled) were recorded as unable to take part in the survey.

Examination

Verbal consent was taken from each participant prior to any examination after a complete explanation of the study.

Each eligible individual had a visual acuity assessment using an illiterate tumbling E chart at six metres. Each eye was examined separately and the individual had to correctly identify four out of five characters on the E chart to achieve a specific category of visual acuity. 'Presenting' visual acuity assessment was conducted with their own distance spectacles if used. A pinhole visual acuity (termed 'corrected' visual acuity) assessment was conducted on all eyes that failed to see 6/18. Every individual then had an ocular examination using a direct ophthalmoscope and/or torch this included a lens assessment with the following categories; no/minimal lens opacity, significant lens opacity, pseudophakia with/without PCO or aphakia.Individuals whose visual acuity in either eye was worse than 6/18 with pinhole, then received, where appropriate, a dilated ocular examination by the ophthalmologist using a direct ophthalmoscope to determine the cause(s) of visual impairment.

Data Collection

Data was collected using a standard proforma. This included information on visual acuity, the status of the lens and the causes of any visual loss. Causes of visual loss (worse than 6/18) were described for each eye and a main cause described for the person. The main cause of visual loss was determined by the ease of treatment, as specified by the WHO [13]. Hence, refractive error is easier to treat than cataract, so if an individual had both refractive error and cataract their main cause of visual loss would be refractive error. Blindness, severe visual impairment and visual impairment were defined according to the WHO categorization [13].

Information was also collected about any cataract surgery that had occurred or, for those with cataract, why cataract surgery had not taken place.

Data Entry

Data was double entered into software developed for RAAB surveys. This allows automated entry cleaning and checking.

Data Analysis

The RAAB software automatically produces reports on the results of the survey. This was supplemented by further analysis in Stata.

Acknowledgments

The authors would like to acknowledge the ophthalmologists, ophthalmic clinical officers, ophthalmic nurses and others in Zambia who collected the data for this survey.

Author Contributions

Conceived and designed the experiments: RL JM. Performed the experiments: RL MM. Analyzed the data: RL UG FB JM. Wrote the paper: RL UG FB MM JM.

References

1. Pascolini D, Mariotti SP (2010) Global estimates of visual impairment. Br J Ophthalmol doi:10.1136/bjophthalmol-2011-300539.
2. Pizzarello L, Abiose A, Ffytche T, Duerksen R, Thulasiraj R, et al. (2004) VISION 2020: The Right to Sight: a global initiative to eliminate avoidable blindness. Arch Ophthalmol 122: 615–20.
3. WHO IAPB. (2006) The VISION 2020 Action Plan, 2006-2011. Geneva.
4. Kalua K, Lindfield R, Mtupanyama M, Mtumodzi D, Msiska V (2011) Findings from a rapid assessment of avoidable blindness (RAAB) in Southern Malawi. PLoS One 6: e19226.
5. Mathenge W, Kuper H, Limburg H, Polack S, Onyango O, et al. (2007) Rapid assessment of avoidable blindness in Nakuru district, Kenya. Ophthalmology 114: 599–605.
6. Mathenge W, Nkurikiye J, Limburg H, Kuper H (2007) Rapid assessment of avoidable blindness in Western Rwanda: blindness in a postconflict setting. PLoS Med 4: e217.
7. Habiyakire C, Kabona G, Courtright P, Lewallen S (2010) Rapid assessment of avoidable blindness and cataract surgical services in Kilimanjaro region, Tanzania. Ophthalmic Epidemiol 17: 90–4.
8. Kuper H, Polack S, Limburg H (2006) Rapid assessment of avoidable blindness. Community Eye Health 19: 68–9.
9. UNDP (2011) National Human Development Reports for Zambia.
10. Resnikoff S, Pascolini D, Etya'ale D, Kocur I, Pararajasegaram R, et al. (2004) Global data on visual impairment in the year 2002. Bull World Health Organ 82: 844–51.
11. Zulu F (2005) A situation analysis of eye care services in Zambia. Lusaka: Sightsavers International.
12. Central Statistical Office (2003) Zambia 2000 Census of population and housing. Populations projections report. Lusaka.
13. WHO Programme for the Prevention of Blindness (1988) Coding instructions for the WHO/PBL eye examination record (version III). World Health Organisation: Geneva. 1–17.
14. WHO (1998) Informal consultation on analysis of blindness prevention outcomes. Geneva.
15. Lindfield R, Kuper H, Polack S, Eusebio C, Mathenge W, et al. (2009) Outcome of cataract surgery at one year in Kenya, the Philippines and Bangladesh. Br J Ophthalmol 93: 875–80.

16

Rapid Assessment of Avoidable Blindness in the Occupied Palestinian Territories

Far Chiang[1], Hannah Kuper[2], Robert Lindfield[2], Tiarnan Keenan[3], Na'el Seyam[4], Denise Magauran[5], Nasrallah Khalilia[1], Habes Batta[1], Ziad Abdeen[6], Nicholas Sargent[1]*

1 St. John Eye Hospital, Jerusalem, Occupied Palestinian Territories, **2** London School of Hygiene and Tropical Medicine, London, United Kingdom, **3** Manchester Royal Eye Hospital, Manchester, United Kingdom, **4** Military Medical Services, Gaza, Occupied Palestinian Territories, **5** Epsom and St. Helier University Hospitals NHS Trust, Sutton, United Kingdom, **6** Al-Quds Nutrition and Health Research Institute, Al Quds University, Jerusalem, Occupied Palestinian Territories

Abstract

Background: There are no recent data on the prevalence and causes of blindness in the Occupied Palestinian Territories. The aim of our study was to estimate the prevalence and causes of blindness and visual impairment in the population aged 50 years and above in the Occupied Palestinian Territories using the Rapid Assessment of Avoidable Blindness (RAAB) survey method.

Methods and Findings: Clusters of 40 people who were 50 years and above were selected with probability proportionate to size using a multistage cluster random sampling method. Participants received a comprehensive ophthalmic examination in their homes, including visual acuity testing by one of three experienced ophthalmologists. The principal cause for visual loss was determined by an experienced ophthalmologist using portable diagnostic instruments. Information about previous cataract surgery, satisfaction with surgery and barriers to cataract surgery were collected. The prevalence of self-reported diabetes was also determined. The prevalence of bilateral blindness (VA<3/60 in the better eye with available correction) was 3.4% (95% CI: 2.7–4.0), 2.0% (95% CI: 1.4–2.5) for severe visual impairment (VA≥3/60 and <6/60), and 7.4% (95% CI: 6.4–8.3) for visual impairment (VA≥6/60 and <6/18). Avoidable causes (i.e. cataract, refractive error, aphakia, surgical complications, corneal scarring and phthysis) accounted for 80.0% of bilateral blindness, severe visual impairment (70.7%) and visual impairment (86.2%). Cataract was the main cause of blindness (55.0%). The prevalence of blindness was higher in Gaza (4.9%, 95% CI: 3.7–6.1%) than in the West Bank (2.5%, 95% CI: 1.9–3.1%) and among women (4.3%,95% CI: 3.3–5.2%) compared to men (2.2%,95%CI:1.5–2.9%). Among people who had undergone cataract surgery in the past, only 54.5% of eyes obtained a good outcome (VA≥6/18), 23.2% had a borderline outcome (VA<6/18 and ≥6/60) and 22.3% had a poor outcome (VA<6/60) with available correction. The prevalence of self-reported diabetes mellitus in ≥50 year age group was 26.4% (95% CI: 24.9–27.9).

Conclusions: The prevalence of blindness suggests that significant numbers of people in the Occupied Palestinian Territories exist who do not access eye care - predominantly women and those residing in Gaza. Programmes need to focus on maximizing the use of current services by these excluded groups.

Editor: Antje Timmer, Helmholtz Zentrum München, Germany

Funding: The funders had no role in study design, data collection and analysis, decision to publish, or preparation of the manuscript. The study was principally funded by The Linbury Trust (www.linburytrust.org.uk). This funding agency did not take part directly nor influenced the conducting of the study in any way and did not take part in the preparation of the manuscript.

Competing Interests: The authors have declared that no competing interests exist.

* E-mail: njsargent@hotmail.com

Introduction

The World Health Organisation (WHO) estimates that there are 45 million people in the world who are blind (vision worse than 3/60 in the better eye with presenting vision). This is expected to rise to 76 million by 2020 if current services are not improved. VISION 2020 is a joint initiative by the WHO and the International Association for the Prevention of Blindness that aims to eliminate avoidable blindness by the year 2020. The first step in achieving this target is to obtain baseline data on visual impairment at country and district levels for planning and monitoring eye care programmes.

The prevalence of blindness differs between countries [1], and may be increased four-fold in areas affected by violent conflict [2]. The WHO estimates that the number of blind people in 2002 in the Eastern Mediterranean Region-B (which includes the Occupied Palestinian Territories) was over 1 million people, and that the prevalence of blindness in adults aged 50 years and above in this region was 5.6% [1].

The Occupied Palestinian Territories comprise East Jerusalem, the West Bank and the Gaza Strip. The total population of the Occupied Palestinian Territories in 2007 (figures available at the time of the study) was estimated at 3,761,600, with 2,345,100 living in East Jerusalem and the West Bank, and 1,416,500 in the

Gaza Strip [3–4]. Military occupation means that people with an identity card recognising them as Palestinians from the West Bank or Gaza can enter Jerusalem via military checkpoints only with a special permit. Such permits are not always granted thus restricting access to secondary and tertiary referral centres in East Jerusalem [5–8].

No robust or comprehensive study of blindness in Palestinians has been conducted for over 20 years. The most recent population-based study of blindness in the OPT was conducted in 1984 and included 9,054 people selected by cluster random sampling [9]. The estimated prevalence of blindness for all ages (including refractive error) was 1.7% and for visual impairment was 6.8%. The major causes of blindness were cataract (31.6%) and trachoma (13.4%). However, substantial demographic changes have occurred in the Occupied Palestinian Territories over the past 20 years, including a large increase in the Palestinian population. A study conducted in 1990 by the visiting Russian ophthalmologist, Golychev, reviewed people presenting at clinics set up in both the West Bank and Gaza [10]. The main cause of blindness was found to be corneal opacification of all types. As this was a sample of convenience, selection bias prevents the results from being assumed to be reflective of the population. Surveys conducted in nearby countries have produced prevalence estimates for blindness from 0.6% and 0.7% in Lebanon and Saudi Arabia, to 3.2% in Pakistan and Oman [1,11–12].

Current ophthalmic services for Palestinians include clinics and hospitals run by the Palestinian Authority hospitals, non-governmental organisations (NGOs) and the private sector. The St John Eye Hospital network is a NGO that includes the main hospital in East Jerusalem, permanent clinics in Gaza, Hebron and Anabta, and two mobile outreach services operating in the West Bank. Established in 1882 as a charitable organisation, St John Eye Hospital is the largest single provider of ophthalmic care in the Occupied Palestinian Territories, which it provides to all people irrespective of race, religion or ability to pay. The Palestinian Authority delivers ophthalmic services in the West Bank through Rafidia Hospital (located in Nablus), and in the Gaza Strip through Nasser Hospital and European Gaza Hospital. There is financial cover for treatment of members in the Palestinian Authority national medical insurance scheme in non-governmental centres [8]. Other NGO service providers include the Bethlehem Arab Society for Rehabilitation (located in Beit Jala), which conducts intraocular surgery for the Bethlehem area. Finally, many private clinics operate in the West Bank and Gaza Strip. The Palestinian Society of Ophthalmologists has 68 licensed ophthalmologists in the West Bank, and 74 in the Gaza Strip, though the majority of these do not perform cataract surgery largely due to a lack of training. Those needing services also seek eye care in Israel and neighbouring Arab countries including Egypt and Jordan.

The aim of this study was to conduct a Rapid Assessment of Avoidable Blindness (RAAB) in people aged 50 years and above in the Occupied Palestinian Territories, in order to estimate the magnitude and causes of blindness and visual impairment, and to provide information that would enhance the impact of services and resources for this area.

Methods

Sample Size Calculation

At the time of the survey, approximately 9% (338,400) of the total Palestinian population in the Occupied Palestinian Territories (3,761,600) was over 50 years old [3,13]. To estimate the required sample size we assumed the following: expected prevalence of blindness 4%, desired precision 20% (worst acceptable result 4.8%), confidence level 95%, and non-response rate 15%. In addition, the required sample size was increased because of the use of cluster rather than simple random sampling, and we used a design effect of 1.4 for this purpose. The sample size required calculated using the RAAB software (http://www.cehjournal.org/files/s0701.html) was 3,800 individuals, corresponding to 95 clusters of 40 people.

Sampling Frame

Data from the Palestinian Central Bureau of Statistics 1997 were used as the sampling frame, updated with 2007 growth rates (by governorate) to generate up-to-date population estimates for each enumeration area [13–15]. From the enumeration areas, 95 clusters were selected using probability proportionate to size, including 3 clusters located in East Jerusalem from neighbourhoods included in the Palestinian Authority census. In the conflict area of Beit Hanoun, Gaza, 3 clusters were replaced with locations in the West Bank (due to the logistical constraints of working in Gaza it was not possible to replace these with clusters from Gaza).

The examination team sequentially visited households until 40 people ≥50 years were identified. If an eligible person was absent, the examination team returned twice to the household on the same day to examine the individual before leaving the area. For eligible individuals who could not be examined on the day, information on visual status was collected from relatives or neighbours. Non-responders were not included in the analyses nor in the estimates of prevalence of blindness, but information was collected on their visual status to allow assessment of whether non-attendance introduced bias in the estimate of blindness. If 40 people were not found in the segment, then sampling was continued in the most adjacent segment until the target number of 40 people was reached. The survey was carried out over an eight-week period (June-July in the West Bank, late June to mid-August in the Gaza Strip) in 2008.

Ophthalmic evaluation and data collection

The standardised set of questions was completed for each eligible person. They were divided into seven parts including: general demographic information; whether known to have diabetes mellitus; visual acuity and lens assessment; principal cause of visual impairment; reasons why cataract surgery had not been done; and information about cataract surgery done including time, place and level of patient satisfaction.

VA was measured using a Snellen tumbling 'E' chart, which had an optotype size 6/18 on one side and 6/60 on the other side at a 6 or 3 metre distance, and was measured in full daylight with available correction. Pinhole VA was measured when the VA was <6/18 in either eye. The lens was examined in both eyes using a direct ophthalmoscope or portable slit-lamp and was graded into the following categories; 'normal lens', 'obvious lens opacity', 'lens absent (aphakia)' or 'IOL implantation'. If corneal opacification precluded lens examination then 'no view of lens' was recorded.

If the VA improved to 6/18 or better with pin-hole, then refractive error was assigned as the cause of visual impairment. If it was found that the vision in either eye was <6/18 with a pinhole, a more detailed examination was performed of the anterior segment to elicit the cause. If the cause was not in the anterior segment, the ophthalmologist proceeded to perform fundoscopy with a mydriatic eye drop. Glaucoma was defined as the principal cause of visual impairment if the optic cup-to-disc ratio was greater than 0.6, in the absence of another cause of reduced vision.

The principal cause of visual impairment was based on the WHO convention whereby the principal cause is attributed to the primary disorder. If there are multiple causes, then following this convention, the cause that can be most easily treated was assigned as the principal cause [16].

Categories of visual impairment

This study used the WHO categories for visual impairment. Based on presenting visual acuity (VA) with available correction in the better eye, the three categories are defined as follows: Blindness, VA<3/60 in the better eye; severe visual impairment, VA<6/60 but≥3/60 in the better eye; visual impairment, VA<6/18 but ≥6/60 [19].

Training and intervariability testing of survey teams

The RAAB methodology required three teams, each comprising an experienced ophthalmologist, an ophthalmic assistant and a driver. Two teams were assigned to the West Bank, and one to the Gaza Strip. All teams received one week of training in both theoretical and practical aspects of the RAAB methodology by certified RAAB trainers. Inter-observer variation between all teams was measured using repeat examination of 40 participants. The assessment of VA, lens examination and assigned cause of blindness were compared to ensure a high degree of consistency between teams. The kappa statistic was >0.60 for all these measures and so the teams were deemed to be consistent in their assessments. The training programme also included a pilot visit to a field location with the trainers.

Statistical Analysis

The survey software program 'RAAB version 4.02' (Health Information Services and Tax Software) was used. This software allows data entry, sample size calculation and inter-observer variability testing as well as standardised data analysis. The prevalence estimates took account of the design effect when estimating the confidence intervals because cluster sample was used rather than simple random sampling.. The cataract surgical coverage of people was defined as the proportion of people needing surgery who had undergone cataract surgery. This is calculated as:

Cataract Surgical Coverage

$$= \frac{\text{Number of people who have undergone cataract surgery}}{\text{Number of people needing cataract surgery}}$$

$$= \frac{\begin{array}{l}\text{(No.people with bilateral pseudophakia/aphakia)}\\ +\text{(No. people with unilateral pseudophakia/aphakia and}\\ \text{visual impairment in other eye)}\end{array}}{\begin{array}{l}\text{(No. people with bilateral pseudophakia/aphakia)}\\ +\text{(No. people with unilateral pseudophakia/aphakia and}\\ \text{visualimpairment in other eye)}\\ +\text{(No. people with bilateral visual impairment from}\\ \text{cataract)}\end{array}}$$

For these purposes visual impairment was defined using pinhole vision. Cataract surgical coverage was also calculated for eyes. Since the VA prior to surgery was not known, we assumed, in turn, that only patients with VA below a certain threshold (<3/60, <6/60, <6/18 respectively) received surgery for their cataract. Estimates of the number of cases with blindness, severe visual impairment and visual impairment were obtained by extrapolating the age-sex-specific prevalence estimates to the age-sex structure of the population and these were rounded to the nearest 10.

Ethical approval

The study was approved and endorsed by the Palestinian Ministry of Health. Ethics approval was granted by the St John Eye Hospital Ethics Committee and the research followed the tenets of the Declaration of Helsinki. Informed verbal consent was obtained for each person included in the study. This method of consent was specifically approved by the same ethics committee in light of a two day pilot showing many Palestinians refuse to sign any paperwork to unknown visitors. Claims exist that Jewish settlement groups have tricked Palestinians into signing away property rights under false pretences. An explanation of the nature and the aims of the nature and possible consequences of the study were provided to participants. All participants received feedback about their eyes and were advised to seek ophthalmic attention if they had any concerns. People who were discovered to have eye problems were given relevant counseling and advice. Those whom it was thought would benefit from further management, including those with operable cataracts, were referred to a St. John facility for a free consultation unless they were already receiving treatment from an ophthalmologist.

Results

Of the 3,800 selected participants aged ≥50 years, 3,579 were examined (response rate of 94.2%). Of the 221 non-respondents, 177 (4.7%) were not available, 29 (8%) refused to participate and 15 (0.4%) were not capable of being examined. Those examined were representative of the population of the Occupied Palestinian Territories in terms of age and sex distribution (Table 1). The majority who were not available were men (72.3%). More women refused participation (62.1%) compared to men (37.9%). Among the non-responders, 9 were reported to be believed to be blind (4%).

The prevalence of blindness, based on presenting vision, in the ≥50 years age group was 3.4% (95% CI: 2.7–4.0%). The prevalence was 2.6% (95% CI: 2.0–3.1%) for severe visual impairment and 10.7% (95% CI: 9.4–12.0%) for visual impairment (Table 2). Bilateral blindness was twice as prevalent in Gaza (4.9%, 95% CI: 3.7–6.1%) as in the West Bank (2.5%, 95% CI: 1.9–3.1%). In addition, both severe visual impairment and visual impairment were more prevalent in Gaza (3.2% and 12.5%) than the West Bank (2.2% and 9.7%). Unilateral blindness was more than twice as common as binocular blindness (8.2%, 95% CI: 7.3–9.1%). Compared to men women had a higher prevalence of blindness, severe visual impairment and visual impairment, but this only reached statistical significance for blindness ($p = 0.0007$) and not for severe visual impairment ($p = 0.58$) or visual impairment ($p = 0.50$). The prevalence of self-reported diabetes mellitus in ≥50 years age group was 26.4% (95% CI: 24.9–27.9%).

Avoidable causes of blindness (cataract, refractive error, corneal scar, surgical complications, trachoma and phthysis) accounted for 80.0% of the total amount of blindness, 70.7% of severe visual impairment and 86.2% of visual impairment in the Occupied Palestinian Territories (Table 3). Cataract was the dominant cause of blindness (55.0%), severe visual impairment (56.5%), and visual impairment (45.2%). Corneal scarring was also an important cause of blindness (14.2%) and severe visual impairment (7.6%).

Table 1. Composition of population in sample and in survey area, by age and sex for the Occupied Palestinian Territories.

	Occupied Palestinian Territories		West Bank		Gaza	
	Survey area (N)*	Examined (n)	Survey area(N)*	Examined(n)	Survey area(N)*	Examined(n)
Age group						
50–59 y	141,900 (42.5%)	1,625 (45.4%)	94,500 (42.1%)	1,052 (45.9%)	47,400 (43.6%)	573 (44.4%)
60–69 y	110,600 (33.2%)	1,002 (28.0%)	73,500 (32.8%)	612 (26.7%)	37,100 (34.1%)	390 (30.2%)
70–79 y	57,000 (17.1%)	674 (18.8%)	39,500 (17.6%)	432 (18.9%)	17,500 (16.1%)	242 (18.8%)
80+ y	23,900 (7.2%)	278 (7.8%)	17,000 (7.6%)	194 (8.5%)	6,900 (6.3%)	84 (6.5%)
Men	148300 (44.5%)	1,618 (45.2%)	100,400 (44.8%)	1,036 (45.2%)	47,800 (43.9%)	582 (45.1%)
Women	185100 (55.5%)	1,961 (54.8%)	124,000 (55.2%)	1,254 (54.8%)	61,100 (56.1%)	707 (54.8%)
Total	333,400	3,579	224,000	2,290	109,000	1,289

*Source: Palestinian Central Bureau of Statistics [4,16].

Diabetic retinopathy accounted for 8.3% of blindness, 14.1% of severe visual loss and 5.5% of visual impairment. Glaucoma was responsible for 5.8% of blindness. Refractive error was an important cause of visual impairment (36.3%), but not severe visual impairment or blindness. The prevalence of blindness from bilateral cataract for the Occupied Palestinian Territories was 1.23% (95%CI 0.86%–1.60%) with the prevalence being higher in Gaza (1.86%, 95%CI 1.11%–2.61%) compared to the West Bank (0.87%, 95%CI 0.49%–1.25%)

The cataract surgical coverage was high with 86% of people requiring surgery at VA<3/60 level having received surgery (Table 4). This was even higher in men (91.5%) than in women (82.5%). For people with VA<6/60 and VA<6/18, 80.7% and 61.8% of those needing surgery had received it, respectively.

The vast majority of people who had undergone cataract surgery (94.3%) had received an intraocular lens. However, only 54.5% of eyes obtained a good post-operative outcome (VA≥6/18), 23.2% had a borderline outcome (VA<6/18 and≥6/60) and 22.3% had a poor outcome (VA<6/60) with available correction (Table 5). This fails to meet the WHO target >80% of eyes having good vision with available correction. The proportion of eyes that had a good outcome was slightly higher in those eyes that were operated within 5 years of the survey (58.3%) compared to those eyes operated over 5 years before the survey (50.2%). Outcomes were a little higher in the West Bank than in Gaza (57.5% had good outcome compared to 50.2% respectively). In those eyes with a poor outcome (VA<6/60 with available correction), the single largest cause was attributable to ocular co-morbidity (e.g. ARMD, glaucoma, diabetic retinopathy) in 59.5%, followed by surgical complications in 28.1%. This contrasted with the single largest cause of visual impairment (VA<6/18) in eyes following cataract surgery, which was lack of spectacles (35.7%). Despite the poor results, most of the people who received cataract surgery in the Occupied Palestinian Territories were very satisfied (54%) or partially satisfied (30%).

Up to two reasons could be given for not obtaining cataract surgery. The most common reasons cited by people with bilateral vision ≤6/60 due to cataract (were "Old age and need not felt" (33%), "Could not afford" (20%), "Contraindication" (15%), "Fear of operation (14%) and "Unaware of treatment" (6%). Women were more likely than men to cite "Cannot afford" (21% and 17% respectively) and "Fear of operation" (19% and 0% respectively). The problem of obtaining permits to pass through military checkpoints within the West Bank (including East Jerusalem) was cited by 11% as a barrier to obtaining cataract surgery.

Table 2. Prevalence of Blindness, Severe Visual Impairment, and Visual Impairment in the Occupied Palestinian Territories (with available correction in the better eye in adults aged 50 years and above).

Area	Sex	Total number	Bilateral blindness (VA<3/60)		Bilateral severe visual impairment (VA<6/60 and VA≥3/60)		Bilateral visual impairment (VA<6/18 and VA≥6/60)	
			Number	Prevalence (95% CI)	Number	Prevalence (95% CI)	Number	Prevalence (95% CI)
Occupied Palestinian Territories	Men	1618	36	2.2% (1.5–2.9%)	39	2.4% (1.6–3.2%)	167	10.3% (8.7–12.0%)
	Women	1961	84	4.3% (3.3–5.2%)	53	2.7% (1.9–3.5%	216	11.0% (9.5–12.6%)
	Total	3579	120	3.4% (2.7–4.0%)	92	2.6% (2.0–3.1%)	383	10.7% (9.4–12.0%)
West Bank	Men	1036	19	1.8% (1.0–2.7%)	24	2.3% (1.4–3.3%)	104	10.0% (7.8–12.3%)
	Women	1254	38	3.0% (2.1–4.0%)	27	2.1% (1.4–3.0%)	118	9.4% (7.7–11.1%)
	Total	2,290	57	2.5% (1.9–3.1%)	51	2.2% (1.6–2.9%)	222	9.7% (8.1–11.3%)
Gaza	Men	582	17	2.9% (1.6–4.2%)	15	2.6% (1.3–3.9%)	63	10.8% (8.6–13.1%)
	Women	707	46	6.5% (4.6–8.4%)	26	3.7% (2.2–5.2%)	98	13.9% (11.0–16.8%)
	Total	1,289	63	4.9% (3.7–6.1%)	41	3.2% (2.1–4.2%)	161	12.5% (10.4–14.6%)

Table 3. Proportion of Blindness, Severe Visual Impairment, and Visual Impairment due to specific causes in the Occupied Palestinian Territories.

Cause	Blindness (VA<3/60 with available correction)			Severe visual impairment (VA<6/60 to 3/60 with available correction)			Visual impairment (VA<6/18 to 6/60 with available correction)		
	Occupied Palestinian Territories	**West Bank**	**Gaza**	**Occupied Palestinian Territories**	**West Bank**	**Gaza**	**Occupied Palestinian Territories**	**West Bank**	**Gaza**
	n = 120	**n = 57**	**n = 63**	**n = 92**	**n = 51**	**n = 41**	**n = 383**	**n = 222**	**n = 161**
Avoidable causes									
Refractive error	1.7%	1.8%	1.6%	2.2%	0	4.9%	36.3%	37.8%	34.2%
Cataract	55.0%	56.1%	54.0%	56.5%	62.7%	48.8%	45.2%	43.7%	47.2%
Aphakia (uncorrected)	0	0	0	0	0	0	0.3%	0	0.6%
Surgery related	5.0%	3.5%	6.3%	4.3%	2.0%	7.3%	2.3%	1.8%	3.1%
Corneal Scar (non-trachomatous)	14.2%	19.3%	9.5%	7.6%	7.8%	7.3%	1.8%	2.7%	0.6%
Phthysis	2.5%	3.5%	1.6%	0	0	0	0	0	0
Trachoma	1.7%	1.8%	1.6%	0	0	0	0.3%	0	0.6%
Total Avoidable*	80.0%	86.0%	74.6%	70.7%	72.5%	68.3%	86.2%	86.0%	86.3%
Potentially avoidable and other causes**									
Diabetic retinopathy	8.3%	7.0%	9.5%	14.1%	11.8%	17.1%	5.5%	4.5%	6.8%
Glaucoma	5.8%	1.8%	9.5%	3.3%	3.9%	2.4%	0.3%	0.5%	0
ARMD	2.5%	3.5%	1.6%	4.3%	7.8%	0	2.3%	2.7%	1.9%
Other posterior segment/CNS	3.3%	1.8%	4.8%	6.5%	2.0%	12.2%	5.5%	5.9%	5.0%
Globe abnormality	0	0	0	1.1%	2.0%	0	0.3%	0.5%	0

*Refractive error, cataract, aphakia (uncorrected), surgical complications, corneal scar, phthysis, trachoma.

**Diabetic retinopathy, glaucoma, age-related macular degeneration (ARMD), other posterior segment and central nervous system diseases, globe abnormalities.

Table 4. *Cataract Surgical Coverage (CSC) by person and eyes in the Occupied Palestinian Territories.

	Occupied Palestinian Territories		West Bank		Gaza	
	CSC-Persons	CSC-Eyes	CSC-Persons	CSC-Eyes	CSC-Persons	CSC-Eyes
VA<3/60						
Men	91.5%	69.0%	90.9%	67.7%	91.6%	70.4%
Women	82.5%	59.5%	87.6%	63.0%	77.0%	56.3%
Total	86.0%	63.4%	89.9%	65.0%	82.6%	61.6%
VA<6/60						
Men	86.1%	61.3%	85.3%	60.0%	87.1%	62.9%
Women	77.0%	53.8%	80.1%	56.9%	74.0%	51.0%
Total	80.7%	56.9%	82.2%	58.2%	79.2%	55.5%
VA<6/18						
Men	65.1%	44.9%	64.5%	44.6%	65.4%	44.5%
Women	59.5%	37.7%	65.4%	42.0%	54.1%	34.0%
Total	61.8%	40.6%	65.0%	43.1%	58.5%	37.9%

*with pin-hole vision in the better eye in adults aged 50 years and above.

Population estimates

Extrapolating the survey estimates to the age and sex distribution of the Occupied Palestinian Territories from the updated census data suggests that in the ≥50 years age group, there are an estimated 10,870 blind people (95% CI: 8,560–12,850), 8,810 (95% CI: 7,120–10,850) severely visually impaired people and 36,010 (95% CI: 31,670–40,340) visually impaired people (Table 6). The all-age prevalence of blindness for the Occupied Palestinian Territories is estimated to be 0.4%, based on the WHO estimate that 82% of blindness occurs in ≥50 years. This equates to 13,300 people out of a population of 3.7 million.

Using the estimates of the prevalence of cataract in the Occupied Palestinian Territories, it is expected that in the ≥50 years group, cataract accounts for 6,000 blind, 5,000 severely visually impaired, and 16,300 visually impaired. To reach the Vision 2020 target of operating on 20% of the prevalence of cataract per year causing VA<6/60 bilaterally; 2,200 cataract operations on separate people would need to be performed per year.

Discussion

RAAB surveys have been conducted in several countries [18–24]. This was the first to be completed in the Middle East, providing an essential baseline for Vision 2020 programmes in the Occupied Palestinian Territories. The prevalence of bilateral blindness (VA<3/60 in the better eye with available correction) was 3.4% (95% CI: 2.7–4.0) in those people aged ≥50 years. This gave rise to an estimate of blindness for the total population of 0.4%, which was half of that previously estimated for the EMR-B (0.8%) [1]. The prevalence of blindness was higher in Gaza (4.9%, 95% CI: 3.7–6.1%) than in the West Bank (2.5%, 95% CI: 1.9–3.1%) and among women (4.3%,95% CI: 3.3–5.2%) compared to men (2.2%,95% CI:1.5–2.9%).

Avoidable causes (i.e. cataract, refractive error, aphakia, surgical complications, corneal scarring and phthysis) accounted for 80.0% of bilateral blindness and cataract was the main cause of blindness (55.0%). This dispels the conclusions of a previous clinic-based study that suggested that corneal scarring was the main cause of blindness in the region [10]. A smaller proportion of the cases of

Table 5. Visual acuity in eyes following cataract surgery in the Occupied Palestinian Territories.

Post-operative visual acuity	Occupied Palestinian Territories	West Bank	Gaza	WHO recommended standard
	n = 543	n = 320	N = 223	
Available correction				
Good (VA 6/6–6/18)	296 (54.5%)	184 (57.5%)	112 (50.2%)	>80%
Borderline (VA 6/18–6/60)	126 (23.2%)	70 (21.9%)	56 (25.1%)	<15%
Poor (VA<6/60)	121 (22.3%)	66 (20.6%)	55 (24.7%)	<5%
Best correction				
Good (VA 6/6–6/18)	357 (65.7%)	220 (68.8%)	137 (61.4%)	>90%
Borderline (VA 6/18–6/60)	87 (16.0%)	42 (13.1%)	45 (20.2%)	<5%
Poor (VA<6/60)	99 (18.2%)	58 (18.1%)	41 (18.4%)	<5%

Table 6. Extrapolated estimates for the number of Blind, Severe Visually Impaired and Visually Impaired in the Occupied Palestinian Territories.

VA with available correction	Bilateral blindness		Bilateral severe visual impairment		Bilateral visual impairment	
	Number	(95% CI)	Number	(95% CI)	Number	(95% CI)
Occupied Palestinian Territories						
Men	3,180	(2,120–4,230)	3,570	(2,430–4,710)	15,210	(12,760–17650)
Women	7,700	(5,920–9,470)	5,240	(3,830–6,650)	20,800	(17,910–23,690)
Total	10,870	(8,770–12,970)	8,810	(6,910–10,720)	36,010	(31,770–40,240)
West Bank						
Men	1,740	(900–2,570)	2,330	(1,370–3,300)	10,050	(7,780–12,220)
Women	3,730	(2,590–4,870)	2,790	(1,800–3,790)	11,810	(9,700–13,920)
Total	5,470	(4,080–6,860)	5,130	(3,640–6,610)	21,860	(19,620–24,110)
Gaza						
Men	1,370	(740–2,000)	1,140	(520–1,770)	5,170	(4,100–6,250)
Women	3,540	(2,390–4,690)	2,300	(1,390–3,220)	8,480	(6,720–10,250)
Total	4,910	(3,600–6,220)	3,450	(2,360–4,540)	13,660	(11,340–15,970)

blindness were attributable to trachoma (1.7%) compared with the results of a previous study (13.4%) [9]. Outcome after cataract surgery was found to be inadequate as only half of eyes that had undergone surgery had achieved a good outcome (VA≥6/18).

Unlike the Occupied Palestinian Territories, neighbouring Israel (not included in the Eastern Mediterranean Region, but included in the 'European Region' by the WHO) has a much lower estimated prevalence of blindness in the population (0.3%) compared to the Eastern Mediterranean Region (0.8%), and has a profile for causes of blindness similar to relatively wealthy nations such as the UK with age-related macular degeneration and glaucoma being the two main causes of blindness [25–26]. In neighbouring Lebanon, a national survey including people who were three years and above gave a slightly higher estimate compared to the Occupied Palestinian Territories for the prevalence of blindness of 0.6% and similarly found cataract as the leading cause of blindness (41%) [11]. Refractive errors, however, were the second largest cause (13%) followed by non-trachomatous corneal opacification (7.5%). Oman, located in the Arabian Peninsula, is much wealthier than the Occupied Palestinian Territories, yet was estimated to have a higher prevalence of blindness in a survey including all age groups of 1.1% [12]. However, the two largest causes of blindness were also cataract (30.5%) and trachomatous corneal scarring (24%).

The results of the survey suggest that approximately 6,000 people in the Occupied Palestinian Territories are blind due to cataract. The reasons given for not attending for cataract surgery suggest education and beliefs play the largest factor in the under-utilisation of services by the blind and that merely increasing the number of cataract surgeons and operations may not in itself effectively reduce the number of blind people in the population. Any expansion of surgical services need to be coupled with education programmes that raise public awareness and support health services to provide early identification and referral.

Those participants with visual impairment due to cataract regarded the process of obtaining permits and getting through military checkpoints (where access can still be refused with or without a permit), as a barrier. The prevalence of blindness in Gaza was twice that of the West Bank, where unemployment, poverty, and access to outside health services (such as Egypt and Jerusalem are worse than in the West Bank.

Our study points to inequity between the sexes with women having a greater prevalence of blindness and lower cataract surgical coverage. This has been found in other RAAB surveys in other countries [19–22]. Women in our study were only marginally more likely to express poverty as a reason not to have cataract surgery compared to men. Studies from Egypt have discussed and suggested that such gender disparity may be partly due to the preference of women to seek opinions for eye care no further than other family members and traditional healers [27–28]. Further anthropological studies may confirm if a similar pattern occurs in the Palestinian population.

The high proportion of participants with a poor outcome after surgery is of concern and requires further research and auditing of surgical cases to identify possible ways of reducing it. Post-operative refractive error was a major cause of poor and borderline outcome. The provision of glasses will reduce the proportion of visually impaired people after cataract surgery.

The number of people with diabetes mellitus in the Middle East is expected to grow from the 2000 estimate of 20 million to just under 60 million in 2030 [29]. The prevalence of self-reported diabetes in the >50 years age group was high (26.4%, 95% CI: 24.9–27.9), and the real estimate is likely to be higher still when considering the number of undiagnosed cases in the community. Our estimate is comparable to the prevalence of diabetes obtained from routine data of the UN Relief and Works Agency (19.1% at 50–59 years and 24.8% at ≥60 years) [7]. The high proportion of people with <6/60 visual acuity due to diabetic retinopathy points to an urgent need to plan future diabetic eye services.

Our study highlights the problem of conducting population-based studies in areas of conflict and military occupation. The decision to carry out reselection of three clusters in Gaza due to security reasons was not taken lightly but was deemed necessary. Since the prevalence of blindness was higher in Gaza than in the West Bank this could have caused a slight under-estimation of the overall prevalence of blindness. Although East Jerusalem was included in the sampling frame, no clusters in East Jerusalem were selected in the randomised selection process. Estimation of the proportion of people with posterior segment disease and glaucoma may have been imprecise because detailed examination was not always possible. Applanation tonometry was abandoned at the trial stage when it was realised that written consent for the procedure aroused suspicion in a population experiencing problems with land rights.

Confidence in the estimates for our study can be based on several strengths. All teams received organised training and were regularly monitored in the field. Selection bias was likely to be low as we achieved a high response rate and the prevalence of blindness was similar in responders compared to non-responders. Information bias including observer bias was reduced by all teams receiving training using experienced ophthalmologists and by having inter-observer variability tested objectively. Further quality control in the field was ensured by monitoring.

In conclusion, our study shows that despite the lower than predicted level of blindness, most blindness in the Occupied Palestinian Territories is avoidable. Raising health awareness, gender equity, better outcomes of cataract surgery and improving accessibility should be targeted. The implementation of strategic and sustainable interventions in the delivery of eye services must be made a high priority.

Acknowledgments

The authors wish to thank all the staff based at the St. John facilities in Jerusalem and Gaza for their contributions as well as the study participants. We would like to thank Anthony Chignell, Steven James and Charles Kanawati for initiating this study, Philip Mann for his assistance with the original proposal, and Assad Yousef Hussein and Jom'a El Jazzar for initiating the study in Gaza. We greatly appreciated the support and permission given by the Palestinian Authority Ministry of Health and local municipalities.

Author Contributions

Analyzed the data: FC HK RL NJS. Wrote the paper: FC HK RL TK NK NJS. Contributed to the design of the study: NJS FC HK NK ZA. A principal investigator: NJS FC. Helped with the preliminary analyses of the data: NJS FC. Helped collect data in the field: NJS FC. Helped initiate the survey in the Occupied Palestinian Territories: NJS. One of the principal coordinators for the implementation of the study: NJS FC. Reviewed the draft manuscript: NJS FC HK RL TK NS DM NK HB ZA. Contributed to writing the paper: NJS FC HK RL TK NS DM NK HB ZA. Contributed to calculating the sample size and selecting clusters: FC HK RL. Contributed to initiating the survey in the Occupied Palestinian Territories: HK ZA. Contributed to the training of the survey teams in the survey protocol and procedures: HK RL. Contributed to collecting data in the field: TK NS DM NK HB.

References

1. Resnikoff S, Pascolini D, Etya'ale D, Kocur I, Pararajasegaram R, et al. (2004) Global data on visual impairment in the year 2002. Bull World Health Organ 82: 844–851.
2. Ngondi J, Ole-Sempele F, Onsarigo A, Matende I, Baba S, et al. (2006) Prevalence and causes of blindness and low vision in Southern Sudan. PloS Medicine 3: e478. doi:10.1371/journal.pmed.0030478.
3. Palestinian Central Bureau of Statistics (2008) Census final results in The West Bank summary (population and housing), Available: http://www.pcbs.gov.ps/Portals_PCBS/Doanloads/book1487.pdf. Accessed 2nd May 2009.
4. Palestinian Central Bureau of Statistics (2008) Census final results in Gaza Strip summary (population and housing). Available: http://www.pcbs.gov.ps/Portals/_PCBS/Downloads/books1509.pdf. Accessed 2nd May 2009.
5. The humanitarian impact of the West Bank Barrier on Palestinian communities. Update No 7 (2007) United Nations-Office for the Coordination of Humanitarian Affairs. Jerusalem.
6. Access to Health Services Survey: 2003 (2004) Palestinian Central Bureau of Statistics. Ramallah, Palestine.
7. Husseini A, Abu-Rmeileh NM, Mikki N, Ramahi TM, Ghosh HA, et al. (2009) Cardiovascular diseases, diabetes mellitus, and cancer in the Occupied Palestinian Territory. Lancet 373: 1041–1049.
8. Mataria A, Khatib R, Donaldson C, Bossert T, Hunter DJ, et al. (2009) The health-care system: an assessment and reform agenda. Lancet 373: 1207–1217.
9. Thomson IM, Chumbley LC (1984) Eye disease in the West Bank and Gaza strip. British Journal of Ophthalmology 68(8): 598–602.
10. Golychev VN (1991) [Ocular morbidity in Palestine]. Vestn Oftalmol 107: 63–65.
11. Mansour AM, Kassak K, Chaya M, Hourani T, Sibai A (1997) National survey of blindness and low vision in Lebanon. British Journal of Ophthalmology 81: 905–906.
12. Khandekar R, Mohammed AJ, Negrel AD, Al Riyami A (2002) The prevalence and causes of blindness in the Sultanate of Oman: the Oman Eye Study (OES). British Journal of Ophthalmology 86: 957–962.
13. Palestinian Central Bureau of Statistics (2008) Palestine in Figures 2007. Available: http://www.paltrade.org/en/about-palestine/Figures.pdf. Accessed 28th April 2008.
14. Palestinian Central Bureau of Statistics (2007) Palestine in Figures 2006. Available: http://www.pcbs.gov.ps/Portals/_PCBS/Downloads/book1342.pdf. Accessed 28th April 2008.
15. Palestinian Central Bureau of Statistics (2007) Statistical Abstract of Palestine No.8. Available: http://www.pcbs.gov.ps/DesktopDefault.aspx?tabID=4121&lang=en. Accessed 28th April 2008.
16. World Health Organisation. Programme for the Prevention of Blindness and Deafness (1988) Coding instructions for the WHO/PBL eye examination record (version iii). 1–17. Geneva.
17. Thylefors B, Negrel AD, Pararajasegaram R, et al. (1995) Global data on blindness. Bull World Health Organ 73: 115–121.
18. Amansakhatov S, Volokhovskaya Z, Afanasyeva A, Limburg H (2002) Cataract blindness in Turkmenistan: results of a national survey. British. J Ophthalmol 86: 1207–1210.
19. Oye J, Kuper H, Dineen B, Befidi-Mengue R, Foster A (2006) Prevalence and causes of blindness and visual impairment in Muyuka: a rural health district in South West Province, Cameroon. British. J Ophthalmol 90: 538–542.
20. Wadud Z, Kuper H, Polack S, Lindfield R, Akm MR, et al. (2006) Rapid assessment of avoidable blindness and needs assessment of cataract services in Satkhira District, Bangladesh. British J Ophthalmol.
21. Mathenge W, Kuper H, et al, Limburg H, Polack S, Onyango O, et al. (2007) Rapid assessment of avoidable blindness in Nakuru District, Kenya. Ophthalmology 114: 599–606.
22. Mathenge W, Nkurikiye J, Limburg H, Kuper H (2007) Rapid assessment of avoidable blindness in Western Rwanda: blindness in a postconflict setting. PLoS Med 4(7): e217.
23. Wu M, Yip J, Kuper H (2008) Rapid assessment of avoidable blindness in Kunming, China. Ophthalmology 115: 969–974.
24. Habiyakire C, Kabona G, Courtright P, Lewallen S (2010) Rapid assessment of avoidable blindness and cataract surgical services in Kilimanjaro Region, Tanzania. Ophthamic Epidemiol 17: 90–94.
25. Avisar R, Bahar I, Weinberger D (2003) [Causes of blindness in the year 2000 in Israel]. Harefuah 142: 94–96, 160.
26. Avisar R, Friling R, Snir M, Avisar I, Weinberger D (2006) Estimation of prevalence and incidence rates and causes of blindness in Israel, 1998–2003. Isr Med Assoc J 8: 880–881.
27. Fouad D, Mousa A, Courtright P (2004) Sociodemographic characteristics associated with blindness in a Nile Delta governate of Egypt. British Journal of Ophthalmology 88: 614–618.
28. Lane SD, Millar MI (1987) The "Hierarchy of Resort" reexamined: status and class differentials as determinants of therapy for eye disease in the Egyptian delta. Urban Anthropol 16: 151–82.
29. WHO (2005) Prevention of blindness from diabetes mellitus: a report of a WHO consultation in Geneva, Switzerland, November. pp 9–11.

The Relationship between the Disability Prevalence of Cataracts and Ambient Erythemal Ultraviolet Radiation in China

Yang Wang[1], Jiaming Yu[2], Qian Gao[1], Liwen Hu[1], Na Gao[1], Huizhi Gong[1], Yang Liu[1]*

1 School of Public Health, China Medical University, Shenyang, People's Republic of China, 2 Ophthalmology Department, The Fourth Affiliated Hospital of China Medical University, Shenyang, People's Republic of China

Abstract

In Western countries, ultraviolet (UV)-induced skin cancer has been studied extensively regarding the high incidence of skin cancers in the white population; however, for people of color, cataracts are the main public health issue in relation to increased ambient ultraviolet radiation (UVR). To our knowledge, few studies have been conducted examining the relationship between cataracts and ambient UVR in China. In this study, we aimed to explore the relationship between and the factors influencing the disability prevalence of cataracts and annual ambient erythemal UVR exposure in 31 regions of China. The data used to determine the disability prevalence of cataracts was obtained from the Second China National Sample Survey on Disability. The regional annual erythemal UVR was calculated using Geographic Information System (GIS) methods based on data from the National Aeronautics and Space Administration (NASA) database. The relationship between the disability prevalence of cataracts and the annual ambient erythemal UVR was examined by using logistic regression. Both the age-standardized disability prevalence of cataracts (OR = 3.97, 95%CI 1.30–12.13, per 100KJ/m^2 increase in annual ambient erythemal UVR) and the disability prevalence of cataracts among a population ≥65 years old (OR = 3.97, 95%CI 1.30–12.13, per 100KJ/m^2 increase in annual ambient erythemal UVR) were higher in association with higher ambient erythemal UVR. Regions with higher urbanization and educational levels had lower disability prevalence of cataracts. We found positive associations of the age-standardized disability prevalence of cataracts and the disability prevalence of cataracts among a population ≥65 years old with ambient erythemal UVR in 31 regions of China.

Editor: Pedro Gonzalez, Duke University, United States of America

Funding: The Chinese National Natural Science Foundation supported this study (No.81273034, No. 30800895 and No.30700652). The funders had no role in study design, data collection and analysis, decision to publish, or preparation of the manuscript.

Competing Interests: The authors have declared that no competing interests exist.

* E-mail: cmuliuyang@yahoo.com

Introduction

Since the hole in the ozone layer in the South Pole was firstly reported in 1985 [1], ozone depletion has become an important environmental issue that has attracted worldwide attention. Two main public health issues in relation to ozone depletion, increased ultraviolet (UV)-induced skin cancer and cataracts, have been studied by researchers from different countries over the past two decades [2–8]. In Western countries, UV-induced skin cancer is more well studied than cataracts due to the high incidence of skin cancer among the white population. For people of color, however, cataracts have been the main public health concern due to increased ambient UVR [3–5,9] because this population is less likely to develop skin cancer due to the protective properties of their skin.

The relationship between cataracts and ambient UVR or UV exposure has been established in previous studies [7,10–12]. For example, West et al. reported that the odds of cortical opacity increased with increasing ocular exposure to ultraviolet radiation-B (UVB) [10]. Additionally, West et al. estimated that 167,000–830,000 additional cases of cortical cataracts would be identified by 2050 in the U.S. with 5–20% ozone depletion resulting in an increase of UVB rays [7]. However, to our knowledge, few studies have been conducted on the relationship between cataracts and ambient UVR or UV exposure in China.

The unique geographic condition and epidemiological characteristics of cataracts make China an ideal country to study the relationship between cataracts and ambient UVR. From a geographic point of view, from the southernmost region to northernmost region, China extends across nearly 50 degrees latitude, and the altitude of the western and eastern regions differs by nearly 4,000 meters. China's wide ranges in latitude and altitude provide a broad environmental gradient for estimating UV exposure.

In 2007, China's cataract patients numbered more than 60 million, and the population with a disability caused by cataracts numbered more than 7 million [13]. Today, cataracts are the leading cause of visual disability in China [14,15]. When taken together, the enormous public health burden attributed to cataracts along with the country's geographic conditions make studying the relationship between the prevalence of cataracts and ambient UVR in China an urgent and suitable endeavor. Because up-to-date national data on the prevalence of cataracts was not available due to the lack of recent national epidemiological surveys, in the present study, we used the disability prevalence due to cataracts obtained from the Second China National Sample Survey on Disability as the index of UV-induced health effects on eyes.

The present study used data from the Second China National Sample Survey on Disability in 2006 to calculate the age-standardized disability prevalence of cataracts in 31 regions of China and used estimated daily ambient erythemal UVR from National Aeronautics and Space Administration (NASA) satellites, together with ArcGIS software, to calculate annual ambient erythemal UVR in corresponding regions. The main objectives of this study were (1) to estimate the disability prevalence of cataracts and the annual ambient erythemal UVR in 31 regions of China; (2) to evaluate the relationship between the disability prevalence of cataracts and annual ambient erythemal UVR in China; and (3) to compare the disability prevalence of cataracts and annual ambient erythemal UVR by latitude and altitude, respectively.

Methods

1. Ethics Statement

The Second China National Sample Survey on Disability was a government-organized survey, and was conducted by the China Disabled Persons' Federation and approved by the State Council of the People's Republic of China. The procedures of this survey satisfied the requirements of the Statistics Law of the People's Republic of China. All survey subjects completed the written informed consent provided by the Chinese government.

2. Measurement of the disability prevalence of cataracts

The Second China National Sample Survey on Disability was carried out on April 1, 2006 in 31 regions, including 22 provinces, 5 autonomous regions, and 4 municipalities in Mainland China. The geographic distribution of the 31 regions is shown in Figure 1. A stratified, multi-phased cluster random sampling design was applied in this survey. Sampling was conducted at three levels. The offices at the provincial level randomly selected 734 counties (cities or districts) based on economic development in each region. Each county then randomly selected 4 towns (with the exception of Beijing, Tianjin, and Shanghai, which selected more than 4 towns each) for a total of 2,980 towns (townships or streets). Finally, each town and street randomly selected 2 communities for a total of 5,964 communities represented in this survey [13]. The nation-wide participation rate was 1.93‰. The investigation was conducted in two stages. The first stage consisted of residential family investigation. The 771,797 sampled families and 2,526,145 people within the included families were asked to report the disabled individuals who suffer from abnormalities such as a loss in function (psychologically or physiologically) or anatomical structure of a certain organ and whether they have totally or partially lost the ability to perform an activity in a way considered to be normal based on the guidelines provided in the screening table of the Second China National Sample Survey on Disability. The second stage involved the investigation of the identified disabled persons. All candidates received medical tests and were graded according to the Grading Standard of Disabilities of the Second China National Sample Survey on Disability. Of those selected, there were 142,112 families with disabled persons and 161,479 people with disabilities within the included families.

This survey targeted populations within the People's Republic of China who were permanent residents of the sampled residential quarters. Three types of survey forms were used: household questionnaires, disability questionnaires and community questionnaires. There were 52 survey items in all that included family and personal information on the sample group, focusing on the causes of disability, living conditions and major needs of the disabled population.

In this survey, "visual disability" referred to poor vision or the constriction of visual field in both eyes that may have been caused for various reasons and is uncorrectable. Visual disability consisted of two categories: blindness and low vision. The grading standard of visual disability is shown in Table 1 [13]. In the Second China National Sample Survey on Disability, "visual disability" was measured first and the reason of visual disability was examined by ophthalmologist for each visually disabled subject. If the subject was diagnosed as cataract, this subject was categorized as "visual disability due to cataract".

3. Measurement of ambient erythemal UVR

Erythemal UVR is commonly calculated by weighing the solar UV radiation with the erythemal action spectrum to reflect the erythemal effect of UVB radiation to the human skin. The estimated daily ambient erythemal UVR, expressed in joules per meter squared (J/m^2), was obtained on a 1° of latitude (89.5S to 89.5N) by 1° of longitude (180W to 180E) grid for all of China. The grid was generated from the NASA Goddard Space Flight Center Data Archive Center database of readings from the Total Ozone Mapping Spectrometer mounted on the Nimbus-7 satellite [16] and Earth Probe satellite [17]. We estimated the erythemal UVR measurement by averaging daily estimates from 1980 through 2005 and calculated the annual erythemal UVR based on the assumption that the relative distribution of annual UVR was stable over time. As the NASA database did not provide a complete dataset of estimated daily erythemal UVR from 1993 to 1996, data from these years were not included in this study. ArcGIS 9.2 (http://www.esri.com/software/arcgis/index.html) software was used for spatial modeling of the erythemal UVR data, and the selection function was used to obtain region-level average daily erythemal UVR. Then annual erythemal UVR was calculated based on the regional average daily erythemal UVR.

4. Statistical analysis

We calculated the number of patients with visually disabling cataracts of different age groups in each of the 31 regions (0–14 years, 15–64 years and ≥65 years) based on the survey data. We calculated the total and age-specific disability prevalence of cataracts for each region by dividing the number of patients with visually disabling cataracts in each age group by the surveyed population in each age group.

To control for the effect of age on the disability prevalence of cataracts, we age-standardized the disability prevalence of cataracts using an direct standardization method. Several steps were included in this method: (1) the disability prevalences of cataracts for each of the three age groups (0–14,15–64, ≥65) were obtained from the surveyed population in each region; (2) the disability prevalence of cataracts in each of the three age groups in each region was multiplied by the number of people representing the standard population (the entire population of the survey) in each of the three age groups, and the three products were then summed to obtain the expected disability population of cataracts for each region; (3) the standard population was divided by the expected disability population of cataracts in each region to obtain the age-standardized disability prevalence for each region.

We also calculated the annual ambient erythemal UVR in three different decades (1980 s, 1990 s, and 2000 s) and the average annual ambient erythemal UVR of 31 regions in China.

SPSS 17.0 software was used to perform a logistic regression analysis to establish the relationship between the age-standardized disability prevalence of cataracts and the annual erythemal UVR.

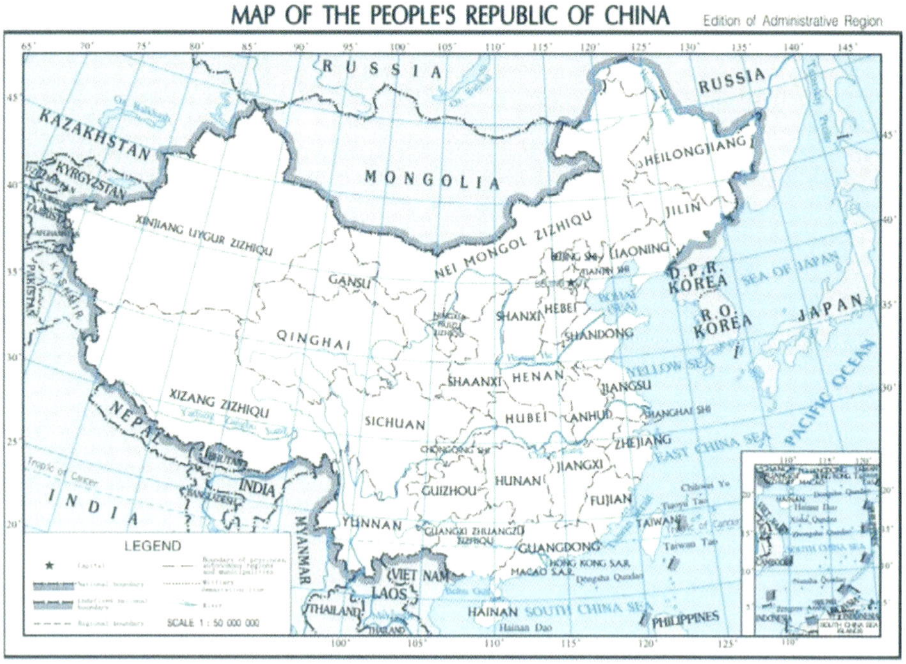

Figure 1. Map of China with the 31 regions included in the present study. Note: Taiwan, Hong Kong, and Macau were not included in the Second China National Sample Survey on Disability and thus were not included in our analyses. Cited from the National Administration of Surveying, Mapping and Geoinformation website, 2007. Standard map service. Available: http://www.sbsm.gov.cn/article/zxbs/dtfw// [Accessed 31 August 2011].

The age-standardized disability prevalence of cataracts was defined as "1" if it was larger than the median and as "0" if it was equal or smaller than the median, and it was analyzed as the binominal dependent variable. The annual erythemal UVR was the independent variable in the model. Similarly, the relationship between the annual ambient erythemal UVR and the disability prevalence of cataracts among a population ≥65 years old was established using the same method. In these two models, the unit of the annual ambient erythemal UVR was transferred from KJ/m^2 to $100KJ/m^2$.

Thirty-one regions were divided into three groups based on latitude and altitude. Regions with an average latitude below or including 30°N were allocated to latitude group 1; regions with an average latitude between 30°N and 40°N were allocated to latitude group 2; and regions with an average latitude above or including 40°N were allocated to latitude group 3 (Figure 2). Regions are divided into three altitude groups based on the unique geographic feature of China, which Chinese geographers name "three-step ladder". Regions with an average altitude higher or equal to 4,000 meters were allocated to altitude group 1; regions with an average altitude between 500 meters and 2,000 meters were allocated to altitude group 2; and regions with an average altitude less than 500 meters were allocated to altitude group 3 (Figure 3). Regions with an average altitude between 2,000 meters and 4,000 meters don't exist in China. Kruskal-Wallis test was used to compare the age-standardized disability prevalence of cataracts, disability prevalence of cataracts among a population ≥65 years old, and the ambient erythemal UVR among the three latitude groups and among the three altitude groups. Wilcoxon rank sum test was performed to do pairwise comparisons by adjusting α level to 0.017 (0.05/3).

To roughly reflect the effect of urbanization and educational levels on the amount of time people spent outdoors and further on the disability prevalence of cataracts, we compared the age-

Table 1. Grading standard of visual disability.

Category	Degree	Optimum corrected vision
Blindness	Degree 1	<0.02 (no light perception or visual field radius less than 5 degrees)
	Degree 2	0.02–0.05 (or visual field radius less than 10 degrees)
Low vision	Degree 3	0.05–0.1
	Degree 4	0.1–0.3

Cited from Documentation of the Second China National Sample Survey on Disability, 2007.

Notes: (1) Blindness or low vision refers to both eyes. In the event that the degree of the two eyes were different, only the eye with better vision was considered. If a person had one eye that was considered to be blind or to have low vision but the other eye was not recognized as visually disabled (greater than 0.3), then that person was excluded from this analysis. (2) The optimum corrected vision referred to the best vision after appropriate eyeglass rectification or vision measured by pinhole glass. (3) Persons with field of vision less than 10 degrees were recognized as visually disabled.

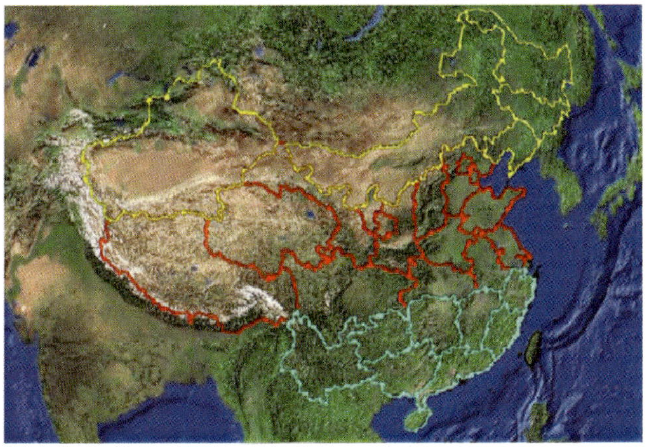

Figure 2. Illustration of the divisions of the three latitude groups. Note: Regions with green, red, and yellow borders are defined as latitude group 1, latitude group 2 and latitude group 3, respectively.

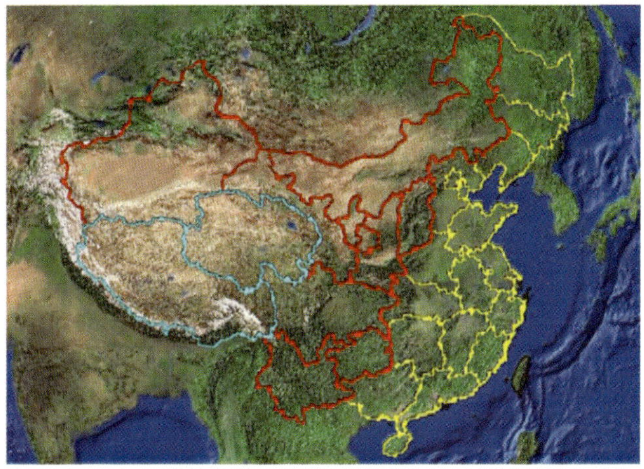

Figure 3. Illustration of the divisions of the three altitude groups. Note: Regions with green, red, and yellow borders are defined as altitude group 1, altitude group 2 and altitude group 3, respectively.

standardized disability prevalence of cataracts and the disability prevalence of cataracts among a population ≥65 years old between Beijing and Hebei as well as between Shanghai and Zhejiang. Beijing (longitude 115°24′E-117°30′E and latitude 39°28′N-41°05′N; altitude≈43 meters) and Shanghai (longitude 120°51′E-122°12′E and latitude 30°40′N-31°53′N; altitude≈4 meters) are two municipalities that are self-governed. These two cities have high population densities, high urbanization levels, and high education levels, resulting in a high proportion of indoor workers in these two cities. Hebei Province (longitude 113°04′E-119°53′E and latitude 36°01′N-42°37′N; altitude≈50 meters) and Zhejiang Province (longitude 118°24′E-122°24′E and latitude 27°30′N-31°00′N; altitude≈350 meters) are located at geographic positions where the latitude and altitude are similar to those of Beijing and Shanghai, respectively. The data in Table 2 showed that the annual ambient erythemal UVR in Beijing and Heijing were similar and that the exposure in Shanghai and Zhejiang were also similar. Compared to Beijing and Shanghai, the urbanization and education levels of the population in Hebei Province and Zhejiang Province were lower. In 2005, the proportion of the urban population in Beijing was 83.62%, whereas in Hebei province, the urban population was 37.69%. The proportion of the urban population in Shanghai was 89.09%, whereas 56.02% in Zhejiang Province represented the urban population [18]. The proportion of people with a college education or above was 12.13% in Beijing, but only 1.15% in Hebei. The proportion of people with a college education or above was 8.23% in Shanghai, but only 1.83% in Zhejiang [12]. We compared the age-standardized disability prevalence of cataracts and the disability prevalence of cataracts among a population ≥65 years old between Beijing Province and Hebei Province and between Shanghai Province and Zhejiang Province to observe the influence of outdoor time on the actual UV exposure among the population and its influence on the disability prevalence of cataracts.

Results

1. Distribution of the disability prevalence of cataracts

The Second China National Sample Survey on Disability surveyed 2,525,145 people, and the total number with a visual disability caused by cataracts was 18,085. As shown in Table 2, the average age-standardized disability prevalence of cataracts in the country was 749 per 100,000. Beijing had the lowest age-standardized disability prevalence of cataracts at 213 per 100,000, while Xizang (Tibet) had the highest age-standardized disability prevalence of cataracts at 1,651 per 100,000. The national average age-standardized disability prevalence of cataracts among a population ≥65 years old was 6,984 per 100,000. The lowest disability prevalence of cataracts among a population ≥65 years old was observed in Beijing (2,018 per 100,000), while the highest was observed in Xizang (15,148 per 100,000).

2. Distribution of the ambient erythemal UVR

The lowest ambient erythemal UVR was recorded in Heilongjiang province with a daily exposure of 1728.94 J/m^2 and an annual exposure of 631.06 KJ/m^2. The highest ambient erythemal UVR was recorded in Xizang with a daily exposure of 4688.54 J/m^2 and an annual exposure of 1776.29 KJ/m^2. The annual ambient erythemal UVR of the surveyed regions in different decades are shown and sorted by the average ambient erythemal UVR in Table 3.

3. Relationship between the disability prevalence of cataracts and the annual ambient erythemal UVR

As shown in Figures 4 and 5, the age-standardized disability prevalence of cataracts and the disability prevalence of cataracts among a population ≥65 years both increased with increases in the annual exposure to erythemal UV. The age-standardized disability prevalence of cataracts and the disability prevalence of cataracts among a population ≥65 years were found to be associated with the annual ambient erythemal UVR in the logistic regression models [$OR_{\text{age-standardized disability prevalence of cataracts}} = 3.97$, 95%CI 1.30–12.13, per 100KJ/m^2 increase in annual ambient erythemal UVR; $OR_{\text{disability prevalence of cataracts among a population} \geq 65 \text{ years}} = 3.97$, 95%CI 1.30–12.13, per 100 KJ/m^2 increase in annual ambient erythemal UVR].

4. The influence of latitude and altitude

As shown in Table 4, the median annual ambient erythemal UVR of latitude group 1 was 288.13 KJ/m^2 higher than that of latitude group 3 ($P = 0.005$). Compared to latitude group 3, the median age-standardized disability prevalence of cataracts was 652/100,000 higher ($P<0.001$), and the median disability prevalence of cataracts among a population ≥65 years old was

Table 2. Disability prevalence of cataracts in 31 regions of China (sorted by the age-standardized disability prevalence of cataracts).

Region	Surveyed population	Age-standardized disability prevalence of cataracts (%)	Disability prevalence of cataracts among a population ≥65 years (%)
Beijing	74,795	0.213	2.018
Tianjin	72,351	0.325	3.016
Heilongjiang Province	70,405	0.371	3.139
Liaoning Province	83,857	0.407	3.635
Shanghai Province	73,864	0.408	3.750
Inner Mongol Autonomous Region	65,247	0.476	4.327
Shanxi Province	75,016	0.488	4.486
Xinjiang Autonomous Region	51,775	0.494	4.497
Jilin Province	76,408	0.532	4.899
Hebei Province	104,713	0.566	5.274
Guizhou Province	104,169	0.568	5.353
Shaanxi Province	82,460	0.576	5.324
Zhejiang Province	75,636	0.600	5.645
Hunan Province	73,425	0.610	5.144
Chongqing	95,392	0.619	5.307
Jiangsu Province	106,065	0.620	5.851
Shandong Province	127,567	0.648	6.206
Hubei Province	101,674	0.713	6.448
Anhui Province	105,201	0.819	7.317
Henan Province	125,641	0.920	8.671
Qinghai Province	130,415	0.925	8.838
Jiangxi Province	83,088	0.937	8.811
Sichuan Province	30,395	0.965	8.460
Ningxia Autonomous Region	45,882	0.982	9.765
Guangdong Province	63,249	1.059	10.313
Gansu Province	41,214	1.064	10.160
Hainan Province	71,484	1.075	10.390
Fujian Province	125,442	1.076	10.423
Guangxi Autonomous Region	80,712	1.180	11.081
Yunnan Province	86,032	1.336	12.798
Xizang Autonomous Region	22,571	1.651	15.148
Average	74,795	0.749	6.984

6,678/100,000 higher ($P<0.001$) in latitude group 1. The median annual ambient erythemal UVR of latitude group 2 was 151.76 KJ/m^2 higher than that of latitude group 3 ($P=0.002$). Compared to latitude group 3, the median age-standardized disability prevalence of cataracts was 306/100,000 higher ($P<0.001$), and the median disability prevalence of cataracts among a population ≥65 years old was 2,813/100,000 higher in latitude group 2 ($P<0.001$).

As shown in Table 5, the medians of the age-standardized disability prevalence of cataracts and the medians of the disability prevalence of cataracts among a population ≥65 years old were not significantly different for any of the altitude groups. The median annual ambient erythemal UVR of altitude group 1 was 747.57 KJ/m^2 higher than that of altitude group 3 ($P=0.009$).

5. Influence of urbanization level and educational level

Age-standardized disability prevalence of cataracts and the disability prevalence of cataracts among a population ≥65 years old in Hebei Province were 566 per 100,000 and 5,274 per 100,000, respectively, while in Beijing, these values were 213 per 100,000 and 2,018 per 100,000, respectively. The disability prevalence of cataracts in Hebei was higher when compared to that in Beijing. The age-standardized disability prevalence of cataracts and the disability prevalence of cataracts among a population ≥65 years old in Zhejiang Province were 600 per 100,000 and 5,645 per 100,000, respectively, while in Shanghai, these values were 408 per 100,000 and 3,750 per 100,000, respectively. The age-standardized disability prevalence of cataracts and the disability prevalence of cataracts among a population ≥65 years old were higher in Zhejiang Province compared with Shanghai.

Table 3. Annual ambient erythemal UVR of 31 regions in different decades in China [sorted by the average ambient erythemal UVR (KJ/m^2)].

Region	1980s	1990s	2000s	Average
Heilongjiang Province	603.87	652.66	636.66	631.06
Jilin Province	719.85	758.46	739.85	739.39
Liaoning Province	796.06	818.29	813.66	809.33
Inner Mongol Autonomous Region	818.05	862.52	854.91	845.16
Tianjin	871.57	872.80	862.74	869.04
Beijing	864.66	876.80	869.87	870.44
Hebei Province	893.34	907.27	896.31	898.97
Chongqing	944.77	920.81	929.89	931.82
Shandong Province	964.15	955.71	942.13	954.00
Henan Province	995.68	994.67	965.63	985.33
Jiangsu Province	1013.14	973.48	979.03	988.55
Hubei Province	1004.06	996.56	979.05	993.22
Shanxi Province	989.98	1012.00	988.64	996.87
Anhui Province	1017.54	988.30	984.92	996.92
Shaanxi Province	994.66	1019.63	1010.50	1008.27
Hunan Province	1062.59	1003.81	972.12	1012.84
Guizhou Province	1067.72	1004.04	991.32	1021.03
Shanghai	1057.67	1002.70	1002.86	1021.08
Zhejiang Province	1095.34	1034.29	1010.12	1046.58
Jiangxi Province	1117.50	1050.13	1021.50	1063.04
Ningxia Autonomous Region	1088.52	1113.60	1111.28	1104.47
Fujian Province	1189.63	1114.35	1095.88	1133.29
Guangxi Autonomous Region	1195.32	1108.11	1098.18	1133.87
Xinjiang Autonomous Region	1138.64	1178.44	1170.82	1162.63
Guangdong Province	1248.23	1178.36	1166.28	1197.63
Gansu Province	1200.5	1225.31	1216.96	1214.26
Sichuan Province	1426.37	1381.64	1380.06	1396.02
Hainan Province	1534.21	1414.96	1336.03	1428.40
Yunnan Province	1516.06	1397.98	1423.23	1445.75
Qinghai Province	1696.85	1696.97	1708.08	1700.63
Xizang Autonomous Region	2026.67	1977.06	1325.13	1776.29

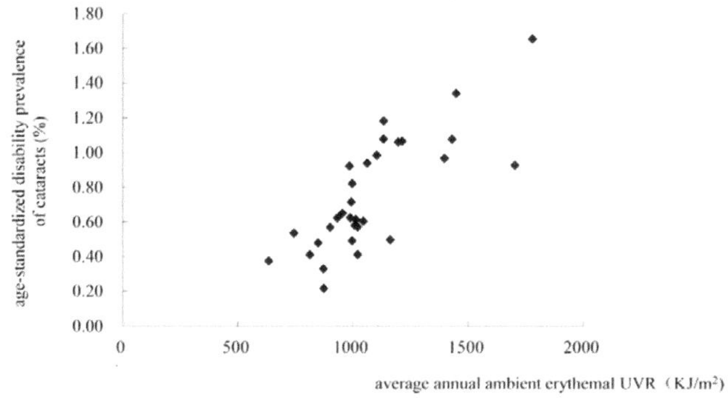

Figure 4. Scatter plot of the relationship between the age-standardized disability prevalence of cataracts (y) and the average annual ambient erythemal UVR (x) in 31 regions in China.

Discussion

The results in the present study demonstrated that Xizang (Tibet) had the highest ambient erythemal UVR (annual exposure: 1776.29 KJ/m^2) and the highest age-standardized disability prevalence of cataracts (1,651 per 100,000). Xizang has an average altitude of over 4,000 meters, which makes the air much thinner than in the lower, plains regions. Additionally, the long duration of sunshine and the intense reflection and scattering of UV radiation due to rocks and snow on the Xizang Plateau also contribute to the high ambient erythemal UVR in Xizang. Hainan Province (which is located at the southernmost part of China and has the lowest average latitude and a low altitude) also had a very high annual ambient erythemal UVR and a high disability prevalence of cataracts. Conversely, regions of the northeastern part of China (which has the highest latitudes, low altitudes, and shorter hours of sunshine) had the lowest ambient erythemal UVR and the lowest disability prevalence of cataracts.

Notably, the present study found that when we controlled the effect of age structure of populations by age-standardizing, there was a strong correlation between the age-standardized disability prevalence of cataracts and the disability prevalence of cataracts among a population ≥65 years old. The reason would be that cataract is generally a disease of older age and the age-standardized disability prevalence was largely made up of the disability prevalence of cataracts among a population ≥65 years old.

In the present study, we found that the age-standardized disability prevalence of cataracts and the disability prevalence of cataracts among a population ≥65 years old were both associated with the annual ambient erythemal UVR in 31 regions of China. A 100KJ/m^2 increase in the annual ambient erythemal UVR was associated with a 397% increase in the log odds of having a regional age-standardized disability prevalence of cataracts or a disability prevalence of cataracts among a population ≥65 years above the median level.

Latitude and altitude are two main determinants of both ambient erythemal UVR level and disability prevalence of cataracts. Javitt and Taylor identified UVB (280–320 nm)

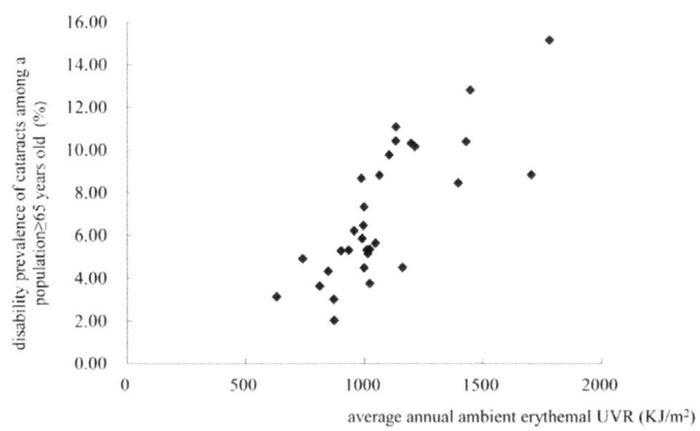

Figure 5. Scatter plot of the relationship between the disability prevalence of cataracts among a population ≥65 years old (y) and the average annual ambient erythemal UVR (x) in 31 regions in China.

Table 4. Comparison of the age-standardized disability prevalence of cataracts, the disability prevalence of cataracts among a population ≥65 years old and the ambient erythemal UVR among the three latitude groups.

Latitude group	n	Average latitude	Age-standardized disability prevalence of cataracts (%) Median	Disability prevalence of cataracts among a population ≥65 years old (%) Median	Annual ambient erythemal UVR (KJ/m²) Median
1	9	25.1°N	1.059*	10.313**	1133.29**
2	15	33.9°N	0.713*	6.448**	996.92*
3	7	43.4°N	0.407	3.635	845.16

*Difference is statistically significant compared to group 3, P<0.017.
**Difference is statistically significant compared to group 3, P<0.001.

exposure as inversely correlated with latitude and showed that the probability of cataract surgery in the U.S. increased by 3% for each 1-degree decrease in latitude [19]. Our findings also showed that the age-standardized disability prevalence of cataracts, the disability prevalence of cataracts among a population ≥65 years old, and the ambient erythemal UVR were significantly higher in low and middle latitude regions than in high latitude regions. Blumthaler et al. found that UVB irradiance increased with altitude in and over the UVB band: 24% per 1,000 m at 300 nm and 11% per 1,000 m at 320 nm inside the UVB band and 9% per 1,000 m at 370 nm(UVA 320–400 nm) outside the UVB band [20]. The present study showed that the ambient erythemal UVR in regions with an average altitude above 4000 m (including Xizang and Qinghai Provinces) were significantly higher than that in regions with an average altitude between 500–2000 m. However, the age-standardized disability prevalence of cataracts and the disability prevalence of cataracts among a population ≥65 years in the three altitude groups were not significantly different. The lack of significance in these results could be the small sample size in each altitude group.

Beijing and Shanghai had a lower age-standardized disability prevalence of cataracts and disability prevalence of cataracts among a population ≥65 years old compared to Hebei and Zhejiang, which are geographically similar to Beijing and Shanghai respectively, but with a much lower population density. The findings are consistent with a lower level of outdoor exposure in the more urbanized regions, and thus with the findings that higher UVR exposure (a combination of ambient UVR and time outdoors) increases the likelihood of having a disabling cataract.

Several strengths were presented in this study. First, this is the first study to investigate the relationship between the disability prevalence of cataracts and ambient erythemal UVR in China. A very large sample size from the Second China National Sample Survey on Disability provided this study with a good representation of people of color. Second, we included 31 regions of China in this study. A wide range in latitude and altitude in these regions provides a broad environmental gradient for estimating ambient erythemal UVR and the disability prevalence of cataracts. Third, vision disability not only devalues the quality of life of cataract patient, especially among the elderly, but also brings serious economic and disease burden to individuals, families and communities. The results of this study can provide scientific support to further research on the prevention of cataracts, especially for people of color, thus help to decrease the disease burden of cataracts and improve cataract patients' quality of life.

However, several limitations in the present study must be mentioned. First, we used the average ambient erythemal UVR in each region to describe the ambient UVR. It did not reflect the actual UV exposure of individual populations. The geographic environment and population distribution in some regions were so complicated that we may have masked the affect of these characteristics by using the average value. For example, the average altitude in the eastern part of Sichuan Province is below 500 meters, whereas the average altitude in the western part is between 4,000 and 4,500 meters. It is possible there was a substantial difference in ambient erythemal UVR between these two regions. Most of the population in Sichuan Province was located in the eastern part; thus, when we used the average ambient erythemal UVR in each region, we may have overestimated the actual UV exposure of the local population and masked

Table 5. Comparison of the age-standardized disability prevalence of cataracts, the disability prevalence of cataracts among a population ≥65 years old and the ambient erythemal UVR among the three altitude groups.

Altitude group	n	Average altitude (meters)	Age-standardized disability prevalence of cataracts (%) Median	Disability prevalence of cataracts among a population ≥65 years (%) Median	Annual ambient erythemal UVR (KJ/m²) Median
1	2	4000	1.288	11.993	1738.46
2	9	500–2000	0.576	5.353	1104.47
3	20	<500	0.619	5.748	990.89*

*Difference is statistically significant compared to group 1, P<0.017.

the affect related to the differences in geographic characteristics and population density. Second, many factors influence the actual UV exposure of a population, such as activity time outdoors and air quality. To roughly reflect the influence of activity time outdoors on the disability prevalence of cataracts, we compared the disability prevalence of cataracts between regions with similar latitude and altitude (Beijing vs. Hebei; Shanghai vs. Zhejiang); however, precise estimation of the activity time outdoors of the population is difficult to achieve. Additionally, air quality (smog or dust) in urban areas could have a major effect on actual UV exposure. For example, the number of smog days in Beijing might have a major effect on individual UV exposure. Third, some factors that can influence the disability prevalence of cataracts, such as cataract surgery frequency, diabetes, medications and smoking were not included in the present study. For example, patients who had surgery would have normal vision and would not have been detected in the screen for disability. It is plausible, for example, that people who live in Beijing or Shanghai have much better access to cataract surgery and have a much higher volume of surgery performed. This would result in lower rates of visually disabling cataracts in these areas. Finally, studies have shown that UVR was mainly related to the prevalence of cortical cataracts [10]. However, the disability prevalence of cortical cataracts is difficult to obtain in 31 regions because the Second China National Sample Survey on Disability did not capture details on the types of cataracts. Although the survey was not designed for our study, the national data of disability prevalence was still very valuable in studying the health effects of increased ambient UVR.

Acknowledgments

We thank all the study participants and dedicated personnel. We grateful acknowledge Professor Ge Wang from Virginia Tech, United States for his important comments and editorial help.

Author Contributions

Conceived and designed the experiments: YW YL. Performed the experiments: YW JMY QG LWH YL. Analyzed the data: YW NG. Contributed reagents/materials/analysis tools: HZG. Wrote the paper: YW.

References

1. Farman JC, Gardiner BG, Shanklin JD (1985) Large losses of total ozone in Antarctica reveal seasonal ClOx/NOx interaction. Nature 315: 207–210.
2. Rosmini F, Stazi MA, Milton RC, Sperduto RD, Pasquini P, et al. (1994) A dose-response effect between a sunlight index and age-related cataracts. Italian-American Cataract Study Group. Ann Epidemiol 4: 266–270.
3. Sasaki K, Ono M, Aoki K, Katou N, Morine M, et al. (1995) Cataract epidemiology survey in the three different areas in Japan – prevalence of cataracts and types of lens pacification. J Jpn Ophthalmol Soc 99: 204–211.
4. Sasaki K, Sasaki H, Kojima M, Shui YB, Hockwin O, et al. (1999) Epidemiological studies on UV-related cataract in climatically different countries. J Epidemiol 9: S33–S38.
5. Dandona L, Dandona R, Naduvilath TJ, McCarty CA, Srinivas M, et al. (1999) Burden of moderate visual impairment in an urban population in southern India. Ophthalmol 106: 497–504.
6. Elwood JM, Jopson J (1997) Melanoma and sun exposure: an overview of published studies. Int J Cancer 73: 198–203.
7. West SK, Longtreth JD, Mañoz B, Pitcher HM, Duncan DD (2005) Model of risk cortical cataract in the US population with exposure to increased ultraviolet radiation due to stratospheric ozone depletion. Am J Epidemiol 162: 1080–1088.
8. Lucas RM (2011) An epidemiological perspective of ultraviolet exposure-public health concerns. Eye Contact Lens 37: 168–175.
9. Vajpayee RB, Joshi S, Saxena R, Gupta SK (1999) Epidemiology of cataract in India: combating plans and strategies. Ophthalmic Res 31: 86–92.
10. West SK, Duncan DD, Mañoz B, Rubin GS, Fried LP, et al. (1998) Sunlight exposure and risk of lens opacities in a population-based study: the Salisbury Eye Evaluation project. JAMA 280: 714–718.
11. United Nations Environment Program (2002) Environmental Effects of Ozone Depletion and its Interactions with Climate Change: 2002 Assessment. In: De Gruijl FR, Longstreth J, Norval M, Cullen AP, Slaper H, et al. editors. Health Effects from Stratospheric Ozone Depletion and interactions with Climate Change. Nairobi, Kenya: United Nations Environment Program. pp. 25–53.
12. Cullen AP (2011) Ozone depletion and solar ultraviolet radiation: ocular effects, a United nations environment programme perspective. Eye Contact Lens 37: 185–190.
13. Office of the Second China National Sample Survey on Disability (2007) Documentation of the Second China National Sample Survey on Disability. Beijing: China Statistics Press. 1380 p.
14. Xu L, Cui T, Yang H, Hu AL, Ma K, et al. (2006) Prevalence of visual impairment among adults in China: the Beijing Eye Study. Am J Ophthalmol 141: 591–593.
15. Huang SS, Zheng YF, Foster PJ, Huang WY, He MG. (2009) Prevalence and causes of visual impairment in Chinese adults in urban Southern China. Arch Ophthalmol 127: 1362–1367.
16. Nimbus 7 data. NASA Goddard Space Flight Center Data ArchiveCenter database. Available: ftp://toms.gsfc.nasa.gov/pub/nimbus7/data/uv_ery_4_wavelengths/ery_dose/Accessed 27 April 2006.
17. Earth Probe data. NASA Goddard Space Flight Center Data ArchiveCenter database. Available: ftp://toms.gsfc.nasa.gov/pub/eptoms/data/uv_ery_4_wavelengths/ery_dose/. Accessed 15 May 2006.
18. National Bureau of Statistics of China (2005) Statistical communique on regional census in 2005. Available: http://www.stats.gov.cn/tjgb/rkpcgb/. Accessed 27 August 2011.
19. Javitt JC, Taylor HR (1994–1995) Cataract and latitude. Doc Ophthalmol 88: 307–325.
20. Blumthaler M, Ambach W, Ellinger R (1997) Increase in solar UV radiation with altitude. J Photochem Photobiol B 39: 130–134.

Entropic Imaging of Cataract Lens: An *In Vitro* Study

Zhuhuang Zhou[1]⁹, Chih-Chung Huang[2]⁹, K. Kirk Shung[3], Po-Hsiang Tsui[4,5]*, Jui Fang[6], Hsiang-Yang Ma[4,7], Shuicai Wu[1], Chung-Chih Lin[8]

1 Biomedical Engineering Center, College of Life Science and Bioengineering, Beijing University of Technology, Beijing, China, **2** Department of Biomedical Engineering, National Cheng Kung University, Tainan, Taiwan, **3** NIH Resource on Medical Ultrasonic Transducer Technology, Department of Biomedical Engineering, University of Southern California, Los Angeles, California, United States of America, **4** Department of Medical Imaging and Radiological Sciences, College of Medicine, Chang Gung University, Taoyuan, Taiwan, **5** Institute for Radiological Research, Chang Gung University and Chang Gung Memorial Hospital, Taoyuan, Taiwan, **6** Ph.D. Program in Biomedical Engineering, Chang Gung University, Taoyuan, Taiwan, **7** Graduate Institute of Clinical Medical Sciences, College of Medicine, Chang Gung University, Taoyuan, Taiwan, **8** Department of Computer Science and Information Engineering, Chang Gung University, Taoyuan, Taiwan

Abstract

Phacoemulsification is a common surgical method for treating advanced cataracts. Determining the optimal phacoemulsification energy depends on the hardness of the lens involved. Previous studies have shown that it is possible to evaluate lens hardness via ultrasound parametric imaging based on statistical models that require data to follow a specific distribution. To make the method more system-adaptive, nonmodel-based imaging approach may be necessary in the visualization of lens hardness. This study investigated the feasibility of applying an information theory derived parameter – Shannon entropy from ultrasound backscatter to quantify lens hardness. To determine the physical significance of entropy, we performed computer simulations to investigate the relationship between the signal-to-noise ratio (SNR) based on the Rayleigh distribution and Shannon entropy. Young's modulus was measured in porcine lenses, in which cataracts had been artificially induced by the immersion in formalin solution in vitro. A 35-MHz ultrasound transducer was used to scan the cataract lenses for entropy imaging. The results showed that the entropy is 4.8 when the backscatter data form a Rayleigh distribution corresponding to an SNR of 1.91. The Young's modulus of the lens increased from approximately 8 to 100 kPa when we increased the immersion time from 40 to 160 min (correlation coefficient $r = 0.99$). Furthermore, the results indicated that entropy imaging seemed to facilitate visualizing different degrees of lens hardening. The mean entropy value increased from 2.7 to 4.0 as the Young's modulus increased from 8 to 100 kPa ($r = 0.85$), suggesting that entropy imaging may have greater potential than that of conventional statistical parametric imaging in determining the optimal energy to apply during phacoemulsification.

Editor: Edathara Abraham, University of Arkansas for Medical Sciences, United States of America

Funding: This work was supported by the National Science Council (Taiwan) under Grant No. NSC 102-2221-E-182-008 and the Chang Gung Medical Research Program (CMRP) for Proton Therapy Basic Research (Grant No. CMRPD1C0661). This work was also supported by the Doctoral Fund of Innovation of Beijing University of Technology and in part by the National Natural Science Foundation of China (Grant No. 81127006). KKS was supported partially by National Institutes of Health (NIH) Grant # P41-EB002182. The funders had no role in study design, data collection and analysis, decision to publish, or preparation of the manuscript.

Competing Interests: The authors have declared that no competing interests exist.

* E-mail: tsuiph@mail.cgu.edu.tw

⁹ These authors contributed equally to this work.

Introduction

A cataract is a clouding of the normally transparent crystalline lens of the eye, resulted from factors such as aging, lens damage, and heredity. The formation of a cataract can be considered a process of lens fibrosis, whereby both protein aggregation and fiber coemption occur inside the lens causing the lens hardness to increase [1,2]. The initial stage of cataract formation can generally be mitigated by applying a medical eyewash. However, advanced cataracts require treatment with phacoemulsification to replace the turbid lens with an artificial one, thereby restoring clear vision. Lens hardness exerts a marked effect on the optimal ultrasonic energy in phacoemulsification, in which optimizing the energy improves the efficiency of the surgery and reduces the injury to the lens capsule and corneal endothelium. Therefore, evaluating the lens hardness is critical to facilitate successful phacoemulsification surgery.

Ultrasound, an acoustic wave with a frequency exceeding 20 kHz, has been widely used for imaging the eye in ophthalmic applications. In addition to morphology analysis, ultrasound can be applied to evaluate the hardness of a lens. Previous studies have demonstrated that acoustic attenuation and the speed of sound tend to increase as the hardness of a cataract lens increases [1,3–5]. The major shortcoming of applying quantitative ultrasound parameters is that the local variation in lens hardness is difficult to estimate. Employing high-frequency ultrasound B-mode imaging to image a cataract lens is a feasible method for addressing this problem. In principle, the echo intensity of a cataract lens differs from that of a normal lens; specifically, optical opacities produce acoustic inhomogeneity inducing high echogenicity [6]. However, relying on echo intensity alone as a criterion for grading and staging of lens hardening has been shown to be problematic because of the poor reproducibility. Our previous studies, which investigated cataracts of porcine eyes in vitro with high-frequency ultrasound, showed that the B-mode image revealed only the structures of the cataract lens, and it was difficult to assess lens hardness merely from the echo intensity [7,8]. In addition, compared with the conventional B-mode imaging, which shows the backscatter intensity, ultrasound parametric imaging capable of providing additional information associated with scatterer arrangements [9] based on the statistical distribution of the backscatter envelope was found to perform satisfactorily in characterizing the degree of lens hardening [7]. Several studies have shown that high-frequency statistical parametrical imaging could distinguish both global and local variations in lens hardness [7,8].

Although the hardness of the cataract lens can be characterized by applying statistical distributions to model the envelope statistics, one constraint in employing a statistical model is that the backscatter data must be assumed to follow a specific distribution [10]. This requirement may not always be satisfied because adjusting the settings in an ultrasound system can alter the statistical distribution of raw data, rendering these statistical models inapplicable. To address this limitation and ensure that the method is more system-adaptive, developing a nonmodel-based imaging approach for visualizing lens hardness is preferred.

Among all possibilities, an information theory derived parameter, entropy, is a suitable candidate for developing a system-adaptive imaging method based on analyzing backscatter statistics. Entropy is a measure of uncertainty in a random variable. An increase in entropy indicates a change in the properties of backscatter signals from regular, random, to complex, corresponding to an increase in signal uncertainty. Entropy is not a model-based measure but rather is a function of the variable's probability density function (PDF); therefore, it may reflect the physical significance associated with the backscatter statistics to a degree. This also explains why the entropy 1) increases as the density of scatterers in the resolution cell increases, 2) increases as the scatterer spacing decreases, and 3) is independent of scattering amplitude [11]. Moreover, this parameter does not require the backscatter data to follow a specific distribution, providing a chance to construct methods that are more flexible in practical applications.

Shannon entropy is the most frequently used entropy in information theory. Therefore, this study examined the feasibility of applying the Shannon entropy of ultrasound backscatter data to image the cataract lens. The Shannon entropy $H(X)$ of a continuous random variable X with the PDF $f(x)$ is defined in [12] and is expressed as follows:

$$H(X) = -\int_{-\infty}^{\infty} f(x)\ln f(x)dx \equiv -E(\ln f(x)), \tag{1}$$

where $E(.)$ is the expected value operator. Initially, we investigated the relationship between the signal-to-noise ratio (SNR) and Shannon entropy by conducting computer simulations to better understand the physical meaning of Shannon entropy. In particular, we determined the Shannon entropy threshold for classifying regular (a partially developed speckle), random (a fully developed speckle), and complex (a fully developed speckle with clustered scatterers). Next, we measured the Young's modulus in cataracts at different stages that were artificially induced in porcine lenses in vitro. The samples were scanned with a high-frequency ultrasound transducer to obtain the B-mode and entropy images, and the entropy parameters in the regions of interest (ROI) were compared with the Young's modulus to evaluate the performance of the entropy image in quantifying the lens hardness.

Materials and Methods

Computer Simulations

To explore the physical meaning of Shannon entropy, the entropy value under the condition of a fully developed speckle image was estimated, according to the simulation procedure in Figure 1. A system-based model was used to simulate ultrasonic signals. The backscatter radiofrequency (RF) signals can be modeled as [13].

$$RF(x,y,z) = H(x,y,z) \otimes Z(x,y,z) + N, \tag{2}$$

where x and z respectively denote the axes along the lateral and elevation dimensions, y is the axial direction along which the incident ultrasonic wave propagates, H represents the transducer transfer function, Z is the spatial distribution function of the scatterers, and N is signal-independent white noise.

The simulated sampling rate was set at 50 MHz, and the speed of sound was 1540 m/s. To simplify computational complexity, the elevation direction was not considered, and only 2D simulations were performed. First, a homogeneous computer phantom was constructed. A computer phantom is a 2D matrix with randomly positioned delta functions that describe the spatial arrangement of M scatterers in a medium, which can be expressed as

$$Z(x,y) = \sum_{n=1}^{M} \delta(x - x_n, y - y_n). \tag{3}$$

The phantom was of the size 3 cm × 3 cm having a scatterer concentration of 32 scatterers/mm^2. A 5-MHz Gaussian incident pulse in the y direction with a pulse length of 0.45 mm and a beam width of 0.9 mm was produced using

$$Hg\,(t) = -t\,\exp\left(-4\beta^2 t^2\right)\sin\left(2\pi f_0 t\right), \tag{4}$$

where f_0 is the center frequency and β is the bandwidth. The beam width along the x direction was determined according to the far-field power density, as provided in [14] and expressed as

$$Hc(x) = \left(\frac{2J_1(k_w a x / z_R)}{k_w a x / z_R}\right)^2, \tag{5}$$

where J_1 denotes a first order Bessel function, a and z_R respectively represent the radius and focal length of the transducer, and k_w is the wave number. Consequently, simulated ultrasonic RF signals were obtained according to the convolution of an incident wave with the computer phantom, and then demodulated using the Hilbert transform.

It is known that the backscatter statistics of a fully developed speckle follow the Rayleigh distribution corresponding to a speckle SNR of 1.91. In a previous study [9], we demonstrated that the simulation settings used in the current study can produce the envelope statistics of the Rayleigh distribution and an SNR value of 1.91. The histogram (described using bins = 40) of the envelope data was used for estimating Shannon entropy by using

$$H(X) = -\sum_{i=1}^{bins} f(x_i)\ln f(x_i), \tag{6}$$

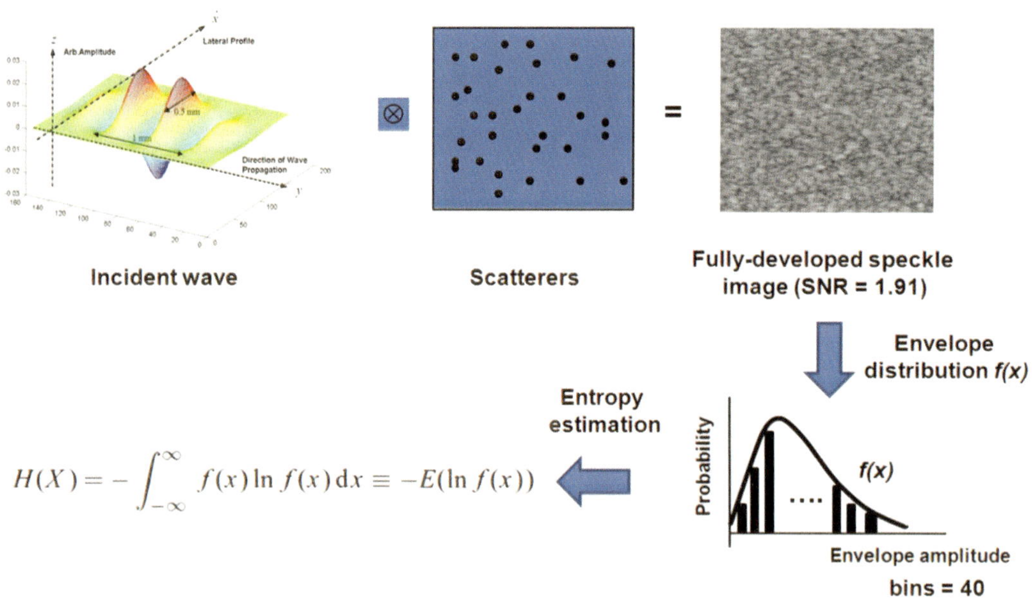

Figure 1. Simulation procedure for determining the threshold of Shannon entropy to classify regular (partially developed speckle), random (fully developed speckle), and complex (fully developed speckle with clustered scatterers).

where $f(x_i)$ is the PDF of the ith bin. A total of 1000 simulation tests were performed to compare the relationships between the SNR and the entropy. The results revealed that the entropy equals 4.8 when the backscatter statistics form a Rayleigh distribution corresponding to an SNR of 1.91, meaning that the property of the backscatter data is random. Because an increase in the entropy means a change in the signal properties from regular, random, to complex, it can be inferred that entropy <4.8 represents a partially developed speckle (regular), and that entropy >4.8 indicates a fully developed speckle with clustered scatterers (complex).

Acquisition of Backscatter Data from a Lens

In this study, we used the experimental raw image data acquired in our previous study [7] to validate the proposed concept. A brief introduction to sample preparation and the procedure of backscatter data acquisition is described as follows. Five lenses from porcine eyes collected from a local slaughterhouse were used. To induce the cataract, the lenses were immersed in a solution of ethanol, 2-propanol, and formalin at a ratio of 3:3:4 [15]. The hardness of the cataract lens was evaluated by measuring the Young's modulus and using a commercial mechanical device (ElectroForce 3100 Test Instrument, Bose Corporation, Minnesota). The Young's modulus for each specimen at the immersion times of 40, 80, 120, and 160 min was computed based on the slope of the stress-strain curve.

An ultrasonic transducer (NIH Ultrasonic Transducer Resource Center, USC, CA) was used at a central frequency of 35 MHz. Both the transducer and lens samples were immersed in a saline buffer solution at a room temperature of approximately 25°C. The transducer movement was controlled using a motor stage and controller (Parker Hannifin Corp., Cleveland, OH) to scan the lens samples. An ultrasonic pulser (AVB2-TB-C, Avtech Electrosystems Ltd., Ottawa, Ontario, Canada) was used to drive the transducer. The image RF signals received from the lens were subsequently amplified using a low-noise amplifier (Miteq 1166, Miteq Inc., Hauppauge, NY), filtered using a bandpass filter (Model BIF-50, Mini-Circuits, Brooklyn, NY), and digitalized using an analog-to-digital converter (CS14200, Gage Applied Technologies, Inc., Lachine, Quebec, Canada) at a sampling rate of 200 MHz. For each lens at the immersion times of 40, 80, 120, and 160 min, the image scanning was performed to acquire 1000 A-lines of backscatter signals from the lens; the distance between each scan-line was 12 μm. Each scan-line was then demodulated to obtain the envelope image of the lens. The B-mode image is displayed based on the log-compressed envelope image with a dynamic range of 40 dB. Figures 2 (a) and (c) show a normal and cataract lens, respectively. The B-mode images of normal and cataract lens are shown in Figures 2 (b) and (d), respectively.

Using the *in vitro* cataract model, cortical cataract was induced along the capsule of a lens. During ultrasound scanning, the focal zone of the transducer was located at the lens capsule so that the major portions of the lens with cataract were scanned. The thickness of the cataract layer generated beneath the capsule was approximately 1 mm, as shown in Figure 2. Therefore, the beam divergence effect of the transducer may not have a significant effect on the ultrasound backscattered signals.

Entropy Image Formation

The entropy image was constructed using a square sliding window to process the envelope image with no log-compression (Figure 3). A square window within the lens envelope image was used to collect the local backscatter envelopes for estimating the local entropy e_w. The parameter e_w was assigned as the new pixel located in the center of the window. The window was moved throughout the entire envelope image in steps of one pixel, and the above step was repeated. The entropy image of the cataract lens was subsequently constructed using the map of the parameter e_w. Based on the recommendations of a previous study [9], the size of the sliding window was set as the square with a sidelength corresponding to three times the transducer pulse length (i.e., 231 μm) to collect enough numbers of envelope data points for a stable parameter estimation. In the entropy image, the parameters e_w < 4.8 were assigned blue shades varying from deep to shallow with

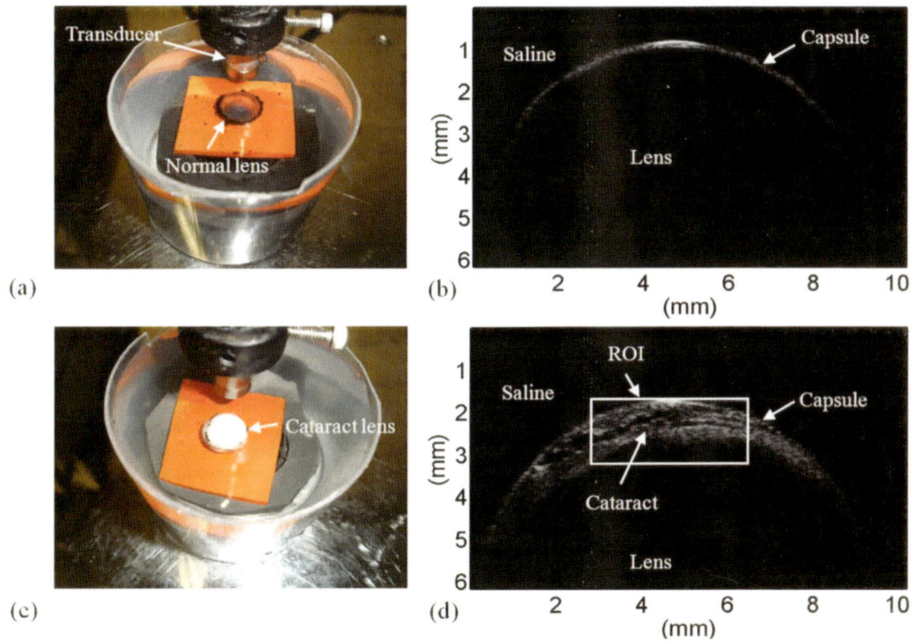

Figure 2. A normal and a cataract lens are shown in (a) and (c), respectively. The B-mode images corresponding to (a) and (c) are shown in (b) and (d), respectively.

an increasing parameter value, representing various regular characteristics of the scatterers. When $e_w = 4.8$, the shade was yellow to express the random property of the scatterers, and those higher than 4.8 were assigned the shades of progressive red in accordance with the increasing parameter value, indicating the incremental degree of clustering in the scatterers.

Results

Figure 4 shows the results of the lens stiffness during cataract induction. The Young's modulus of the lens increased from approximately 8 to 100 kPa as the immersion time was increased from 40 to 160 min (correlation coefficient $r = 0.99$), indicating that cataract induction increases the stiffness of the lens. Figure 5 shows the B-mode images of the lens for different immersion times. Figure 6 shows the entropy images corresponding to the B-mode images. Most of the deep blue shadings in the entropy images corresponded to the background (saline buffer solution) and the transparent portions of the lens. The light blue shading was more evident in the cataract regions in the entropy images for shorter immersion times, and increasing the immersion time resulted in more red shading in the ROIs of the entropy images. This indicated that the entropy image has the ability to describe different stages of lens cataracts.

To confirm the experimental results, we calculated the mean value of e_w in the ROI, $\overline{e_w}$ as a function of immersion time (Figure 7

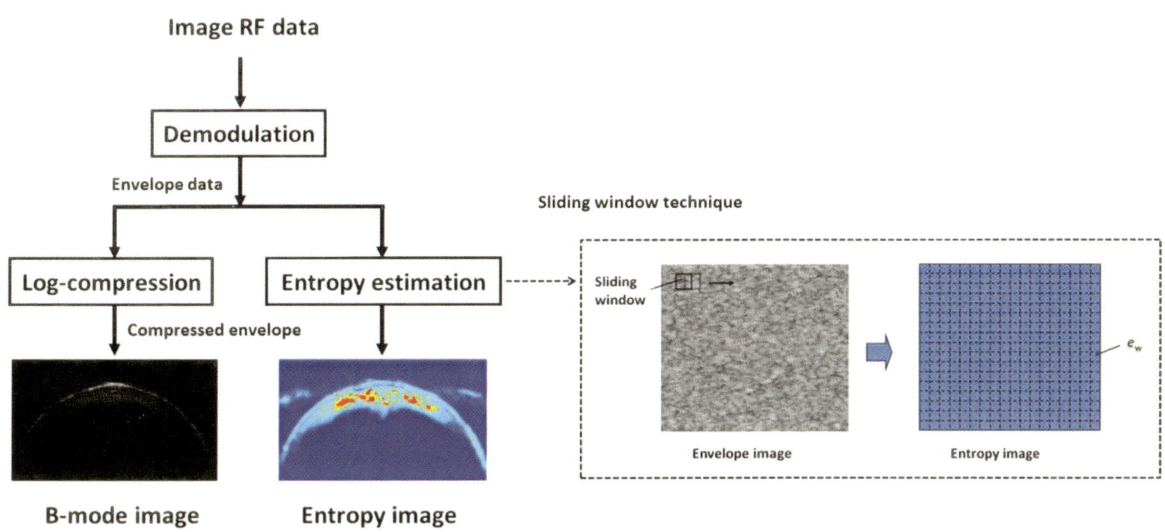

Figure 3. The algorithmic procedure for the construction of ultrasound entropy images.

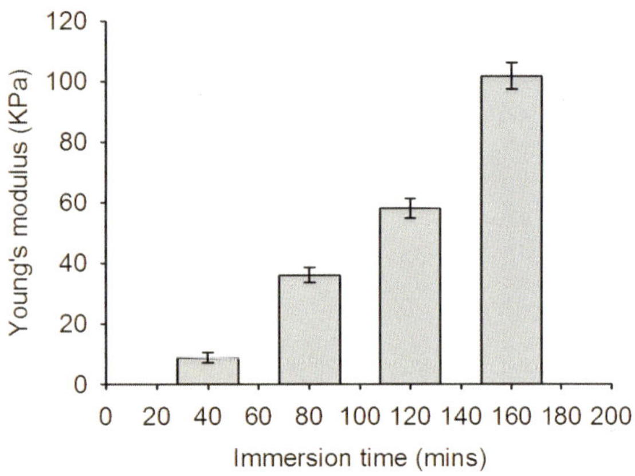

Figure 4. Average Young's modulus as a function of the immersion time. This result indicates a successful induction of cataract lens.

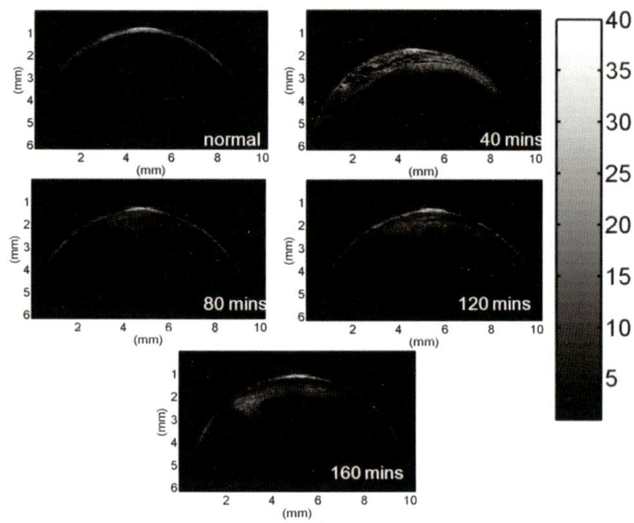

Figure 5. Representative B-mode images of the porcine lens at different stages of cataract formation.

(a)). The value of $\overline{e_w}$ increased from approximately 2.7 to 4.0 as the immersion time was increased from 40 to 160 min ($r = 0.88$). This indicated that the speckle patterns varied from a partially developed speckle to a fully developed speckle, and that the scatterer properties changed from regular to random as the immersion time was increased. Figure 7 (b) shows that $\overline{e_w}$ increased from 2.7 to 4.0 as the Young's modulus increased from 8 to 100 kPa ($r = 0.85$). The high correlation coefficient shows that the entropy image is suitable for locally distinguishing variations in the hardness of a cataract lens. Moreover, the overall lens hardness can be determined by calculating the mean of the $\overline{e_w}$ values in the ROI in an entropy image.

Discussion

Change in entropy during cataract formation

The protein aggregation and fiber coemption that occur in a lens in the presence of a cataract increase the lens hardness. The current results demonstrate that ultrasound entropy imaging is promising for identification of lens stiffness during cataract induction. Because an entropy image is constructed using the envelope of raw backscatter signals, the mechanism that enables an entropy image to detect the variation of lens hardness can be explained based on the interaction between an ultrasound wave and the scatterers in the scattering medium.

In general, a biological tissue can be modeled as a collection of scatterers. Cataract formation involves changing the arrangements and concentrations of the scatterers (i.e., protein and fibers). Therefore, detecting the variation in the scatterer structures of a lens is integral to determining the hardness of a cataract lens (Figures 6 and 7). For a normal lens, the entropy of backscatter envelope is very small. The global and local entropies of the backscatter envelope in the early stage of cataract formation (i.e., with a short immersion time) have significant regular characteristics ($\overline{e_w}$ <3.0 in the ROI, with e_w <3.0 mostly). This is because the scatterer concentration is comparatively low in the cataract region of the lens, which corresponds to minor protein aggregation and fiber coemption being present at the initial stage of cataract formation. For cataracts at later stages, the global entropy of the backscatter envelope of the ROI gradually approaches a Rayleigh distribution ($\overline{e_w}$ ≈4.8 in the ROI), with the local entropy of the backscatter envelope represented by different degrees of clustered characteristics (e_w >4.8 mostly). Evidently, the long immersion time required to form a cataract lens induces more pronounced protein aggregation and fiber coemption, and reduces the scatterer spacing, generating a clustered structure of the scatterers in the lens.

Comparison between entropy and model-based statistical parametric images

We compared the entropy image and ultrasound statistical parametric image based on the Nakagami distribution model that was previously proposed to detect lens cataract [7]. According to the previous study and the current findings, both the entropy image and Nakagami statistical parametric image can reflect different degrees of a lens cataract. However, they have different physical meanings. Ultrasound Nakagami imaging is constructed using the Nakagami parameter map. The Nakagami parameter is the shape parameter of the Nakagami statistical distribution estimated according to the second and fourth moments of

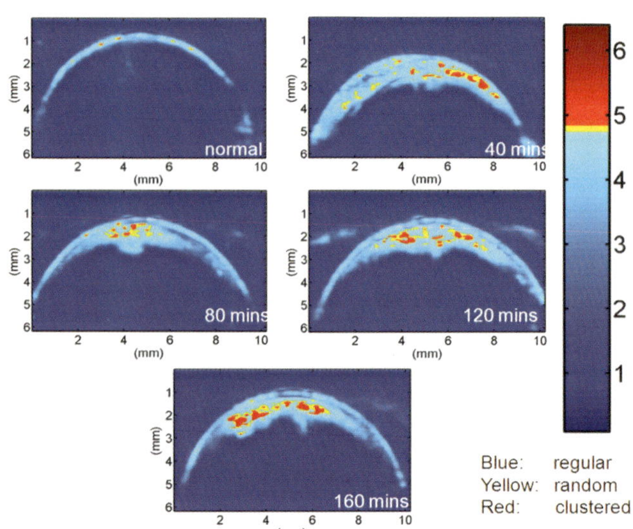

Figure 6. Representative entropy images of the porcine lens at different stages of cataract formation.

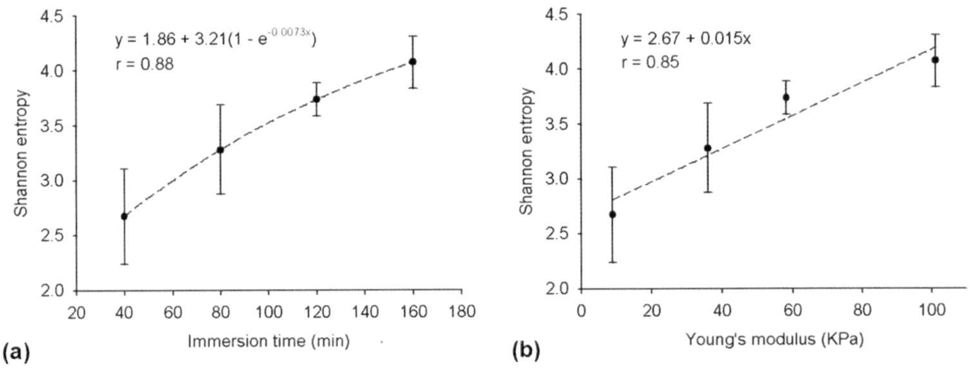

Figure 7. Average entropy as a function of immersion time is shown in (a), and average local entropy as a function of Young's modulus is shown in (b).

backscatter envelopes, thus providing an estimate of backscatter statistics for characterizing tissues. Using an ultrasound Nakagami image to visualize backscatter statistics has been demonstrated to characterize tissue effectively in several medical applications [16–19]. Compared with the Nakagami image, the entropy image is constructed using the backscatter envelopes to estimate the entropy value, which is a measure of signal complexity and uncertainty. The entropy itself is not a model-based parameter, although it increases as the density of scatterers in the resolution cell increases [11]. In other words, the entropy may reflect the physical meaning of the backscatter statistics to a degree. In our simulation tests, we determined that the entropy threshold corresponding to the backscatter statistics of the Rayleigh distribution is 4.8, thereby enabling the classification of regular, random, and complex properties of the backscatter data. More importantly, the prerequisite for using the Nakagami distribution or other statistical models in scatterer characterization is that data must follow the used distribution. The superiority of the entropy over the statistical parameters is that the entropy can be estimated using any type of data (e.g., backscatter data after log-compression or nonlinear processing), to provide a more flexible operation in practical applications.

Subresolvable effect

Refer to the previous study again [7]. The subresolvable effect at an interface or a tissue boundary is an unavoidable issue when using the sliding window algorithm to construct an ultrasound statistical parametric image. When the sliding window moves onto the capsule, the window not only covers the signals from the front interface but also contains those from partial background or lens. Because the front interface contributes stronger echoes than the background and lens do, the parameter value of the backscattered envelopes acquired by the window would tend to be smaller, making a window-shaped artifact occur in the parametric image. However, compared with the previous study [7], the window-shaped artifact caused by the subresolvable effect in entropy images is less evident, although it still makes the center of the cataract layer have relatively higher entropy values and the peripheral proportions corresponded to lowers ones (Figure 6). Actually, to further reduce the window-shaped artifact and its possible effects on entropy imaging, a smaller window may be used. This is because entropy is not a model-based parameter, and therefore entropy imaging may have a broader flexibility than the conventional statistical parametric imaging does to use a smaller window to construct a high-resolution parametric image. It should be noted that the entropy threshold for classifying regular, random, and complex should be recalibrated when using different window sizes.

Considerations of the proposed entropy image

In addition to Shannon entropy, many other entropy definitions have been introduced for quantifying the scattering characteristics, such as the Renyi or Tsallis entropy measures. Furthermore, numerous algorithms have been developed to facilitate robust entropy estimation [20–23]. Thus far, no appropriate entropy approach has been proposed for constructing parametric imaging techniques to characterize tissues. The definition of the Shannon entropy used in this study is the easiest method to implement in practical applications. However, the major limitation of using the proposed Shannon entropy is that the number of bins affects the value of entropy. According to Equation (6), it can be expected that using different bins to describe the histogram of envelope data will result in different values of Shannon entropy. Additional studies are necessary to explore the effects of bin numbers in future applications when using the Shannon entropy defined in Equation (6). When using a different bin number, the entropy corresponding to SNR = 1.91 may have a different value. The entropy threshold for identifying the fully developed speckle may be obtained by conducting calibrations when using different numbers of bins to describe the probability distribution of envelope signals.

Conclusion

In this study, we explored the usefulness of information-theory derived entropic imaging in characterizing cataract lenses in porcine eyes at 35-MHz. The results show that entropy imaging can be used to distinguish both global and local variations in lens hardness. This is because the scatterer concentration of the fiber coemption, which is mainly responsible for the increase in lens hardness during cataract formation, can be quantified using the entropy technique to describe the uncertainty of ultrasound backscatter data. In contrast to the conventional ultrasound parametric imaging based on the statistical models, constructing the entropy image does not require the backscatter data to follow a specific statistical distribution. Entropy imaging may have greater potential than that of the statistical parametric images in evaluating the structure and elastic properties of a lens and providing a more flexible and feasible approach in determining the optimal energy to apply during phacoemulsification.

Author Contributions

Conceived and designed the experiments: CCH KKS PHT. Performed the experiments: CCH PHT. Analyzed the data: ZZ JF HYM CCL. Contributed reagents/materials/analysis tools: KKS PHT. Wrote the paper: ZZ KKS PHT SW. Simulations: PHT.

References

1. Tabandeh H, Wilkins M, Thompson G, Nassiri D, Karim A (2000) Hardness and ultrasonic characteristics of human crystalline lens. J Cataract Refract Surg 26: 838–841.
2. Kanski JJ (2006) Clinical diagnosis in ophthalmology. London: Elsevier Mosby.
3. Huang CC, Ameri H, DeBoer C, Rowley AP, Xu X, et al. (2007) Evaluation of lens hardness in cataract surgery using high frequency ultrasonic parameters *in vitro*. Ultrasound Med Biol 33: 1609–1616.
4. Huang CC, Zhou Q, Ameri H, Wu D, Sun L, et al. (2007) Determining the acoustic properties of the lens using a high-frequency ultrasonic needle transducer. Ultrasound Med Biol 33: 1971–1977.
5. Huang CC, Chen R, Tsui PH, Zhou Q, Humayun MS, et al. (2009) Measurements of attenuation coefficient for evaluating the hardness of cataract lens by a high frequency ultrasonic needle transducer. Phys Med Biol 54: 5981–5994.
6. Coleman DJ, Silverman RH, Lizzi FL, Rondeau MJ (2006) Ultrasonography of the eye and orbit. Philadelphia: Lippincott Williams & Wilkins.
7. Tsui PH, Huang CC, Chang CC,Wang SH, Shung KK (2007) Feasibility study of using high-frequency ultrasonic Nakagami imaging for characterizing the cataract lens *in vitro*. Phys Med Biol 52: 6413–6425.
8. Tsui PH, Huang CC, Zhou Q, Shung KK (2011) Cataract measurement by estimating the ultrasonic statistical parameter using an ultrasound needle transducer: an *in vitro* study. Physiol Meas 32: 513–522.
9. Tsui PH, Chang CC (2007) Imaging local scatterer concentrations by the Nakagami statistical model. Ultrasound Med Biol 33: 608–619.
10. Shankar PM (2000) A general statistical model for ultrasonic backscattering from tissues. IEEE Trans Ultrason Ferroelectr Freq Control 47: 727–736.
11. Smoliková R, Wachowiak MP, Zurada JM (2004) An information-theoretic approach to estimating ultrasound backscatter characteristics. Comput Biol Med 34: 355–370.
12. Kapur JN, Kesavan HK (1992) Entropy optimization principles with applications. New York: Academic Press.
13. Fontaine I, Bertrand M, Cloutier G (1999) A system-based approach to modeling the ultrasound signal backscattered by red blood cells. Biophys J 77: 2387–2399.
14. Christensen DA (1988) Ultrasonic bioinstrumentation. New York: Wiley.
15. Sugiura T, Kurosaks D, Uezuki Y, Eguchi S, Obata H, et al. (1999) Creating cataract in pig eye. J Cataract Refract Surg 25: 615–621.
16. Tsui PH, Huang CC, Sun L, Dailey SH, Shung KK (2011) Characterization of lamina propria and vocal muscle in human vocal fold tissue by ultrasound Nakagami imaging. Med Phys 38: 2019–2026.
17. Ho MC, Lee YH, Jeng YM, Chen CN, Chang KJ, et al. (2013) Relationship between ultrasound backscattered statistics and the concentration of fatty droplets in livers: an animal study. PLoS One 8: e63543.
18. Ho MC, Lin JJ, Shu YC, Chen CN, Chang KJ, et al. (2012) Using ultrasound Nakagami imaging to assess liver fibrosis in rats. Ultrasonics 52: 215–222.
19. Zhang S, Zhou F, Wan M, Wei M, Fu Q, et al. (2012) Feasibility of using Nakagami distribution in evaluating the formation of ultrasound-induced thermal lesions. J Acoust Soc Am 131: 4836–4844.
20. Hughes MS (1993) Analysis of digitized waveforms using Shannon entropy. J Acoust Soc Am 93: 892–906.
21. Hughes MS (1994) Analysis of digitized waveforms using Shannon entropy. II. High speed algorithms based on Green's functions. J Acoust Soc Am 95: 2582–2588.
22. Hughes MS, McCarthy JE, Marsh JN, Arbeit JM, Neumann RG, et al. (2007) Properties of an entropy-based signal receiver with an application to ultrasonic molecular imaging. J Acoust Soc Am 121: 3542–3557.
23. Hughes MS, McCarthy JE, Marsh JN, Wickline SA (2013) Joint entropy of continuously differentiable ultrasonic waveforms. J Acoust Soc Am 133: 283–300.

Prevalence and Outcomes of Cataract Surgery in Adult Rural Chinese Populations of the Bai Nationality in Dali: The Yunnan Minority Eye Study

Wei Shen[1,2], Yongming Yang[1], Minbin Yu[3], Jun Li[2], Tao Wei[4], Xun Li[4], Juanjuan Li[1], Xiaodan Su[1], Hua Zhong[1]*, Yuansheng Yuan[1]*

1 The First Affiliated Hospital of Kunming Medical University, Kunming, China, **2** Yunnan Red Cross Hospital, Kunming, China, **3** State Key Laboratory of Ophthalmology, Zhongshan Ophthalmic Center, Sun Yat-sen University, Guangzhou, China, **4** Kunming Medical University, Kunming, China

Abstract

Purpose: To investigate the prevalence and visual acuity (VA) outcomes of cataract surgery in adults of the Bai Nationality populations in rural China.

Methods: We conducted a population-based cross-sectional survey (from randomly selected block groups) of Chinese Bai Nationality aged ≥50 years in southwestern China. Presenting visual acuity (PVA), best corrected visual acuity (BCVA) were recorded and a detailed eye examination was carried out. For all aphakic and pseudophakic subjects identified, information on the date, setting, type, and complications of cataract surgery were recorded. In eyes with VA <20/63, the principal cause of visual impairment was identified.

Results: Of 2133 (77.8% of 2742) subjects, 99 people (129 eyes) had undergone cataract surgery. The prevalence of cataract surgery was 4.6%. Surgical coverage among those with PVA <20/200 in both eyes because of cataract was 52.8%. Unoperated cataract was associated with older age. The main barrier to cataract surgery was lack of awareness and knowledge, cost, and fear. Among the 129 cataract-operated eyes, 22.5% had PVA of ≥20/32, 25.6% had PVA of 20/40 to 20/63, 23.3% had PVA <20/63 to 20/200, and 28.7% had PVA<20/200. With BCVA, the percentages were 42.6%, 23.3%, 10.9%, and 23.3%, respectively. Aphakia (odds ratio [OR], 8.49; P<0.001) and no education (OR, 10.18; P = 0.001) or less education (OR, 6.49; P = 0.014) were significantly associated with postoperative visual impairment defined by PVA, while aphakia (OR, 8.49; P<0.001) and female gender (OR, 4.19; P = 0.004) were significantly associated with postoperative visual impairment by BCVA. The main causes of postoperative visual impairment were refractive error, retinal disorders and glaucoma.

Conclusions: Half of those with bilateral visual impairment or blindness because of cataract remain in need of cataract surgery in Bai population. Surgical uptake and visual outcomes should be further improved in the future.

Editor: Yingfeng Zheng, Zhongshan Ophthalmic Center, China

Funding: Supported by the National Natural Science Foundation of China under grant No. 30860309, No. 81160121 and Yunnan Province Science and Technology Project under grant No. 2009CA007. The funders had no role in study design, data collection and analysis, decision to publish, or preparation of the manuscript.

Competing Interests: The authors have declared that no competing interests exist.

* E-mail: zhoculist@163.com (HZ); 1119abcd@163.com (YY)

Introduction

Although cataract is avoidable, it remains the leading cause of blindness worldwide, and is responsible for 47.8% or 17.7 million blind people [1]. Cataract surgery is the only currently available and effective method of restoring vision for those with visual impairment due to cataract. Population-based studies in different regional, racial and ethnic groups have suggested significant differences in cataract prevalence, surgical uptake and the quality of cataract surgeries. People in developing countries have had limited access to cataract surgery, but even if this is available the uptake of surgery can still be low. Recent population studies have reported that barriers such as cost, fear, ageism, and lack of awareness and knowledge restrict the uptake of available services [2–9]. Moreover, where services are available, there are concerns that they are often of poor quality [10]. Poor outcome may be due to other ocular pathology, surgical complications and uncorrected refractive error [10].

Cataract is also the leading cause of vision loss in China. However,the cataract surgical rate (CSR, cataract operations per million population per year) in China is only 446. It was almost the lowest cataract surgical rates in Asia [11]. Cataract surgical coverage (CSC) also continues to remain low [8,9,12–19]. And the quality of surgery remains a problem that should be addressed. The effect of age-related cataract can be expected to grow as the Chinese population continues to age. It is estimated that 2.5 million people in China will be blind from cataract, accounting for half of China's blind by 2020 [20].

In recent years several population-based cross-sectional eye care studies in China have been reported [8,9,12–19], however, none focused on the Chinese ethnic minorities, whose culture, socioeconomic status, health care services accessibility, and the quality of eye care service providers may be quite different from that of the Han population.

Yunnan has a total of 26 different recognized ethnic groups. Yunnan is among the ethnically most diverse regions not only of China but also of all of Asia. The Yunnan Minority Eye Study (YMES) was designed to determine the prevalence and impact of eye diseases among rural south-western Chinese populations of the minority nationality (including the Bai, Dai, and Yi Nationality) [21,22].

The Bai people are one of the dominant ethnic groups of Yunnan. We have recently reported the results of a 2010 survey of prevalence and causes of blindness and visual impairment in elderly Bai ethnic group in rural China [21]. The prevalence of visual impairment and blindness was 15.22% and 3.59%, respectively; Cataract accounted for 53.0% of visual impairment and 64.5% blindness. As a part of YMES, the purpose of this study was to report the prevalence of cataract surgery, surgical coverage among those visually impaired or blind as a result of cataract, risk factors for unoperated cataract, self-reported barriers to cataract surgery, visual acuity outcomes of cataract surgery, and risk factors and causes contributing to poor outcomes in adult rural Chinese populations of the Bai nationality in Dali.

Patients and Methods

The methodology used in the YMES has been described in detail elsewhere [21,22]. In brief, the decision to select Dali for the survey was due to the fact that more than 80% of the population of Bai nationality in China live in Dali Prefecture and it is a socioeconomic profile that is representative of Bai nationality as a whole. The subjects were identified by cluster random sampling. Those aged 50 years and older who resided in the selected study clusters for more than 6 months were considered eligible. The eligible subjects were invited for a comprehensive eye examination in the local community facilities. Written informed consent was obtained from the subjects at the examination site. A structured questionnaire was used to obtain information based on demographic data (age, gender, locality, marital status, and education), personal ophthalmic and medical history, and lifestyle (smoking and alcohol intake). Participants' self-reported demographic data were assessed. Level of education (no school, primary school without diploma, primary school with diploma, secondary school, higher education, and higher education or above) was categorized as follows: (1) 0 year: no school; (2) 1–6 years: primary school without diploma or with diploma; (3) >6 years: secondary school or higher education or above. Subjects were asked about marital status (married, divorced, widowed, and not married). Personal ophthalmic history was investigated by means of a checklist. The subjects were asked whether they had been diagnosed with ophthalmic diseases such as cataract, glaucoma, uveitis, keratitis, ocular injury, vitreoretinopathy, and so on by a ophthalmologist. Personal medical history was also investigated by means of a checklist. The subjects were asked whether they had been diagnosed with a chronic disease such as hypertension and diabetes by a physician.

Detailed study procedures have been reported elsewhere [21,22]. Distance VA was measured using a retroilluminated logarithm of the minimum angle of resolution tumbling E chart (wh06, Wehen Vision Technology Co., Ltd.). Each eye was measured separately, with glasses if worn for distance correction. The PVA with habitual correction was recorded. In those presenting with VA<20/25 in either eye, best-corrected visual acuity (BCVA) was assessed using the results of autorefraction and subjective refinement. For those in whom subjective refraction was not performed, BCVA was assumed to be the same as pinhole vision. The detailed examination of the eyelid, globe, pupillary reflex, lens and fundus was carried out by an experienced ophthalmologist using a slitlamp (model SL-1E; Topcon, Tokyo, Japan), a +90 diopter lens at×16 magnification and direct ophthalmoscopy.

Those with cataract surgery were queried as to the year and type of surgical facility for each operated eye. The type of cataract surgery, posterior capsule status, and signs of surgical complications were noted in the examination of cataract-operated eyes.

Table 1. Cataract Surgery by Age, Gender, and Education.

Variables	Examined	Post-operative Persons		Adjusted OR	P Value
	No. (%)	No.	% Prevalence(95% CI)	(95% CI)	
Age(yrs)					
50–59	715(33.5)	7	1.0 (0.3–1.7)	Reference	
60–69	775(36.3)	21	2.7 (1.6–3.9)	2.96(1.24–7.05)	0.014
70–79	525(24.6)	50	9.5 (7.0–12.0)	10.97(4.76–25.30)	0.000
80+	118(5.5)	21	17.8 (10.0–24.7)	22.36(8.93–55.99)	0.000
Gender					
Male	769(36.1)	35	4.6 (3.1–6.0)	Reference	
Female	1364(63.9)	64	4.7 (3.6–5.8)	1.06(0.65–1.74)	0.817
Education(yrs)					
>6	506(23.7)	17	3.4 (1.8–4.9)	Reference	
1–6	868(40.7)	29	3.3 (2.2–4.5)	0.68(0.36–1.28)	0.234
0	759(35.6)	53	7.0 (5.2–8.8)	0.86(0.44–1.69)	0.661
Total	2133(100)	99	4.6 (3.8–5.5)		

OR: odds ratios; CI: Confidence Interval.

Table 2. Post-operative and Unopreted Persons with Cataract-Related Severe Visual Impairment or Blindness (<20/200) by Age, Gender, and Education.

Variables	Examined	Post-operative Persons				Unopreted Persons				Surgical Coverage (%)
		All Operated		Presumed Severe Visual Impairment or Blindness*‡		Cataract Severe Visual Impairment or Blindness*		Cataract Social Burdon		
	No.	No.	Prevalence†	No.	Prevalence†	No.	Prevalence†	No	Prevalence†	
Age(yrs)										
50–59	715	7	1.0	4	0.6	3	0.4	7	1.0	57.1
60–69	775	21	2.7	13	1.7	9	1.2	22	2.8	59.1
70–79	525	50	9.5	41	7.8	38	7.2	79	15.0	51.9
80+	118	21	17.8	18	15.3	18	15.3	36	30.5	50.0
Gender										
Male	769	35	4.6	27	3.5	25	3.3	52	6.8	51.9
Female	1364	64	4.7	49	3.6	43	3.2	92	6.7	53.3
Education(yrs)										
>6	506	17	3.4	10	2.0	5	1.0	15	3.0	66.7
1–6	868	29	3.3	20	2.3	22	2.5	42	4.8	47.6
0	759	53	7.0	46	6.1	41	5.4	87	11.4	52.9
Total	2133	99	4.6	76	3.6	68	3.2	144	6.8	52.8

*Visual acuity <20/200.
†Prevalence per 100 examined participants.
‡Includes all bilaterally operated persons and unilaterally operated persons with a severely visually impaired or blind fellow eye.

Table 3. Association of Age, Gender, and Education with Cataract-Related Severe Visual Impairment or Blindness (<20/200) by Multiple Logistic Regression Analysis.

Variables	Post-operative Presumed Severely Impaired or Blind		Unoperated Cataract Severely Impaired or Blind		Cataract Social Burdon		Cataract Surgical Coverage	
	Adjusted OR (95% CI)	**P Value**	**Adjusted OR (95% CI)**	**P Value**	**Adjusted OR (95% CI)**	**P Value**	**Adjusted OR (95% CI)**	**P Value**
Age(yrs)								
50–59	Reference		Reference		Reference		Reference	
60–69	3.01 (0.97–9.34)	0.057	2.51 (0.67–9.37)	0.171	2.80 (1.18–6.62)	0.019	1.18 (0.21–6.77)	0.855
70–79	13.19 (4.53–38.37)	0.000	14.54 (4.33–48.80)	0.000	14.75 (6.59–33.00)	0.000	0.77 (0.15–3.97)	0.753
80+	27.63 (8.86–86.16)	0.000	33.28 (9.36–118.40)	0.000	36.16 (15.25–85.73)	0.000	0.72 (0.13–4.02)	0.704
Gender								
Male	Reference		Reference		Reference		Reference	
Female	0.88 (0.50–1.55)	0.657	0.81 (0.44–1.46)	0.477	0.83 (0.54–1.28)	0.403	1.20 (0.52–2.76))	0.677
Education(yrs)								
>6	Reference		Reference		Reference		Reference	
1–6	0.81(0.37–1.78)	0.594	1.82(0.67–4.96)	0.240	1.15(0.61–2.16)	0.663	0.41(0.11–1.49)	0.177
0	1.34(0.59–3.02)	0.481	2.37(0.84–6.70)	0.104	1.76(0.91–3.38)	0.093	0.56(0.41–2.24)	0.415

OR: odds ratios; CI: Confidence Interval.

Table 4. Presenting and Best-Corrected Acuity of Post-operative Eyes by Age, Gender, Education, Intraocular lens Status, and Year of Surgery.

Variables	NO.(%) of Eyes	NO. (%) by Presenting Visual Acuity				NO. (%) of Best-Corrected Visual Acuity			
		≥20/32	20/40–20/63	<20/63–20/200	<20/200	≥20/32	20/40–20/63	<20/63–20/200	<20/200
Age(yrs)									
50–59	9 (7.0)	5 (55.6)	2 (22.2)	1 (11.1)	1 (11.1)	8 (88.9)	0 (0)	0 (0)	1 (11.1)
60–69	25 (19.4)	8 (32.0)	7 (28.0)	5 (20.0)	5 (20.0)	16 (64.0)	3 (12.0)	1 (4.0)	5 (20.0)
70–79	70 (54.3)	16 (22.9)	19 (27.1)	15 (21.4)	20 (28.6)	28 (40.0)	21 (30.0)	8 (11.4)	13 (18.6)
80+	25 (19.4)	0 (0)	5 (20.0)	9 (36.0)	11 (44.0)	3 (12.0)	6 (24.0)	5 (20.0)	11 (44.0)
Gender									
Male	47 (36.4)	13 (27.7)	15 (31.9)	10 (21.3)	9 (19.1)	24 (51.7)	14 (29.8)	2 (4.3)	7 (14.9)
Female	82 (63.6)	16 (19.5)	18 (22.0)	20(24.4)	28 (34.1)	31 (37.8)	16 (19.5)	12 (14.6)	23 (28.0)
Education									
0	68 (52.7)	11 (16.2)	14 (20.6)	18 (26.5)	25 (36.8)	21 (30.9)	17 (25.0)	11 (16.2)	19 (27.9)
1–6	39 (30.2)	6 (15.4)	13 (33.3)	11 (28.2)	9 (23.1)	17 (43.6)	10 (25.6)	3 (7.7)	9 (23.1)
>6	22 (17.1)	12 (54.5)	6 (27.3)	1 (4.5)	3 (13.6)	17 (77.3)	3 (13.6)	0 (0)	2 (9.1)
IOL status									
Aphakic	26 (20.2)	1 (3.8)	1 (3.8)	5 (19.2)	19 (73.1)	1 (3.8)	7 (26.9)	4 (15.4)	14 (53.8)
Pseudophakic	103 (79.8)	28 (27.2)	32 (31.1)	25 (24.3)	18 (17.5)	54 (52.4)	23 (22.3)	10 (9.7)	16 (15.5)
Year of surgery									
≥2001	93 (72.1)	26 (28.0)	28 (30.1)	22 (23.7)	17 (18.3)	48 (51.6)	22 (23.7)	9 (9.7)	14 (15.1)
≤2000	27 (20.9)	3 (11.1)	5 (18.5)	6 (22.2)	13(48.1)	6 (22.2)	8 (29.6)	4 (14.8)	9 (33.3)
Missing	9 (7.0)	0 (0)	0 (0)	2 (22.2)	7 (77.8)	1 (11.1)	0 (0)	1 (11.1)	7 (77.8)
Total	129 (100)	29 (22.5)	33 (25.6)	30 (23.3)	37 (28.7)	55 (42.6)	30 (23.3)	14 (10.9)	30 (23.3)

IOL: intraocular lens.

Subjects with unoperated cataract were questioned about the main reason of not having had cataract surgery. The questionnaire presented several alternative common reasons for not having had an operation in Chinese, such as "unaware of cataract", "could not afford to undergo cataract surgery", "fear of further loss of vision after surgery", "fear of surgery", "no need to have cataract surgery", "being told to wait until the cataract gets mature", "not accompanied by others for surgery", "being told that there was a contraindication", and "undetermined".

A principal cause of visual impairment or blindness for eyes with PVA of 20/40 or worse at presentation was determined by the examining ophthalmologist's clinical judgment using a 15-item list (refractive error, cataract, posterior capsule opacification, phthisical/disorganized/absent globe, glaucoma, high myopic maculopathy, diabetic retinopathy, diabetic macular edema, corneal opacity/scar, age-related macular degeneration, vascular occlusion, other optic atrophy, amblyopia, other cause, undetermined cause). Refractive error was assigned as the cause for eye with of VA 20/40 or worse that could be subsequently improved to better than 20/40 with refractive correction, or with pinhole vision when subjective refraction was not possible because of age or disability. Cataract was assigned when lens opacity was commensurate with BCVA<20/25 and no other abnormality could account for the decrease in VA.

Post-operative cataract severe visual impairment or blindness was defined as cataract-operated persons who were presumed to have been bilaterally severely visually impaired or blind (PVA<20/200) when first operated on for cataract, including all bilaterally operated persons and unilaterally operated persons with a severely visually impaired or blind fellow eye. Because the indications for cataract surgery adopted by many health care facilities in rural China were cataract-induced severely visual impairment, so we presumed that the cataract-operated eyes were severe visual impairment or blindness in present study. Unoperated cataract severe visual impairment or blindness was defined as unoperated persons who were bilaterally severely visually impaired or blind (PVA<20/200) due to cataract in one or both eyes. The social burden of cataract-related visual impairment and blindness (PVA<20/200) was defined as the sum of (1) the number of persons who already had undergone surgery and who were presumed to have been bilaterally impaired or blind when first operated on for cataract, and (2) the number of unoperated persons who were bilaterally impaired or blind because of cataract in one or both eyes [15]. Cataract surgical coverage (CSC) among the cataract-related severe visual impairment or blindness (PVA<20/200) was calculated as the ratio of the post-operative presumed severe visual impairment or blindness to unoperated severe visual impairment or blindness plus the post-operative presumed severe visual impairment or blindness.

Data Management and Analysis

The prevalence of cataract surgery in the study population was calculated by age, gender, and education. Both univariate analysis and multiple logistic regression were used to investigate the association of age, gender, and education with operated cataract, post-operative cataract with severe visual impairment or blindness,

Table 5. Effect of Variables on Presenting and Best-Corrected Visual Acuity <20/63 in Post-operative Eyes by Multiple Logistic Regression Analysis.

Variables	Presenting Visual Acuity				Best-Corrected Visual Acuity			
	P Value	Regression Coefficient	OR	95% CI	P Value	Regression Coefficient	OR	95% CI
Age(yrs)								
50–59	Reference				Reference			
60–69	0.910	0.114	1.12	0.16–8.03	0.742	0.407	1.50	0.13–17.03
70–79	0.964	−0.046	0.96	0.13–6.92	0.980	0.031	1.03	0.09–12.51
80+	0.298	1.147	3.15	0.36–27.36	0.329	1.267	3.55	0.28–45.29
Gender								
Male	Reference				Reference			
Female	0.807	0.131	1.14	0.40–3.26	0.004	1.432	4.19	1.59–11.04
Education								
>6	Reference				Reference			
1–6	0.014	1.870	6.49	1.46–28.89	0.494	0.658	1.93	0.29–12.73
0	0.001	2.320	10.18	2.43–42.61	0.204	1.263	3.54	0.50–24.81
IOL status								
Pseudophakia	Reference				Reference			
Aphakia	<0.001	3.028	20.66	4.06–105.14	<0.001	2.139	8.49	3.01–23.95
Year of surgery								
≤2000	Reference				Reference			
≥2001	0.577	−0.352	0.70	0.20–2.42	0.547	−0.374	0.69	0.20–2.33

OR: odds ratios; CI: Confidence Interval; IOL: intraocular lens.

unoperated cataract with severe visual impairment or blindness, the social burden of cataract-related severe visual impairment and blindness, and CSC among the cataract-related severely visually impaired or blind population.

PVA and BCVA in cataract-operated eyes were tabulated by age, gender, and education, intraocular lens (IOL) status, and year of surgery. Visual acuity was categorized as: normal vision, ≥20/32; mild visual impairment, 20/40 to 20/63; moderate visual

Table 6. Principal Cause of Presenting and Best-Corrected Visual Acuity <20/63 in Post-operative Eyes.

Principal Cause	Presenting Visual Acuity			Best-Corrected Visual Acuity
	Aphakia	Pseudophakia	Total	
Refractive error/uncorrected aphakia	5(20.8)	17(39.5)	22 (32.8)	0 (0.0)
Retinal disorder	7(29.1)	5(11.6)	12 (17.9)	12(27.3)
AMD	4(16.7)	4(9.3)	8 (11.9)	8 (18.2)
Retinal detachment	1(4.2)	0(0.0)	1 (1.5)	1 (2.3)
Macular hole	0(0.0)	1(2.3)	1 (1.5)	1 (2.3)
Vitreous haze	2(8.3)	0(0.0)	2 (3.0)	2 (4.5)
Glaucoma	2(8.3)	8(18.6)	10 (14.9)	10 (22.7)
Optic atrophy	6(25.0)	2(4.7)	8 (11.9)	8 (18.2)
PCO	1(4.2)	4(9.3)	5 (7.5)	5 (11.4)
pterygium	2(8.3)	2(4.7)	4(6.0)	4 (9.0)
High myopic retinopathy	1(4.2)	2(4.7)	3(4.5)	2 (4.5)
Corneal opacity/scar	0(0.0)	1(2.3)	1 (1.5)	1 (2.3)
Other cause	0(0.0)	1(2.3)	1 (1.5)	1 (2.3)
Undetermined	0(0.0)	1(2.3)	1 (1.5)	1 (2.3)
All	24(100)	43(100)	67 (100)	44 (100)

AMD: age-related macular degeneration; PCO: posterior capsule opacification.
Data are presented as No. (%) of eyes.

impairment, <20/63 to 20/200; severe visual impairment, <20/200 to 20/400; and blindness, <20/400. The association of age, gender, education, IOL status, and year of surgery with PVA and BCVA of <20/63 (considered a poor visual outcome) in post-operative eyes was investigated with univariate analysis and multiple logistic regression. Principal causes of cataract-induced visual impairment or blindness in eyes with PVA and BCVA <20/63 were tabulated.

Statistical analyses were performed using SPSS 17.0 for Windows (SPSS, Inc., Chicago, IL, USA). Confidence intervals (CIs) and P values (considered significant at the P<0.05 levels) were calculated with adjustment for clustering effects and stratification associated with the sampling design.

Ethical approval was obtained from the Kunming Medical University Ethics Review Board. The study was conducted in accordance with the tenets of the World Medical Association's Declaration of Helsinki.

Results

A total of 2742 subjects aged ≥50 years were enumerated, and a total of 2133 (77.8%) subjects were successfully examined. 99 persons (129 eyes) had undergone cataract surgery in one (69 subjects, 69.7%) or both eyes (30 subjects, 30.3%), representing a cataract surgery prevalence of 4.6% (95% CI, 3.8%–5.55%) (Table 1), age- and sex-standardized prevalence 3.7%. In univariate analysis, cataract surgery was significantly associated with older age and higher education. Multiple logistic regression analysis revealed that the prevalence of cataract surgery remained significantly associated with older age.

Of the 99 post-operative subjects, 76 were presumed to have had severe visual impairment or blindness (PVA<20/200) in both eyes at the time of initial surgery (Table 2). An additional 68 subjects were severely impaired or blind because of unoperated cataract. Thus, the social burden of cataract-related severe visual impairment or blindness included 144 (6.8%) of the study participants. CSC within this cohort of post-operative and unoperated subjects was 52.8%.

In univariate analysis, post-operative cataract with presumed severe visual impairment or blindness, unoperated cataract with severe visual impairment or blindness and the burden of cataract-related severe visual impairment or blindness was significantly associated with older age and less education. In multiple logistic regression (Table 3), post-operative severe visual impairment or blindness, unoperated cataract severe visual impairment or blindness and the social burden of cataract-related severe visual impairment or blindness was associated with older age. However, there was no statistically significant difference between age, gender or educational status for CSC.

Subjects severely visually impaired or blind because of unoperated cataract cited that the most common reason for not having cataract surgery was that they were "unaware of cataract" (31 person, 45.6%), followed by "could not afford to undergo cataract surgery" (12 persons, 17.6%), "fear of further loss of vision after surgery" (5 persons, 7.4%), "fear of surgery" (4 persons, 5.9%), "no need to have cataract surgery" (4 persons, 5.9%), "being told to wait until the cataract gets mature" (4 persons, 5.9%), "not accompanied by others for surgery" (1 person, 1.5%), "being told that there was a contraindication" (1 person, 1.5%), and "undetermined" (6 person, 8.8%).

As shown, of the 129 cataract-operated eyes, 72.1% were operated on during the interval between 2001 and the time of the survey (early 2010), 20.9% were operated before 2000, and the others (7%) were uncertain. The percentage of cases that were pseudophakic was 79.8% of the 129 post-operative eyes (Table 4). The proportion of pseudophakic in cataract-operated eyes in the past 10 years was 93.5%, compared with 44.4% before 2000.

Of the 99 post-operative subjects, 30 were operated in both eyes: 21 were pseudophakic in both eyes, 5 were aphakic in both eyes, and 4 were pseudophakic in one eye and aphakic in the fellow eye. For the 69 with unilateral cataract surgery, 57 were pseudophakic and 12 were aphakic. Five (5.1%) of the 99 post-operative subjects were wearing glasses for distance correction at the time of the examination.

PVA and BCVA for the 129 post-operative eyes by age, gender, education, IOL status, and year of surgery are shown in Table 4. Overall, a reasonably good vision outcome (VA ≥20/63) was found in 48.1% of eyes with PVA and in 65.9% with BCVA. In univariate analysis, higher prevalence of visual impairment (VA <20/63) defined by both PVA and BCVA was significantly associated with older age, female, less education, aphakia, and year of surgery. In multiple logistic regression (Table 5), aphakia (odds ratio [OR], 8.49; P<0.001) and no education (OR, 10.18; P=0.001) or less education (OR, 6.49; P=0.014) were significantly associated with postoperative visual impairment by PVA, while aphakia (OR, 8.49; P<0.001) and female gender (OR, 4.19; P=0.004) were significantly associated with postoperative visual impairment by BCVA. Age or year of surgery was not significantly associated with either PVA or BCVA, in part because of its correlation with IOL status.

Table 6 identifies the principal cause of impairment for the 67 cataract-operated eyes with VA worse than 20/63. The main causes of post-operative visual impairment were refractive error, retinal disorders and glaucoma. Potentially treatable diseases, including refractive error, PCO, and pterygium accounted for 46.3% of impaired cataract-operated eyes.

Discussion

This study provides the first population-based data on the prevalence of cataract surgery, surgical coverage, risk factors for unoperated cataract, self-reported barriers to cataract surgery, visual acuity outcomes of cataract surgery, and risk factors and causes contributing to poor outcomes in the elderly Bai ethnic population in rural China. Although the sample size chosen for the survey was calculated according to estimates of prevalence of glaucoma, we have no reason to suspect that the sample of operated cases was not representative of the Bai as a whole.

The prevalence of cataract surgery of 4.6% as found among the Bai people in current study was considerably higher than that found earlier in China [8,9,12–15], in Sri Lanka (3.9%) [3], and lower than Brazil (6.28%) [23], Nepal (7.0%) [24], India (17.6%) [25]. These figures suggest a pronounced increase in the prevalence of cataract surgery in the past 15 years in rural China. Since minorities reside in the remote area and usually poor, the Chinese government has a preference policy to provide funding and training for the minorities to progress, govern and manage. The encouraging prevalence of cataract surgery may be attributed to rapid economic growth in Dali, and sustained successful effort on sight-restoring cataract surgery by training cataract surgeons, inputting surgical equipment, and offering free surgeries in Yunnan in recent years.

CSC of 52.8% as found among the Bai people in current study was generally comparable to that reported in Shunyi (47.8%) [12], Kunming (46.4%) [9], Tibet (56%) [8], and higher than that reported in Doumen (40.3%) [13] and the China Nine-Province Survey (35.7%) [15], but lower than Beijing (82.1%) [14]. CSC found in Dali was also at the moderate level, compared with previous studies in other developing countries [3–7,23–27]. The moderate CSC in Bai people reveals that combating cataract blindness just now gained a preliminary victory and that sustained efforts are needed to reach the remaining half of Bai people with bilateral visual impairment or blindness because of cataract. Findings also suggest that the CSC showed a more equitable distribution of cataract surgical service delivery by gender and educational status. A similar trend was observed for CSC in Harbin [16].

The social burden of cataract-related severe visual impairment or blindness of 6.8% as found among the Bai people in current study was remarkably higher than that found among the Han people in Beijing (3.48%) [14] and the China Nine-Province Survey (3.83%) [15]. A greater social burden of cataract-related severe visual impairment or blindness is suggestive a great incidence of cataract-related severe visual impairment or blindness, which may be due to a greater risk of cataract development. The elderly were particularly affected by severe visual impairment or blindness because of both unoperated and post-operative cataract. However, CSC differentially favored younger people, although not at level of statistical significance. The rapidly ageing population of Bais and the higher altitude (1974 m) with increased exposure to ultraviolet light in Dali may account for the higher burden of visual impairment or blindness resulting from cataract that was seen in our study. Education of the elderly within the community may therefore bring about a more considerable reduction in the burden of visual impairment or blindness in the region.

Current findings suggest the most commonly self-reported barriers to surgery in Bai population were lack of awareness and knowledge, cost and fear. Public health education to raise public awareness of the importance of eye health will need to take account of the very high levels of illiteracy found among the Bai people with unoperated cataract visual impairment or blindness (60.5%). By improving health education on cataract, reducing the price of cataract surgery for those who cannot afford it, and ensuring a high surgical quality, the uptake of cataract surgery could be increased considerably.

According to World Health Organization guidelines [28], visual outcome of cataract surgery among Bai people in our study was generally poor. The proportion of eyes with PVA and BCVA of 20/63 or better was 48.1% and 65.9%, respectively. The visual outcome in our study is comparable that found in the China Nine-Province Survey [15] and India [25], is better than that in earlier China [9,12,13,16] and Pakistan [29], and is worse than that in economically developed areas [14,17,18]. This result is partly due to differences in the study population and quality of eye care service.

The risk factors associated with visual impairment in post-operative adult Bai people include aphakia, illiteracie and female. The strongest association of poor visual acuity outcomes was aphakia; in multiple logistic regression, aphakia was 20 times more likely than pseudophakia to have poor outcome. Findings suggest that aphakia was more likely to suffer from surgical complications. Although no other abnormality could account for the decrease in VA, uncorrected aphakia were not fully correctable with corrective spectacles due to underlying surgical complications or optical weaknesses present in spectacles. We also found the presence of optic atrophy in 7 subjects (8 eyes) who had poor outcome after cataract surgery. Of the 7 such cases, 1 was bilateral aphakia in eyes with cataract surgery, while 6 was unilateral in eyes with cataract surgery, 4 aphakia, and 2 pseudophakic. Dandona et al. [30] suspect that the unilateral optic atrophy after cataract surgery with no other obvious cause may result from anesthesia or poor surgical technique. Fortunately, the proportion of IOL implantation in Dali was much higher than some that have been reported in similar surveys in China [8,9,12,13,15,16], and the value in the past 10 years was markedly higher than that before 2000. This may reflect the improvement of surgical technique in the region. The relatively poor PVA outcomes in illiteracies were the result of more cases with refractive error, retinal disorders, glaucoma, and other ocular comorbidities. And the relatively poor BCVA outcomes in females were the result of more cases with retinal disorders, glaucoma, and PCO. Illiteracy and female gender were used as disadvantage groups for socioeconomic status and members of these groups may mistakenly attribute poor visual acuity to failure of cataract surgery and may not seek future treatment for refractive error, PCO, or other ocular disease.

The main causes of visual impairment in post-operative eyes of the Bai people were refractive error, retinal disorders, and glaucoma. Similar findings were reported from surveys from Doumen [13], Liwan [17], and Hong Kong [18]. Potentially treatable diseases, including refractive error, PCO, and pterygium accounted for 46.3% of impaired eyes. Refractive error was the most common cause. The use of spectacles was only 5.1% among cataract-operated subjects. Pseudophakia accounted for more than three fourths of those with refractive error. The differences in PVA and BCVA after operation highlight the importance of appropriate preoperative IOL power estimation and postoperative adequate spectacle provision. PCO is a well-recognized, vision-impairing complication of cataract surgery and can be treated easily with laser capsulotomy. Pterygium, the prevalence of which was high in the Bais, can also be diagnosed and resolved easily with out-patient surgery. We could not determine whether retinal disorders and glaucoma had coexisted at the time of cataract surgery or developed after cataract surgery. Some pathologic features may be surgery-related, such as retinal detachment, partial AMD, which presented in aphakic eyes. To avoid these problems, more attention should be given to thorough pre-operative screening, high cataract surgical quality, regular post-operative follow-up, and timely treatment of complications and comorbidities.

There still remain some limitations in our study. Firstly, the relatively low response rate of the youngest group (aged 50–59 years, 63.7%) and male (58.5%) [22] was a source of potential bias. Younger men who were more healthy and mobile may have been less likely to participate because they were busy with working. Under-representation in younger men might result in over-estimation of the true burden of cataract-related severe visual impairment and blindness. Secondly, similar to previous studies in China, cataract was diagnosed not using a standardized cataract classification system. We adopted the clinical diagnostic criteria of cataract for which does not affect the analysis of cataract surgical coverage among the cataract severely impaired or blind population.

In conclusion, cataract surgery is reaching more than half of those with bilateral severe visual impairment or blindness because of cataract in the elderly Bai population living in rural south-western China. Surgical uptake is still low, and the social burden of cataract-related severe visual impairment or blindness is heavy, especially in the elderly. A significant degree of poor outcomes remains after cataract surgery. Many of the potential causes of visual impairment are treatable to improvement or correction by careful postoperative follow-up. Surgical uptake and visual outcomes should be further improved by creating a program that facilitates access to ophthalmic healthcare services by Bai people would address many of the risk factors and causes associated with visual impairment in cataract-operated adult Bai people.

Acknowledgments

The authors thank Geoffrey Arden, City University London for paper revises.

Author Contributions

Conceived and designed the experiments: HZ YSY MBY. Performed the experiments: WS YMY JL XL JJL XDS HZ. Analyzed the data: TW WS. Wrote the paper: WS HZ MBY YSY.

References

1. Resnikoff S, Pascolini D, Etya'ale D, Kocur I, Pararajasegaram R,et al. (2004) Global data on visual impairment in the year 2002. Bull World Health Organ 82: 844–851.
2. Sapkota YD, Pokharel GP, Dulal S, Byanju RN, Maharjan IM (2004) Barriers to up take cataract surgery in Gandaki Zone, Nepal. Kathmandu Univ Med J (KUMJ) 2: 103–112.
3. Athanasiov PA, Edussuriya K, Senaratne T, Sennanayake S, Selva D, et al. (2009) Cataract in central Sri Lanka: cataract surgical coverage and self-reported barriers to cataract surgery. Clin Experiment Ophthalmol 37: 780–784.
4. Jadoon Z, Shah SP, Bourne R, Dineen B, Khan MA, et al. (2007) Pakistan National Eye Survey Study Group. Cataract prevalence, cataract surgical coverage and barriers to uptake of cataract surgical services in Pakistan: the Pakistan National Blindness and Visual Impairment Survey. Br J Ophthalmol 91: 1269–1273.
5. Athanasiov PA, Casson RJ, Newland HS, Shein WK, Muecke JS, et al. (2008) Cataract surgical coverage and self-reported barriers to cataract surgery in a rural Myanmar population. Clin Experiment Ophthalmol 36: 521–525.
6. Wadud Z, Kuper H, Polack S, Lindfield R, Akm MR, et al. (2006) Rapid assessment of avoidable blindness and needs assessment of cataract surgical services in Satkhira District, Bangladesh. Br J Ophthalmol 90: 1225–1229.
7. Rabiu MM, Muhammed N (2008) Rapid assessment of cataract surgical services in Birnin-Kebbi local government area of Kebbi State, Nigeria. Ophthalmic Epidemiol 15: 359–365.
8. Bassett KL, Noertjojo K, Liu L, Wang FS, Tenzing C, et al. Cataract surgical coverage and outcome in the Tibet Autonomous Region of China. Br J Ophthalmol. 2005; 89: 5–9.
9. Wu M, Yip JL, Kuper H (2008) Rapid assessment of avoidable blindness in Kunming, China. Ophthalmology 115: 969–974.
10. Johnson GJ (2000) Improving outcome of cataract surgery in developing countries. Lancet 355: 158–159.
11. China Disabled Person's Federation (CDPF) (2005) Statistics Yearbook on the Undertakings of People with Disabilities in China. Beijing: CDPF Information Center.
12. Zhao J, Jia L, Sui R, Ellwein LB (1998) Prevalence of blindness and cataract surgery in Shunyi County, China. Am J Ophthalmol 126: 506–514.
13. Li S, Xu J, He M, Wu K, Munoz SR, et al. (1999) A survey of blindness and cataract surgery in Doumen County, China. Ophthalmology 106: 1602–1608.
14. Liu B, Xu L, Wang YX, Jonas JB (2009) Prevalence of cataract surgery and postoperative visual outcome in Greater Beijing: the Beijing Eye Study. Ophthalmology 116: 1322–1331.
15. Zhao J, Ellwein LB, Cui H, Ge J, Guan H, et al. (2010) Prevalence and outcomes of cataract surgery in rural China the China nine-province survey. Ophthalmology 117: 2120–2128.
16. Li Z, Cui H, Zhang L, Liu P, Yang H (2009) Cataract blindness and surgery among the elderly in rural southern Harbin, China. Ophthalmic Epidemiol 16: 78–83.
17. Huang W, Huang G, Wang D, Yin Q, Foster PJ, et al. (2011) Outcomes of cataract surgery in urban southern China: the Liwan Eye Study. Invest Ophthalmol Vis Sci 52: 16–20.
18. Lau J, Michon JJ, Chan WS, Ellwein LB (2002) Visual acuity and quality of life outcomes in cataract surgery patients in Hong Kong. Br J Ophthalmol 86: 12–17.
19. Hsu WM, Cheng CY, Liu JH, Tsai SY, Chou P (2004) Prevalence and causes of visual impairment in an elderly Chinese population in Taiwan: the Shihpai Eye Study. Ophthalmology 111: 62–69.
20. Vision 2020 launched in the Western Pacific [press release]. Geneva: World Health Organization; September 6, 1999. Available: http://www.who.int/inf-pr-1999/en/pr99-46.html. Accessed 16 May 2012.
21. Li J, Zhong H, Cai N, Luo TH, Li JJ, et al. (2012) The Prevalence and Causes of Visual Impairment in an Elderly Chinese Bai Ethnic Rural Population: The Yunnan Minority Eye Study. Invest Ophthalmol Vis Sci 53: 4498–4504.
22. Zhong H, Li J, Li C, Wei T, Cha X, et al. (2012) The prevalence of glaucoma in adult rural Chinese populations of the Bai nationality in Dali: the Yunnan Minority Eye Study. Invest Ophthalmol Vis Sci 53: 3221–3225.
23. Salomão SR, Soares FS, Berezovsky A, Araújo-Filho A, Mitsuhiro MR, et al. (2009) Prevalence and outcomes of cataract surgery in Brazil: the São Paulo eye study. Am J Ophthalmol 148: 199–206.
24. Sherchan A, Kandel RP, Sharma MK, Sapkota YD, Aghajanian J, et al. (2010) Blindness prevalence and cataract surgical coverage in Lumbini Zone and Chetwan District of Nepal. Br J Ophthalmol 94: 161–166.
25. Murthy GV, Vashist P, John N, Pokharel G, Ellwein LB (2009) Prevalence and vision-related outcomes of cataract surgery in Gujarat, India. Ophthalmic Epidemiol 16: 400–409.
26. Limburg H, Silva JC, Foster A. (2009) Cataract in Latin America: findings from nine recent surveys. Rev Panam Salud Publica 25: 449–455.
27. Limburg H, Barria von-Bischhoffshausen F, Gomez P, Silva JC, Foster A (2008) Review of recent surveys on blindness and visual impairment in Latin America. Br J Ophthalmol 92: 315–319.
28. World Health Oganization (1998) Informal consultation on analysis of blindness prevention outcomes. WHO/PBL/98.68.Geneva: WHO.
29. Bourne R, Dineen B, Jadoon Z, Lee PS, Khan A, et al. (2007) Outcomes of cataract surgery in Pakistan: results from The Pakistan National Blindness and Visual Impairment Survey. Br J Ophthalmol 91: 420–426.
30. Dandona L, Dandona R, Naduvilath TJ, McCarty CA, Mandal P, et al. (1999) Population-based assessment of the outcome of cataract surgery in an urban population in southern India. Am J Ophthalmol 127: 650–658.

Body Mass Index and Risk of Age-Related Cataract: A Meta-Analysis of Prospective Cohort Studies

Juan Ye*, Li-Xia Lou, Jin-Jing He, Yu-Feng Xu

Department of Ophthalmology, the Second Affiliated Hospital of Zhejiang University, College of Medicine, Hangzhou, Zhejiang, China

Abstract

Background: Age-related cataract (ARC) is the leading cause of blindness in the world. The relationship between body mass index (BMI) and risk of ARC is controversial across observational studies. We therefore performed this meta-analysis to evaluate the association between BMI and risk of ARC.

Methods: Eligible studies were identified through an electronic search of PubMed, Embase and the Cochrane Library. We pooled study-specific relative risks (RRs) and 95% confidence intervals (CIs) to determine the risk of ARC associated with BMI categories and per 1 kg/m^2 increase in BMI.

Results: A total of 17 prospective cohort studies were included in the meta-analysis. The pooled RRs of ARC were 1.08 (95% CI, 1.01–1.16) for overweight and 1.19 (95% CI, 1.10–1.28) for obesity compared with normal weight. These findings were robust when stratified by sex, sample source, outcome types and confounders, while significantly differed by assessment of BMI and ARC, and duration of follow-up. The summary RR suggested that per 1 kg/m^2 increase in BMI was associated with a 2% increased risk of ARC (RR 1.02, 95% CI 1.01–1.03). Pooled estimates of RRs consistently indicated a trend for subjects with a high BMI to develop posterior subcapsular cataracts (RR 1.19, 95% CI 1.06–1.35, for overweight; RR 1.50, 95% CI 1.24–1.81, for obesity; RR 1.04, 95% CI 1.01–1.06, per 1 kg/m^2 increase in BMI) other than nuclear or cortical cataracts.

Conclusions: The overall findings suggest that elevated BMI may increase the risk of ARC, especially posterior subcapsular cataracts. Further trials are needed to investigate the effect of weight reduction in obese populations on the risk of ARC.

Editor: Ram Nagaraj, Case Western Reserve University, United States of America

Funding: This study was funded by: 1. Natural Science Foundation of China (No. 81070756); 2. National "Twelfth Five-Year" Plan for Science & Technology Support of China (No. 2012BAI08B01); 3. Program for New Century Excellent Talents in University, China (No. NCET-11-0161); 4. Zhejiang Provincial Program for Cultivation of High-Level Innovative Health Talents; 5. The Specialized Key Science & Technology Foundation of Zhejiang Provincial S & T Department (No. 2012C13023-2); 6. Zhejiang Provincial Key Project of Medical and Health (No. 2011ZDA014). The funders had no role in study design, data collection and analysis, decision to publish, or preparation of the manuscript.

Competing Interests: The authors have declared that no competing interests exist.

* E-mail: yejuan@zju.edu.cn

Introduction

Age-related cataract (ARC) is a common ocular disease characterized by lens opacities and visual impairment, which develops slowly as a consequence of aging. Opacities originate in the nucleus, cortex or the posterior pole of the lens, resulting in nuclear, cortical or posterior subcapsular cataracts (PSCs), respectively [1]. Visual impairment and blindness caused by ARC remain major public health problems throughout the world [2]. Although cataract extraction is an effective treatment, many people in developing countries still suffer from cataracts due to high surgery costs and inadequate medical care [3]. The pathogenesis of ARC is multifactorial and not completely understood yet. A number of epidemiologic studies have identified several factors associated with an increased risk of ARC among population worldwide, such as age, smoking, alcohol consumption and ultraviolet radiation [4–6].

Compared with normal weight, defined by World Health Organization (WHO) as body mass index (BMI) of 18.5-<25 kg/m^2, excess body weight (overweight defined as BMI of 25-<30 kg/m^2, and obesity as BMI of ≥30 kg/m^2) [7], is recognized as a well-known risk factor for some common diseases, such as diabetes mellitus and cardiovascular diseases [8,9]. The relationship between BMI and risk of cataract is controversial across observational studies, with reports of positive linear relationship [10–12], reduced risk in heavier people [13,14], and no significant relationship [4,15,16]. Prospective data from several large population-based studies demonstrate that obesity was associated with an increased risk of ARC, especially PSC [17,18]. To our best knowledge, a meta-analysis on the association between obesity and ARC does not exist to date. We have therefore performed a meta-analysis to quantitatively summarize the results of existing prospective cohort studies concerning the effect of BMI on the risk of ARC.

Materials and Methods

Searching Strategy

A comprehensive literature search of PubMed (1950 to May 2013), Embase (1900 to May 2013) and the Cochrane Library (up to May 2013) was conducted to identify relevant epidemiological studies. We combined a set of search terms, truncated with wildcard characters if necessary: ("cataract" OR "lens opacity" OR "cataract extraction" OR "cataract surgery") AND ("body mass index" OR "BMI" OR "obesity" OR "adiposity" OR "overweight" OR "fat" OR "body weight") with language restricted to English. The titles and abstracts were scanned to exclude any clearly irrelevant studies. The full texts of the remaining articles were read to determine whether they contained information on the topic of interest. We contacted the authors of retrieved articles if additional data were needed. In order to find additional references, we also checked the reference lists of the retrieved publications.

Study Selection

Two investigators (L.X.L. and J.J.H.) independently evaluated all retrieved studies for possible inclusion. To be included, the study had to meet the following criteria: (1) had a prospective cohort study design; (2) reported BMI categories identical or similar to the WHO recommended classifications of body weight [7]; (For Asian populations, WHO suggests categories as follows: 18.5-<23 kg/m^2 normal weight; 23-<27.5 kg/m^2 overweight; and ≥27.5 kg/m^2 obesity [19].) (3) the outcome measure was incident cataract or cataract extraction; (4) reported effect estimates (relative risks (RRs), odds ratios (ORs) or hazard ratios (HRs)) with corresponding 95% confidence intervals (CIs) for BMI categories associated risk of ARC, provided effect estimates per unit (in kg/m^2) increase in BMI, or allowed for calculation from raw data contained in the article. If more than one study used the same cohort, the one with the most comprehensive population or longest follow-up time was included. We excluded any article with inconsistent or erroneous data. Conference abstracts or unpublished reports were not considered.

Data Extraction and Study Quality Assessment

Two investigators (L.X.L. and J.J.H.) independently extracted data from each included study. Any disagreements were resolved through discussion with the senior investigator (J.Y.). We collected the following information, including last name of first author, year of publication, study location, mean follow-up time, sample size, age range of subjects, BMI determinants, case definitions of ARC, outcome types (incident cataract including nuclear cataract, cortical cataract and PSC, or cataract extraction), covariates adjusted in multivariable analysis, and effect estimates for BMI categories or per unit increase in BMI. The BMI categories that were closest to the WHO definition of weight status were applied if non-standard categories were used in individual studies included in this meta-analysis. If a study had several adjustment models, we extracted the one that reflected the maximum extent of adjustment for potentially confounding variables. If no adjusted estimates were available, unadjusted estimates were used. We extracted sex-specific data *if* they were available in individual studies.

Study quality assessment was performed using the Newcastle-Ottawa scale [20], which is validated for non-randomised studies in a meta-analysis. This scale awards a maximum of nine points to each study: four for selection of participants and measurement of exposure (BMI); two for comparability of cohorts on the basis of the design or analysis; and three for assessment of outcomes (incident cataract or cataract extraction) and adequacy of follow-up.

Statistical Analysis

The RRs with corresponding 95% CIs were considered as the effect estimates for all included studies. Any results stratified by sex were treated as two separate reports. If a study only reported results specific for ARC subtypes, the subtype-specific RRs were pooled as an estimate for ARC of any type. Study-specific RRs were pooled using fixed-effects models with the Mantel-Haenszel method when heterogeneity was negligible, or random-effects models with the DerSimonian-Laird method when heterogeneity was significant [21]. We evaluated the risk of ARC in overweight and obese subjects in contrast to normal weight subjects. Also, we analysed the linear relationship between BMI and risk of ARC. Several studies included in this meta-analysis reported RRs for cataracts associated with per 1 kg/m^2 increase or per 5 kg/m^2 increase in BMI. If the RR was on the 5 kg/m^2 increase scale, the log RR and its standard error were divided by 5 to derive the corresponding 1 kg/m^2 increase estimate [22].

Statistical heterogeneity among studies was evaluated using the Cochran's *Q* test and I^2 statistic [23]. Heterogeneity was confirmed with a significance level of $P<0.10$. I^2 values of <25%, 25%-<50%, 50%-<75% and ≥75% were considered as no, low, moderate and high heterogeneity, respectively. Sensitivity analysis was performed to investigate the contribution of each study to the heterogeneity by sequentially removing one study and reanalyzing the pooled estimate for the remaining studies. We also conducted subgroup analyses investigating whether sex, sample source, BMI and ARC ascertainments, duration of follow-up, outcome types, ARC subtypes, and adjustment for confounders influenced the results [24]. Publication bias assessment was done using the Egger regression asymmetry test and the Begg adjusted rank correlation test [25,26]. All statistical analyses were performed with Stata 12.0 (Stata Corporation, College Station, TX). For all analyses, except heterogeneity, *a value of* $P<0.05$ was regarded as statistically significant, and all tests were two-sided.

Results

Literature Search and Characteristics of Included Studies

The literature search yielded 4340 articles from the electronic database. After removing 391 duplicate publications, 3949 studies were considered of potential relevance (Fig. 1). In total, 28 articles were retrieved for full-text review, 19 of which met all the predefined inclusion criteria. However, we excluded studies that were limited to non-generalizable patients, including 2 studies of ARC in diabetic patients [27,28]. Finally, 17 prospective cohort studies were included in this meta-analysis. 11 studies were eligible for the categorical relationship between BMI and ARC [4,12,15–18,29–33], 1 of which only evaluated nuclear cataract [18]. 7 studies were eligible for the linear relationship [10–13,34–36], 2 of which only reported incident nuclear cataract [13,34].

Characteristics of the included studies are summarized in Table 1. ARC definitions and assessment varied among the studies. Diagnosis of cataract or cataract surgery was ascertained by standardized criteria in 9 studies [4,13,16–18,31,34–36], and self-reported by questionnaire or interview in 6 studies [10–12,30,32,33], while in 2 studies cases were determined based on a national register [15,29]. 15 studies reported incident cataract as the measure of outcome and 5 studies evaluated cataract extraction. For studies which reported both of the outcome measures [4,17,18,32], we considered incident cataract as the primary outcome. BMI was calculated by measured weight and height in 7 studies [4,13,16,17,31,34,36], and identified by self-reports of anthropometric measurements in 10 studies [10–12,15,18,29,30,32,33,35]. Results of quality assessment yielded a score range from 5 to 9 for the included studies with an average score of 6.7. The influences of the indicators of study quality on the relationship between BMI and ARC, such as sample source, exposure and outcome determinants, duration of follow-up, and

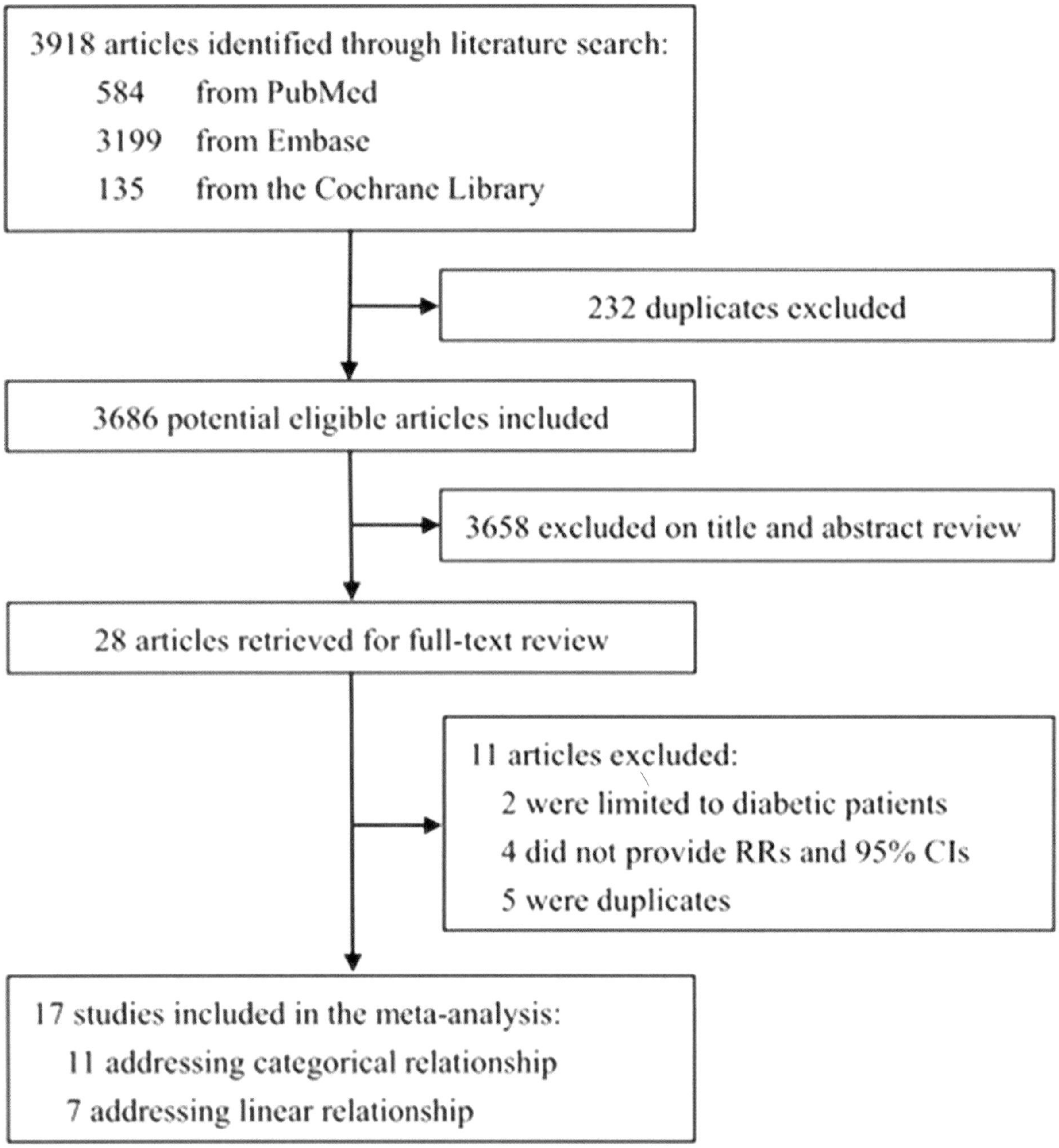

Figure 1. Flow diagram of study selection process.

adjustment for confounders, were then investigated in subgroup analyses.

The Association between BMI Categories and Risk of ARC

The pooled results of 10 studies showed that overweight subjects had a statistically significantly increased risk of ARC (RR 1.08, 95% CI 1.01–1.16; $I^2 = 67.6\%$, $P_{heterogeneity} < 0.001$) when compared to normal weight subjects (Fig. 2). Sensitivity analyses indicated that the pooled RR was not excessively changed by any individual studies, ranging from 1.05 (95% CI 1.00–1.11) to 1.10 (95% CI 1.02–1.18). Table S1 shows the results of sensitivity analyses. Egger's and Begg's test confirmed the absence of publication bias (Egger's test = 0.614, Begg's test = 0.945). Obese subjects also had a higher risk of ARC (RR 1.19, 95% CI 1.10–1.28; $I^2 = 55.7\%$, $P_{heterogeneity} = 0.010$). Omission of individual studies revealed that no single study had a particular influence on the pooled estimate, detected by pooled RR ranging from 1.15 (95% CI 1.07–1.24) to 1.21 (95% CI 1.12–1.30). No publication bias was detected by Egger's and Begg's test (Egger's test = 0.823, Begg's test = 1.000).

We performed subgroup analyses to investigate the effect of sex, sample source, BMI and ARC ascertainments, duration of follow-up, outcome types, ARC subtypes, and selected confounders (alcohol use, diabetes and hypertension) on the relationship between BMI categories and ARC (Table 2). Similar risk estimates were found in both genders. Likewise, there was no evidence that

Table 1. Characteristics of Studies Included in the Meta-Analysis.

Authors (published year, location)	Years of follow-up	Participants	Age range, y	Sample size	BMI determinants	ARC definitions	Outcome types	Study quality
Schaumberg et al.[32] (2000, USA)	13.7	Volunteers	40–84	20271 men	Self-reported	Self-reported with confirmation	Any type, NC, CC, PSC, Extraction	6
Tan et al.[17] (2008, Australia)	10.5	Population-based	≥49	2564	Measured	Standard criteria	NC, CC,PSC, Extraction	9
Weintraub et al.[12] (2002, USA)	10 (male) 16 (female)	Volunteers	≥45	45549 men 87682 women	Self-reported	Self-reported with confirmation	Extraction (Any type, NC,PSC)	6
Yoshida et al.[33] (2000, Japan)	5	Population-based	≥50	35365 men 40825 women	Self-reported	Self-reported	Any type	6
Lindblad et al.[15] (2008, Sweden)	8.2	Population-based	49–83	35369 women	Self-reported	National register	Extraction	6
Hiller et al.[31] (1998, USA)	12.5	Population-based	52–80	714	Measured	Standard criteria	Any type, NC, CC, PSC	8
Richter et al.[16] (2012, USA)	4	Population-based	≥40	3471	Measured	Standard criteria	NC, CC, PSC	6
Chang et al.[4] (2011, USA)	9.8	Hospital-based	55–80	4425	Measured	Standard criteria	Any type, NC, CC, PSC, Extraction	7
Appleby et al.[29] (2011, UK)	11.4	Population-based	≥40	27670	Self-reported	National register	Any type	7
Chodick et al.[30] (2008, USA)	20	Volunteers	23–44	35705	Self-reported	Self-reported	Any type	6
Mares et al.[18] (2010, USA)	6	Population-based	50–79	1808 women	Self-reported	Standard criteria	NC	7
Glynn et al.[10] (2009, USA)	13	Volunteers	40–84	20599 men	Self-reported	Self-reported with confirmation	NC, CC, PSC	6
Klein et al.[35] (2003, USA)	5	Population-based	43–84	4926	Self-reported	Standard criteria	NC, CC, PSC	7
Williams.[11] (2009, USA)	7	Volunteers	38–44	29025 men 11967 women	Self-reported	Self-reported	Any type	5
Zhang et al.[36] (2011, China)	5	Population-based	≥45	3251	Measured	Standard criteria	NC, CC, PSC	6
Leske et al.[13] (2002, Barbados)	4	Population-based	40–84	3427	Measured	Standard criteria	NC	8
Karppi et al.[34] (2012, Finland)	4	Population-based	61–80	1689	Measured	Standard criteria	NC	8

ARC: age-related cataract; BMI: body mass index; CC: cortical cataract; NC: nuclear cataract; PSC: posterior subcapsular cataract.

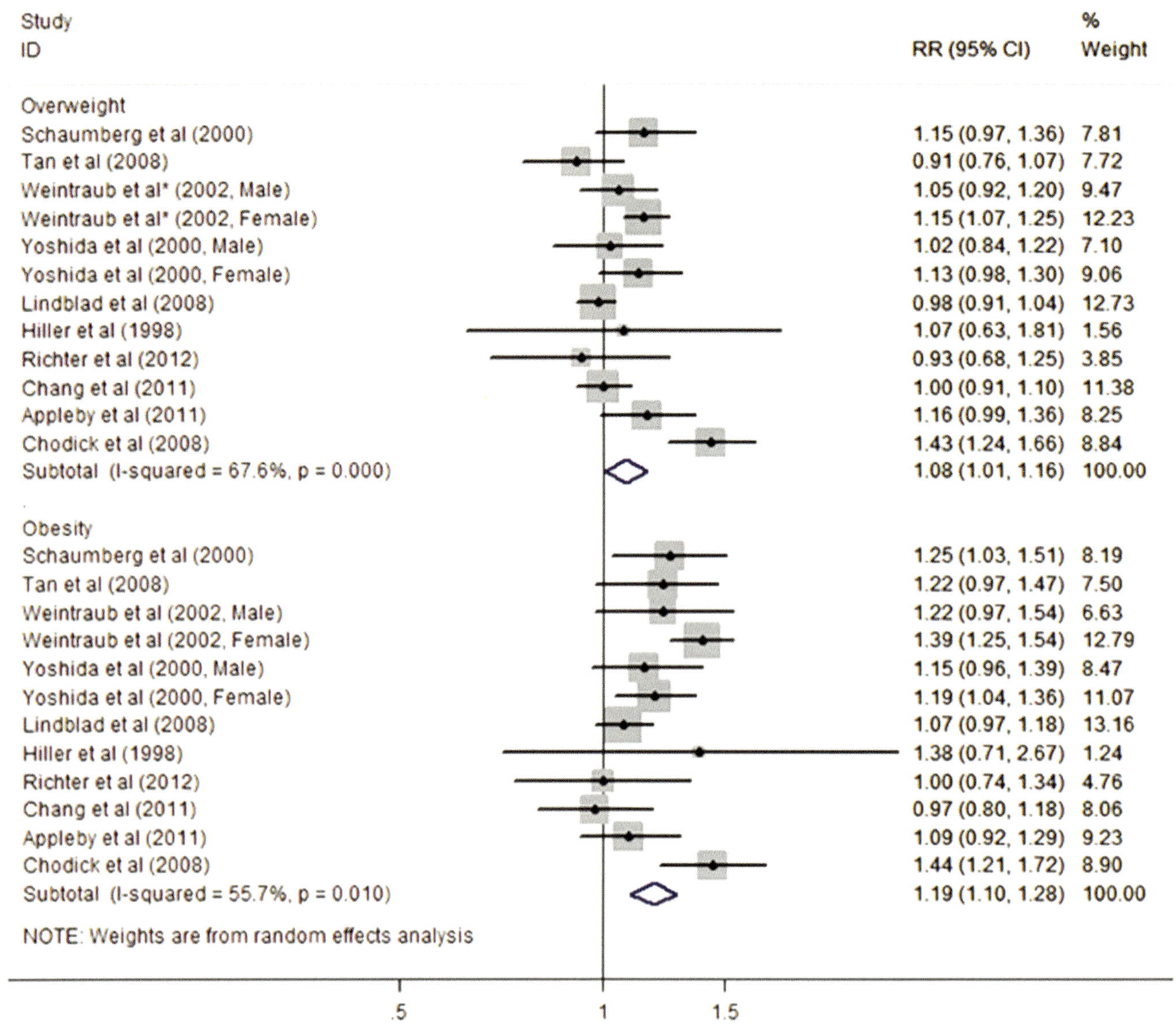

Figure 2. Forest plot of risk estimates of age-related cataract associated with overweight and obesity. *Derived by combining BMI categories of 25–<27.9 kg/m^2 and 28-<29.9 kg/m^2.

the pooled RRs differed significantly by sample source, outcome types or adjustment of confounders. However, ascertainments of exposure and outcome were found to significantly modify the association between ARC and overweight, but not obesity. The pooled RR from studies with measured BMI and standard diagnosis of cataract (overweight: RR 0.98, 95% CI 0.90–1.06) was lower than from studies with self-reported BMI and non-standard definition of cataract (overweight: RR 1.12, 95% CI 1.03–1.22). When pooling results from studies with more than 10 years of follow-up, the RRs were significantly higher than from studies with less than 10 years of follow-up (overweight: RR 1.13, 95% CI 1.03–1.25 versus RR 1.00, 95% CI 0.96–1.05; obesity: RR 1.28, 95% CI 1.19–1.39 versus RR 1.09, 95% CI 1.02–1.17). There was no evidence for significant relationship between BMI categories and cortical or nuclear cataract. However, BMI was strongly associated with PSC (overweight: RR 1.19, 95% CI 1.06–1.35; obesity: RR 1.50, 95% CI 1.24–1.81).

The Association between per 1 kg/m^2 Increase in BMI and Risk of ARC

We performed fixed-effects meta-analysis of 5 studies to determined the risk of ARC associated with per 1 kg/m^2 increase in BMI. Figure 3 shows that an increase in BMI of 1 kg/m^2 was statistically significantly associated with ARC (RR 1.02, 95% CI 1.01–1.03; $I^2 = 19.5\%$, $P_{heterogeneity} = 0.281$). Egger's and Begg's test confirmed no evidence of publication bias. Stratified analyses by ARC subtypes revealed differences among the three subtypes (RR 1.00, 95% CI 0.98–1.02, for nuclear cataract, 6 cohorts; RR 1.01, 95% CI 0.99–1.02, for cortical cataract, 3 cohorts; RR 1.04, 95% CI 1.01–1.06, for PSC, 4 cohorts).

Discussion

This meta-analysis of 11 prospective cohort studies addressing the categorical relationship between BMI and ARC revealed that overweight and obesity were significantly associated with an

Table 2. Subgroup Analyses of Body Mass Index (BMI) Categories and Risk of Age-Related Cataract (ARC).

		Overweight			**Obesity**		
Subgroup	**N of studies**	**Pooled RR (95% CI)**	$P_{heterogeneity}$	$P_{difference}$	**Pooled RR (95% CI)**	$P_{heterogeneity}$	$P_{difference}$
All	10	1.08 (1.01–1.16)	<0.001		1.19 (1.10–1.28)	0.010	
Gender							
Male	3	1.08 (0.99–1.18)	0.466	Reference	1.22 (1.09–1.36)	0.711	Reference
Female	3	1.08 (0.96–1.21)	0.006	1.000	1.21 (1.03–1.42)	0.002	0.934
Sample source							
Population-based	5	1.02 (0.95–1.10)	0.165	Reference	1.12 (1.05–1.19)	0.701	Reference
Other	5	1.14 (1.02–1.26)	0.003	0.090	1.26 (1.11–1.43)	0.034	0.102
BMI & ARC ascertainments							
Measured & Standard criteria	4	0.98 (0.90–1.06)	0.775	Reference	1.08 (0.94–1.23)	0.352	Reference
Self-reported & Non-standard	6	1.12 (1.03–1.22)	<0.001	0.026	1.22 (1.12–1.33)	0.010	0.134
Duration of follow-up							
≥10 yrs	6	1.13 (1.03–1.25)	0.007	Reference	1.28 (1.19–1.39)	0.246	Reference
<10 yrs	4	1.00 (0.96–1.05)	0.482	0.025	1.09 (1.02–1.17)	0.433	0.002
Outcome type							
Incident cataract	7	1.08 (0.97–1.21)	0.002	Reference	1.19 (1.08–1.30)	0.151	Reference
Cataract extraction	5	1.04 (0.95–1.15)	0.002	0.613	1.16 (0.99–1.34)	<0.001	0.778
ARC subtype							
Nuclear cataract	7	1.00 (0.90–1.11)	0.131	Reference	1.08 (0.94–1.24)	0.066	Reference
Cortical cataract	5	1.04 (0.92–1.18)	0.364	0.637	1.12 (0.93–1.35)	0.246	0.759
PSC	6	1.19 (1.06–1.35)	0.589	0.033	1.50 (1.24–1.81)	0.224	0.006
Adjustment for confounders							
Alcohol use							
Yes	4	1.13 (0.98–1.30)	<0.001	Reference	1.20 (1.08–1.33)	0.059	Reference
No	6	1.05 (0.98–1.13)	0.102	0.363	1.17 (1.03–1.32)	0.021	0.759
Diabetes							
Yes	5	1.09 (0.94–1.25)	0.001	Reference	1.19 (1.07–1.33)	0.104	Reference
No	5	1.07 (0.99–1.16)	0.030	0.824	1.18 (1.05–1.32)	0.008	0.917
Hypertension							
Yes	3	1.11 (0.92–1.35)	0.001	Reference	1.24 (1.13–1.37)	0.284	Reference
No	7	1.06 (0.99–1.13)	0.058	0.656	1.15 (1.03–1.28)	0.006	0.309

CI: confidence interval; PSC: posterior subcapsular cataract; RR: relative risk.

increased risk of ARC, especially PSC. This positive relationship is independent of sex, sample source, outcome types, and selected confounders, such as alcohol intake, diabetes and hypertension, while significantly differed by assessment of BMI and ARC, and duration of follow-up. However, one must be wary of generalizing results from subgroup analyses because of relatively fewer studies involved.

There was evidence of moderate heterogeneity among the studies included in the categorical analysis. Adjustment of confounders was different among the studies and residual confounding may have affected the individual effect estimates and thus the pooled RR. All these studies, except the study by Richter et al [16], evaluated the relationship between BMI and ARC after adjusting for potential confounders, such as age and smoking. When removing the study by Richter et al [16], the risk estimates were essentially unchanged (Table S1).A wide variation existed among the cohorts with regard to the duration of follow-up. Studies with more than 10 years of follow-up showed a stronger positive association between BMI and risk of ARC than studies with shorter follow-up duration (Table 2). Considering that catarcts progress at various rates in different individuals to the point where they are detected and require extraction, achieving adequate follow-up in cohorts is essential to establish the validity of the findings. We noticed that a large proportion of the studies were conducted in non-Asian regions, in keeping with the high prevalence of obesity in these regions and associated research efforts. After exclusion of the only study conducted in Asia, the summary RR remained stable (Table S1) [33].

We also found a linear positive association between BMI and risk of ARC. Per 1 kg/m^2 increase in BMI was associated with a 2% increased risk of ARC, with no heterogeneity detected ($I^2 = 19.5\%$). Caution must be taken in the interpretation of this pooled estimate. Although the pooled effect size represents only a weak positive association, its interpretation depends on the unit of measurement. A 5 kg/m^2 increase in BMI equates to a much stronger association (RR 1.10). Similarly, subgroup analyses found

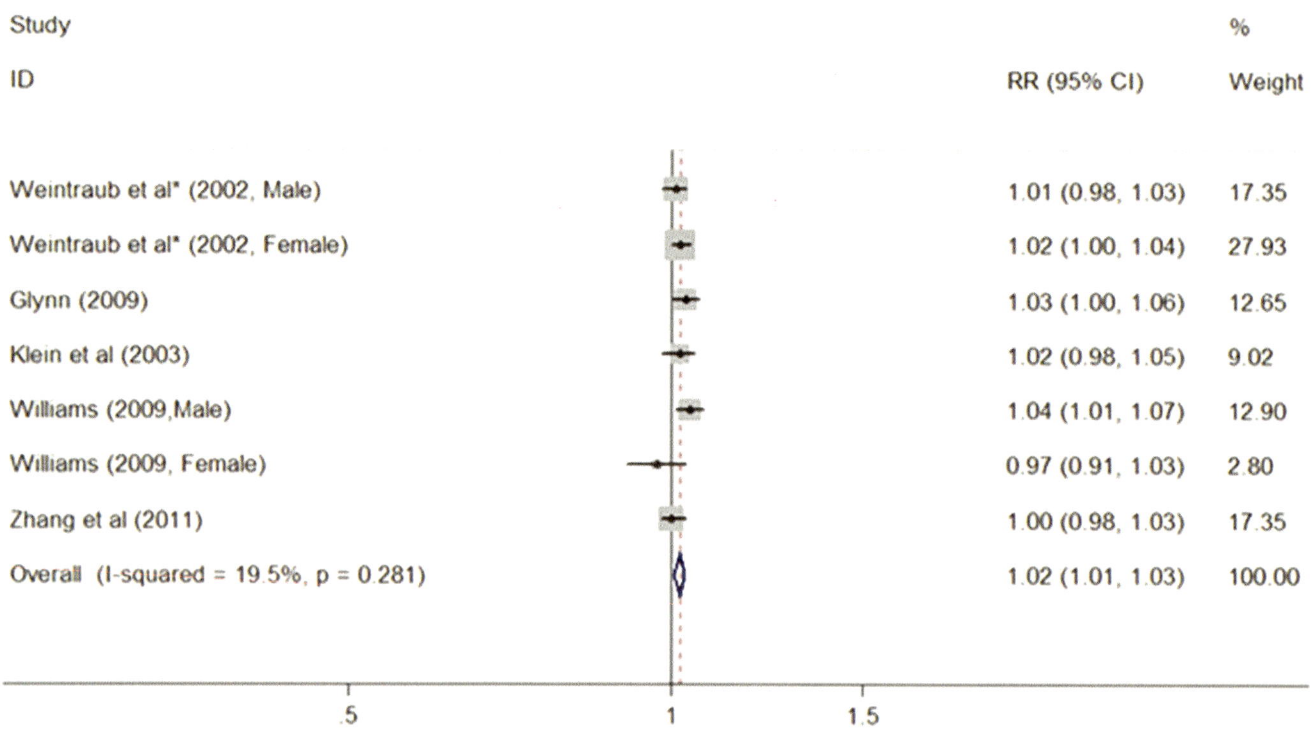

Figure 3. Forest plot of risk estimates of age-related cataract associated with per 1 kg/m^2 increase in BMI. *Derived from RRs associated with per 5 kg/m^2 increase in BMI.

that per 1 kg/m^2 increase in BMI was more strongly associated with the risk of PSC than other types of ARC, as well as the results of BMI categorical analysis. Likewise, we cannot exclude type I error, because the sample size was small in these subgroups.

Strengths of our meta-analysis included the quantitative analyses based on prospective cohort studies, which tend to be less susceptible to recall and selection bias than retrospective case-control studies. Moreover, most cohorts were population-based with findings being more generalizable. The large number of included studies allowed us to investigate both the categorical and linear relationship between BMI and ARC, and to better explore the effect of excess weight on various subgroups.

However, our meta-analysis has several limitations that may affect the interpretation of the results. First, the included studies exhibited wide differences in outcome definition. Because several studies relied on participants to self-report their diagnoses of cataract, underestimates of the number of cases might have occurred due to a few false-negative cases. Besides, cataract surgery depends on health services provision and access, which would produce bias if different between normal weight and excess weight individuals. Second, in some studies BMI determinants were dependent on self-reporting questionaires. A downward bias in self-reported BMI especially of heavier individuals has been found to result in misclassification of weight status [37]. However, a few included studies had validated self-reported information with correlation of self-reported weight versus measured weight ranging from 0.96 to 0.97 [12,32]. Third, as in any meta-analysis, the possibility of publication bias is of concern because studies which have results that are not statistically significant or have been previously published may be less likely to be published. However, statistical tests did not provide evidence of publication bias in our meta-analysis.

There are several plausible pathophysiological pathways through which increased BMI might promote cataract formation. First, obese individuals have elevated plasma levels of leptin [38], which might be involved in lens opacity for enhancing accumulation of reactive oxygen species [39–41]. Second, individuals with obesity have more intense systemic inflammation with elevated levels of C-reactive protein and pro-inflammatory cytokines [42], both of which could promote the development of cataract [43,44]. Third, obesity might be linked to cataract by its complications such as diabetes, hyperlipidemia and hypertension [8,38,45], which are all known risk factors for cataract [46,47]. The stronger association between BMI and PSC might be due to the different patterns of formation and progression of ARC subtypes. Although less common than nuclear and cortical opacities, PSCs are more likely to result in visual disability, and are highly overrepresented among extracted cataracts [41].

In summary, findings from our meta-analysis indicate that high BMI may increase the risk of ARC in both sexes, especially PSC. As obesity prevalence continues to be on an upward trajectory worldwide [48], the contribution of obesity to the development of ARC might constitute a proportion of the global burden of ARC. The results of our meta-analysis imply that beneficial lifestyle changes to reduce body weight, which clearly have other health benefits as well, might help to lessen the incidence and associated costs of cataract. In future research, randomized trials are needed to examine the effect of weight reduction in obese populations on the risk of ARC.

Acknowledgments

The authors are grateful to Birgitta Ejdervik Lindblad, from Department of Ophthalmology, Sundsvall Hospital; the writing team and the members of the AREDS Research Group, especially Emily Y. Chew and Elvira Agrón, from National Eye Institute, National Institutes of Health, USA; Jing Shang Zhang, from Beijing Institute of Ophthalmology, China, for providing data in statistical analyses. We also thank Yunxian Yu, from Department of Epidemiology & Health Statistics, School of Public Health, Zhejiang University, for his comments and advice on the manuscript.

Author Contributions

Conceived and designed the experiments: JY LL. Performed the experiments: LL JH. Analyzed the data: JY LL JH YX. Contributed reagents/materials/analysis tools: JY LL JH YX. Wrote the paper: JY LL JH.

References

1. Asbell PA, Dualan I, Mindel J, Brocks D, Ahmad M, et al. (2005) Age-related cataract. Lancet 365: 599–609.
2. Pascolini D, Mariotti SP (2012) Global estimates of visual impairment: 2010. Br J Ophthalmol 96: 614–618.
3. Ono K, Hiratsuka Y, Murakami A (2010) Global inequality in eye health: country-level analysis from the Global Burden of Disease Study. Am J Public Health 100: 1784–1788.
4. Chang JR, Koo E, Agron E, Hallak J, Clemons T, et al. (2011) Risk factors associated with incident cataracts and cataract surgery in the Age-related Eye Disease Study (AREDS): AREDS report number 32. Ophthalmology 118: 2113–2119.
5. Pastor-Valero M, Fletcher AE, de Stavola BL, Chaques-Alepuz V (2007) Years of sunlight exposure and cataract: a case-control study in a Mediterranean population. BMC Ophthalmol 7: 18–25.
6. Kanthan GL, Mitchell P, Burlutsky G, Wang JJ (2010) Alcohol consumption and the long-term incidence of cataract and cataract surgery: the Blue Mountains Eye Study. Am J Ophthalmol 150: 434–440.
7. Tauber WB (1992) Clinical consequences of Thorotrast in a long-term survivor. Health Phys 63: 13–19.
8. Radzeviciene L, Ostrauskas R (2012) Body mass index, waist circumference, waist-hip ratio, waist-height ratio and risk for type 2 diabetes in women: A case-control study. Public Health 127: 241–246.
9. Friedemann C, Heneghan C, Mahtani K, Thompson M, Perera R, et al. (2012) Cardiovascular disease risk in healthy children and its association with body mass index: systematic review and meta-analysis. BMJ 345: 4759–4774.
10. Glynn RJ, Rosner B, Christen WG (2009) Evaluation of risk factors for cataract types in a competing risks framework. Ophthalmic Epidemiol 16: 98–106.
11. Williams PT (2009) Prospective epidemiological cohort study of reduced risk for incident cataract with vigorous physical activity and cardiorespiratory fitness during a 7-year follow-up. Invest Ophthalmol Vis Sci 50: 95–100.
12. Weintraub JM, Willett WC, Rosner B, Colditz GA, Seddon JM, et al. (2002) A prospective study of the relationship between body mass index and cataract extraction among US women and men. Int J Obes Relat Metab Disord 26: 1588–1595.
13. Leske MC, Wu SY, Nemesure B, Hennis A (2002) Risk factors for incident nuclear opacities. Ophthalmology 109: 1303–1308.
14. Nirmalan PK, Robin AL, Katz J, Tielsch JM, Thulasiraj RD, et al. (2004) Risk factors for age related cataract in a rural population of southern India: the Aravind Comprehensive Eye Study. Br J Ophthalmol 88: 989–994.
15. Lindblad BE, Hakansson N, Philipson B, Wolk A (2008) Metabolic syndrome components in relation to risk of cataract extraction: a prospective cohort study of women. Ophthalmology 115: 1687–1692.
16. Richter GM, Choudhury F, Torres M, Azen SP, Varma R, et al. (2012) Risk factors for incident cortical, nuclear, posterior subcapsular, and mixed lens opacities: the Los Angeles Latino eye study. Ophthalmology 119: 2040–2047.
17. Tan JS, Wang JJ, Mitchell P (2008) Influence of diabetes and cardiovascular disease on the long-term incidence of cataract: the Blue Mountains eye study. Ophthalmic Epidemiol 15: 317–327.
18. Mares JA, Voland R, Adler R, Tinker L, Millen AE, et al. (2010) Healthy diets and the subsequent prevalence of nuclear cataract in women. Arch Ophthalmol 128: 738–749.
19. Consultation WHOE (2004) Appropriate body-mass index for Asian populations and its implications for policy and intervention strategies. Lancet 363: 157–163.
20. Wells GA, Shea B, O'Connell D, Peterson J, Welch V The Newcastle-Ottawa Scale (NOS) for assessing the quality of nonrandomized studies in meta-analyses. Available: http://www.ohri.ca/programs/clinical_epidemiology/oxford.htm. Accessed April 25, 2013.
21. DerSimonian R, Kacker R (2007) Random-effects model for meta-analysis of clinical trials: an update. Contemp Clin Trials 28: 105–114.
22. Sherwin JC, Reacher MH, Keogh RH, Khawaja AP, Mackey DA, et al. (2012) The association between time spent outdoors and myopia in children and adolescents: a systematic review and meta-analysis. Ophthalmology 119: 2141–2151.
23. Higgins JP, Thompson SG, Deeks JJ, Altman DG (2003) Measuring inconsistency in meta-analyses. BMJ 327: 557–560.
24. Altman DG, Bland JM (2003) Interaction revisited: the difference between two estimates. BMJ 326: 219.
25. Egger M, Davey Smith G, Schneider M, Minder C (1997) Bias in meta-analysis detected by a simple, graphical test. BMJ 315: 629–634.
26. Begg CB, Mazumdar M (1994) Operating characteristics of a rank correlation test for publication bias. Biometrics 50: 1088–1101.
27. Janghorbani M, Amini M (2004) Cataract in type 2 diabetes mellitus in Isfahan, Iran: incidence and risk factors. Ophthalmic Epidemiol 11: 347–358.
28. Janghorbani MB, Jones RB, Allison SP (2000) Incidence of and risk factors for cataract among diabetes clinic attenders. Ophthalmic Epidemiol 7: 13–25.
29. Appleby PN, Allen NE, Key TJ (2011) Diet, vegetarianism, and cataract risk. Am J Clin Nutr 93: 1128–1135.
30. Chodick G, Bekiroglu N, Hauptmann M, Alexander BH, Freedman DM, et al. (2008) Risk of cataract after exposure to low doses of ionizing radiation: a 20-year prospective cohort study among US radiologic technologists. Am J Epidemiol 168: 620–631.
31. Hiller R, Podgor MJ, Sperduto RD, Nowroozi L, Wilson PW, et al. (1998) A longitudinal study of body mass index and lens opacities. The Framingham Studies. Ophthalmology 105: 1244–1250.
32. Schaumberg DA, Glynn RJ, Christen WG, Hankinson SE, Hennekens CH (2000) Relations of body fat distribution and height with cataract in men. Am J Clin Nutr 72: 1495–1502.
33. Yoshida M, Inoue M, Iwasaki M, Tsugane S (2010) Association of body mass index with risk of age-related cataracts in a middle-aged Japanese population: the JPHC Study. Environ Health Prev Med 15: 367–373.
34. Karppi J, Laukkanen JA, Kurl S (2012) Plasma lutein and zeaxanthin and the risk of age-related nuclear cataract among the elderly Finnish population. Br J Nutr 108: 148–154.
35. Klein BE, Klein R, Lee KE, Moore EL (2003) Do multiple families alter estimates of risk for age-related cataract in a population-based study? The Beaver Dam Eye Study. Ophthalmic Epidemiol 10: 97–106.
36. Zhang JS, Xu L, Wang YX, You QS, Wang JD, et al. (2011) Five-year incidence of age-related cataract and cataract surgery in the adult population of greater Beijing: the Beijing Eye Study. Ophthalmology 118: 711–718.
37. Hattori A, Sturm R (2013) The obesity epidemic and changes in self-report biases in BMI. Obesity (Silver Spring) 21: 856–860.
38. Muoio DM, Newgard CB (2006) Obesity-related derangements in metabolic regulation. Annu Rev Biochem 75: 367–401.
39. Yamagishi S, Amano S, Inagaki Y, Okamoto T, Takeuchi M, et al. (2003) Pigment epithelium-derived factor inhibits leptin-induced angiogenesis by suppressing vascular endothelial growth factor gene expression through anti-oxidative properties. Microvasc Res 65: 186–190.
40. Bouloumie A, Marumo T, Lafontan M, Busse R (1999) Leptin induces oxidative stress in human endothelial cells. FASEB J 13: 1231–1238.
41. Beebe DC, Holekamp NM, Shui YB (2010) Oxidative damage and the prevention of age-related cataracts. Ophthalmic Res 44: 155–165.
42. Ritchie SA, Connell JM (2007) The link between abdominal obesity, metabolic syndrome and cardiovascular disease. Nutr Metab Cardiovasc Dis 17: 319–326.
43. Schaumberg DA, Ridker PM, Glynn RJ, Christen WG, Dana MR, et al. (1999) High levels of plasma C-reactive protein and future risk of age-related cataract. Ann Epidemiol 9: 166–171.
44. Klein BE, Klein R, Lee KE, Knudtson MD, Tsai MY (2006) Markers of inflammation, vascular endothelial dysfunction, and age-related cataract. Am J Ophthalmol 141: 116–122.
45. Spiegelman D, Israel RG, Bouchard C, Willett WC (1992) Absolute fat mass, percent body fat, and body-fat distribution: which is the real determinant of blood pressure and serum glucose? Am J Clin Nutr 55: 1033–1044.
46. Leske MC, Wu SY, Hennis A, Connell AM, Hyman L, et al. (1999) Diabetes, hypertension, and central obesity as cataract risk factors in a black population. The Barbados Eye Study. Ophthalmology 106: 35–41.
47. Younan C, Mitchell P, Cumming R, Rochtchina E, Panchapakesan J, et al. (2003) Cardiovascular disease, vascular risk factors and the incidence of cataract and cataract surgery: the Blue Mountains Eye Study. Ophthalmic Epidemiol 10: 227–240.
48. Haidar YM, Cosman BC (2011) Obesity epidemiology. Clin Colon Rectal Surg 24: 205–210.

Vitreous Hyper-Reflective Dots in Optical Coherence Tomography and Cystoid Macular Edema after Uneventful Phacoemulsification Surgery

Jong-Hyun Oh[1], Roy S. Chuck[2], Jae Rock Do[1], Choul Yong Park[1]*

1 Department of Ophthalmology, Dongguk University Ilsan Hospital, Goyang, South Korea, 2 Department of Ophthalmology and Visual Sciences, Montefiore Medical Center, Albert Einstein College of Medicine, Bronx, New York, United States of America

Abstract

Purpose: To report the observation of hyper-reflective dots in the vitreous cavity using spectral domain optical coherence tomography (SD-OCT) after uneventful phacoemulsification cataract surgery and to investigate their association with cystoid macular edema (CME).

Materials and Methods: Medical records of consecutive Asian patients who had no preoperative retinopathy and underwent uneventful phacoemulsification cataract surgery from March 2012 through February 2013 were reviewed. SD-OCTs were performed before, 1 week, and 1 month after surgery. The number of vitreous hyper-reflective dots (VHDs) was counted in 5 OCT images of high-definition 5-line raster scans. The development of CME was assessed using postoperative 1-month OCT.

Results: In 74 eyes of 74 patients, all of three SD-OCTs with a signal to noise ratio of 0.6 or more were available and were analyzed in this study. In preoperative OCT, the VHD was observed in 2 (2.7%) of 74 eyes; one eye had 1 VHD and the other eye had 2 VHDs. In 72 eyes with no preoperative VHD, VHDs were observed in 40 (55.6%) eyes at 1 week after the surgery. In the multivariate analysis, the number of VHDs measured at 1 week after the surgery was significantly associated with CME development at 1 month after the surgery (odds ratio = 1.93, 95% confidence interval = 1.15 to 3.24, $P = 0.012$).

Conclusions: VHDs were frequently observed in OCT after uneventful phacoemulsification cataract surgery. VHDs observed at 1 week after the surgery may be a risk factor for the development of pseudophakic CME. Further studies are needed to identify the source of the VHDs.

Editor: Demetrios Vavvas, Massachusetts Eye & Ear Infirmary, Harvard Medical School, United States of America

Funding: The funders had no role in study design, data collection and analysis, decision to publish, or preparation of the manuscript' in the financial disclosure.

Competing Interests: The authors have declared that no competing interests exist.

* E-mail: oph0112@gmail.com

Introduction

Pseudophakic cystoid macular edema (CME) is a common cause of unexpected visual loss after cataract surgery. The exact pathogenesis of CME is unclear; however, increased vascular permeability by inflammatory mediators may play a critical role. [1] Various preoperative and postoperative factors are proposed to increase CME after cataract surgery; iris trauma or posterior capsule rupture, vitreous loss, diabetic retinopathy, retinal vein occlusion, epiretinal membrane, or uveitis are some of those factors. [2–6] It is not uncommon; however, to encounter CME in otherwise healthy eyes after uneventful phacoemulsification surgery [7,8].

Optical coherence tomography (OCT) can obtain high-resolution cross-sectional images of various parts of the eye. It was initially utilized to evaluate the retina and the optic nerve head, but with the advance of the technology, OCT is now used to evaluate additionally other parts of the eye including cornea, tear film, choroid and vitreous body. [9–14] Using high-resolution, spectral domain (SD) OCT, we observed some hyper-reflective dots in the vitreous cavity after uneventful phacoemulsification cataract surgery (Figure 1).

In the present study, we analyzed the incidence of these vitreous hyper-reflective dots (VHDs) and their association with the development of CME after uneventful phacoemulsification surgery.

Materials and Methods

This study was designed as a retrospective case series. Written consent was given by the patients for their information to be stored in the hospital database and used for research. Institutional review board approval was obtained from the Dongguk University Ilsan Hospital, Goyang, South Korea. All research adhered to the tenets of the Declaration of Helsinki.

Patients and Data Collection

We retrospectively reviewed the medical records of consecutive patients who underwent phacoemulsification cataract surgery by a single surgeon (C.Y.P.) from March 2012 through February 2013 at Dongguk University Ilsan Hospital, Goyang, South Korea. Patients who underwent OCT examinations before, 1 week, and 1 month after surgery were included in this study. If data from both eyes were available, only the first operative eyes were included. Eyes with retinopathy including diabetic retinopathy, retinal vein occlusion, epiretinal membrane, and age-related macular degeneration, were excluded from the study. Cases with intraoperative complications, such as posterior capsule rupture, were also excluded.

Data including age, sex, history of diabetes, laterality of the eye, best-corrected Snellen visual acuity (BCVA), and biometric values were obtained. SD-OCTs with a signal to noise ratio of 0.6 or more were assessed for the study.

Patient Managements and Surgical Technique

Before cataract surgery, patients were subjected to ophthalmic examinations including BCVA measurements, biomicroscopic examination, applanation tonometry, indirect ophthalmoscopy, SD-OCT, and when needed, fluorescein angiography. In addition, partial coherence interferometry or ultrasound biometry, and Scheimpflug imaging were performed to obtain ocular biometric values. Postoperative medication included topical 1% prednisolone applied as 1 drop 4 times per day for 4 weeks, and 0.5% levofloxacin applied 4 times per day for 4 weeks. In addition to BCVA measurements, patients underwent SD-OCT 1 week and 1 month after surgery. Fundus examination was routinely performed 1 month after surgery.

The same surgical techniques were used by a single surgeon (C.Y.P.) in all cases. Under topical anesthesia, a corneal paracentesis was made with a 1-mm diamond knife and then a temporal clear corneal incision was made with a 2.8-mm diamond knife. After the anterior chamber was filled with 4% chondroitin sulfate–3% sodium hyaluronate (Viscoat, Alcon Laboratories, Fort Worth, TX), a continuous curvilinear capsulorhexis of 5 to 5.5 mm was created with a forceps followed by hydrodissection with balanced salt solution using a hydration cannula. Phacoemulsification was performed with the Stellaris phacoemulsification machine (Bausch and Lomb, Rochester, NY). A phaco chop technique was used with the following parameters: 400 mmHg vacuum, 20% initial power, and 110 cm bottle height. Phacoemulsification power was adjusted depending on the density of the lens nucleus. Automated aspiration of the remaining soft lens matter was set at 500 mmHg vacuum and 110 cm bottle height and then followed by capsule polish with a 15 mmHg vacuum and 80 cm bottle height. A single-piece hydrophobic acrylic intraocular lens (Tecnis, Abbott Medical Optics, Inc. Santa Ana, CA) was implanted in the capsular bag with an injector system and residual viscoelastic material was removed from the anterior chamber. After the hydro-sealing technique with a balanced salt solution was applied to the temporal corneal incision, the anterior chamber was reformed with balanced salt solution.

Optical Coherence Tomography

SD-OCT was performed using the Cirrus™ HD-OCT (Model 4000, software version 6.0, Carl Zeiss Meditec, Dublin, CA) using a wavelength of 840 nm and an axial resolution of 5 μm. All SD-OCT included a macular cube scan and a high-definition 5-line raster scan. The 512×128 macular cube scan produced 128 horizontal scan lines, each comprising 512 A-scans per line, of a 6 mm×6 mm area. Central subfield retinal thickness (CRT) was assessed at the macular center (1 mm diameter) using a topographic map of the macular cube scan. The high-definition 5-line raster scan, which is less affected by ocular movement due to the short scanning time, produced 5 horizontal scan lines that were 6 mm long separated by 250 μm; each scan line comprised 4096 A scans.

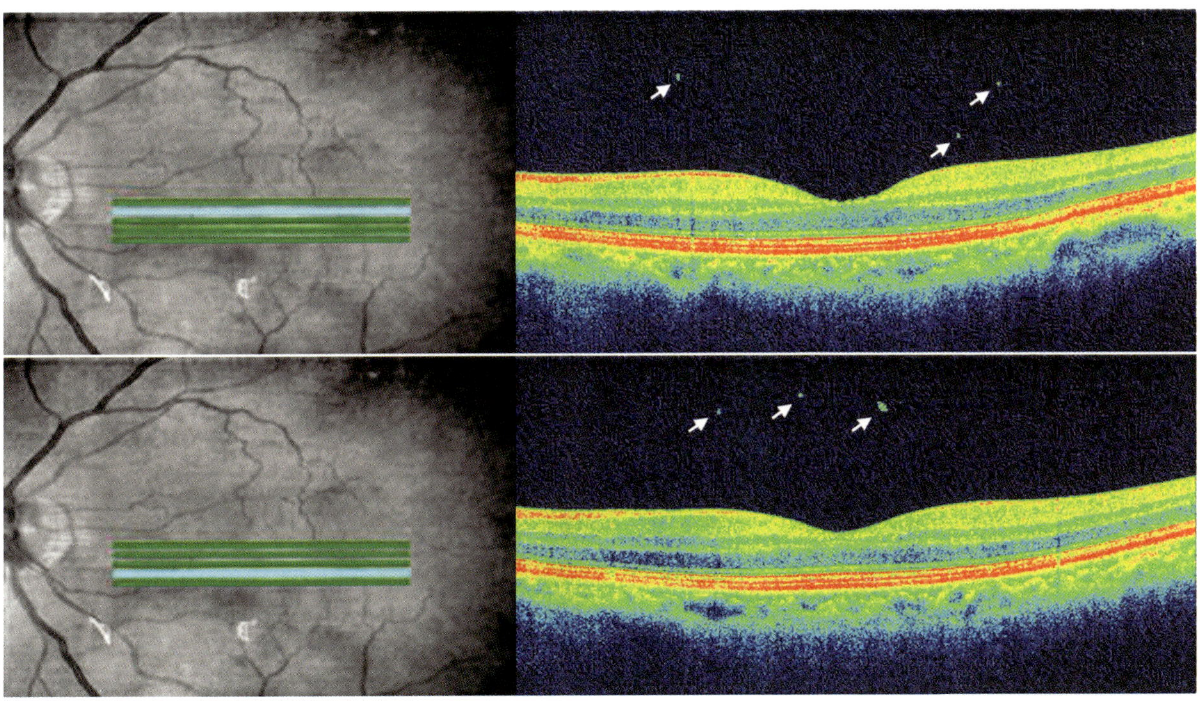

Figure 1. OCT images of an eye 1 month after uneventful phacoemulsification cataract surgery. In the vitreous cavity, hyper-reflective dots (arrows) are observed on OCT images of a high-definition 5-line raster scan images.

VHDs were identified in 5 color images of the high-definition 5-line raster scan. A VHD was defined as a hyper-reflective round- or rod-shaped dot in the vitreous cavity with a vertical length of a least 20 μm (Figure 1). The number of VHDs was counted in each image and summed twice by each of two independent observers (J.-H.O., J.R.D.). Vertical and horizontal lengths of each VHD were measured respectively with OCT software. The diameter of VHD was calculated from the average of vertical and horizontal lengths. CME was defined based on OCT as increased CRT of at least 300 μm or the presence of intraretinal cystoid spaces, defined as relative hypo-reflective areas with a surrounding hyper-reflective boundary and with the shortest diameter of at least 50 μm in macular cube scan images [2,15].

Ocular Biometric Values

Keratometric values, anterior chamber depth (ACD), and anterior chamber angle were measured with Scheimpflug imaging (Pentacam, version 1.17r24, Oculus Inc., Wetzlar, Germany). The ACD was measured from the endothelium to the anterior surface of the lens. Axial length was measured with partial coherence interferometry (IOLMaster, version 5.0, Carl Zeiss Meditec) or when needed, ultrasound biometry (Compact II, Quantel Medical, Cedex, France).

Statistical Analyses

All data were analyzed using SPSS software version 20.0 (SPSS Inc., Chicago, IL, USA). Mean, standard deviation, median, and proportion were used, as appropriate, as descriptive statistics. The Kolmogorov-Smirnov test was used to verify the normality of the distribution of continuous variables. Intra-observer reproducibilities for counting the number of VHDs were assessed using an intraclass correlation coefficient (ICC). Inter-observer ICC also measured using the number of VHDs first counted by each of two independent observers. The number of VHDs first counted by J.-H.O. was used for other analyses. For comparison between groups, the chi-square analysis or Fisher's exact test was used for categorical variables and the t-test or Mann-Whitney U test was used for continuous variables. The changes in CRT or BCVA were analyzed using a paired t-test. To identify factors for predicting CME development, multivariate logistic regression analyses were used. Odds ratios (ORs) and 95% confidence intervals (CIs) were calculated. The correlation between the number of VHD at 1week after surgery and CME development was assessed with Chi-square test for trend. All statistics were two-tailed, and a P value less than 0.05 was considered significant.

Results

One hundred ninety-six eyes of 147 Asian patients who underwent phacoemulsification cataract surgery were retrospectively reviewed. Seven eyes with diabetic retinopathy, 4 eyes with retinal vein occlusion, 4 eyes with epiretinal membrane, 2 eyes with age-related macular degeneration, and 3 eyes with an intraoperative complication of posterior capsule rupture were excluded from the study. No eyes had a history of uveitis or previous intraocular surgery such as filtering surgery or pars plana vitrectomy. Of the remaining 176 eyes, 100 eyes of 74 patients were performed all of three SD-OCTs with a signal to noise ratio of 0.6 or more before, 1 week and 1 month after surgery. Seventy-four eyes of 74 patients (33 men and 41 women) were analyzed for the study. Mean age was 68.5±9.85 years (range, 47–89), and there were 37 (50%) right eyes and 37 (50%) left eyes. In all 74 eyes, there were no serious postoperative complications, including retinal tear, retinal detachment, or endophthalmitis.

Vitreous Hyper-reflective Dots in OCT

Intra-observer ICCs for counting the number of VHDs were 0.995 [95% confidence interval (CI) = 0.993 to 0.997, $P<0.001$] and 0.991 (95% CI = 0.986 to 0.994, $P<0.001$) respectively, and inter-observer ICC was 0.989 (95% CI = 0.982 to 0.993, $P<0.001$).

In preoperative OCT, 2 (2.7%) of 74 eyes had the VHD; one eye had one VHD and the other eye had two VHDs. The median diameter of preoperative VHDs was 32 μm (range, 25–32). The remaining 72 eyes had no VHDs detected preoperatively. We performed further analysis using these 72 eyes. At 1 week after the surgery, VHDs were observed in 40 (55.6%) eyes; 18 (25.0%) eyes had one VHD, 8 (11.1%) eyes had two VHDs, and the other 14 (19.4%) eyes had at least three VHDs. Median diameter of VHDs was measured as 40 μm (range, 20–72). At 1 month after the surgery, OCTs of 72 eyes revealed VHDs in 41 (56.9%) eyes; 12 (16.7%) eyes had one VHD, 8 (11.1%) eyes had two VHDs, and the other 21 (29.2%) eyes had at least three VHDs. Median diameter of VHDs was measured as 40 μm (range, 20–78).

Factors Associated with the Presence of VHDs at 1 Week after the Surgery

Seventy two eyes with no preoperative VHD were divided into two groups according to the existence of VHD at 1 week after surgery. The characteristics of the two groups are shown in Table 1. Mean axial length in eyes with VHDs was significantly shorter than eyes without VHDs ($P = 0.039$).

The Change of CRT and BCVA in Eyes with or without VHDs

In 72 eyes with no preoperative VHD, mean CRT increased from 242±21.9 μm to 257±29.6 μm and mean BCVA improved from 0.31±0.264 logMAR to 0.10±0.158 logMAR at 1 month after surgery ($P<0.001$ and $P<0.001$ respectively). Mean postoperative CRT and BCVA showed no significant difference between eyes with or without VHDs at 1month after surgery ($P = 0.476$ and $P = 0.766$ respectively, Table 1).

VHDs and Cystoid Macular Edema

OCT-proven CME developed in 10 (13.9%) of 72 eyes at 1 month after surgery. On OCT, 4 eyes had both intraretinal cystoid spaces and increased CRT of at least 300 μm, 5 eyes showed only intraretinal cystoid spaces, and the other one eye showed only increased CRT (317 μm). The characteristics of the groups with or without CME are shown in Table 2. Age, sex, history of diabetics, laterality, preoperative BCVA, and preoperative biometric values did not differ between two groups with or without CME. The mean postoperative CRT measured at 1 month after surgery was significantly thicker in the group with CME than that in the group without CME ($P = 0.002$); however, the mean postoperative BCVA did not differ between two groups ($P = 0.811$). The number of VHDs at 1 week and 1 month postoperatively was significantly greater in the group with CME than in the group without CME ($P = 0.025$ and $P = 0.004$, respectively). In the multivariate analysis, age (OR = 1.14, 95% CI = 1.01 to 1.28, $P = 0.032$) and the number of postoperative 1-week VHDs (OR = 1.93, 95% CI = 1.15 to 3.24, $P = 0.012$) were significantly associated with CME development at 1 month after surgery (Table 3 and Figure 2). The number of postoperative 1-week VHDs was significantly correlated with CME development ($P = 0.001$, Table 4).

Table 1. Characteristics of eyes with or without VHDs at 1 week after the surgery.

Factor		Eyes		
		without VHD	With VHD(%)*	
		(n = 32)	(n = 40)	*P* value
Age, years		67.2±10.74	69.6±9.16	0.314
Sex, n				
	male	14	18 (56.3%)	0.916
	female	18	22 (55.0%)	
History of diabetes, n				
	no	27	34 (55.7%)	0.999†
	yes	5	6 (54.5%)	
Laterality, n				
	OD	13	23 (63.9%)	0.155
	OS	19	17 (47.2%)	
Preoperative BCVA, logMAR		0.33±0.273	0.30±0.258	0.565
Snellen equivalent		20/43	20/40	
Biometric values				
Mean keratometric value, D		42.6±1.21	43.0±1.60	0.278
Anterior chamber depth, mm		2.71±0.439	2.59±0.340	0.172
Anterior chamber angle, degrees		34.2±5.92	31.8±6.44	0.121
Axial length, mm		24.2±1.14	23.6±1.04	0.039
Preoperative CRT, μm		243±21.6	242±22.3	0.727
Postoperative 1-month BCVA, logMAR		0.11±0.137	0.10±0.175	0.766
Snellen equivalent		20/26	20/25	
Postoperative 1-month CRT, μm		254±24.9	259±33.0	0.476

VHD = vitreous hyper-reflective dot; BCVA = best-corrected visual acuity; logMAR = the logarithm of the minimum angle of resolution; D = diopters; CRT = central subfield retinal thickness.
Results are expressed a mean ± standard deviation.
*Incidence of VHDs in total cases of stated condition.
P values were calculated with the chi-square analysis or Fisher exact test† for categorical variables and t-test for continuous variables.

Discussion

In the present study, we found that VHDs were frequently observed in OCT after uneventful phacoemulsification surgery. In addition, the number of VHDs detected at 1 week after the surgery was significantly associated with the development of CME at 1 month. The exact nature of VHDs in this study is a key feature that can explain the relation between VHDs and CME. However, it is not feasible to perform a pathologic analysis using a sample obtained from a functioning eye. Therefore, we estimated the etiology of VHDs based on a review of previous studies. The possible nature of VHDs includes, but not limited to, lens fragments, denatured proteins, and clumps of intraocular cells.

Ang et al. [16] reported that retrocapsular lens fragments are present in 17% of patients, suggesting the entry into the retrolenticular space via weak zonules. In the present study, VHDs may be retrocapsular lens fragments that sank into the posterior vitreous cavity over time. However, Liu et al. [17,18] reported that all anterior vitreous specimens were negative for lens matter in a cytopathologic study of patients undergoing combined phacoemulsification and vitrectomy. Therefore, there is debate about the lenticular fragment access into vitreous cavity.

Yoshimoto et al. [19] demonstrated that vitreous collagen fibrils are condensed by laser-induced heat in bovine and pig eyes. The heat generated during phacoemulsification may denature vitreous fibrils and appear as VHDs in postoperative period.

Inflammatory cells usually infiltrate eyeball after surgery trauma. Saito et al. [12] previously reported that vitreous cavity cells could be visualized as hyper-reflective dots in OCT in uveitic eyes. However, it is noteworthy that their hyper-reflective dots ranged from 15 μm to 20 μm whereas the VHDs in our study were a least 20 μm in size in the definition. During phacoemulsification, zonular stress may cause epithelial cells to be released from the ciliary body. [20] These cells are another candidate for VHDs. Although the exact nature of VHDs is unclear, the significant association of VHDs with postoperative CME suggests that the VHD may be related to the postoperative inflammation and vascular permeability which are known as the most potent inducers of CME.

It is interesting that VHDs were also observed in the preoperative OCT. The nature of preoperative VHDs can be aggregation of collagen fibrils [21] or asteroid bodies presenting as hyper-reflective lesions in OCT. [22,23] The vitreous body contains hyalocytes and fibroblasts, although the number is small. [24] Hyalocytes range from 10 to 15 μm in diameter, and fibroblasts are usually localized in the cortex near the ciliary processes, vitreous base, and adjacent to the optic disc. [24,25] Therefore, these cells are not likely to be detected as VHD (vertical length of a least 20 μm) in our study.

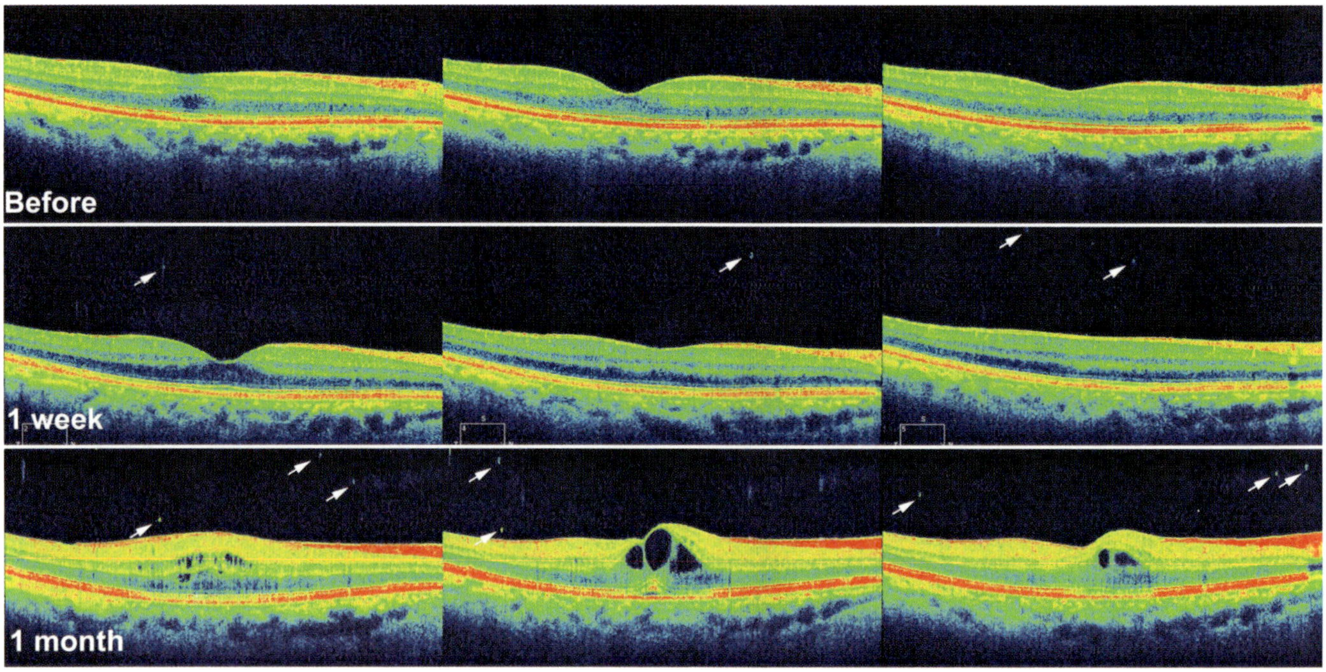

Figure 2. Serial OCT images of an eye with cystoid macular edema at 1 month after uneventful phacoemulsification cataract surgery. VHDs (arrows) are observed at 1 week and 1 month after the surgery in OCT and intraretinal cystoid spaces are observed in OCT at 1 month after the surgery.

The incidence of pseudophakic CME ranges from 4% to 11% in OCT after uneventful phacoemulsification cataract surgery, [6,8,26] and peaks at approximately 4 to 6 weeks. [2,7] In the present study, the incidence of CME at 1 month after surgery was 13.9%. The incidence is slightly higher; however, it is difficult to compare due to different study designs, surgical techniques, subject characteristics, and definitions of CME. Currently in the literature, there is no validated or universally accepted method for reporting pseudophakic CME. [15,27] Although fluorescein angiography remains the gold standard, [2] CME was defined based on OCT, but without reference to the vision loss in the present study. In addition, our definition of CME included not only the thickening of the retina, but also subtle intraretinal cystoid abnormalities without substantial increase in retinal thickness. It is known that intraretinal cystoid change without retinal thickening may be more common pattern in the macular changes which can be detected with OCT after cataract surgery. [15] With recent advance in technology, SD-OCT allows us to detect subtle changes of the macula. [28] Our definition of CME may result in not-significant difference in the mean postoperative BCVA between the groups with and without CME.

Using multivariate analyses, we found that the number of VHDs at 1 week after the surgery was significantly associated with the development of CME at 1 month. Therefore, VHDs observed at 1 week after surgery may be used as a risk factor (OR = 1.93) for CME development after routine cataract surgery. Intensive CME prevention using anti-inflammatory topical drugs may be helpful in the patients with high number of VHDs at 1 week after cataract surgery. It is noteworthy that the presence of VHDs at 1 week did not influence CRT and BCVA at 1 month in this study. These findings may be related to low incidence (17.5%) of CME in eyes with postoperative 1-week VHDs and the small difference of CRT between eyes with or without CME (mean CRT 296 μm vs. 251 μm, table 2). In addition, the same BCVA does not necessarily translate to identical functional vision. [29] For example, macular edema can affect lower more than higher contrast visual acuity. [30,31] As expected, age was significantly associated with CME development in this study. Previous studies reported a positive correlation of CME with age, demonstrating an increased incidence of CME in older patients [3,32].

This study has several limitations. Nuclear density and surgical techniques (phaco duration and power) may affect the presence of VHDs after surgery. However, retrospective study design prevented further analysis. Second, poor image quality due to cataract could interrupt the detection of VHDs in preoperative OCT. Even though we analyzed only SD-OCT with a signal to noise ratio of 0.6 or more, removal of the cataract will increase signal transmission of SD-OCT to the vitreous and may increase the detection of pre-existing VHDs. Another limitation of our study is that VHDs were manually counted. A VHD was at least 20 μm in size by definition in order to differentiate it from noise. However, ICCs for counting the number of VHDs were all >0.9. Another limitation is that VHDs were counted only in the posterior vitreous cavity near the retina. Therefore, the incidence of VHDs in the whole vitreous cavity was likely underestimated in the present study. If the source of VHDs were something migrating from the anterior part to the posterior part of the vitreous cavity after the surgery, it is unlikely in eyes with a longer axial length that VHDs would reach the posterior vitreous cavity and be detected with OCT. The finding that axial length of eyes with VHDs was significantly shorter, although the mean difference was measured only 0.6 mm, may be understood in the same context. In addition, high-definition 5-line raster scan images of the Cirrus™ HD-OCT were used to detect VHDs even though macular cube scan images show a more extensive region. The high-definition 5-line raster scan images with higher resolution allowed us to more reliably detect VHDs. Further study is needed to confirm whether images from other OCT devices can be used

Table 2. Characteristics of groups with or without CME in OCT 1 month after surgery.

		CME development		
		no	yes (%)*	
Factor		**(n = 62)**	**(n = 10)**	***P* value**
Age, years		67.9±10.05	72.4±8.25	0.189
Sex, n				
	male	26	6 (18.8%)	0.317
	female	37	4 (9.8%)	
History of diabetes, n				
	no	53	9 (14.5%)	0.999
	Yes	10	1 (9.1%)	
Laterality, n				
	OD	32	5 (13.5%)	0.999
	OS	31	5 (13.9%)	
Preoperative BCVA, logMAR		0.31±0.272	0.35±0.216	0.337
Snellen equivalent		20/41	20/45	
Biometric values				
Mean keratometric value, D		42.8±1.38	42.9±1.88	0.968
Anterior chamber depth, mm		2.65±0.394	2.58±0.375	0.563
Anterior chamber angle, degrees		33.1±6.50	31.2±4.61	0.449
Axial length, mm		23.9±1.07	23.8±1.41	0.654
Preoperative CRT, μm		241±20.0	249±31.6	0.479
Postoperative 1-month BCVA, logMAR		0.11±0.160	0.09±0.151	0.811
Snellen equivalent		20/26	20/25	
Postoperative 1-month CRT, μm		251±21.1	296±44.6	0.002
Median number of 1-week VHDs, n (range)		1.0 (0–8)	2.5 (0–18)	0.025
Median number of 1-month VHDs, n (range)		1.0 (0–10)	5.0 (0–11)	0.004

CME = cystoid macular edema; OCT = optical coherence tomography; BCVA = best-corrected visual acuity; logMAR = the logarithm of the minimum angle of resolution; D = diopters; CRT = central subfield retinal thickness; VHD = vitreous hyper-reflective dot.
Results are expressed a mean ± standard deviation.
*Incidence of CME in total cases of each condition.
P values were calculated with the Fisher exact test for categorical variables and the Mann-Whitney U test for continuous variables.

Table 3. Multivariate logistic regression results for predicting CME development.

Factor	**OR**	**95% CI**	***P* value**
Age, years	1.136	1.011 to 1.276	0.032
Sex, male	2.664	0.412 to 17.226	0.304
History of diabetes	0.174	0.010 to 3.142	0.236
Laterality, OD	0.495	0.068 to 3.595	0.487
Preoperative BCVA, logMAR	0.918	0.040 to 21.1651	0.957
Mean keratometric value, D	0.847	0.416 to 1.723	0.646
Anterior chamber depth, mm	3.185	0.181 to 55.992	0.428
Anterior chamber angle, degrees	0.958	0.789 to 1.163	0.665
Axial length, mm	1.562	0.515 to 4.735	0.431
Preoperative CRT, μm	0.995	0.952 to 1.041	0.836
Postoperative 1-week VHDs, n	1.934	1.154 to 3.242	0.012

CME = cystoid macular edema; OR = odds ratio, CI = confidence interval; BCVA = best-corrected visual acuity; logMAR = the logarithm of the minimum angle of resolution; D = diopters; CRT = central subfield retinal thickness; VHD = vitreous hyper-reflective dot.

Table 4. The correlation between the number of postoperative 1-week VHD and the development of CME.

	CME		
Number of VHDs	**no**	**yes (%)**	***P* value***
0	29	3 (9.4%)	0.001
1	18	0 (0%)	
2	6	2 (25.0%)	
3	4	1 (20.0%)	
4	2	1 (33.3%)	
5	1	0 (0%)	
6	1	1 (50%)	
8	1	1 (50%)	
18	0	1 (100%)	

VHD = vitreous hyper-reflective dot; CME = cystoid macular edema.
*chi-square test for trend (linear-by-linear association).

comparably to detect VHD. Another limitation relates to the lack of follow-up. Long-term prospective studies are needed to identify how long the VHDs remain and to understand the pathophysiology of VHDs.

In conclusion, the emergence of VHDs was frequently observed in OCT at 1 week and at 1 month after uneventful phacoemulsification surgery. The VHD observed at 1 week after the surgery was a risk factor for the CME development. To the best of our knowledge, this study is the first to report VHDs after phacoemulsification surgery and their clinical significance. Further studies to investigate the etiology of VHDs after cataract surgery are warranted.

Acknowledgments

We thank Chiyeon Lim, PhD, at the Department of Biostatistics, Dongguk University Ilsan Hospital, for providing statistical assistance.

Author Contributions

Conceived and designed the experiments: CYP RSC. Performed the experiments: CYP J-HO JRD. Analyzed the data: CYP J-HO. Contributed reagents/materials/analysis tools: J-HO JRD. Wrote the paper: J-HO CYP RSC.

References

1. Benitah NR, Arroyo JG (2010) Pseudophakic cystoid macular edema. Int Ophthalmol Clin 50: 139–153.
2. Yonekawa Y, Kim IK (2012) Pseudophakic cystoid macular edema. Curr Opin Ophthalmol 23: 26–32.
3. Lobo C (2012) Pseudophakic cystoid macular edema. Ophthalmologica 227: 61–67.
4. Hayashi K, Igarashi C, Hirata A, Hayashi H (2009) Changes in diabetic macular oedema after phacoemulsification surgery. Eye (Lond) 23: 389–396.
5. Henderson BA, Kim JY, Ament CS, Ferrufino-Ponce ZK, Grabowska A, et al. (2007) Clinical pseudophakic cystoid macular edema. Risk factors for development and duration after treatment. J Cataract Refract Surg 33: 1550–1558.
6. Belair ML, Kim SJ, Thorne JE, Dunn JP, Kedhar SR, et al. (2009) Incidence of cystoid macular edema after cataract surgery in patients with and without uveitis using optical coherence tomography. Am J Ophthalmol 148: 128–135.
7. Kusbeci T, Eryigit L, Yavas G, Inan UU (2012) Evaluation of cystoid macular edema using optical coherence tomography and fundus fluorescein angiography after uncomplicated phacoemulsification surgery. Curr Eye Res 37: 327–333.
8. Vukicevic M, Gin T, Al-Qureshi S (2012) Prevalence of optical coherence tomography-diagnosed postoperative cystoid macular oedema in patients following uncomplicated phaco-emulsification cataract surgery. Clin Experiment Ophthalmol 40: 282–287.
9. Li Y, Meisler DM, Tang M, Lu AT, Thakrar V, et al. (2008) Keratoconus diagnosis with optical coherence tomography pachymetry mapping. Ophthalmology 115: 2159–2166.
10. Ibrahim OM, Dogru M, Takano Y, Satake Y, Wakamatsu TH, et al. (2010) Application of visante optical coherence tomography tear meniscus height measurement in the diagnosis of dry eye disease. Ophthalmology 117: 1923–1929.
11. Margolis R, Spaide RF (2009) A pilot study of enhanced depth imaging optical coherence tomography of the choroid in normal eyes. Am J Ophthalmol 147: 811–815.
12. Saito M, Barbazetto IA, Spaide RF (2013) Intravitreal cellular infiltrate imaged as punctate spots by spectral-domain optical coherence tomography in eyes with posterior segment inflammatory disease. Retina 33: 559–565.
13. Orefice JL, Costa RA, Scott IU, Calucci D, Orefice F (2013) Spectral optical coherence tomography findings in patients with ocular toxoplasmosis and active satellite lesions (MINAS Report 1). Acta Ophthalmol 91: e41–47.
14. Diniz B, Regatieri C, Andrade R, Maia A (2011) Evaluation of spectral domain and time domain optical coherence tomography findings in toxoplasmic retinochoroiditis. Clin Ophthalmol 5: 645–650.
15. Kim SJ, Bressler NM (2009) Optical coherence tomography and cataract surgery. Curr Opin Ophthalmol 20: 46–51.
16. Ang A, Menezo i Rallo V, Shepstone L, Burton RL (2004) Retrocapsular lens fragments after uneventful phacoemulsification cataract surgery. J Cataract Refract Surg 30: 849–853.
17. Liu DT, Lee VY, Li CL, Choi PC, Lam PT, et al. (2008) Retrocapsular lens matter in uneventful phacoemulsification: does it really exist? Clin Experiment Ophthalmol 36: 31–35.
18. Liu DT, Choi PC, Chan WM, Lam DS (2005) Retrocapsular lens fragments after uneventful phacoemulsification cataract surgery. J Cataract Refract Surg 31: 1856–1857.
19. Yoshimoto H, Kampik A, Birngruber R, Gabel VP (1984) Vitreous morphology after carbon dioxide laser irradiation. Graefes Arch Clin Exp Ophthalmol 221: 276–281.
20. Raviola G (1971) The fine structure of the ciliary zonule and ciliary epithelium. With special regard to the organization and insertion of the zonular fibrils. Invest Ophthalmol 10: 851–869.
21. Sebag J, Balazs EA (1989) Morphology and ultrastructure of human vitreous fibers. Invest Ophthalmol Vis Sci 30: 1867–1871.
22. Mochizuki Y, Hata Y, Kita T, Kohno R, Hasegawa Y, et al. (2009) Anatomical findings of vitreoretinal interface in eyes with asteroid hyalosis. Graefes Arch Clin Exp Ophthalmol 247: 1173–1177.
23. Hwang JC, Barile GR, Schiff WM, Ober MD, Smith RT, et al. (2006) Optical coherence tomography in asteroid hyalosis. Retina 26: 661–665.
24. Ponsioen TL, Hooymans JM, Los LI (2010) Remodelling of the human vitreous and vitreoretinal interface–a dynamic process. Prog Retin Eye Res 29: 580–595.
25. Bloom GD, Balazs EA (1965) An electron microscopic study of hyalocytes. Exp Eye Res 4: 249–255.
26. Perente I, Utine CA, Ozturker C, Cakir M, Kaya V, et al. (2007) Evaluation of macular changes after uncomplicated phacoemulsification surgery by optical coherence tomography. Curr Eye Res 32: 241–247.

27. Kim SJ, Belair ML, Bressler NM, Dunn JP, Thorne JE, et al. (2008) A method of reporting macular edema after cataract surgery using optical coherence tomography. Retina 28: 870–876.
28. Gabriele ML, Wollstein G, Ishikawa H, Kagemann L, Xu J, et al. (2011) Optical coherence tomography: history, current status, and laboratory work. Invest Ophthalmol Vis Sci 52: 2425–2436.
29. Ibanez HE, Lesher MP, Singerman LJ, Rice TA, Keep GF (1993) Prospective evaluation of the effect of pseudophakic cystoid macula edema on contrast sensitivity. Arch Ophthalmol 111: 1635–1639.
30. Ginsburg AP, Cheetham JK, DeGryse RE, Abelson M (1995) Effects of flurbiprofen and indomethacin on acute cystoid macular edema after cataract surgery: functional vision and contrast sensitivity. J Cataract Refract Surg 21: 82–92.
31. Sukha AY, Rubin A (2009) High, medium, and low contrast visual acuities in diabetic retinal disease. Optom Vis Sci 86: 1086–1095.
32. Stern AL, Taylor DM, Dalburg LA, Cosentino RT (1981) Pseudophakic cystoid maculopathy: a study of 50 cases. Ophthalmology 88: 942–946.

22

Inhibition of Pirfenidone on TGF-beta2 Induced Proliferation, Migration and Epithlial-Mesenchymal Transition of Human Lens Epithelial Cells Line SRA01/04

Yangfan Yang, Yiming Ye, Xianchai Lin, Kaili Wu, Minbin Yu*

State Key Laboratory of Ophthalmology, Zhongshan Ophthalmic Center, Sun Yat-sen University, Guangzhou, China

Abstract

Background: Posterior capsular opacification (PCO) is a common complication of cataract surgery. Transforming growth factor-β2 (TGF-β2) plays important roles in the development of PCO. The existing pharmacological treatments are not satisfactory and can have toxic side effects.

Methodologies/Principal Findings: We evaluated the effect of pirfenidone on proliferation, migration and epithlial-mesenchymal transition of human lens epithelial cell line SRA01/04 (HLECs) in vitro. After treatment with 0, 0.25, and 0.5 mg/ml pirfenidone, cell proliferation was measured by MTT assay. Cell viability was determined by trypan blue exclusion assay and measurement of lactate dehydrogenase (LDH) activity released from the damaged cells. And cell migration was measured by scratch assay in the absence or presence of transforming growth factor-β2 (TGF-β2). The expressions of TGF-β2 and SMADs were evaluated with real-time RT-PCR, western blot, and immunofluorescence analyses. The mesenchymal phenotypic marker fibronectin (FN) was demonstrated by Immunocytofluorescence analyses. The cells had high viability, which did not vary across different concentrations of pirfenidone (0 [control] 0.3, 0.5 or 1.0 mg/ml) after 24 hours. Pirfenidone (0~0.5 mg/ml) had no significant cytotoxicity effect on SRA01/04 by LDH assay. Pirfenidone significantly inhibited the proliferation and TGF-β2-induced cell migration and the effects were dose-dependent, and inhibited TGF-β2-induced fibroblastic phenotypes and TGF-β2-induced expression of FN in SRA01/04 cells. The cells showed dose-dependent decreases in mRNA and protein levels of TGF-β2 and SMADs. Pirfenidone also depressed the TGF-β2-induced expression of SMADs and blocked the nuclear translocation of SMADs in cells.

Conclusion: Pirfenidone inhibits TGF-β2-induced proliferation, migration and epithlial-mesenchymal transition of human lens epithelial cells line SRA01/04 at nontoxic concentrations. This effect may be achieved by down regulation of TGF-β/SAMD signaling in SRA01/04 cells.

Editor: Ed Manser, Astar-Neuroscience Research Partnership (NRP) and Institute of Medical Biology (IMB), Singapore

Funding: This study was funded by Guangdong Science and Technology Fund (Grant No. 2009B030801193), Medical Scientific Research Foundation of Guangdong Province (Grant No.B2012128) and Fundamental Research Funds of State Key Laboratory of Ophthalmology, People's Republic of China. The funders had no role in study design, data collection and analysis, decision to publish, or preparation of the manuscript.

Competing Interests: The authors have declared that no competing interests exist.

* E-mail: yuminbin@mail.sysu.edu.cn

Introduction

Posterior capsular opacification (PCO) is the most frequent complication of cataract surgery and mainly caused by fibrosis on lens capsular bag and/or posterior capsule [1]. Previous studies have shown that many growth factors, especially transforming growth factor-β2 (TGF-β2), play important roles in the development of PCO, which may trigger a series of events (including cell proliferation, differentiation, migration and capsular fibrosis) during wound healing process [2–5]. Blockage of TGF-β2 signaling may represent a means to prevent the development of PCO.

Many methods have previously been developed to prevent the development of such fibrosis. These include topical administration of anti-inflammation medications (e.g., dexamethasone, heparin, diclofenac) [6–8] or anti-metabolic agents (e.g., 5-fluorouracil, mitomycin) [9,10], improved design of intraocular lens (IOL) [11,12], new IOL materials, and modified surgical procedures (e.g., bag-in-the-lens IOL implantation, optic buttonholing) [13–15]. However, none of the pharmacological therapies is effective and safe enough for the prevention of PCO, and some of them are toxic [16,17]. New IOLs and modified surgical methods have led to a significant reduction of PCO in some, but not all patients[16], and they are costly and may not be readily available in low-income countries.

Pirfenidone (PFD) is a novel broad-spectrum anti-inflammatory and anti-fibrosis agent, and it has been widely used as an oral formulation for systemic treatment of idiopathic pulmonary fibrosis (IPF) [18]. Our research team has previously shown that PFD can prevent the proliferation and migration of cultured human Tenon capsule fibroblasts (HTFs) and reduce fibrosis in a rabbit model of glaucoma filtration surgery, and pharmacokinetic analysis showed that PFD can be used as a topical eye drop.

Table 1. Human Primer Sequences Used for Realtime RT-PCR.

Gene	Sense Primer	Antisense Primer	Probe (bp)
TGFβ2	GAGGGATCTAGGGTGGAAATGG	AGGACCCTGCTGTGCTGAGT	104
SMAD3	TCGAGCCCCAGAGCAATATT	CGTCCATGCTGTGGTTCATC	97
SMAD4	ACATTGGATGGGAGGCTTCA	GATCAGGCCACCTCCAGAGA	95
β-actin	GCATGGGTCAGAAGGATTCCT	TCGTCCCAGTTGGTGACGAT	106

Toxicity assessments showed that PFD did not damage the rabbit eyes [19–21].

In the current study, we hypothesized that PFD can suppress the proliferation and migration of human lens epithelial cells (HLECs). We investigated the effects of PFD on proliferation and migration of HLECs. Considering the important effect of TGF-β2 signaling pathway, we examined the roles of PFD on mRNA or protein expression TGF-β2 and SMADs and the nuclear translocation of SMADs.

Materials and Methods

Cell Culture

The SV40 T-antigen-transformed human lens epithelial cell line [22], SRA01/04, was obtained from Cancer Institute of Chinese Academy of Medical Sciences. Cells were cultured in modified Eagle's medium (α-MEM; Hyclone, Logan, UT) supplemented with 10% fetal bovine serum (FBS) and 1% non-essential amino-acid (NEAA) at 37°C in a humidified atmosphere containing 5% CO2. Culture plates were coated for 30 min at 37°C with gelatin solution before cell inoculation.

MTT Assay

HLECs were seeded in 96-well plates (1.0×10^4 cells/well) for 24 hours in α-MEM/10% FBS/1%NEAA, and were cultured in stationary tubes in serum-free medium for 24 hours. And then the culture medium was removed and cells were bathed in α-MEM with 10% FBS and 1% NEAA supplemented with 0, 0.01, 0.1, 0.2,

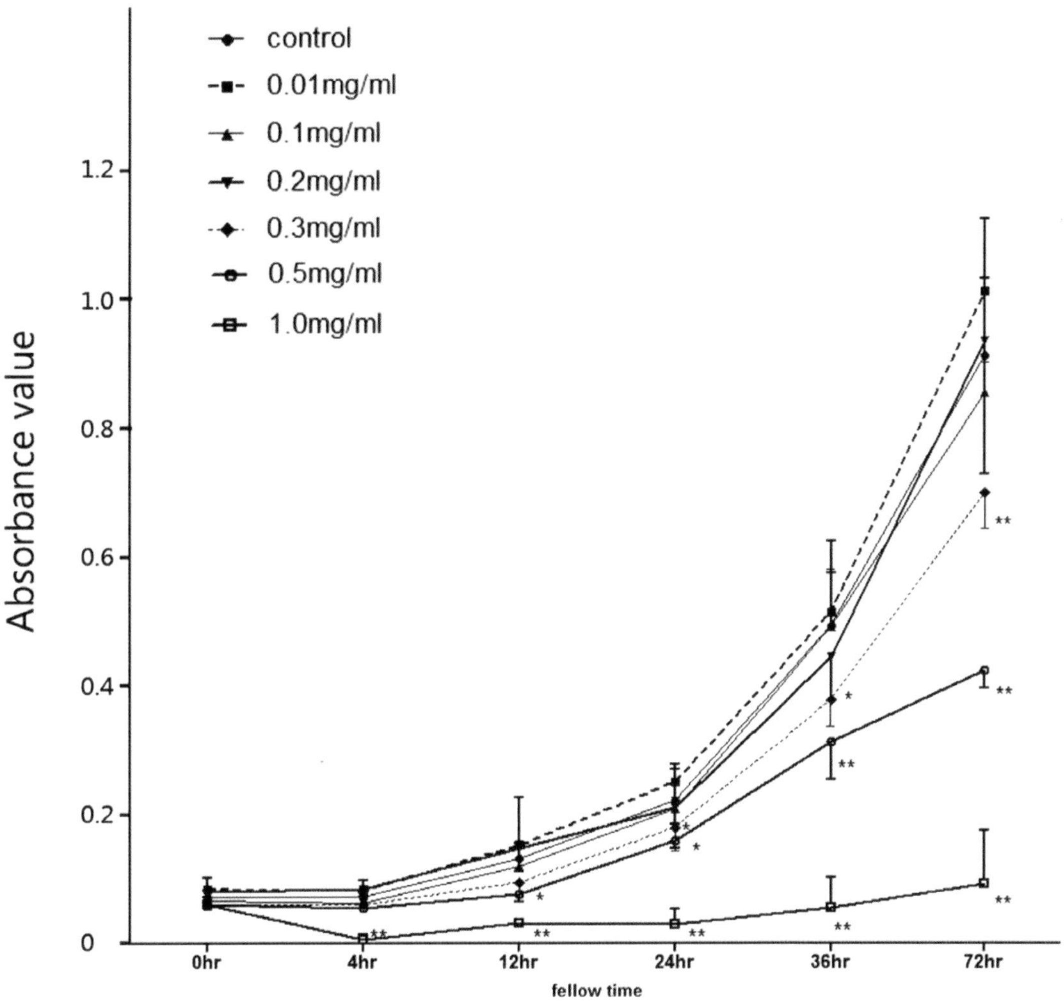

Figure 1. Inhibitory effect of pirfenidone on proliferation of SRA01/04 cells as measured by MTT assay. Cells with 10% FBS were treated with 0, 0.01, 0.1, 0.2, 0.3, 0.5, or 1.0 mg/mL pirfenidone for 0, 4, 12, 24, 48, or 72 hours. Data are derived from the mean ± SD of triplicate results in three independent experiments. *P<0.05, and **P<0.001 from comparisons between cells with treatment and control cells with 10% FBS, at different time points.

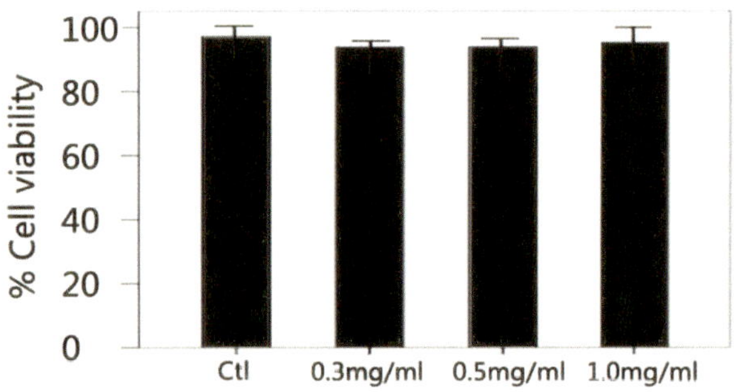

Figure 2. Cell viability of SRA01/04 cells after treated with pirfenidone for 24 hours in a trypan blue exclusion test. After 24 hours' treatment with PFD (0, 0.3, 0.5, and 1 mg/ml), the percentages of living cells were more than 90% in all groups. No statistically significant difference was found between PFD treated and control groups ($P>0.05$). Data are the mean ± SD of triplicates from an experiment that was repeated with similar results.

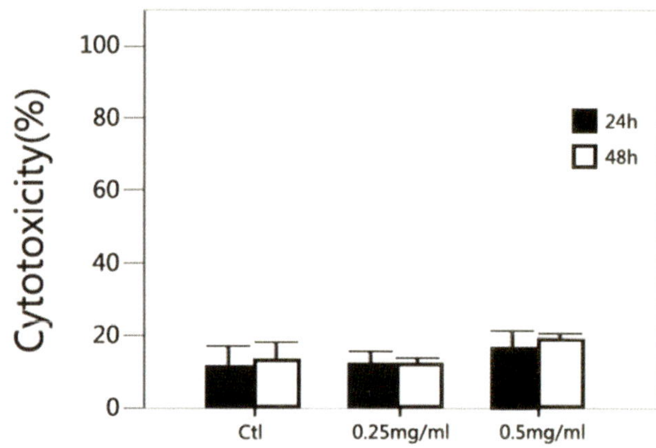

Figure 3. Cytotoxicity of pirfenidone in a LDH assay. After 24 or 48 hours' treatment with PFD (0, 0.25, and 0.5 mg/ml), no statistically significant difference was found between the percentage of cell-mediated lysis in PFD treated groups and control group ($P>0.05$). Data are the mean ± SD of triplicates from an experiment that was repeated with similar results.

0.3, 0.5, or 1 mg/ml PFD (Sigma-Aldrich, St. Louis, MO) for 0, 4, 12, 24, 48, or 72 hours. After incubation with 180 μL α-MEM and 20 μL of 5 mg/ml 3-[4, 5-dimethylthiazol-2-yl] -2, 5-diphenyl tetrazolium bromide (MTT, Amresco, Solon, OH) for 4 hours at 37°C, the MTT solution was discarded. The Formosan precipitates were dissolved in 180 μL DMSO (Amresco, Solon, OH) by agitating the dishes for 10 minutes at 200 rpm on an orbital shaker. The absorbance at 490 nm in each well was read with a micro plate reader (Bio-Tek, Vermont, U.S.A). We further examined the effects of PFD by refining the concentrations at 0.2, 0.25, 0.3, 0.4, 0.5 and 0.6 mg/ml using the MTT assay.

Cell Viability Assay

Cell viability was evaluated by both trypan blue exclusion method and measurement of lactate dehydrogenase (LDH) activity released from the cytosol of damaged cells. In trypan blue exclusion test, HLECs were treated with PFD at the concentrations of 0, 0.3, 0.5 or 1 mg/ml. Cell viability was measured within 24 hours. After dye with trypan blue, stained (dead) and unstained (viable) cells were counted with a hematocytometer. The percentage of living cell was calculated according to the following

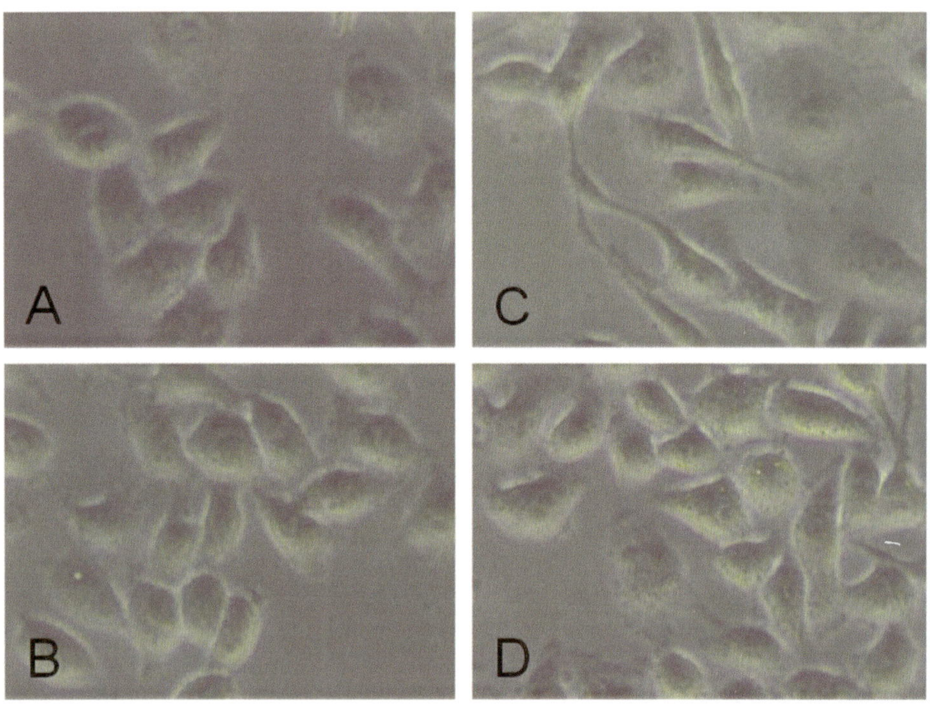

Figure 4. Inhibitory effect of pirfenidone on TGF-β2-induced fibroblastic phenotypes in SRA01/04 cells. There was no apparent morphological change in SRA01/04 cells after 24 hours' treatment with 0.5 mg/ml PFD only (B) compared with control cells(A). In the presence of 12.5 ng/ml TGF-β2, the TGF-β2-induced morphological changes in SRA01/04 cells (C) were detected, including elongated and spindle-like shapes, which were noticeably suppressed by co-treatment with 0.5 mg/ml PFD (D).

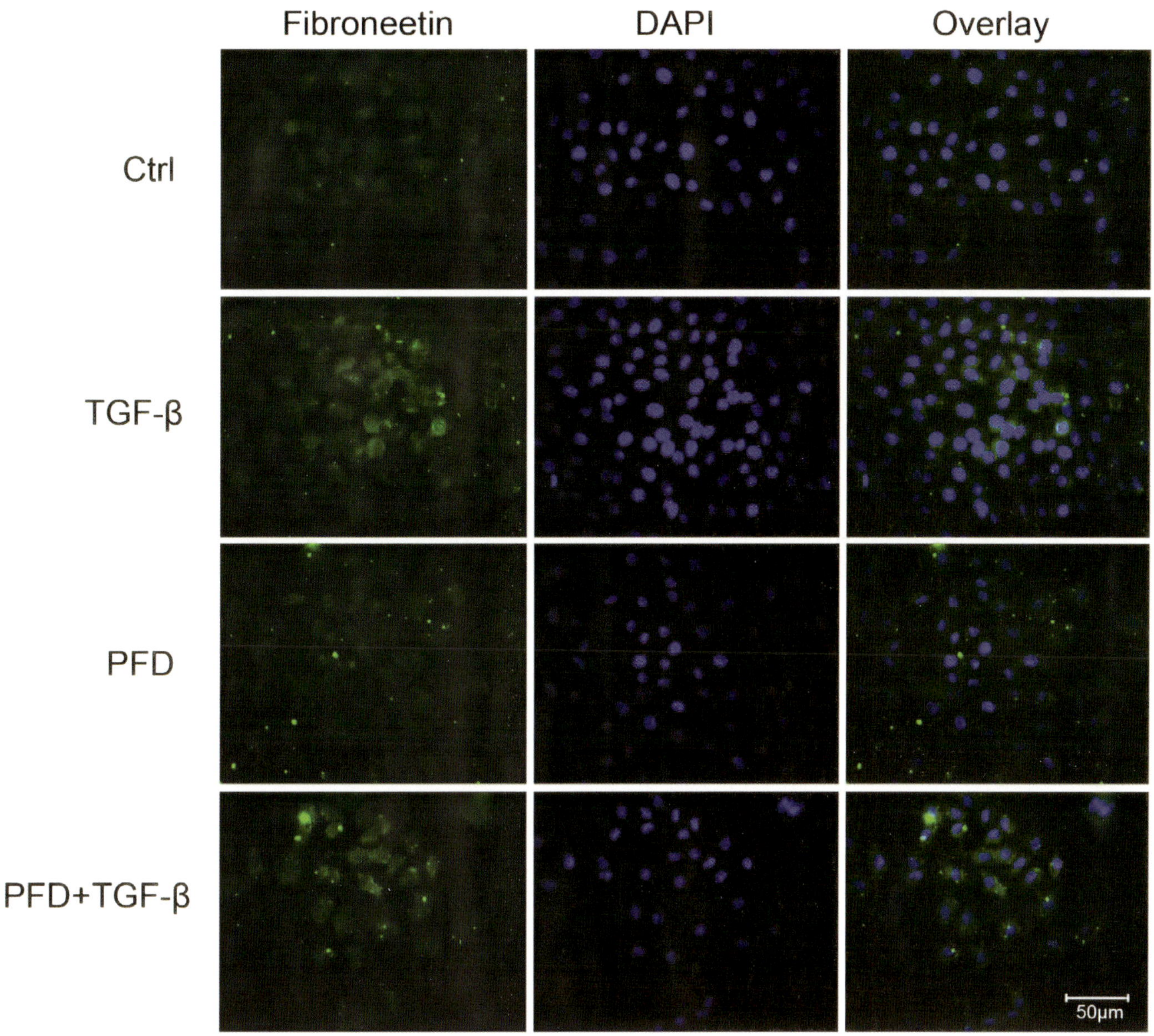

Figure 5. Inhibitory effect of pirfenidone on TGF-β2-induced epithlial-mesenchymal transition in SRA01/04 cells. Compared with control cells (A), immunocytofluorescence demonstrated that the TGF-beta2 significantly up-regulated the mesenchymal phenotypic marker fibronectin (FN, green) in SRA01/04 cells (C). Either in the absence (B) or presence (D) of TGF-beta2, FN was significantly down-regulated after 24 hours' treatment with 0.5 mg/ml PFD. The nuclei stained by DAPI (blue). Magnification, ×400.

formula: % cell viability = (viable cell count/total cell count) × 100. In LDH assay, LDH activity release from the demaged cells was measureed after treatment with 0.25 mg/ml and 0.5 mg/ml PFD. The cultrue medium was collected and a Cytotoxicity Detection Kit (Roche, Penzberg, Germany) was used for the assay. The percentage of cell-mediated lysis was expressed asaccording to the following formula: % cytotoxicity = (exp. value − low control)/(high control − low control).

Cell Migration Assay

We use scarification test to measure the migration ability of the cells. First, the HLECs were grown to a confluent monolayer and then placed in serum-free medium for 24 hours. After the medium was discarded, we make a straight line scratch across the cell layer with a p20 pipette tip and then rinsed with Phosphate buffered saline (PBS) to remove the suspended cells and treated with 0, 0.25 or 0.5 mg/ml PFD in the absence or presence of 12.5 ng/ml TGF-β2 (R&D System, Minneapolis, MN) for 24 hours. The scratch gap was recorded and photographed after 24 hours under a light microscope and analyzed with an image processing software (Photoshop 7.0; Adobe, San Jose, CA).

Real-time Reverse Transcription-polymerase Chain Reaction

HLECs were treated with PFD at the concentrations of 0, 0.25, or 0.5 mg/ml for 24 hours, and then the RNA was isolated from cultured cells with TRIzol reagent (Invitrogen, Carlsbad, CA). Reverse transcription - polymerase chain reaction (RT-PCR) was carried out using the one-step reverse transcription-polymerase

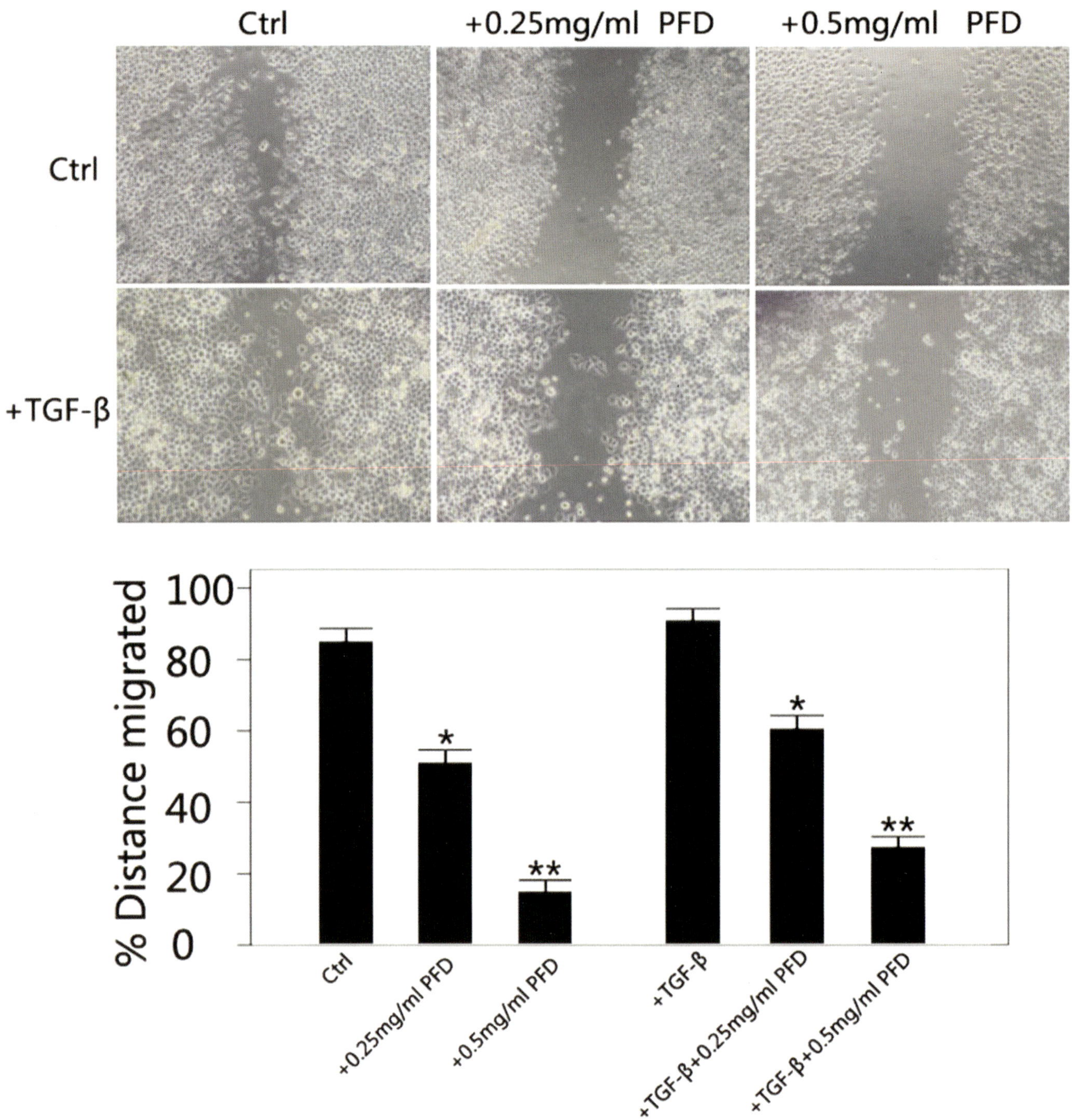

Figure 6. Inhibitory effect of pirfenidone on TGF-β2-induced migration of SRA01/04 cells. Light microscope images show decreased migratory ability of cells at 24 hours, after scratches were applied to the cells with 0, 0.25, or 0.5 mg/mL pirfenidone in the absence or presence of TGF-β2. $^{*}P<0.05$ and $^{**}P<0.01$ versus the corresponding value for control cells. Data in each bar are the mean ± SD of cells that migrated through the membrane in three separate experiments. Magnification, ×40.

chain reaction system (TakaLa, Dalian, China). The primer pairs which we used were listed in **Table 1**.

Western Blot Assay

HLECs were treated with 0, 0.25, or 0.5 mg/ml PFD in the absence or presence of 12.5 ng/ml TGF-β2 for 24 hours. The cells were dispersed in mammalian protein extraction reagent (M-PER; Bioteke, Beijing, China). Final protein concentrations were determined with the BCA protein assay kit (Biocolor, Shanghai, China) according to the manufacturer's instructions. Prepared samples were heated to 100°C for 5 minutes; same amount of protein was added to a well of an 8–12% acrylamide gel according to molecular weight of targeted proteins and resolved by SDS-PAGE. The separate proteins were then transferred to a Polyvinylidene Fluoride membrane (PVDF membrane; Millipore, Billerica, MA). Nonspecific binding was blocked by incubation

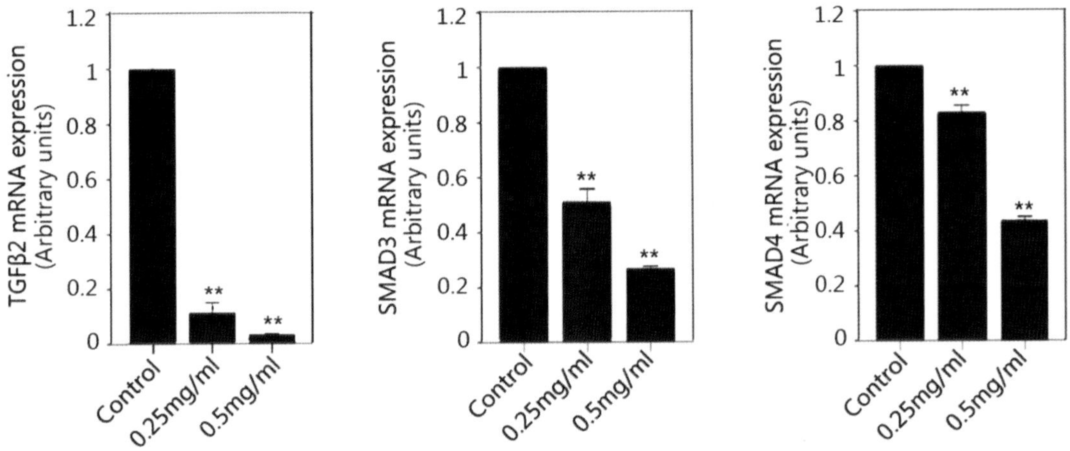

Figure 7. Inhibitory effect of pirfenidone on expression of TGFβ2 and SMADs mRNA in SRA01/04 cells. Real-time RT-PCR showed that pirfenidone reduced the levels of TGFβ2, SMAD3, and SMAD4 when compared with control cells. **$P<0.01$ versus the corresponding value for control cells. Data are the mean ± SD of triplicates from an experiment that was repeated with similar results.

with 5% nonfat milk for 2 hours before overnight incubation with primary antibodies (Abcam, Cambridge, UK) (1:1000 anti-TGF-β2, 1:500 anti-SMADs) at 4°C. After it was washed, the membrane was incubated with 1:5000 dilution of secondary antibody conjugated with horseradish peroxidase (Jetway Biotech, Guangzhou, China) in PBS-Tween. Blots were developed by chemiluminescence, to produce a signal that was captured on Chemi-Smart imaging systems (Vilber Lourmat, Marne-la-Vallée, France) according to the manufacturer's instructions, and were then scanned for densitometric analysis (ImageQuant software, version 5.2; Molecular Dynamics, Sunnyvale, CA).

Immunofluoresence Assay

HLECs were treated with 0, 0.25, or 0.5 mg/ml PFD in the absence or presence of 12.5 ng/ml TGF-β2 on coverslips for 24 hours. They were fixed with pure methanol for 10 minutes at −20°C followed by several rinses in PBS. Nonspecific binding sites were blocked for 30 minutes in PBS with 5% goat serum (Ruite, Guangzhou, China). The cells were incubated overnight at 4°C with primary antibodies (Abcam, Cambridge, UK) at 1:200, and then incubated with secondary antibodies conjugated with Alexa Fluor 488 or Alexa Fluor 594 (Invitrogen, Carlsbad, CA) for 30 minutes in dark at room temperature, followed by incubation with 4′,6-Diamidino-2-phenylindole dihydrochloride (DAPI, Sigma-Aldrich, St. Louis, MO) for 5 minutes. The cells were subsequently scanned with a confocal microscope (Zeiss, LSM 510 META).

Statistical Analysis

All results are expressed as the mean ± SD. Changes in outcome across the various time points in MTT assay were assessed using repeated measure analysis of variance. One-way analysis of variance (ANOVA), the test of homogeneity of variances, and a post hoc test (Bonferroni test) were used to determine significant differences between groups. A $P<0.05$ was considered statistically significant.

Results

Inhibitory Effects of PFD on Cell Proliferation of SRA01/04 Cells

PFD showed its inhibitory effects on the proliferation of HLECs (**Figure 1**). Cell proliferation was attenuated in the 0.3 mg/ml group after 24 hours compared with the control group ($P=0.044$). The effect was more apparent in the 0.5 mg/ml group at 24, 48, and 72 hours ($P<0.05$). The proliferation was almost completely inhibited with 1 mg/ml PFD at all the time-points ($P<0.01$). The assays were repeated by refining the concentration at 0.2, 0.25, 0.3, 0.4 0.5 and 0.6 mg/ml in three independent experiments. After 24 hours treatment, the inhibition started at 0.25 mg/ml and reached a maximum effect at 0.5 mg/ml. The fifty percent inhibiting concentration (IC50) of PFD on HLECs proliferation was 0.47. According to repeated measure analysis of variance, there was significant interaction between the PFD concentration and duration ($P<0.01$). Given these results, the following experiments were carried out with the use of 0.25 and 0.5 mg/ml PFD with 24 hours of observation.

Cell Viability of SRA01/04 Cells after Treated with PFD

In trypan blue exclusion test, after 24 hours' treatment with PFD, the percentages of living cells were 97.06±4.3%, 93.75±1.6%, 93.85±2.9%, and 95.16±4.8% for the control, 0.3, 0.5, and 1 mg/ml PFD groups, respectively (**Figure 2**). There was no statistically significant difference between the groups ($P>0.05$).

In LDH assay, after 24 hours' treatment with PFD, the percentages of cell-mediated lysis were 13.22±5.3%, 14.42±3.9%, and 18.18±3.3% for the control, 0.25 and 0.5 mg/ml PFD groups, and the percentages of cell-mediated lysis after 48 hours' were 16.17±3.1%, 14.51±1.9%, and 20.37±1.6% for the control, 0.25 and 0.5 mg/ml PFD groups. PFD had no significant cytotoxicity effect on SRA01/04 cells ($P>0.05$) (**Figure 3**).

PFD Inhibited TGF-β2-induced Fibroblastic Phenotypes and Epithlial-mesenchymal Transition in SRA01/04 Cells

After 24 hours' treatment with 12.5 ng/ml TGF-β2, the TGF-β2-induced morphological changes in SRA01/04 cells were detected. The cells were elongated and began to be spindle-like shapes. The morphological changes induced by TGF-β2 were noticeably suppressed by co-treatment with 0.5 mg/ml PFD for 24 hours. There was no apparent morphological change in SRA01/04 cells after 24 hours' treatment with 0.5 mg/ml PFD only. (**Figure 4**).

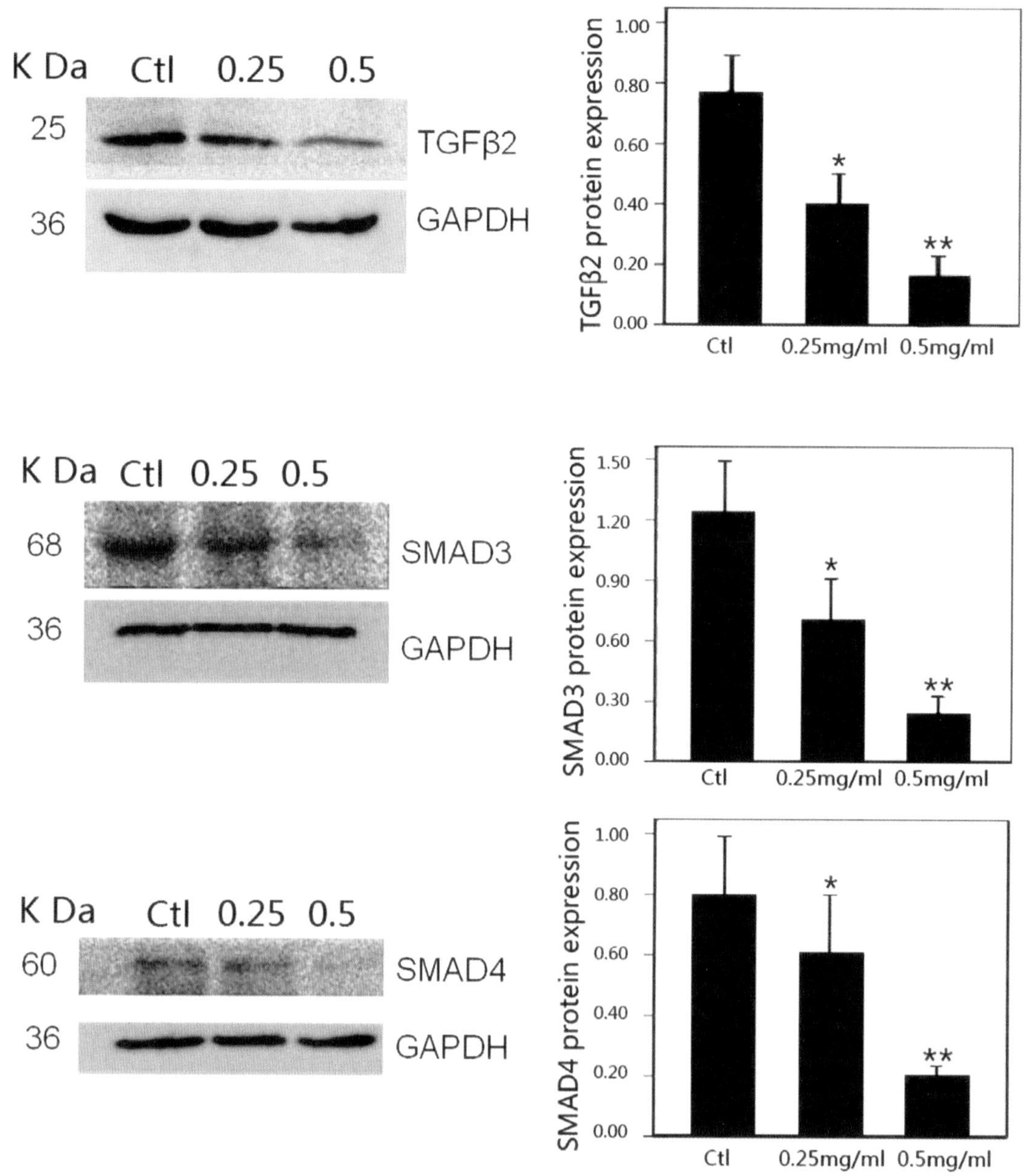

Figure 8. Inhibitory effect of pirfenidone on expression of TGFβ2 and SMADs protein in SRA01/04 cells. Western blot showed that pirfenidone reduced the protein levels of TGFβ2, SMAD3 and SMAD4 when compared with control cells. *$P<0.05$ and **$P<0.01$ versus the corresponding value for control cells. Data are mean ± SD of results from three independent cultures.

Immunocytofluorescence demonstrated that the TGF-beta2 significantly up-regulated the mesenchymal phenotypic marker fibronectin (FN) in SRA01/04 cells compared with control cells. And FN was significantly down-regulated after 24 hours' treatment with 0.5 mg/ml PFD in the absence or presence of 12.5 ng/ml TGF-beta2. (**Figure 5**).

Inhibitory Effect of PFD on the TGF-β2-induced Migration of SRA01/04 Cells

The migration of HLEC was significantly reduced after of the treatment of PFD (0.25 and 0.5 mg/ml) for 24 hours (**Figure 6**) in the absence or presence of 12.5 ng/ml TGF-β2. In the absence of TGF-β2, the migration rates were 84.9%±3.1%, 51.0%±3.4%, and 14.9%±3.4% for the control, 0.25 and 0.5 mg/ml groups, respectively. In the TGF-β2-treated groups, the migration rates were 91.3%±2.8%, 60.9%±3.2%, and 26.1%±2.7% for the control, 0.25 and 0.5 mg/ml groups, respectively ($P<0.05$ between groups).

Effect of PFD on Expression of TGF-β2 and SMADs mRNA and Protein in SRA01/04 Cells

A significant down-regulation of TGF-β2, SMAD3 and SMAD4 mRNA in HLECs was shown in the PFD treated groups ($P<0.01$) compared with the control (**Figure 7**). The expressions of TGF-β2, SMAD3 and SMAD4 protein were inhibited significantly at the concentration of 0.25 ($P<0.05$) and 0.5 mg/ml ($P<0.01$) compared with the control by western blot analyses (**Figure 8**). The effect was dose-dependent. We scanned the expression of TGF-β2, SMAD3

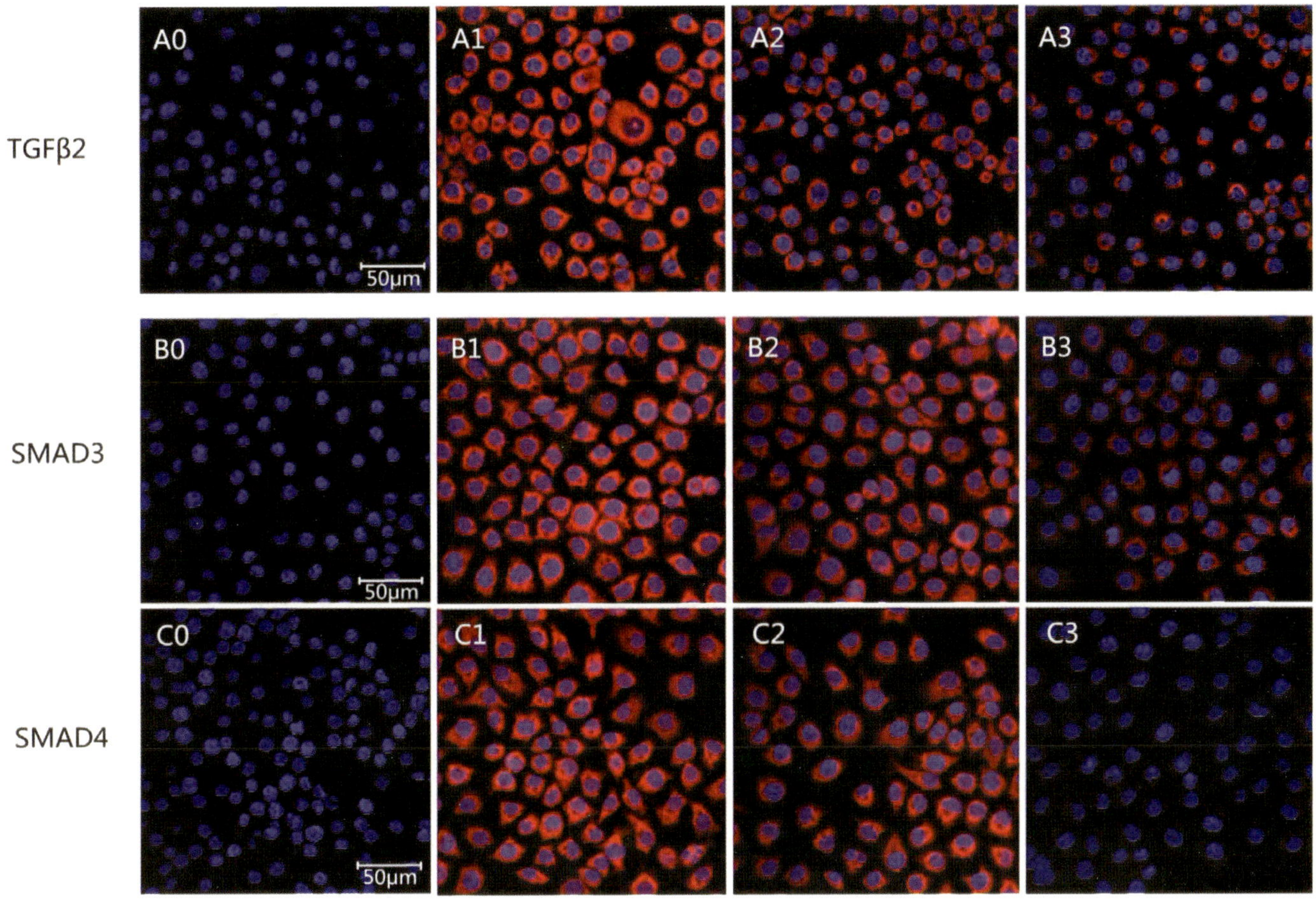

Figure 9. Expression of TGFβ2 and SMADs protein in SRA01/04 cells after treated with pirfenidone by immunocytochemical detection under confocal microscopy. TGFβ2 (A), SMAD3 (B), and SMAD4 (C) in the cytoplasm (red) and nuclei (blue) of HLECs were stained by immunocytochemistry after treatment with 0.25 (A2, B2, C2) and 0.5 mg/mL (A3, B3, C3) pirfenidone, respectively. (A0, B0, C0) Corresponding negative controls. Magnification, ×400.

and SMAD4 protein in HLECs also by immunofluorescence assay under confocal microscopy (**Figure 9**). These proteins could be detected expressing inside the cells and almost in the cytoplasm according to the immunofluorescence assay. After treated with 0.25 and 0.5 mg/ml PFD for 24 hours, TGF-β2, SMAD3 and SMAD4 protein stained by immunocytochemistry in HLECs were very faint under confocal microscopy.

Inhibitory Effect of PFD on TGF-β2-induced Expression of SMADs Protein

In the presence of TGF-β2, PFD reduced the TGF-β2-induced expression of SMAD2 and SMAD3 protein significantly at the concentration of 0.5 mg/ml ($P<0.05$) compared with the control group by western blot analyses. The inhibitory effects could be detected but were not statistically significant in the 0.25 mg/ml PFD groups. (**Figure 10**).

PFD Inhibited TGF-β2-induced Nuclear Translocation of SMADs

In the absence of TGF-β2, staining of nuclei SMAD2/3 and SMAD4 proteins in HLECs were very faint by immunofluorescence assay. After stimulated by 12.5 ng/ml TGF-β2 by 24 hours, nuclear translocation of SMADs could be detected under confocal microscopy: 1.the staining of nuclei SMAD4 enhanced and that of SMAD4 in the cytoplasm were weakened; 2.SMAD2/3 proteins were assembled on the nuclear membrane and some of them entered the nuclei. In the presence of TGF-β2, nuclei SMAD2/3 and nuclei SMAD4 were reduced in the 0.25 and 0.5 mg/ml PFD treated groups compared with the controls under confocal microscopy with magnification of 1000, and the inhibitory effect of 0.5 mg/ml PFD was stronger (**Figure 11**). Therefore, according to our results with immunocytochemistry, PFD could block the TGF-β2-induced nuclear translocation of the Smad2/3 and SMAD4 in HLECs.

Discussion

This is the first study to show an inhibitory effect of PFD on TGF-β2-induced proliferation, migration and epithlial-mesenchymal transition of HLEC (SRA01/04 cells), the pivotal cell being involved in the development of PCO. The effect seemed to follow a dose-dependent manner. Typan blue exclusion test and LDH assay showed that there was no significant toxic effect at the concentration levels (0–0.5 mg/ml) used in this study. These findings raise the possibility that PFD may represent a new therapeutic agent for the prevention of PCO.

PFD is an anti-inflammatory and anti-fibrotic agent and it exhibits the inhibitory effects on a host of cell types in a range of concentration with 0.2 to 2.0 mg/ml with no or few toxic effect

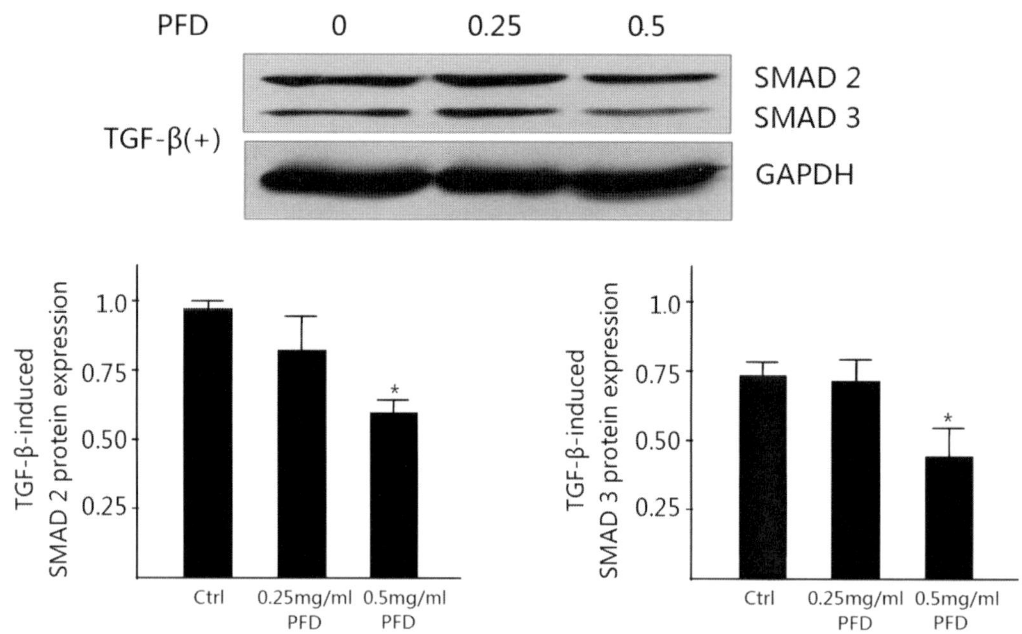

Figure 10. Inhibitory Effect of PFD on TGF-β2-induced Expression of SMADs protein. Western blot showed that pirfenidone (0.5 mg/ml) reduced the TGF-β2-induced Expression of SMAD2 and SMAD3 when compared with control cells. The inhibitory effects could be detected but were not statistically significant in the 0.25 mg/ml PFD groups. *$P<0.05$ versus the corresponding value for control cells. Data are mean ± SD of results from three independent cultures.

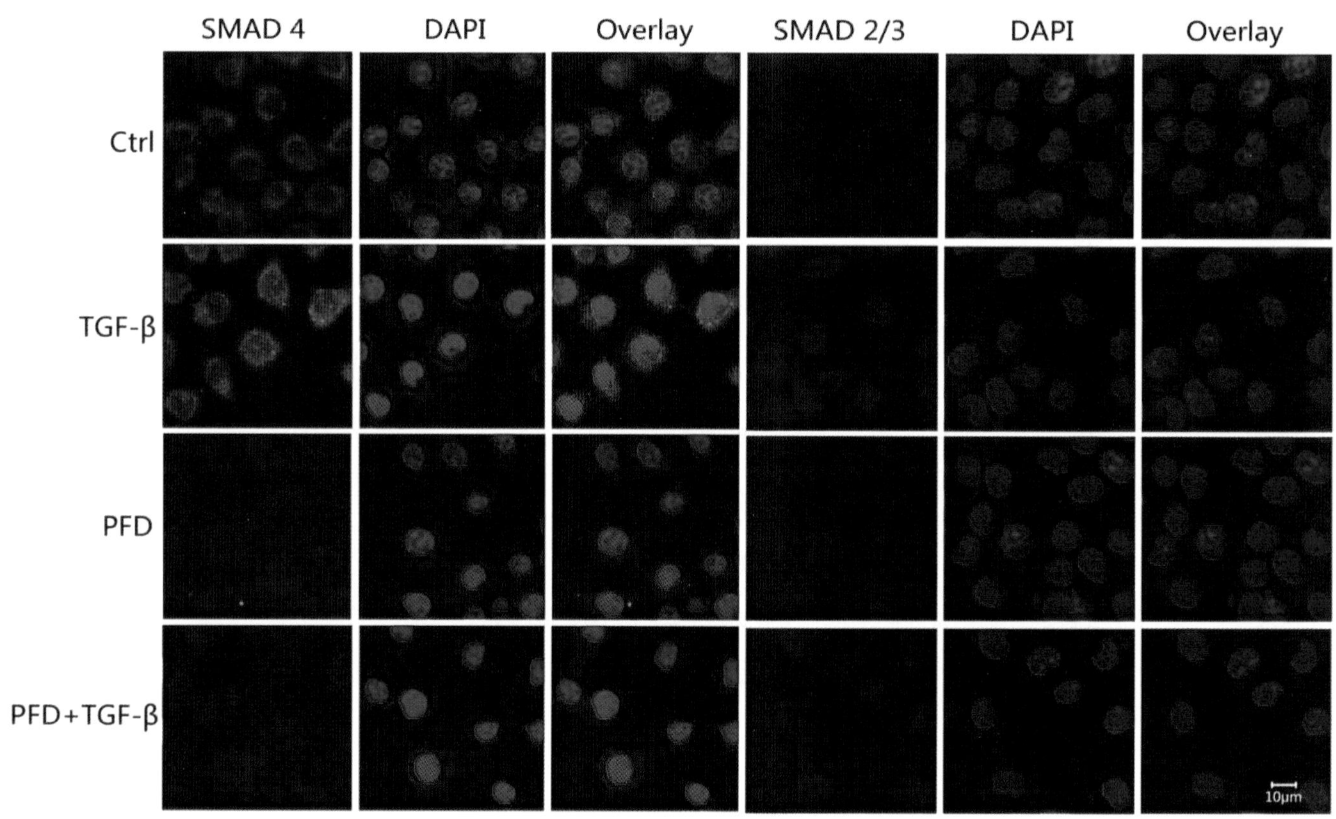

Figure 11. Inhibitory effect of pirfenidone on TGF-β2-induced nuclear translocation of SMADs in SRA01/04 cells under confocal microscopy. After stimulated by 12.5 ng/ml TGF-β2 for 24 hours, the staining of nuclei SMAD4 (green) enhanced when that of SMAD4 in the cytoplasm were weakened, and SMAD2/3 proteins (red) were assembled on the nuclear membrane and some of them entered the nuclei. Expression of nuclei SMAD2/3 and SMAD4 were depressed after treatment with 0.5 mg/ml pirfenidone. The nuclei stained by DAPI (blue). Magnification, ×1000.

in vitro. PFD significantly inhibits proliferation of hepatic stellate cell (with a maximum effect at 0.19 mg/ml) [23], rat renal fibroblasts (at 0.2 mg/ml) [24], myometrial and leiomyoma cells (at 1.0 mg/ml) [25]. PFD also has an inhibition effect on ocular cells. Our previous study indicated that PFD inhibited proliferation, migration, and collagen contraction of HTFs in vitro at the concentrations range from 0.15 to 0.3 mg/ml with no toxic effect [19,20]. Kim H et al. reported that PFD (at 1.9 mg/ml) also inhibited the growth of orbital fibroblasts obtained from patients with thyroid-associated ophthalmopathy (TAO) [26]. Choi K et al. proved the inhibitory effect of PFD (from 0.25 to 0.5 mg/ml) on TGF-β-mediated fibrogenesis in the human RPE cell line ARPE-19 [27]. In the current study, we also found that the maximal inhibitory concentration of PFD on the proliferation, migration of HLECs was 0.5 mg/ml and caused no toxic effect. The infinite cell line (SRA01/04) we used was transfected with plasmid vector DNA containing a T antigen of SV40 from primary cultures of HLECs in 1998 [22], which has been widely used in vitro to investigate the underlying mechanisms of cataract formation.

TGF-β2 signaling plays a key role in the development of PCO after cataract surgery. TGF-β2 can activate its down-streaming SMAD pathways and mediate the regulation of trans-differentiation and matrix contraction, and ultimately contribute to the formation of PCO [28]. our group and others studies have previously shown that PFD can down regulate the expression of TGF-βs in HTFs and many other human cells (e.g., HLECs, hepatic stellate cells, and renal fibroblasts) [19,23,24,29]. Choi K et al. have elucidated the TGF-β signaling pathways as the target of the inhibitory effect of PFD and PFD inhibited TGF-β signaling by preventing nuclear accumulation of active Smad2/3 complexes rather than phosphorylation of Smad2/3 in RPE cells [27]. In the current study, we provided new evidence that PFD exhibited its inhibitory effect by depressing TGF-β-SMAD signaling pathway: PFD inhibited protein and gene expression of TGF-β2, depressed the TGF-β2-induced expression of SMADs proteins, and also prevented the nuclear accumulation and translocation of SMADs proteins in HLECs. As we known, beside SMAD2/3/4 nuclear translocation, TGF-β receptor-induced responses are mediated through numerous signaling pathways, such as TGF-β-induced Erk activation and tyrosine phosphorylation, TGF-β-induced JNK/p38 activation and P13K/Akt pathway, to induce a variety of different responses [30]. And there are cross-talks between TGF-β/SMADs and other cell signaling passways [31]. Futher studies are needed to investigated the other molecular medhanisms of PFD for the inhibitory action for TGF-β2-induced fibrogenesis in lens epithelial cells. Taken together, these findings support the concept that PFD is a broad-spectrum anti-fibrotic agent and the effect may be mediated by the TGF-β/SMAD signaling pathway.

In conclusion, PFD shows an inhibiting effect on the proliferation, migration and epithlial-mesenchymal transition of SRA01/04 cells in vitro even in the presence of TGF-β2 stimulation, and the effect follows a dose-response manner. It is unlikely that the inhibition effect is mediated by toxic effect. The inhibition effect may be related to the regulation of TGF-β2/SMAD mRNA and protein expression. We propose that pirfenidone may be a potential antifibrotic agent to prevent the occurrence of PCO in patients after cataract surgery.

Acknowledgments

The authors thank Yingfeng Zheng (Zhongshan Ophthalmic Center) for edit, Li Xu (Zhongshan Ophthalmic Center) for technical assistance, and Zhongjun Dun (School of Public Health, Sun Yat-sen University) for statistical advices.

Author Contributions

Conceived and designed the experiments: MY. Performed the experiments: Y. Yang Y. Ye XL. Analyzed the data: Y. Yang Y. Ye KW. Contributed reagents/materials/analysis tools: Y. Yang Y. Ye XL KW. Wrote the paper: Y. Yang.

References

1. Wormstone IM, Wang L, Liu CS (2009) Posterior capsule opacification. Exp Eye Res 88: 257–269.
2. Wormstone IM, Tamiya S, Anderson I, Duncan G (2002) TGFβ2-induced matrix modification and cell transdifferentiation in the human lens capsular bag. Invest Ophthalmol Vis Sci 43: 2301–2308.
3. Lee EH, Joo CK (1999) Role of transforming growth factor-beta in transdifferentiation and fibrosis of lens epithelial cells. Invest Ophthalmol Vis Sci 40: 2025–2032.
4. Dawes LJ, Angell H, Sleeman M, Reddan JR, Wormstone IM (2007) TGFbeta isoform dependent SMAD2/3 kinetics in human lens epithelial cells: a cellomics analysis. Exp Eye Res 84: 1009–1012.
5. Wormstone IM, Anderson IK, Eldred JA, Dawes LJ, Duncan G (2006) Shortern exposure to transforming growth factor beta induces long-term fibrotic responses. Exp Eye Res 83: 1238–1245.
6. Wang M, Zhang JJ, Jackson TL, Sun X, Wu W, et al. (2007) Safety and efficacy of intracapsular tranilast microspheres in experimental posterior capsule opacification. J Cataract Refract Surg 33: 2122–2128.
7. Symonds JG, Lovicu FJ, Chamberlain CG (2006) Differing effects of dexamethasone and diclofenac on posterior capsule opacification-like changes in a rat lens explant model. Exp Eye Res 83: 771–782.
8. Wang GQ, Gu HQ, Yuan JQ, Sun HM, Xu YS (2010) F-heparin modified intraocular lenses in Rhesus monkeys. Int J Ophthalmol 3: 141–144.
9. Pandey SK, Cochener B, Apple DJ, Colin J, Werner L, et al. (2002) Intracapsular ring sustained 5-fluorouracil delivery system for the prevention of posterior capsule opacification in rabbits: a histological study. J Cataract Refract Surg 28: 139–148.
10. Kim SY, Kim JH, Choi JS, Joo CK (2007) Comparison of posterior capsule opacification in rabbits receiving either mitomycin-C or distilled water for sealed-capsule irrigation during cataract surgery. Clin Experiment Ophthalmol 35: 755–758.
11. Buehl W, Findl O (2008) Effect of intraocular lens design on posterior capsule opacification. J Cataract Refract Surg 34: 1976–1985.
12. Hazra S, Palui H, Vemuganti GK (2012) Comparison of design of intraocular lens versus the material for PCO prevention. Int J Ophthalmol 5: 59–63.
13. Menapace R (2008) Posterior capsulorhexis combined with optic buttonholing: an alternative to standard in-the-bag implantation of sharp-edged intraocular lenses? A critical analysis of 1000 consecutive cases. Graefes Arch Clin Exp Ophthalmol 246: 787–801.
14. Yazici AT, Bozkurt E, Kara N, Yildirim Y, Demirok A, et al. (2012) Long-term results of phacoemulsification combined with primary posterior curvilinear capsulorhexis in adults. Middle East Afr J Ophthalmol 19: 115–119.
15. Tassignon MJ, Gobin L, Mathysen D, Van Looveren J, De Groot V (2011) Clinical outcomes of cataract surgery after bag-in-the-lens intraocular lens implantation following ISO standard 11979–7: 2006. J Cataract Refract Surg 37: 2120–2129.
16. Findl O, Buehl W, Bauer P, Sycha T (2010) Interventions for preventing posterior capsule opacification. Cochrane Database Syst Rev 41: 507–511.
17. Lukaszewska-Smyk A, Kaluzny J (2011) Prevention of posterior capsule opacification in experimental studies. Klin Oczna 113: 175–179.
18. Hilberg O, Simonsen U, du Bois R, Bendstrup E (2012) Pirfenidone: significant treatment effects in idiopathic pulmonary fibrosis. Clin Respir J 6: 131–43.
19. Lin X, Yu M, Wu K, Yuan H, Zhong H (2009) Effects of pirfenidone on proliferation, migration, and collagen contraction of human Tenon's fibroblasts in vitro. Invest Ophthalmol Vis Sci 50: 3763–3770.
20. Zhong H, Sun G, Lin X, Wu K, Yu M (2011) Evaluation of Pirfenidone as a New Postoperative Anti-scarring Agent in Experimental Glaucoma Surgery. Invest Ophthalmol Vis Sci 52: 3136–3142.
21. Sun G, Lin X, Zhong H, Yang Y, Qiu X, et al. (2011) Pharmacokinetics of pirfenidone after topical administration in rabbit eye. Mol Vis 17: 2191–2196.
22. Ibaraki N, Chen SC, Lin LR, Okamoto H, Pipas JM, et al (1998) Human lens epithelial cell line. Exp Eye Res 67: 577–585.
23. Di Sario A, Bendia E, Svegliati BG, Ridolfi F, Casini A, et al. (2002) Effect of pirfenidone on rat hepatic stellate cell proliferation and collagen production. J Hepatol 37: 584–591.

24. Hewitson TD, Kelynack KJ, Tait MG, Martic M, Jones CL, et al. (2001) Pirfenidone reduces in vitro rat renal fibroblast activation and mitogenesis. J Nephrol 14: 453–460.
25. Lee BS, Margolin SB, Nowak RA (1998) Pirfenidone: a novel pharmacological agent that inhibits leiomyoma cell proliferation and collagen production. J Clin Endocrinol Metab 83: 219–223.
26. Kim H, Choi YH, Park SJ, Lee SY, Kim SJ, et al. (2010) Antifibrotic effect of Pirfenidone on orbital fibroblasts of patients with thyroid-associated ophthalmopathy by decreasing TIMP-1 and collagen levels. Invest Ophthalmol Vis Sci 51: 3061–3066.
27. Choi K, Lee K, Ryu SW, Im M, Kook KH (2012) Pirfenidone inhibits transforming growth factor-β1-induced fibrogenesis by blocking nuclear translocation of Smads in human retinal pigment epithelial cell line ARPE-19. Mol Vis. 18: 1010–1020.
28. Dawes LJ, Sleeman MA, Anderson IK, Reddan JR, Wormstone IM (2009) TGFβ/Smad4-dependent and -independent regulation of human lens epithelial cells. Invest Ophthalmol Vis Sci 50: 5318–5327.
29. Ozes ON, Blatt LM (2006) Development of a high throughput collagen assay using a cellular model of idiopathic pulmonary fibrosis. Chest 130: 230S.
30. Massague J (2000) How cells read TGF-β signals. Nature re Mol. Cell Bio. 1: 169–178.
31. Derynck R, Zhang YE (2003) Smad-dependent and Smad-independent pathways in TGF-beta family signalling. Nature 425: 577–584.

23

Biomechanics of the Cornea Evaluated by Spectral Analysis of Waveforms from Ocular Response Analyzer and Corvis-ST

Sushma Tejwani[1], Rohit Shetty[2], Mathew Kurien[3], Shoruba Dinakaran[1], Arkasubhra Ghosh[4], Abhijit Sinha Roy[5]*

1 Glaucoma Service, Narayana Nethralaya, Bangalore, Karnataka, India, **2** Refractive Surgery, Narayana Nethralaya, Bangalore, Karnataka, India, **3** Cataract Surgery, Narayana Nethralaya, Bangalore, Karnataka, India, **4** Gene, Repair and Regeneration in Ocular Workstation (GROW research lab), Narayana Nethralaya, Bangalore, Karnataka, India, **5** Imaging, Biomechanics and Mathematical Modeling Solutions (IBMS) lab, Narayana Nethralaya, Bangalore, Karnataka, India

Abstract

Purpose: In this study, spectral analysis of the deformation signal from Corvis-ST (CoST) and reflected light intensity from ocular response analyzer (ORA) was performed to evaluate biomechanical concordance with each other.

Methods: The study was non-interventional, observational, cross-sectional and involved 188 eyes from 94 normal subjects. Three measurements were made on each eye with ORA and CoST each and then averaged for each device. The deformation signal from CoST and reflected light intensity (applanation) signal from ORA was compiled for all the eyes. The ORA signal was inverted about a line joining the two applanation peaks. All the signals were analyzed with Fourier series. The area under the signal curves (AUC), root mean square (RMS) of all the harmonics, lower order (LO included 1st and 2nd order harmonic), higher order (HO up to 6th harmonic), CoST deformation amplitude (DA), corneal hysteresis (CH) and corneal resistance factor (CRF) were analyzed.

Results: The device variables and those calculated by Fourier transform were statistically significantly different between CoST and ORA. These variables also differed between the eyes of the same subject. There was also statistically significant influence of eyes (left vs. right) on the differences in a sub-set of RMS variables only. CH and CRF differed statistically significantly between the eyes of subject ($p<0.001$) but not DA ($p=0.65$).

Conclusions: CoST was statistically significantly different from ORA. CoST may be useful in delineating true biomechanical differences between the eyes of a subject as it reports deformation.

Editor: Rajiv R. Mohan, University of Missouri-Columbia, United States of America

Funding: The authors have no funding or support to report.

Competing Interests: The authors have declared that no competing interests exist.

* Email: asroy27@yahoo.com

Introduction

The cornea is responsible for nearly 80% of the total refractive power of the human eye. To achieve good quality vision, the cornea has an intricate structure of collagen fibers arranged in lamellae and interwoven with a cellular matrix to achieve and maintain a specific curvature [1]. Thus, the biomechanical status of the cornea plays a key role in maintaining quality vision [2], [3]. There are several refractive procedures, e.g., Laser-Assisted in situ keratomileusis (LASIK), photorefractive keratectomy (PRK), small incision lenticule extraction (SMILE), where the cornea may have some biomechanical changes after the treatment [4], [5]. Similarly, small incisions in cataract surgery are known to induce unwanted astigmatism in the cornea [6]. There are also several corneal disorders, e.g., keratoconus, pellucid marginal degeneration, where the native lamellar structure is disrupted and the cornea needs transplantation or collagen crosslinking [7], [8], [9]. In all these procedures, the pre-operative biomechanical status, e.g., elastic modulus, of the cornea is not known.

Present clinical evaluation of biomechanics of the cornea is limited to qualitative analysis only as direct measures of moduli are not available. There are presently two clinical devices, the Ocular Response Analyzer or ORA (Reichert Inc., USA) [10] and Corvis-ST or CoST (Oculus Optikgeräte GmbH, Germany) that are capable of measuring the dynamic mechanical properties of the cornea [11]. Both ORA and CoST apply an air-puff on the anterior surface of cornea and cause the cornea to deform. The air-puff technique is commonly used for intraocular pressure measurement. The ORA measures the intensity of the reflected infrared light from the deforming corneal surface and reports several indices for diagnosis [10]. Among them, corneal hysteresis (CH) and corneal resistance factor (CRF) have been investigated extensively in different patient groups [12], [13], [14]. These measures provide qualitative information about the biomechanical state of the cornea and additional waveform analysis has been

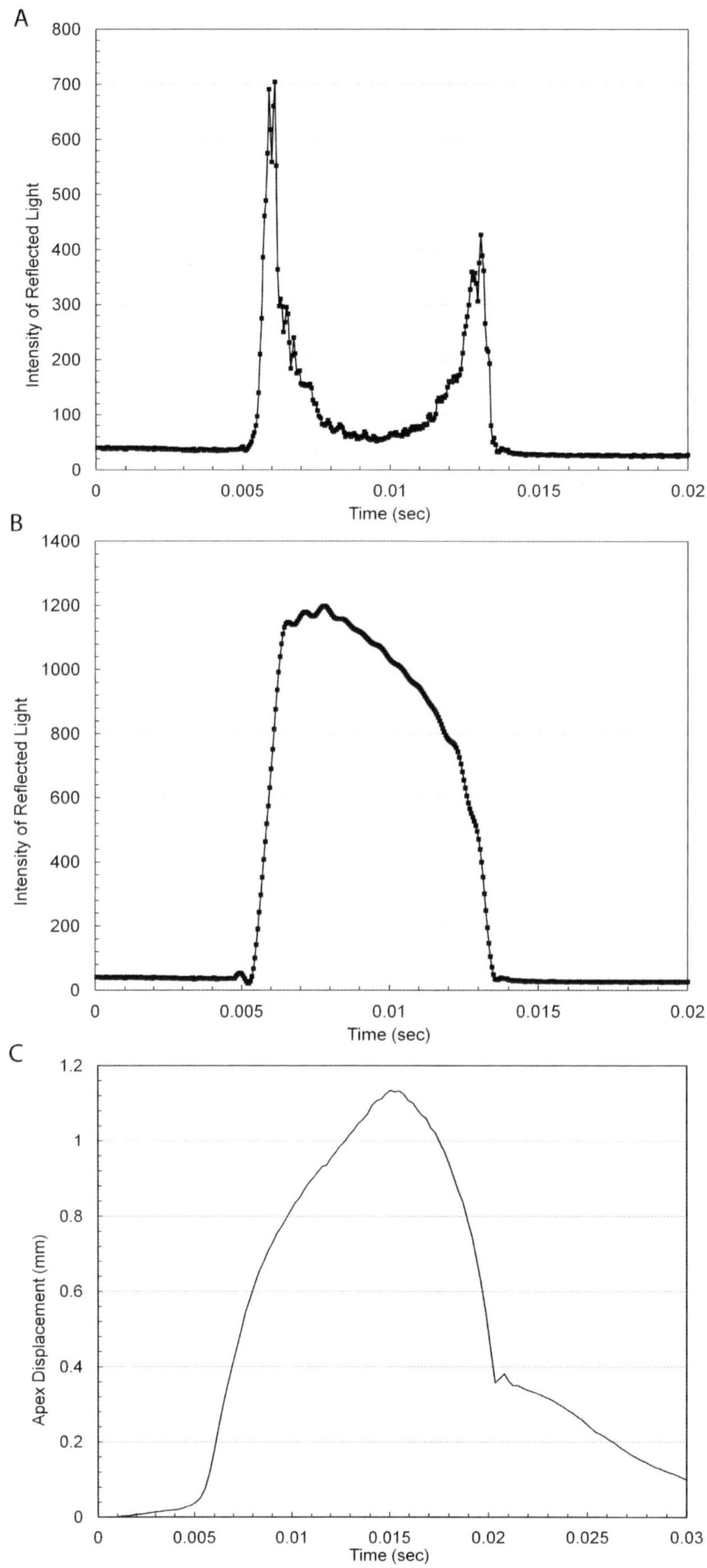
A
800
700
600
500
400
300
200
100
0
Intensity of Reflected Light
0
0.005
0.01
0.015
0.02
Time (sec)
B
1400
1200
1000
800
600
400
200
0
Intensity of Reflected Light
0
0.005
0.01
0.015
0.02
Time (sec)
C
1.2
1
0.8
0.6
0.4
0.2
0
Apex Displacement (mm)
0
0.005
0.01
0.015
0.02
0.025
0.03
Time (sec)

Figure 1. Waveforms reported by Ocular response analyzer (ORA) and Corvis-ST: (a) Example of ORA waveform. The two peaks represent the instant the cornea becomes flat during the forward and backward motion of the cornea; (b) the same OA waveform now inverted about the straight line joining the two peaks in figure 1a; (c) Example of the apex displacement in mm measured by CoST.

investigated [15], [16], [17]. CoST also uses an air-puff to deform the cornea. It uses Scheimpflug imaging and a high-speed camera to record images of a cross-section (the horizontal meridian) of the cornea as it deforms. This enables CoST to provide quantitative information, e.g., displacement of the cornea apex, which may be more relevant for evaluation of corneal biomechanics.

Theoretically, both ORA and CoST measure corneal deformation. However, the ORA output is the signal intensity of the reflected infrared light represented in scalar arbitrary units, i.e., it does not account for direction of corneal motion. On the other hand, CoST reports the corneal displacement (magnitude and direction of motion). Recent studies have shown that spectral analysis of ocular waveforms can provide useful information pertaining to clinical diagnosis of conditions [18], [19]. In this study, spectral analyses of the waveforms reported by ORA and CoST in a cohort of patients with *apparent* normal corneas were conducted. In this study, the biomechanical differences between the devices were evaluated. Further, the influence of fellow eye on differences between the devices was also evaluated. The waveforms were normalized with their respective peak values such that the transformed values of the data points ranged from 0 to 1. Spectral analysis converted these waves into frequency components (harmonics), which were used to define several diagnostic indices.

Methods

The study was a prospective, observational, cross-sectional study performed in Narayana Nethralaya, India. The study was approved by the institutional review board at the Narayana Nethralaya. Informed written consent was obtained from all the subjects and the study adhered to the tenets of the Declaration of Helsinki. Both eyes of 94 subjects were evaluated with the ORA and CoST. The inclusion criteria for the study were age between 18–80 years of age, were either emmetropes or had refractive error between −5D and +3D. Subjects with cataract and pseudophakes that were operated more than a year ago were included. This was done to eliminate any factors that would have affected the corneal biomechanical properties significantly. Similarly subjects with altered corneal biomechanics, e.g., keratoconus, any other cornea problems, e.g., pellucid marginal corneal degeneration, prior refractive surgery, prior cornea surgery, prior retina surgery, cataract surgery done within last one year, aphakia, refractive error between −5.0D and +3.0D, and astigmatism greater than + 3.0D were not included in the study. The screening of the patients was performed based on history, retinoscopy [20], refraction (both objective and subjective) and detailed clinical evaluation by experienced ophthalmologists. Any suspects on clinical grounds underwent corneal topography but all the patients were not subjected to topography to rule out the subclinical disease.

(a) Spectral Analysis of Waveforms from ORA and CoST

The ORA allowed export of the signal intensity waveform (applanation curve) as a comma separated value file. Figure 1a shows a sample measurement by the ORA. The two peaks were the signal intensities at which the cornea becomes flat, the 1st during increasing pressure and the 2nd during decreasing pressure (see figure 1a). The signal intensity decreased between the two peaks because the angle of reflection changes during deformation but the position of beam detector remains fixed. Thus, the region of the waveform between the two peaks was not as accurate as the data collected before the 1st peak and after the 2nd peak. However, some studies have shown statistically significant differences between normal and treated/disease patients in the region between the two peaks of the waveform [15], [16], [17]. Since the intensity was reported as a scalar and does not represent the direction of motion of the cornea during deformation, the region between the two peaks was inverted about a straight line joining the two peaks. Inversion was achieved by adding twice the linear distance of the data point along the y-axis from the straight line. Inversion of the waveform in figure 1a is shown in figure 1b. After inversion, Fourier transform (FT) of the waveform was performed. FT subdivided the wave into its harmonics, each quantified by a phase and magnitude. The magnitude of each harmonic was computed as follows:

$$a_i = \frac{1}{\pi}\int_{-\pi}^{\pi} f(x)\cos(i \times x)dx,\ i \geq 0 \quad (1)$$

Table 1. Mean and SEM of the variables, where SEM is the standard error of the mean.

	CoST				ORA							
OD	**AUC_{CoST}**	**a_i RMS**	**b_i RMS**	**DA**	**AUC_{ORA}**	**a_i RMS**	**b_i RMS**	**IOP_g**	**IOP_{cc}**	**CRF**	**CH**	**Age**
Median	12.4	0.091	0.024	1.08	6.62	0.096	0.042	16	16.9	10.23	10.0	35.7
SEM	0.16	0.0003	0.0003	0.01	0.051	0.0007	0.0009	0.47	0.47	0.18	0.17	1.33
OS												
Median	12.63	0.091	0.023	1.08	6.37	0.09	0.048	15.8	18.1	9.06	8.69	35.7
SEM	0.15	0.001	0.0004	0.01	0.063	0.0009	0.008	0.53	0.53	0.18	0.163	1.33

AUC_{CoST} (Area under CoST curve) has unit of mm-msec. AUC_{ORA} (Area under the ORA curve) has unit of a.u.-msec. a_i and b_i root mean square (RMS) has unit of mm for CoST. a_i and b_i root mean square (RMS) has unit of a.u. for CoST. IOP_g (ORA Goldmann correlated intraocular pressure), IOP_{cc} (ORA Corneal compensated intraocular pressure), CH (Corneal hysteresis) and CRF (Corneal resistance factor) have unit of mmHg. Deformation amplitude (DA) is in mm.

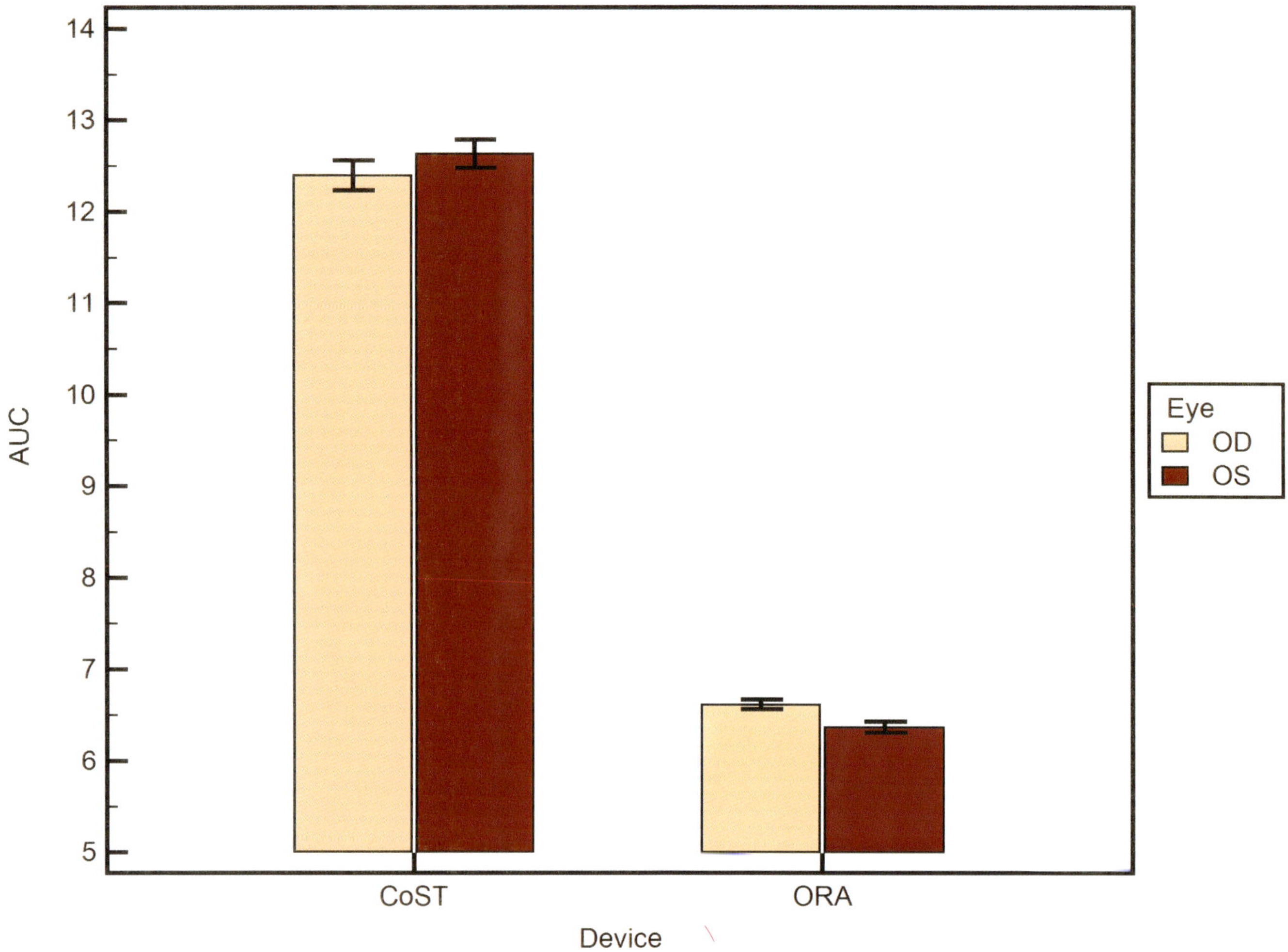

Figure 2. Area under the curve (AUC) from ORA and CoST segregated by the fellow eyes (OD = right and OS = left eye). The mean±SEM is plotted. SEM is the standard error of the mean.

$$b_i = \frac{1}{\pi}\int_{-\pi}^{\pi} f(x)\sin(i \times x)dx,\ i \geq 1 \quad (2)$$

where a_i and b_i were the amplitudes of the cosine and sine components (also called harmonics), x was the non-dimensional time ($= 2\pi \times (t/T - 0.5)$; t and T were the current and cycle time, respectively), and f(x) was the waveform derived after inversion. i represented the ith harmonic of the FT. It was assumed that the cycle time of the ORA was the same as the duration of the applanation test. Similarly, the a_i's and b_i's were computed for the waveform derived from CoST except that no inversion of the CoST waveform was necessary. The FT of the inverted ORA and CoST waveforms are shown in figures 1b and c, respectively. The FT was performed using a custom script written in Python (v.2.7). CoST waveform was extracted from the screen capture of the device computer monitor using Image J (v1.46).

(b) Diagnostic Variables Tested

The area under the curves was computed (AUC_{ORA} and AUC_{CoST}) using a 2nd order accurate numerical integration scheme. However, the ORA and CoST waveform was in arbitrary unit and mm, respectively. To allow comparison of the harmonics of the two curves, each curve was normalized to a range between 0 and 1 by dividing with its' respective peak data point and then the FT was repeated to obtain a_i and b_i for the normalized curves. The FT was performed up to order (n being the total number of harmonics) 31. Thus, the AUC's, a_i's and b_i's were computed using the normalized data points. The following additional variables were defined for statistical comparison of the FT's of each subject:

$$a_i\ RMS = \sqrt{(a_1^2 + a_2^2 + ... + a_{n-1}^2 + a_n^2)/n} \quad (3)$$

$$b_i\ RMS = \sqrt{(b_1^2 + b_2^2 + ... + b_{n-1}^2 + b_n^2)/n} \quad (4)$$

$$a_i\ LORMS = \sqrt{a_1^2 + a_2^2}, \quad (5)$$

$$b_i\ LORMS = \sqrt{b_1^2 + b_2^2} \quad (6)$$

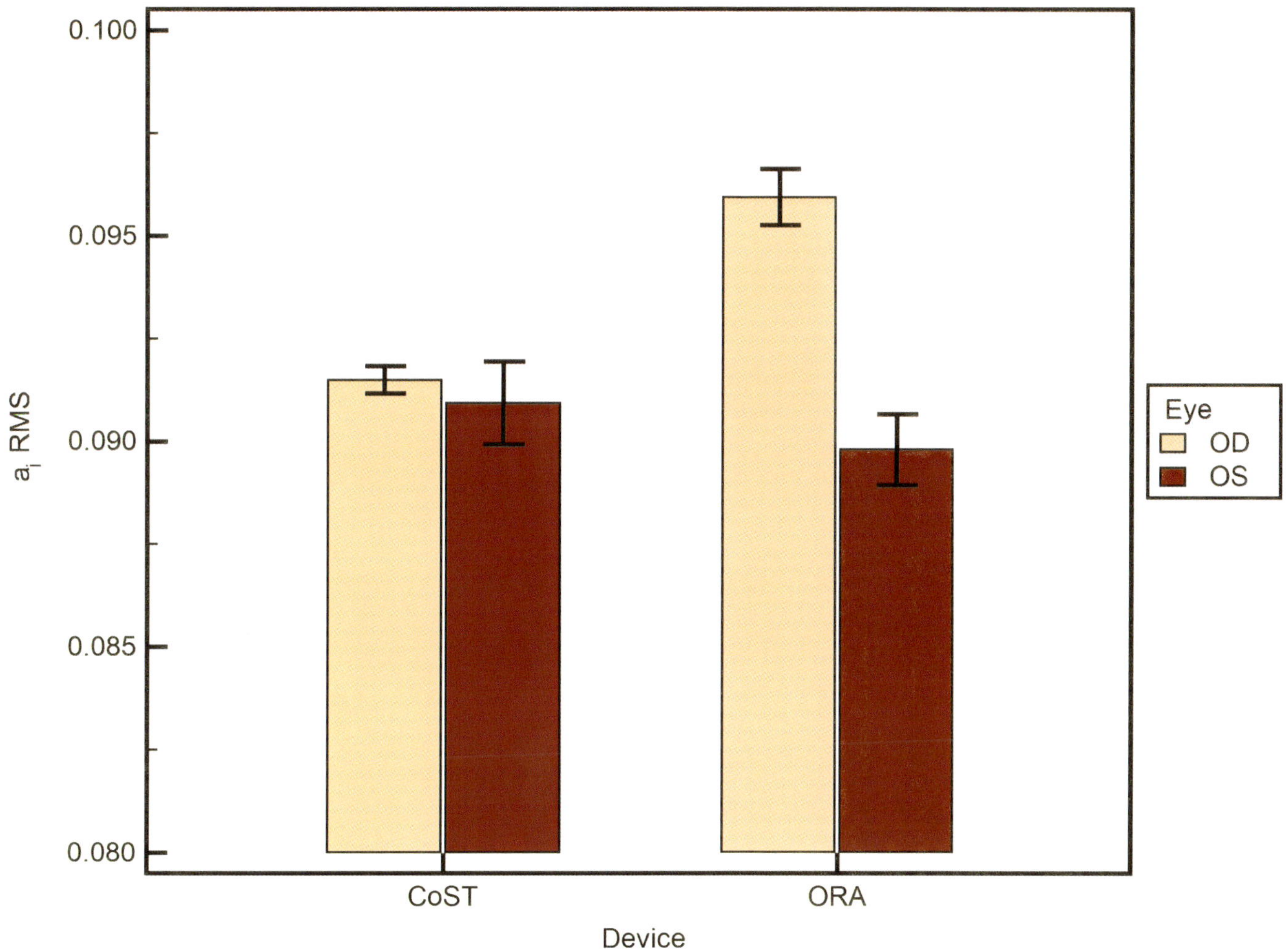

Figure 3. a_i RMS (root mean square) under the curve (AUC) from ORA and CoST segregated by the fellow eyes (OD = right and OS = left eye). The means ± SEM are plotted. SEM is the standard error of the mean.

$$a_i\ \text{HORMS} = \sqrt{a_3^2 + a_4^2 + a_5^2 + a_6^2}, \tag{7}$$

$$b_i\ \text{HORMS} = \sqrt{b_3^2 + b_4^2 + b_5^2 + b_6^2}, \tag{8}$$

RMS was the root mean square. LORMS and HORMS were defined as lower and higher order (or harmonic) root mean square, respectively and were a subset of the corresponding RMS variables. This form of RMS was chosen similar to RMS used in characterizing the corneal and ocular wavefront with Zernike polynomials prior to any refractive surgery. Other variables that were analyzed were corneal hysteresis (CH), corneal resistance factor (CRF) from ORA, and deformation amplitude (DA) from CoST.

(c) Statistical Methods

The normality of the data was evaluated with Chi-square test. Two-way (i.e., difference between devices was the primary factor and effect of the eye measured (left or right) on differences between the devices was the secondary factor) analysis of variance (2-way ANOVA) was used. If 2-way ANOVA resulted in any statistical significance, post-hoc comparison of the effect of factors on group means was performed. All p-values reported from two-way analysis were Bonferroni corrected. 1-way analysis of variance was used to compare differences between measured CH, CRF and DA of the left and right eyes of subjects. Linear regression analysis between the variables and age of the subjects was performed. P-value less than 0.05 was considered statistically significant. The statistical analyses were performed in MedCalc v.12.7.7 (MedCalc Inc., Belgium).

Results

A total of 188 eyes of 94 subjects were analyzed. Table 1 lists the mean of the different variables as mean ± SEM, where SEM is the standard error of mean. The mean age was 35.7 ± 1.33 years. The male to female ratio was 0.85. There was no statistically significant difference between the central corneal thickness of the left and right eyes of the subjects ($p = 0.79$). 2-way ANOVA of AUC was statistically significantly different between the devices (figure 2) ($p < 0.001$). However, AUC did not differ between the eyes of the same subject ($p > 0.05$). There was no influence of eye measured (left or right) on the difference between the two devices ($p > 0.05$). a_i RMS (figure 3) was statistically significantly different between the devices ($p = 0.03$) and between the eyes ($p < 0.001$).

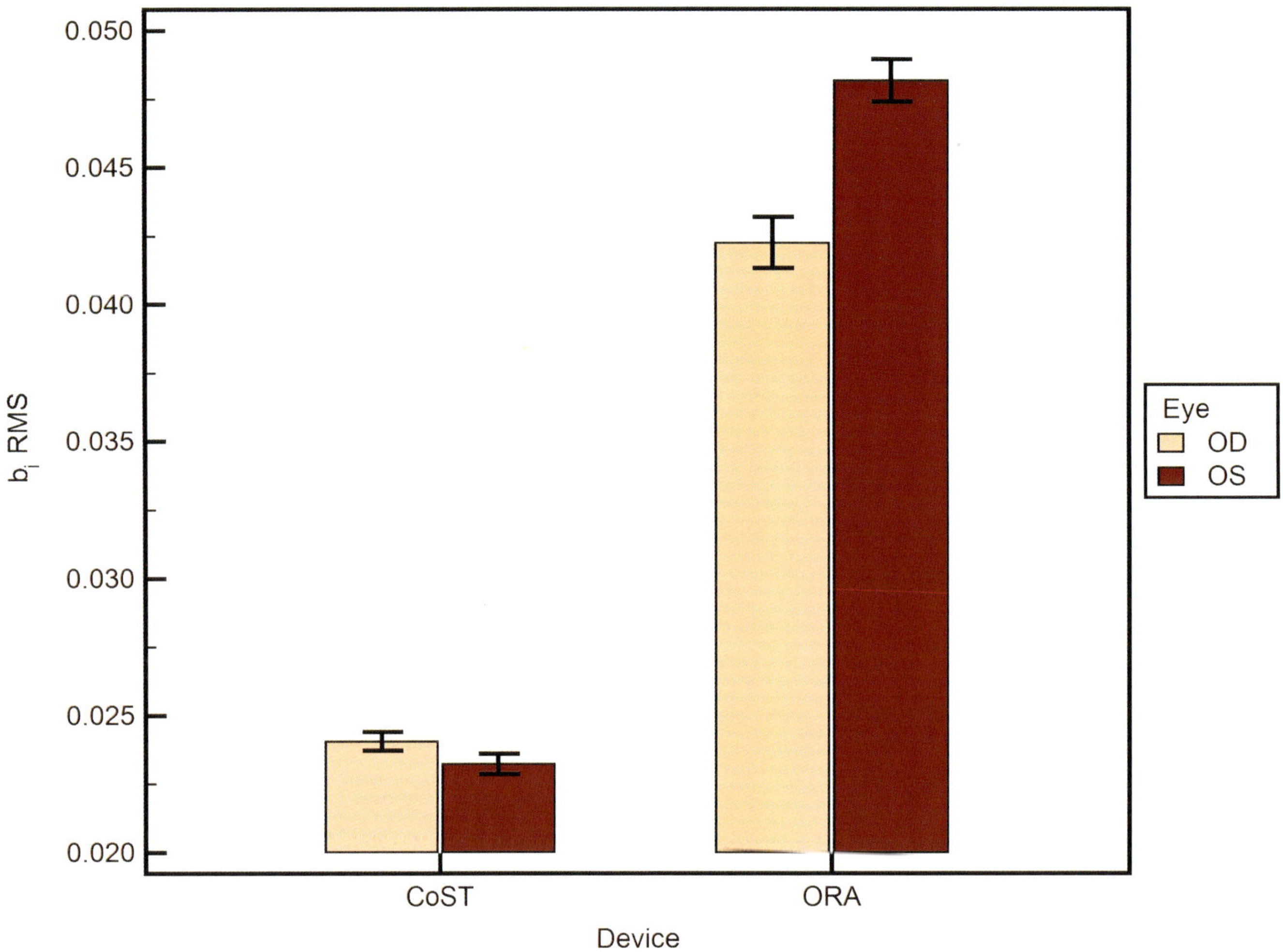

Figure 4. b_i RMS (root mean square) under the curve (AUC) from ORA and CoST segregated by the fellow eyes (OD = right and OS = left eye). The means±SEM are plotted. SEM is the standard error of the mean.

Further, the eye measured (left or right) had a statistically significant influence on the difference between the two devices ($p<0.001$). Similarly, b_i RMS (figure 4) was statistically significantly different between the devices ($p=0.03$), between the eyes ($p<0.001$), and the eye measured (left or right) had a statistically significant influence on the difference between the two devices ($p<0.001$). A similar statistical inference was made from computed values of a_i LORMS and b_i LORMS. However, a_i HORMS was and was not statistically significantly different between the two devices ($p<0.001$) and between the eyes ($p=0.07$), respectively. Further, the eye measured (left or right) did not influence the difference between the two devices ($p=0.17$). Similarly, b_i HORMS was and was not statistically significantly different between the two devices ($p<0.001$) and between the eyes ($p=0.47$), respectively. Further, the eye measured (left or right) did not influence the difference between the two devices ($p=0.22$). CH and CRF (figure 5) differed statistically significantly between the eyes of subjects ($p<0.001$) but not DA (figure 6) ($p=0.65$). Linear regression analysis between age and the all the variables was not statistically significant ($p>0.05$), i.e., slope was not different from zero.

A comparison of magnitudes of cosine harmonic (a_i) up to 6th order in subjects with CCT ranging from 505 to 581 microns has been shown in figures 2 and 3. In figure 7a, the subject had a CCT of 503 micron, AUC_{CoST} was 11.6 mm-msec and DA was 1.01 mm. The 1st and 2nd harmonic had the largest magnitudes compared to other harmonics in both ORA and CoST waveforms. ORA harmonics (3rd and higher) were larger than the corresponding values for CoST. In figure 7b, the subject had a CCT of 525 micron, AUC_{CoST} was 12.52 mm-msec and DA was 1.12 mm. The discrepancy between ORA and CoST was greatest for the 2nd harmonic. In figure 8a, the subject had a CCT of 553 micron, AUC_{CoST} was 9.97 mm-msec and DA was 0.98 mm. The 2nd harmonic showed the most discrepancy between the two devices once again. In figure 8b, the subject had a CCT of 581 micron, AUC_{CoST} was 11.32 mm-msec and DA was 0.97 mm. The magnitude of the harmonics was similar to the subject described in figure 2a. Thus, while the FT distinct different differences between subjects based on harmonics, there were no significant trends between AUC, DA and CCT.

Discussion

The study demonstrated that spectral components of ORA and CoST waveforms can be computed and the harmonics provided additional information about the biomechanical status of the cornea. Waveform analysis of the ORA wave has been performed in both normal and disease corneas [17], [18], [21], [22]. In a

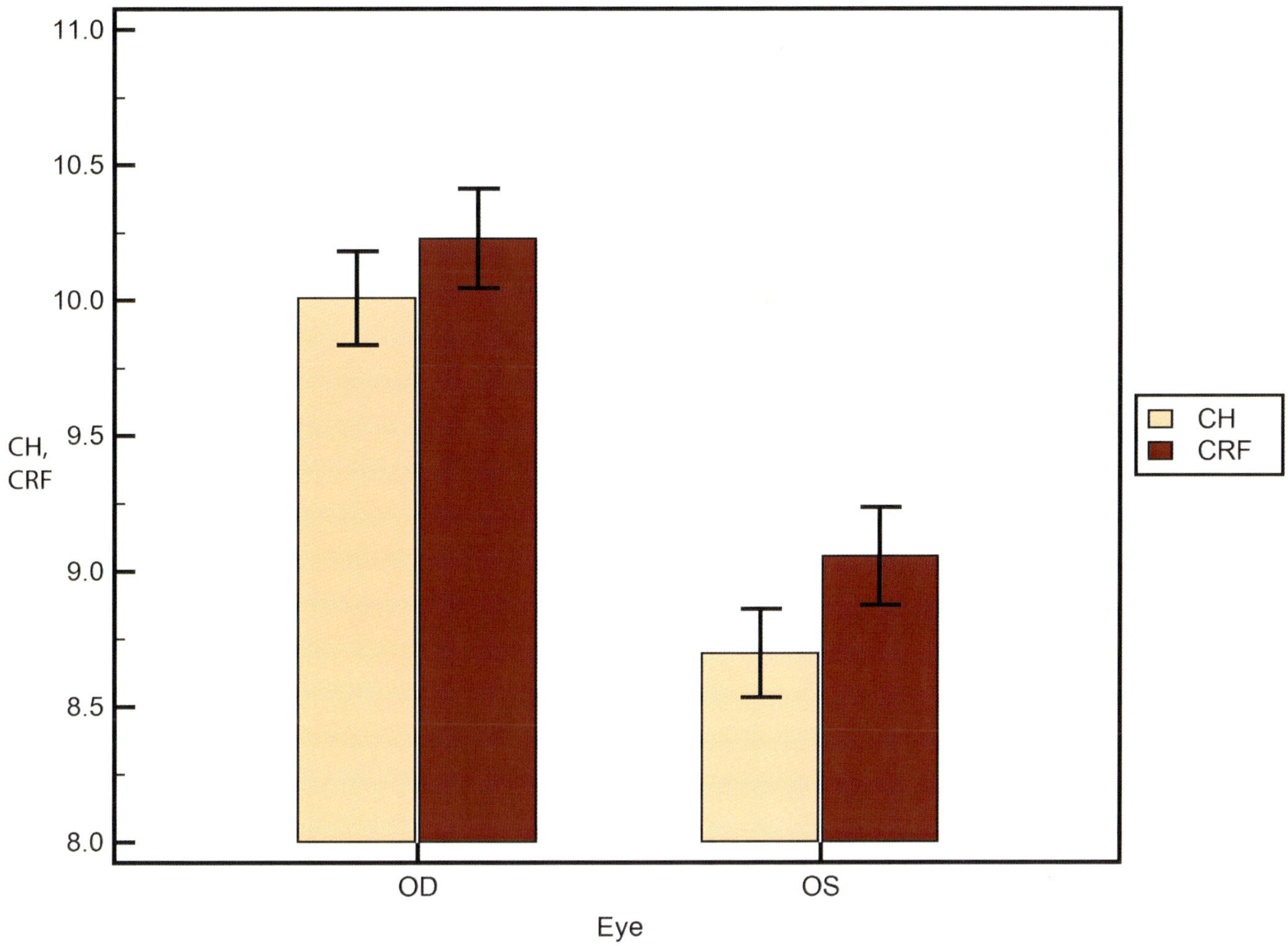

Figure 5. Corneal hysteresis (CH) and corneal resistance factor (CRF) between the fellow eyes of the subjects. The means±SEM are plotted. SEM is the standard error of the mean.

recent study, the ORA pressure was plotted against the applanation signal and then the region of the curve that lay in the "trough" of the ORA signal was inverted [21]. The resulting curve was remarkably similar to curves obtained from viscoelastic measurements of soft tissues on the bench [21]. As per viscoelastic theory, the area enclosed by a stress vs. strain curve (obtained from *ex vivo* testing of tissue) is known as hysteresis. It is the energy dissipated in the tissue when external forces (air-puff) cause deformation of the tissue and this dissipated energy cannot be recovered when the forces are removed. In both CoST and ORA, the applanation pressure can be considered analogous to stress. In CoST, deformation was a measure of strain. In ORA, the reflected light intensity was a measure of strain. However, CoST does not report the pressure signal and therefore, only the deformation signal from CoST and the inverted applanation signal from ORA were compared. The area enclosed by these curves may provide useful information about the viscoelastic status of the cornea, e.g., larger area may correspond to higher viscosity and vice versa.

In our study, the part of the ORA waveform was inverted to make it similar to the CoST waveform. 2-way ANOVA showed statistically significant differences between the devices and between the eyes in most variables. In a few variables (RMS and LORMS variables), there was statistically significant influence of the measured eye on the differences between the devices. Similarly, CH and CRF were statistically significantly different between the left and right eye and not DA and it is generally accepted that the eyes of a subject are biomechanically similar, if they don't have any disease. From a biomechanical perspective, there are structural differences in layout of collagen distribution and orientation between the left and right eye [23]. In contrast, visual parameters, e.g., sphere, cylinder, axis, aberrations, do not appear to correlate between the fellow eyes [24], [25]. In this study, fellow eye differences were evident in a few variables but not all. Individual harmonics (a_i's and b_i's) also differed between the devices and between the eyes. This study cannot establish true differences between the biomechanical differences between the eyes of a patient for lack of a gold standard. However, ORA and CoST are the only clinical devices available and there is potential that CoST may be useful in quantification of biomechanics between the eyes since it reports deformation, which is a fundamental parameter to quantify biomechanics.

The change in CH and CRF reported by ORA in normal, disease and post-treatment corneas has been studied. In post-refractive patients, e.g., LASIK, both CH and CRF decreased after procedure. A combination of thickness reduction and change in the viscoelastic properties of the cornea may be responsible for the decrease in CH and CRF [13], [15], [16], [17]. A few studies had looked at features of the ORA waveform that may have more

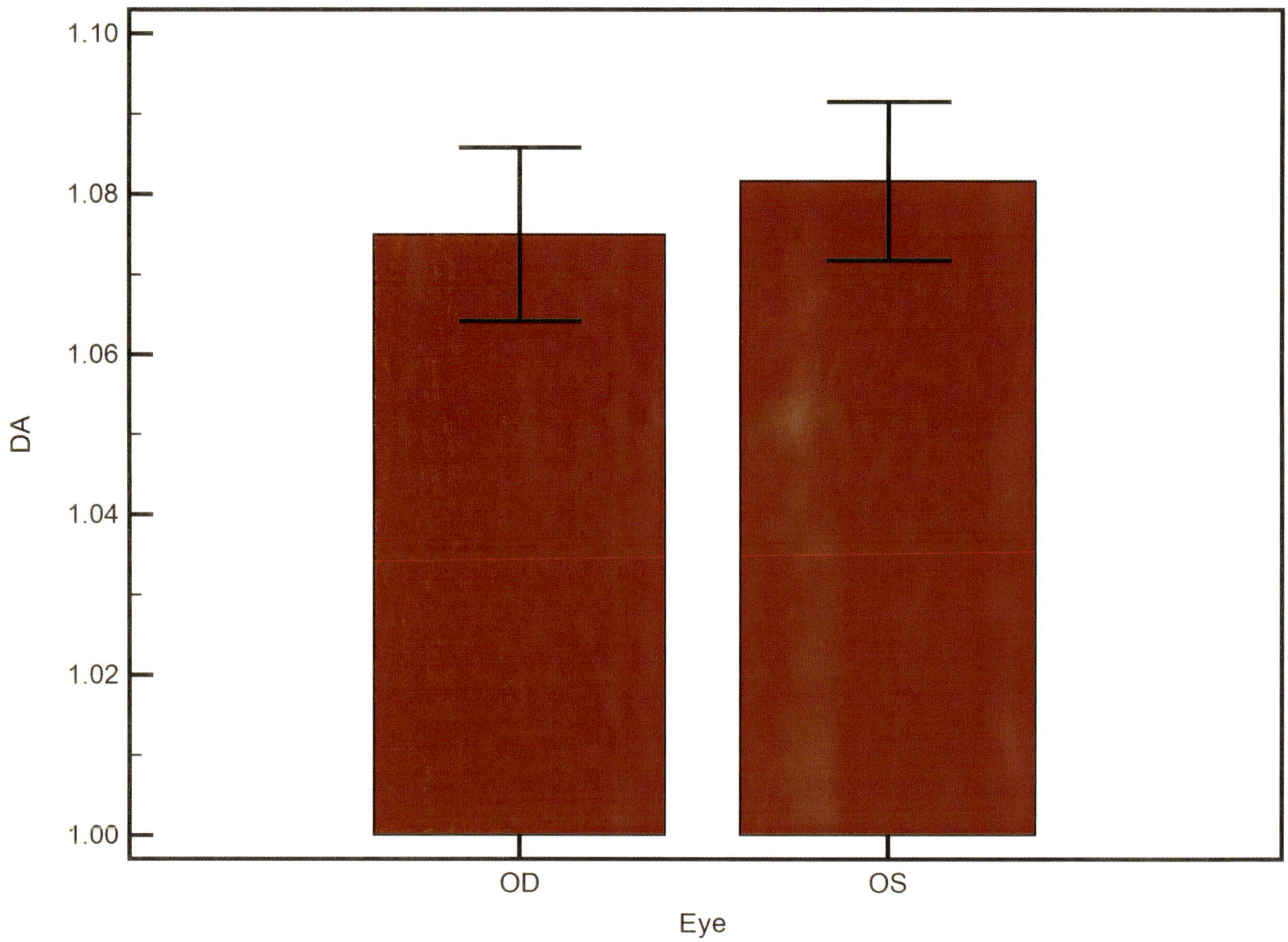

Figure 6. Deformation amplitude (DA) between the fellow eyes of the subjects. The means±SEM are plotted. SEM is the standard error of the mean.

sensitivity to biomechanical changes in the cornea [15], [17], [18], [21]. These studies have highlighted salient features of the ORA waveform that could be useful for diagnosis of disease, e.g., a wider area under 1st or 2nd peak indicated a weaker cornea as the weaker cornea deformed slowly [17], [18]. Spectral analysis of the ocular pulse amplitude reported by dynamic contour tonometry had shown statistical differences between subjects with different types of glaucoma [19], [26]. Statistically significant differences were found between the harmonics of patients with primary open angle glaucoma and normal tension glaucoma, which may lead to newer diagnostic measures for identifying glaucoma suspects [19]. Age was not significantly correlated with any of the variables in this study and in past studies with other variables [27], [28]. This lack of correlation may be due to the diverse ethnic population and varying environmental conditions in India.

Spectral analysis of ocular wavefront has been commonly used in refractive surgery. Zernike polynomials are used to reconstruct the wavefront measured by an aberrometer. The magnitudes of these polynomials has formed the basis for wavefront guided surgery, topography guided surgery in highly aberrated corneas [2], [29]. This study demonstrated a similar form of analysis of the corneal deformation signal with RMS terms so as to identity *suspect* corneas before they are recommended for any corneal surgery. With this method, there may be a possibility to link visual outcomes such as corneal wavefront Zernike magnitudes after surgery to changes in corneal deformation harmonics, e.g., compare spectral analysis of deformation to corneal wavefront zernikes in crosslinked subjects. In keratoconic corneas, aberrations are higher and the Zernike terms also increase in magnitude. Similarly in disease corneas, the ORA and CoST waveforms had more undulations [21] and the Fourier harmonics could be expected to increase in magnitude. Spectral analysis of the deformation curve may also perform better than analyzing distinct features of the signal, e.g., slopes, inflection points.

The air-puff technique also suffers from limitations that may impact accurate determination of the biomechanical status of the cornea. Firstly, CoST recorded only 2-D cross-section images of the cornea. In disease (e.g. keratoconus) or treated (e.g. PRK) corneas, there may be lateral (out-of plane) motion of the cornea, which may not be captured by CoST. Secondly, air-puff technique caused the whole globe to move back when the air pulse impacted the cornea. Thus, the deformation signal and intensity of reflect wave from the anterior corneal surface were affected by it. In a recent study, the impact of orbital muscles was found to have a bigger impact on deformation history than the sclera [30]. Therefore, future studies need to focus on delineating the whole globe motion from the corneal deformation to improve the accuracy of the spectral analysis and to assess changes in the

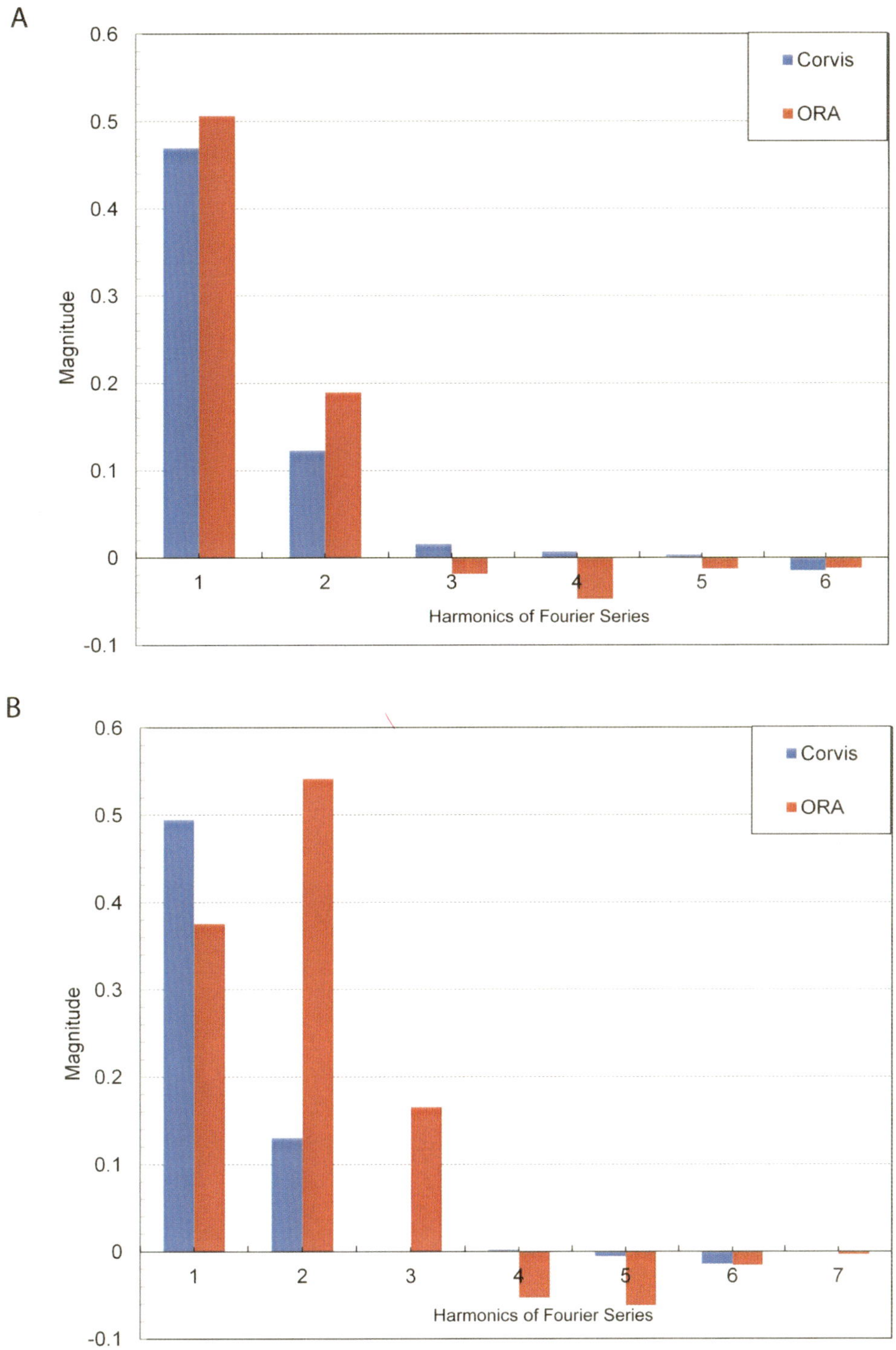

Figure 7. Cosine harmonics from 1st to 6th order in a subject with CCT equal to: (a) 503 micron; (b) 525 micron. The numbers on the horizontal axis represent the order of the harmonics.

harmonics in different diseases and treatments. Another limitation was that the spectral analysis was performed on waveforms obtained from a single perturbation of the cornea and a complete, repeated deformation cycle was not obtained from either device. Therefore, some amount of spectral leakage can occur from Fourier transform. In spectral analysis of ocular pressure pulse wave, several continuous waveforms are available but not in ORA and CoST [19], [21], [22], [27], [28]. This limitation may be overcome to some extent in CoST, if the complete deformation history, i.e., corneal DA reached to zero, was provided. However, it was not possible to obtain multiple periods from either device as only one air-puff can be generated by each device in one measurement. Despite the limitation, the present Fourier transform was conducted with the basic assumption that unique features of the corneal deformation characterized by the harmonics obtained from ORA and CoST may be linked, e.g., whether

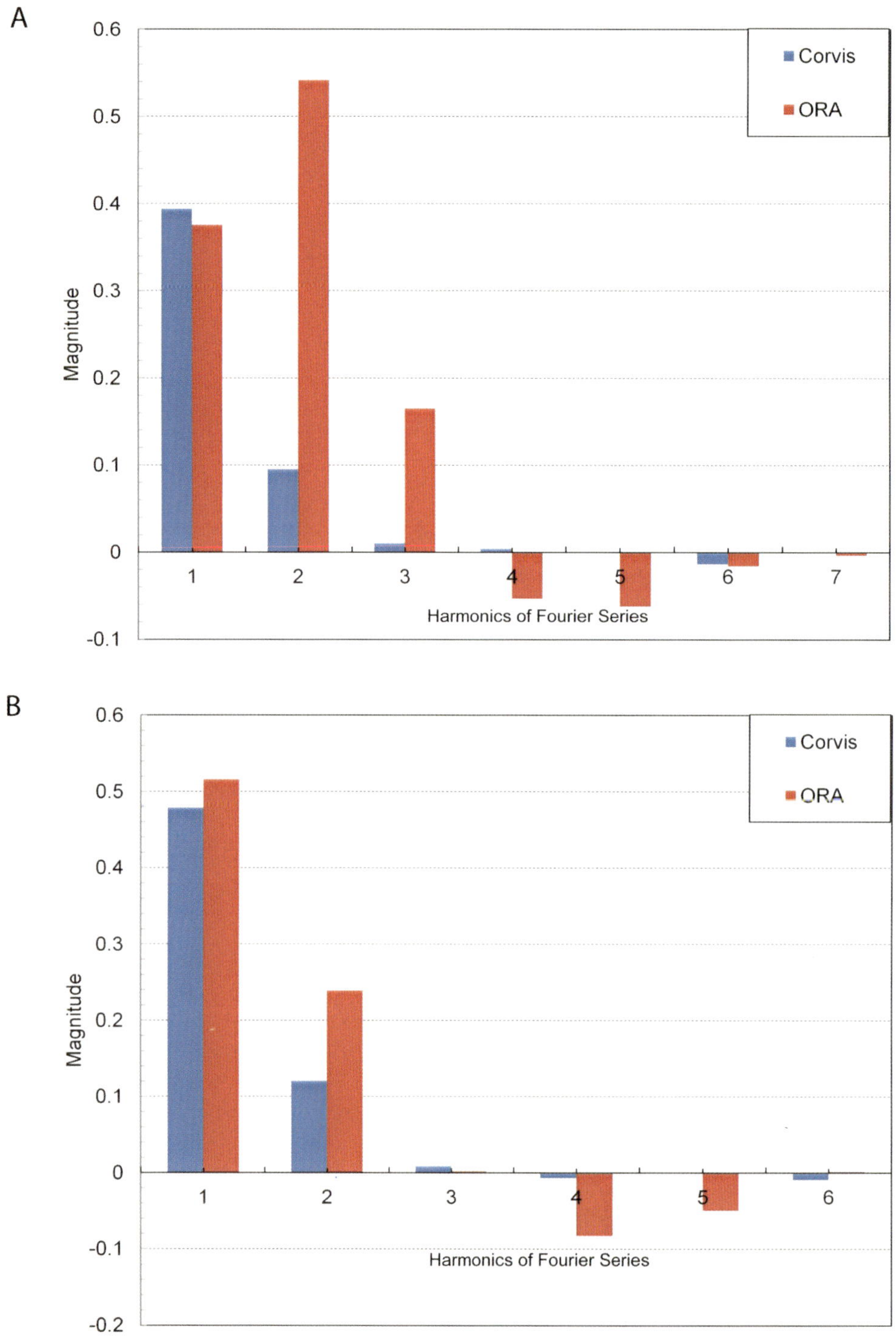

Figure 8. Sine harmonics from 1st to 6th order in a subject with CCT equal to: (a) 553 micron; (b) 581 micron. The numbers on the horizontal axis represent the order of the harmonics.

increased a_i LORMS of subject cornea, when measured by ORA also implied increased a_i LORMS of the same eye when measured by CoST. From this study, it was evident that the two devices did not evaluate a given cornea similarly.

Author Contributions

Conceived and designed the experiments: ST SD RS. Performed the experiments: ST SD RS. Analyzed the data: MK ASR. Contributed reagents/materials/analysis tools: MK ASR. Wrote the paper: AG ASR.

References

1. Kamma-Lorger CS, Boote C, Hayes S, Moger J, Burghammer M, et al. (2010) Collagen and mature elastic fibre organisation as a function of depth in the human cornea and limbus. J Struct Biol 169: 424–30.
2. Roberts C (2000) The cornea is not a piece of plastic. J Refract Surg 16: 407–13.
3. Dupps WJ Jr, Wilson SE (2006) Biomechanics and wound healing in the cornea. Exp Eye Res 83: 709–20.
4. Uzbek AK, Kamburoğlu G, Mahmoud AM, Roberts CJ (2011) Change in biomechanical parameters after flap creation using the Intralase femtosecond laser and subsequent excimer laser ablation. Curr Eye Res 36: 614–9.
5. Kamiya K, Shimizu K, Ohmoto F (2009) Comparison of the changes in corneal biomechanical properties after photorefractive keratectomy and laser in situ keratomileusis. Cornea 28: 765–9.
6. Denoyer A, Ricaud X, Van Went C, Labbé A, Baudouin C (2013) Influence of corneal biomechanical properties on surgically induced astigmatism in cataract surgery. J Cataract Refract Surg 39: 1204–1210.
7. Hayes S, Boote C, Tuft SJ, Quantock AJ, Meek KM (2007) A study of corneal thickness, shape and collagen organisation in keratoconus using videokeratography and X-ray scattering techniques. Exp Eye Res 84: 423–34.
8. Sinha Roy, Dupps WJ Jr (2011) Patient-specific computational modeling of keratoconus progression and differential responses to collagen cross-linking. Invest Ophthalmol Vis Sci 52: 9174–87.
9. Meek KM, Hayes S (2013) Corneal cross-linking–a review. Ophthalmic Physiol Opt 33: 78–93.
10. Luce DA (2005) Determining in vivo biomechanical properties of the cornea with an ocular response analyzer. J Cataract Refract Surg 31: 156–62.
11. Hon Y, Lam AK (2013) Corneal deformation measurement using Scheimpflug noncontact tonometry. Optom Vis Sci 90: e1–8.
12. Zare M, Feizi S, Azimzadeh A, Esfandiari H (2012) Effect of photorefractive keratectomy with mitomycin-C on corneal biomechanical features. Curr Eye Res 37: 457–62.
13. Ambrósio R Jr, Dawson DG, Salomão M, Guerra FP, Caiado AL, et al. (2010) Corneal ectasia after LASIK despite low preoperative risk: tomographic and biomechanical findings in the unoperated, stable, fellow eye. J Refract Surg 26: 906–11.
14. Ruiseñor Vázquez PR, Delrivo M, Bonthoux FF, Pförtner T, Galletti JG (2013) Combining Ocular Response Analyzer Metrics for Corneal Biomechanical Diagnosis. J Refract Surg 17: 1–7.
15. Zarei-Ghanavati S, Ramirez-Miranda A, Yu F, Hamilton DR (2012) Corneal deformation signal waveform analysis in keratoconic versus post-femtosecond laser in situ keratomileusis eyes after statistical correction for potentially confounding factors. J Cataract Refract Surg 38: 607–14.
16. Uzbek AK, Kamburoğlu G, Mahmoud AM, Roberts CJ (2011) Change in biomechanical parameters after flap creation using the Intralase femtosecond laser and subsequent excimer laser ablation. Curr Eye Res 36: 614–9.
17. Kerautret J, Colin J, Touboul D, Roberts C (2008) Biomechanical characteristics of the ectatic cornea. J Cataract Refract Surg 34: 510–3.
18. Terai N (2012) Identification of biomechanical properties of the cornea: The Ocular Response Analyzer. Curr Eye Res 37: 553–62.
19. Božić M, Dukić ML, Stojković M (2012) Spectral analysis of intraocular pressure pulse wave in open angle glaucomas and healthy eyes. Curr Eye Res 37: 1019–24.
20. Rabinowitz YS (2006) Ectatic Disorders of the Cornea. Smolin and Thoft's: The Cornea-Scientific foundations and clinical practice. 889–911: 4th edition.
21. Hallahan KM, Sinha Roy A, Ambrosio R Jr, Salomao M, Dupps WJ Jr (2013) Discriminant Value of Custom Ocular Response Analyzer Waveform Derivatives in Keratoconus. Ophthalmology 121: 459–68.
22. Ventura BV, Machado AP, Ambrósio R Jr, Ribeiro G, Araújo LN, et al. (2013) Analysis of waveform-derived ORA parameters in early forms of keratoconus and normal corneas. J Refract Surg 29: 637–43.
23. Boote C, Hayes S, Abahussin M, Meek KM (2006) Mapping collagen organization in the human cornea: left and right eyes are structurally distinct. Invest Ophthalmol Vis Sci 47: 901–8.
24. Gatinel D, Delair E, Abi-Farah H, Hoang-Xuan T (2005) Distribution and enantiomorphism of higher-order ocular optical aberrations. J Fr Ophtalmol 28: 1041–50.
25. Touzeau O, Gaujoux T, Bullet J, Allouch C, Borderie V, et al. Relationships between refractive parameters: sphere, cylinder and axis. J Fr Ophtalmol 35: 587–98.
26. Evans DW, Hosking SL, Embleton SJ, Morgan AJ, Bartlett JD (2002) Spectral content of the intraocular pressure pulse wave: glaucoma patients versus normal subjects. Graefes Arch Clin Exp Ophthalmol 240: 475–80.
27. Valbon BF, Ambrósio R Jr, Fontes BM, Alves MR (2013) Effects of age on corneal deformation by non-contact tonometry integrated with an ultra-high-speed (UHS) Scheimpflug camera. Arq Bras Oftalmol 76: 229–32.
28. Holland S, Lin DT, Tan JC (2013) Topography-guided laser refractive surgery. Curr Opin Ophthalmol 24: 302–9.
29. Smadja D, Reggiani-Mello G, Santhiago MR, Krueger RR (2012) Wavefront ablation profiles in refractive surgery: description, results, and limitations. J Refract Surg 28: 224–32.
30. Kling S, Marcos S (2013) Contributing factors to corneal deformation in air puff measurements. Invest Ophthalmol Vis Sci 54: 5078–85.

The Long Term Impact of Cataract Surgery on Quality of Life, Activities and Poverty: Results from a Six Year Longitudinal Study in Bangladesh and the Philippines

Lisa Danquah[1], Hannah Kuper[1], Cristina Eusebio[2], Mamunur Akm Rashid[3], Liza Bowen[1], Allen Foster[1], Sarah Polack[1]*

1 Faculty of Infectious and Tropical Diseases, London School of Hygiene & Tropical Medicine, London, United Kingdom, **2** Cataract Foundation of the Philippines, Bacolod, Philippines, **3** Dhaka Community Medical College, Dhaka, Bangladesh

Abstract

Background: Cataract surgery has been shown to improve quality of life and household economy in the short term. However, it is unclear whether these benefits are sustained over time. This study aims to assess the six year impact of cataract surgery on health related quality of life (HRQoL), daily activities and economic poverty in Bangladesh and The Philippines.

Methods and Findings: This was a longitudinal study. At baseline people aged ≥50 years with visual impairment due to cataract ('cases') and age-, sex-matched controls without visual impairment were interviewed about vision specific and generic HRQoL, daily activities and economic indicators (household per capita expenditure, assets and self-rated wealth). Cases were offered free or subsidised cataract surgery. Cases and controls were re-interviewed approximately one and six years later. At baseline across the two countries there were 455 cases and 443 controls. Fifty percent of cases attended for surgery. Response rates at six years were 47% for operated cases and 53% for controls. At baseline cases had poorer health and vision related QoL, were less likely to undertake productive activities, more likely to receive assistance with activities and were poorer compared to controls ($p<0.05$). One year after surgery there were significant increases in HRQoL, participation and time spent in productive activities and per capita expenditure and reduction in assistance with activities so that the operated cases were similar to controls. These increases were still evident after six years with the exception that time spent on productive activities decreased among both cases and controls.

Conclusion: Cataract causing visual loss is associated with reduced HRQoL and economic poverty among older adults in low-income countries. Cataract surgery improves the HRQoL of the individual and economy of the household. The findings of this study suggest these benefits are sustained in the long term.

Editor: Yingfeng Zheng, Zhongshan Ophthalmic Center, China

Funding: This study was supported by grants from Fred Hollows Foundation, CBM, Sightsavers, and ORBIS International. Representatives from the latter three non-governmental organisations were part of the steering committee for the original Cataract Impact Study, which gave guidance towards conduct of the study. They were not involved the data collection, analysis, interpretation of results, preparing the manuscript or the decision to publish. Professor Allen Foster (one of the co-authors) was involved in this study in his position at the London School of Hygiene &Tropical Medicine. At the time of the study Professor Foster was also the Medical Advisor and then President of CBM. He contributed to the conception of the study question, study design, and critically reviewed the draft of the article. He was not involved in the data collection, data analysis or interpretation of results.

Competing Interests: The authors have declared that no competing interests exist.

* E-mail: arah.polack@lshtm.ac.uk

Introduction

Age related cataract is the leading cause of blindness in low-income settings [1]. The aim of cataract surgery is to improve the vision and thereby the quality of the daily lives of people affected. However, relatively little is known about the extent to which this occurs in the long term in low income settings. Blindness and poverty are closely linked; people who are blind may experience restricted opportunities to engage in income generating activities [2,3] and people who are poor are less likely to be able to afford sight restoring cataract surgery [4,5,6]. However, empirical data on whether sight restoration impacts on economic poverty in the long term is lacking.

The 'Cataract Impact Study' was a longitudinal intervention study undertaken to explore the impact of cataract surgery on health related quality of life (HRQoL), daily activities and economic poverty among adults aged ≥50 years in Kenya, the Philippines and Bangladesh [7,8,9]. People with visual impairment from cataract ('cases') and age- gender- matched peers without visual impairment from cataract ('controls') were identified through population based surveys [4,5,6] and interviewed about their HRQoL, daily activities and poverty indicators. All cases were offered free or subsidized surgery. Approximately one year later cases and controls were re-interviewed. At baseline, this study found that compared to people without visual impairment:

- people with cataract had poorer vision specific and generic health related quality of life [10,11,12]
- people with cataract were less likely to engage in and spent less time on productive activities and were more likely to have assistance with daily activities [2]
- people with cataract were poorer in terms of assets, self-rated wealth and household per capita expenditure [13]

One year after cataract surgery this study found that compared to baseline:

- the vision-specific and generic health-related quality of life of people with cataract who had undergone cataract surgery had improved [8]
- people with operated cataract were more likely to undertake and spent more time on productive activities and were less likely to report receiving assistance with activities [7]
- the per capita expenditure of households with people with operated cataract had increased [9]

The cataract impact study highlighted some key benefits of cataract surgery to a population of older adults in low-income countries after one year. However, it is unclear whether these benefits are sustained over time, particularly considering the older age group mainly affected who may be more likely to experience co-morbidities. Few studies have explored the long term impact of cataract surgery on quality of life outcomes [14,15] and no information on long-term impact on time-use or poverty indicators have been identified.

Three different indicators of poverty were included in the Cataract Impact Study: household expenditure, asset ownership and self-rated wealth. While increases in household expenditure were observed among operated cases at one year follow up, asset ownership and self-rated wealth remained largely unchanged. This is unsurprising since they are longer term measures of poverty; more time is needed for households to accumulate additional assets or for perceptions of wealth to change. A longer follow-up is therefore necessary to explore the full impact of cataract surgery on poverty.

In the current study, a six year follow up of the Cataract Impact Study was undertaken in Bangladesh and the Philippines to explore the long term impact of cataract surgery on HRQoL, activities and poverty.

Methods

Study setting

This study was conducted in one district in Bangladesh (Satkhira) and two areas of the Philippines (Negros Island and Antique district, Panay Islay). A third study site (Nakuru, Kenya) included in the original Cataract Impact Study was not included in the six year follow up because of the smaller study numbers recruited at baseline.

Study population

Participants in the Cataract Impact Study were identified primarily through population-based blindness surveys which included >3600 people aged ≥50years in each setting [4,6]. Clusters of 50 people aged ≥50years were selected by probability proportionate to size sampling and within clusters, households were selected using compact segment sampling [16]. Visual acuity was assessed using tumbling E-chart the examination for cataract was conducted by an ophthalmologist using a direct ophthalmoscope. People in the survey with pinhole corrected visual acuity (VA) <6/24 in the better eye due to cataract were eligible to be cases. For each case identified, one (or up to two people in Bangladesh) age and gender matched control without visual impairment was randomly selected from the same cluster. Due to logistical and time constraints, additional case finding was undertaken in the community to increase the number of cases included.

Intervention

All cases were offered cataract surgery at the local hospital. In Bangladesh surgery was free and transport was provided by the hospital. In the Philippines a fee was requested, but those who could not afford the fee were offered free surgery. Patients made their own travel arrangements, but were reimbursed travel costs.

Data collection

Baseline surveys were conducted during 2005–2006. The first follow up was conducted one year later and the current study was conducted in September (Philippines) and November (Bangladesh) 2011 during the same climatic seasons as the baseline. Interviews were conducted in participants' homes by trained interviewers in the local language.

Measures of Health Related Quality of Life. We measured a) vision related QoL and b) generic HRQoL. Vision related quality of life was measured using the WHO/PBD VF20. The scale includes 20 items on overall eyesight, general functioning and psychosocial well-being, each with a 5-point response option. Evidence for reliability and validity of this scale was found at baseline [10,11,12]. Generic HRQL was measured using the European Quality of Life (Euroqol) questionnaire which has shown to be valid and reliable in different settings [17,18,19]. The questionnaire includes two components [20]. The first (EQ-5D) consists of five domains (mobility, self-care, usual activity, pain/discomfort and anxiety/depression) each with three response options (no problem, some problem or extreme problem). The second component measures self-rated health using a visual analogue scale. Participants are asked to rate their 'health today' on a scale ranging from 0 ('worst imaginable health state') to 100 ('best imaginable health state'). Both HRQoL tools were translated into the target languages in each country using standard forward and backward translation methods [10,12]. Translations of the generic HRQoL tool were undertaken independently of the Euroqol group and have not therefore been approved by the Euroqol group.

Measures of activities. Activity data were collected using the 'stylised activity list' developed for the World Bank's Living Standards Measurement Survey [21]. Participants were asked whether they had been involved in each of a preset list of common daily activities during the last week and if they had, whether they had been involved in the activity yesterday. Those who had been involved in an activity 'yesterday' were asked to estimate how much time they had spent on the activity and whether they received any assistance from another person in performing that activity. Activities were grouped as follows:

- Productive activities: household/family activities (cooking/washing dishes, cleaning house/clothes, shopping, looking after children/elderly/sick), paid work (paid employment, commission work, self-employed/own business); work for own use (agriculture, animal rearing, fetching firewood/water, processing agricultural products/food) other
- Leisure outside the home: social visits, attending ceremonies, attending meetings

Table 1. Baseline socio-demographic characteristics of cases and controls included in the one and six year follow-up.

	THE PHILIPPINES			BANGLADESH		
	Operated cases	Controls	P-value	Operated cases	Controls	P-value
	n = 51	n = 91		n = 56	n = 142	
Mean age (years)	69.1 (66.6–71.7)	68.3 (66.4–70.1)	0.58	68.5 (66.1–70.9)	66.7 (65.4–68.1)	0.18
Female	73%	53%	0.02	55%	59%	0.63
Married	49%	63%	0.12	50%	58%	0.28
Education	90%	92%	0.66	18%	39%	0.005
Literate	88%	89%	0.89	9%	30%	0.002
Visual acuity						
≥6/18	0%	100%	N/A	0%	100%	N/A
<6/24–6/60	24%			27%		
<6/60–3/60	20%			20%		
<3/60	56%			53%		

- Leisure inside the home: reading/listening to radio/watching TV; chatting, relaxing with friends/family; prayer (Bangladesh), other
- No activity

Measures of poverty. Three different poverty indicators were measured: a) household per capita expenditure (PCE), b) asset ownership and c)self-rated health. Interviews were conducted with the person primarily responsible for household finances.

a) PCE was measured using methods based on the World Bank's Living Standards Measurement Survey [22]. The household informant was asked to recall the monetary value of food that was purchased, consumed from home production and received as payment in kind or as gifts by all household members. The time period for which this was measured was the past week for frequently consumed items (scaled up to estimate monthly consumption) and the past month for less frequently consumed items. In addition, data were collected about monthly expenditure on education, health, household and personal items and rent paid (or rental equivalent for home owners). In total 90 items were included in the questionnaire for the Philippines and 79 in Bangladesh. The consumption on all items was summed to calculate a monthly household total. PCE was calculated by dividing total consumption by the number of household members.

b) Asset ownership: data were collected on the number and type of different context-specific assets owned by the household (e.g. cattle, furniture, electrical goods, vehicles) and household characteristics (e.g. building materials of the floor, roof and walls; type of toilet and number of rooms). These data were used to develop a relative index of household assets using principal components analysis (PCA) [23].

c) Self-rated wealth: the household informant was asked to rank the household's wealth relative to others in the community from 1(poorest) to 10 (richest)

Covariates

We collected standard socio-demographic variable data including age, gender, education, literacy and marital status.

Ethical considerations

Informed signed or thumb-printed consent was obtained from all cases and controls. All cases with operable cataract (VA<6/24) were referred for surgery. Ethical approval was obtained from the ethics committees of the London School of Hygiene & Tropical Medicine, the Bangladesh Medical Research Council and the University of St. La Salle, Bacolod, Philippines. The use of thumb-printed consent for participants who were unable to write was approved by the ethics committees.

Analysis

Data analyses were restricted to cases and controls included in all three data collection times (baseline, one year and six year follow up). Data on household expenditure were cleaned, excluding gross outliers and imputing rental equivalents based on household characteristics and non-rent expenditure where these estimates were missing or unreasonably low (<$1 per month – 34 in total across the two settings). PCE for the one and six year follow up surveys were deflated by the cumulative inflation rates over that time so that they were comparable to baseline. This adjusted PCE was converted into US dollars using the exchange rate at the time of the baseline survey. The mean proportion of time spent on each activity group was calculated by dividing total minutes on specific activity group by the sum of minutes reported on all activities for that individual, as not all totals were exactly 24 hours. To ease interpretation, the proportion of time was converted into hours and minutes.

We compared the baseline socio-demographic and clinical characteristics of a) cases and controls and b) cases and controls included and lost to follow up using t-tests for continuous variables and chi-squared for categorical variables. Change in outcomes over time were assessed using the paired t-test for continuous variables (log transformed PCE, assets, vision related QoL, self-rated health and time spent) and McNemars test for categorical variables (EQ-5D responses and participation in activities). We compared outcomes between cases and controls at each time point using firstly t-tests and chi square/fishers exact tests and secondly multivariate regression to adjust for age and gender. As the adjusted and unadjusted results were similar only the unadjusted findings will be presented here. PCE data were skewed and so were log transformed for analysis. Vision related QoL and data on amount of time spent on productive activities were also skewed,

Table 2. Vision related quality of life at baseline and one and six year follow up for operated cases and controls.

	THE PHILIPPINES			BANGLADESH		
	Operated cases	Controls		Operated cases	Controls	
	Means (95% CI)	Means (95% CI)	P-value: Cases versus controls	Means (95% CI)	Means (95% CI)	P-value: Cases versus controls
Eyesight rating						
Baseline	18.6 (12.9–24.4)	65.4 (60.1–70.7)	<0.001	12.5 (9.1–15.9)	64.6 (61.6–67.7)	<0.001
1 year follow up	75.5 (69.3–81.7)	75.5 (69.8–81.3)	0.99	75.0 (69.3–80.7)	74.0 (70.7–77.1)	0.74
6 year follow up	70.1 (62.4–77.8)	75.8 (71.0–80.6)	0.19	64.5 (58.5–70.6)	65.6 (61.7–69.5)	0.77
P-value: 1 year versus baseline	<0.001	0.003		<0.001	<0.001	
P-value: 6 year versus 1 year	0.17	0.93		<0.001	<0.001	
General Functioning						
Baseline	27.1 (21.0–33.3)	88.3 (85.4–91.1)	<0.001	16.8 (12.9–20.8)	86.3 (83.8–88.8)	<0.001
1 year follow up	86.1 (81.5–90.7)	85.9 (82.7–89.2)	0.95	82.0 (75.6–88.4)	82.1 (79.2–85.1)	0.95
6 year follow up	79.6 (72.3–87.0)	82.7 (78.7–86.8)	0.43	73.8 (66.8–80.8)	75.8 (71.9–79.7)	0.61
P-value: 1 year versus baseline	<0.001	0.08		<0.001	0.007	
P-value: 6 year versus 1 year	0.02	0.09		<0.001	0.002	
Psychosocial						
Baseline	40.4 (34.4–46.5)	87.4 (84.1–90.6)	<0.001	32.7 (26.0–39.4)	89.9 (87.4–92.4)	<0.001
1 year follow up	83.8 (79.6–88.1)	87.8 (84.3–91.4)	0.16	85.9 (79.8–92.0)	83.0 (79.8–86.2)	0.36
6 year follow up	75.9 (68.6–83.1)	78.1 (73.5–82.7)	0.58	69.9 (63.0–76.7)	69.9 (65.5–74.1)	0.99
P-value: 1 year versus baseline	<0.001	0.72		<0.001	<0.001	
P-value: 6 year versus 1 year	0.02	<0.001		<0.001	<0.001	

but could not be transformed, so analyses of these data were repeated using non-parametric tests (Wilcoxon sign rank and Mann-whitney U test). Findings were essentially unchanged and therefore parametric results are presented.

Results

Study population

The baseline survey included 217 cases and 280 controls in Bangladesh and 238 cases and 163 controls in the Philippines. Uptake of cataract surgery was generally low: 54% of cases (n = 117) identified at baseline attended for surgery by one year in Bangladesh and 47% (n = 112) in the Philippines. Only a small proportion (<5%) of the un-operated cases at one year had received cataract surgery at six years and they were excluded from the analysis. At the six year follow up the response rate in Bangladesh was 48% (n = 56) for operated cases and 51% (n = 142) for controls, and in the Philippines, 45% (n = 51) for operated cases, and 56% (n = 91) for controls. Of those lost to follow up 63% of cases and 56% of controls had died in Bangladesh (p = 0.32) and 75% of cases and 47% of controls had died in the Philippines (p = 0.001).

Operated cases (herein after referred to as 'cases') were similar to controls in terms of socio-demographic variables, with the exception that cases were more likely to be female (p = 0.02) in the Philippines and were less likely to have an education or be literate in Bangladesh (table 1).

There were few differences in socio-demographic, visual acuity, HRQoL, activity and poverty variables between participants included and lost to follow up. The exceptions were that cases lost to follow up (Bangladesh only, p = 0.04) and controls (Bangladesh p = 0.04 and the Philippines p = 0.007) were slightly older than those who were traced, in the Philippines male cases were slightly more likely to be lost to follow up than females (p = 0.03) and in Bangladesh cases lost to follow up spent slightly less time on productive activities (p = 0.02) (data not presented).

Health related Quality of Life

Vision related quality of life. At baseline cases had substantially poorer overall eyesight, general functioning and psychosocial scores compared to controls (p<0.001, table 2). At the one year follow up, all scores among cases increased significantly up to the level of controls and they remained significantly higher compared to baseline after six years (p<0.001). For example in the Philippines mean general functioning scores among cases increased from 27.1 at baseline to 86.1 at one year and was 79.6 at the six year follow up. Among controls scores were 88.3 at baseline, 85.9 at one year and 82.7 at six year follow up. Some reductions in vision related QoL scores were observed between one and six years for both cases and controls, but scores among cases remained substantially higher than at baseline and did not differ significantly from controls at either follow up.

Generic health related quality of life. At baseline in both settings, cases were significantly more likely to report problems in

Table 3. Proportion of respondents reporting some (any/extreme) problem with EQ-5D domains at baseline and one and six year follow up for operated cases and controls.

	THE PHILIPPINES			BANGLADESH		
	Operated cases	Controls		Operated cases	Controls	
	n = 51	n = 91		n = 56	n = 142	
EQ-5D Domain	%	%	P-value: Cases versus controls	%	%	P-value: Cases versus controls
Mobility						
Baseline	82%	57%	0.002	88%	43%	<0.001
1 year follow up	59%	52%	0.41	34%	44%	0.18
6 year follow up	55%	46%	0.32	44%	36%	0.36
P-value: 1 year versus baseline	0.01	0.38		<0.001	<0.001	
P-value: 6 year versus 1 year	0.81	0.38		0.23	0.11	
Self-care						
Baseline	57%	10%	<0.001	66%	18%	<0.001
1 year follow up	31%	23%	0.28	26%	23%	0.60
6 year follow up	41%	34%	0.40	**27%**	**27%**	0.98
P-value: 1 year versus baseline	0.01	0.005		<0.001	0.29	
P-value: 6 year versus 1 year	0.19	0.07		0.78	0.41	
Daily activities						
Baseline	39 (76%)	26 (29%)	<0.001	50 (89%)	60 (42%)	<0.001
1 year follow up	23 (45%)	26 (29%)	0.05	24 (43%)	53 (37%)	0.47
6 year follow up	28 (55%)	37 (41%)	0.10	23 (42%)	46 (33%)	0.24
P-value: 1 year versus baseline	0.01	1.0		<0.001	0.32	
P-value: 6 year versus 1 year	0.28	0.05		0.99	0.40	
Pain/discomfort						
Baseline	49 (96%)	60 (65%)	<0.001	44 (79%)	120 (85%)	0.32
1 year follow up	38 (75%)	65 (71%)	0.69	44 (78%)	117 (82%)	0.53
6 year follow up	38 (75%)	59 (65%)	0.24	49 (89%)	120 (86%)	0.53
P-value: 1 year versus baseline	0.005	0.37		0.99	0.59	
P-value: 6 year versus 1 year	1.0	0.24		0.08	0.40	
Anxiety/depression						
Baseline	71%	52%	0.03	91%	78%	0.03
1 year follow up	61%	41%	0.02	86%	89%	0.46
6 year follow up	37%	44%	0.42	91%	91%	0.91
P-value: 1 year versus baseline	0.25	0.12		0.32	0.01	
P-value: 6 year versus 1 year	<0.001	0.34		0.99	0.004	
Baseline	0.003	0.62		0.32	0.51	

each EQ-5D domain, with the exception of pain/discomfort in Bangladesh (table 3). At the one year follow up the proportion of cases reporting problems reduced significantly by at least 20% in 4 of the 5 domains in the Philippines (mobility, self-care, daily activities, pain/discomfort) and 3 of the 5 domains in Bangladesh (mobility, self-care, daily activities) compared to baseline. These reductions in reported problems among cases remained six years later.

Cases had significantly poorer baseline self-rated health scores compared to controls (Philippines: cases 53.9 vs controls 63.1, p = 0.001; Bangladesh 51.8 vs 59.7, p = 0.02). Self-rated health among cases increased at the one year follow up (Philippines 57.9;

Table 4. Participation in different activities over the past week at baseline and one and six year follow up for operated cases and controls.

	THE PHILIPPINES			BANGLADESH		
	Operated cases	Controls		Operated cases	Controls	
	n = 51	n = 91		n = 56	n = 142	
	%	%	P-value: Cases versus controls	%	%	P-value: Cases versus controls
Productive activities	%					
Baseline	80%	97%	0.002	61%	97%	<0.001
1 year follow up	94%	96%	0.70	88%	94%	0.13
6 year follow up	88%	88%	0.96	79%	83%	0.46
P-value: 1 year versus baseline	0.02	0.65		0.001	0.15	
P-value: 6 year versus 1 year	0.18	0.02		0.09	0.001	
Leisure outside house						
Baseline	47%	45%	0.82	43%	40%	0.73
1 year follow up	67%	77%	0.18	70%	70%	0.99
6 year follow up	65%	70%	0.49	45%	44%	0.90
P-value: 1 year versus baseline	0.03	<0.001		0.007	<0.001	
P-value: 6 year versus 1 year	0.81	0.32		0.01	<0.001	
Assistance with activities						
Baseline	29%	11%	0.008	39%	6%	<0.001
1 year follow up	5%	3%	0.19	14%	9%	0.29
6 year follow up	12%	15%	0.55	11%	10%	0.86
P-value: 1 year versus baseline	<0.001	0.03		0.004	0.35	
P-value: 6 year versus 1 year	0.01	0.002		0.48	0.8	

Bangladesh 70.0) compared to baseline so that they were no longer significantly different to controls. The increase in self-rated health was sustained after six years in Philippines (59.2). In Bangladesh scores decreased among both operated cases (55.7) and controls (50.7) between one and six years, but scores for cases remained significantly higher compared to baseline.

Activities

Participation in activities during the previous week. Nearly all cases and controls (>95%) participated in leisure activities inside the home and 'inactivity' and therefore these categories were not included in the analyses. At baseline cases were significantly less likely to take part in productive activities compared to controls in both settings (80% cases, 97% controls in Philippines, p = 0.002; 61% cases and 97% controls in Bangladesh p = <0.001, Table 4). At both one and six year follow ups the proportion of cases engaged in productive activities was significantly higher compared to baseline (by 14% and 27% at one year and 8% and 18% at six years in Philippines and Bangladesh respectively) so that there were no significant differences between cases and controls at either follow up. For leisure outside of the house, participation was similar for cases and controls at each time point.

Time spent on activities the previous day. At baseline cases spent significantly less time on productive activities (3 hours 57 minutes Philippines, 2 hours 26 minutes Bangladesh) compared to controls (6 hours 02 minutes Philippines, p = 0.002; 5 hours 42 minutes Bangladesh, p = <0.001, figure 1). One year after cataract surgery time spent on productive activities increased significantly among cases (to 6 hours 04 minutes in the Philippines, p = 0.003 and 3 hours 51 minutes in Bangladesh p = 0.004). However, at the six year follow up a significant reduction in productive activity time was observed among both cases and controls in both settings. In the Philippines there was no significant difference between cases and controls at either follow up, but in Bangladesh cases continued to spend significantly less time on productive activities than controls.

Time spent on leisure inside and outside of the house in both settings were similar for cases and controls at each time point (data not shown). In the Philippines, time spent in inactivity did not differ significantly between cases (3 hours 54 minutes) and controls (3 hours 13 minutes) at baseline (p = 0.55). Time in inactivity remained similar among cases at each time point, but increased among controls (to 4 hours 18 minutes at six years, p = 0.02). In Bangladesh, cases spent 2 hours more in inactivity than controls at baseline. At one year, this reduced significantly so that it was similar for cases (3 hours 8 minutes) and controls (2 hours

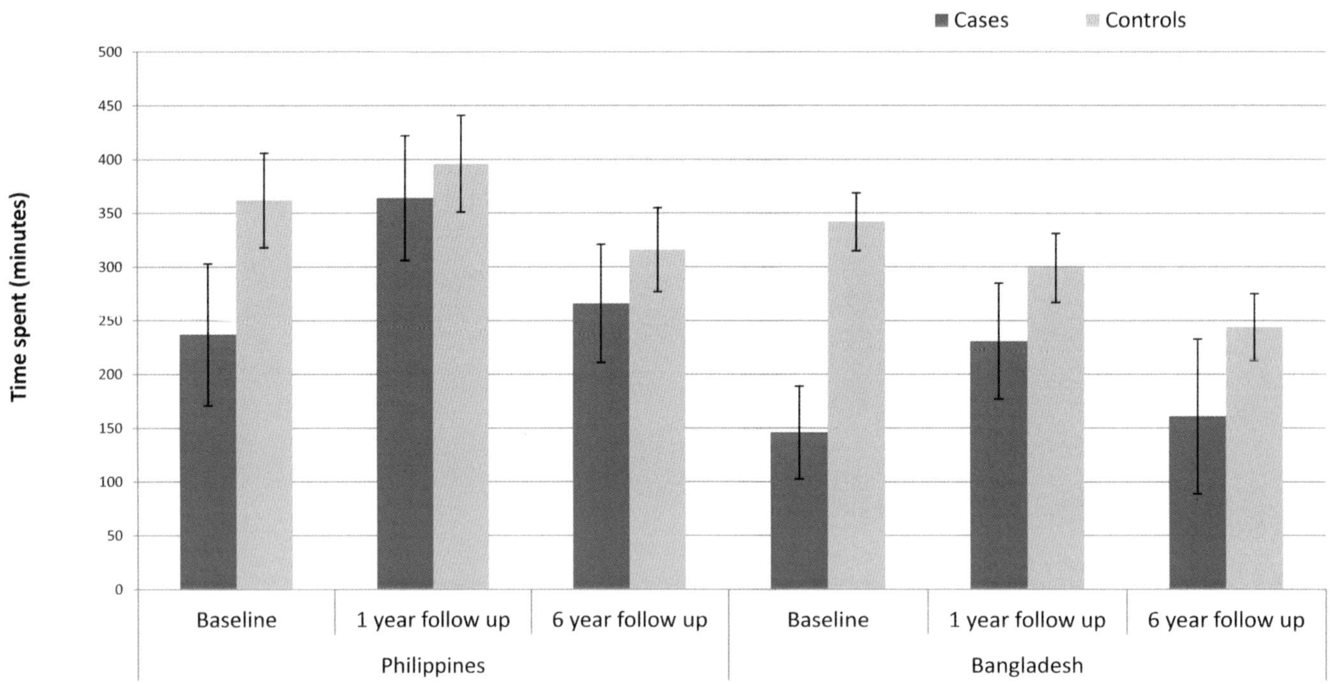

Figure 1. Time (minutes) spent on productive activities at baseline, one year and six year follow up among operated cases and controls.

44 minutes, p = 0.25). However a significant increase was observed for both cases (to 4 hours 32 minutes, p = 0.006) and controls (3 hours 30 minutes, p = 0.007; case vs control p = 0.01) by the six year follow up.

Assistance with activities. At baseline cases compared to controls were two and a half times more likely to receive assistance undertaking activities in the Philippines (p<0.008) and six times more likely in Bangladesh (p<0.001, table 4). At both the one year and six year follow ups the proportion reporting assistance decreased significantly by at least a half so that there were no significant differences between cases and controls.

Poverty

PCE. At baseline, cases had significantly lower PCE compared to controls (Philippines $22 vs $29 per person per month, p = 0.04; Bangladesh $15 vs $27, p = 0.02, table 5). One year after surgery PCE among cases increased compared to baseline to at least the level of the controls. This increase was sustained so that at the six year follow up PCE there were no statistically significant differences between cases and controls (Philippines $39 vs $37 p = 0.85, Bangladesh $23 vs $24 p = 0.85). In the Philippines there was a significant increase in expenditure between one and six years among both cases and controls (p<0.05).

Assets. At baseline, cases had lower asset scores compared to controls although this difference was only borderline significant in Bangladesh (−0.50 vs 0.33p = 0.06, table 5) and non-significant in the Philippines (−0.25 vs 0.32, p = 0.20, Table 2). Scores remained similar at the one year follow up. At the six year follow up, assets scores among cases had increased slightly so that they were similar to controls (Philippines 0.13 cases vs 0.15 controls, p = 0.96 Bangladesh 0.10 vs 0.14,p = 0.85).

Self-rated wealth. In Bangladesh at baseline, self-rated wealth was significantly lower among cases (3.7) compared to controls (4.5, p = 0.01) and this remained similar at the one year follow up (table 5). At the six year follow up, there was a small increase in scores among cases so that mean self-rated wealth was the same for cases and controls (4.1 for both, p = 0.86). In the Philippines there were no significant differences between cases and controls at any of the time points.

Un-operated cases

Among cases who did not attend for surgery ('un-operated cases') the economic and activity variables either stayed similar or worsened over the two follow ups (data not presented). For vision related Qol there were some small increases in scores for un-operated cases, although these were considerably smaller than for the operated cases. The proportion reporting problems with EQ-5D scores remained similar over time, with the exception of mobility and activities in Bangladesh in which there were some reductions in reported problems.

Discussion

The cataract impact study explored the effect of cataract surgery on three different but interlinked outcomes: health related quality of life, daily activities and economic poverty, in Bangladesh and the Philippines. Prior to surgery people with cataract visual impairment had poorer vision and health related QoL, were less likely to undertake and spent less time on productive activities, were more likely to receive assistance with activities and were economically poorer compared to controls without vision impairment. One year after surgery there were improvements in each of these outcomes so that the operated cases were similar to controls. However, it was unclear whether these benefits would be sustained in the long term, particularly considering the older age group of the study population who may be more likely to experience other co-morbidities. The current study has indicated that the increases in vision and health related QoL, participation in productive activities and PCE and reduction in reported assistance with daily

Table 5. Per capita expenditure (PCE), assets and self-rated wealth at baseline and one and six year follow up for operated cases and controls.

	THE PHILIPPINES			BANGLADESH		
	Operated cases	Controls		Operated cases	Controls	
	Means (95% CI)	Means (95% CI)	P-value: Cases versus controls	Means (95% CI)	Means (95% CI)	P-value: Cases versus controls
PCE (US$)						
Baseline	21.73 (3.97–57.51)	29.01 (2.54–184.17)	0.04	14.95 (12.34–17.56)	26.90 (13.21–40.60)	0.02
1 year follow up	27.1 (5.37–134.39)	28.13 (3.27–108.14)	0.50	23.05 (16.55–29.56)	21.24 (19.42–23.07)	0.37
6 year follow up	38.9 (3.9–246.62)	37.4 (3.53–197.36)	0.85	23.29 (17.88–30.09)	24.29 (20.84–27.73)	0.85
P-value: 1 year versus baseline	0.14	0.96		0.001	0.02	
P-value: 6 year versus 1 year	0.008	0.004		0.52	0.74	
ASSETS						
Baseline	−0.25 (−0.97–0.46)	0.32 (−0.20–0.81)	0.20	−0.50 (−1.17–1.18)	0.33 (−0.16–0.82)	0.06
1 year follow up	−0.27 (−1.01–4.64)	0.27 (−0.23–0.77)	0.21	−0.52 (−1.20–0.15)	0.34 (−0.13–0.80)	0.05
6 year follow up	0.13 (−0.58–0.84)	0.15 (−0.37–0.66)	0.97	0.1 (−0.66–0.86)	0.14 (−0.36–0.64)	0.94
P-value: 1 year versus baseline	0.74	0.57		0.54	0.95	
P-value: 6 year versus 1 year	0.97	0.43		0.005	0.26	
Self-rated wealth						
Baseline	4.7 (4.3–5.0)	4.6 (4.3–5.0)	0.94	3.7 (3.1–4.2)	3.8 (3.3–4.3)	0.01
1 year follow up	4.5 (4.1–4.9)	5.1 (4.0–6.1)	0.46	3.8 (3.3–4.3)	4.4 (4.1–4.7)	0.06
6 year follow up	5.4 (3.2–7.7)	4.8 (4.4–5.3)	0.55	4.1 (3.5–4.6)	4.1 (3.8–4.4)	0.85
P-value: 1 year versus baseline	0.34	0.41		0.46	0.35	
P-value: 6 year versus 1 year	0.43	0.72		0.31	0.10	

activities were still evident after six years. Average daily time spent on productive activities decreased among both cases and controls.

We measured three different indicators of poverty: PCE, asset ownership and self-rated wealth. One year after cataract surgery increases in PCE were observed among operated cases, but asset ownership did not change. However, after six years there were some increases in asset scores in both settings among operated cases. This finding is intuitive as asset ownership is a longer term measure of poverty than expenditure and therefore more time is needed for households to accumulate possessions. Improvements in self-rated wealth were not observed. This may be because as it is a measure of perceived wealth relative to other households in the community which might be harder to change or because there was a limited variation in this variable so that we were under-powered to detect a change.

The activity data collected in this study provide possible explanatory routes for the observed improvements in PCE and assets. One route is through the increased productivity of the individual operated for surgery: six years after surgery a higher proportion of cases remained engaged in productive activities than at baseline. Productive activities included paid work and also non-paid activities which can make significant economic contributions [24]. There were some reductions in participation in and time spent on productive activities among both cases and controls between one and six years. This is not surprising in a population of older adults (approximately half of participants were aged 70 years and above in both settings) where health may be deteriorating over time. A second possible route is through increased productivity of other household members as a result of increased independence of the operated case. This is supported by the sustained reduction in reported assistance from others with daily activities six years after surgery. Further research on the impact of cataract surgery on the daily activities of other household members is needed to confirm this.

There are a limited number of longitudinal studies with which to compare these findings. Our findings support two studies in India which showed increased household income [25] (Finger, 2012) and engagement in income generating [25,26] and household activities [26] within a year following surgery. Our current study provides additional evidence that this positive impact is sustained in the longer term.

We also found evidence of substantial sustained benefits of cataract surgery on vision and generic health related quality of life. There were some small reductions in quality of life measures between the one and six year follow up among cases and controls, however this is unsurprising for this age group where deteriorations in vision and health may be expected. The improvements in vision related QoL one year after surgery are consistent with two studies in India [25,27]. Previous studies on generic HRQoL are more mixed, with some studies in high-income settings finding evidence of improvement [28,29] and others showing no change following cataract surgery [15,30,31]. Few studies of the long term impact could be identified. However, our study supports findings by Lundqvist et al that visual function scores remained stable 10 years after cataract surgery [14]. A study in Australia found long term improvements in mental but not physical domains of the SF-36 health related quality of life instrument [15].

There were a number of limitations to this study. Uptake of surgery was lower than expected and loss to follow up was around 50% at the six year follow up. The sample size was therefore small which has implications for the tests of statistical significance (of which there were many) as the study may have had insufficient power to detect statistically significant true differences in the outcome variables. There were few differences in socio-demographic characteristics between operated and unoperated cases and those included/lost to follow up reducing possible impact on external validity. The exception was that the participants who did not attend for surgery (both settings) and cases who were lost to follow up (Bangladesh only) were slightly older. We therefore cannot rule out the possibility that if more of the unoperated cases had attended surgery and if fewer participants were lost to follow up the increases in PCE and productive activities might have been smaller.

There were some improvements in vision and generic HRQoL among unoperated cases over time although this was considerably smaller than for operated cases. The reason for this is unclear, but may reflect adaptation to their level of vision loss over time or that having decided against surgery they under reported difficulties with visual functioning at the follow up to discourage survey team members from trying to suggest they should attend.

Finally there were potential limitations with the activities data in terms of the reliance on recall and the collection of data for a single day which may not represent a typical day. Further although data were collected during the same climatic season at the three time points, they were not always collected during the same month and time of year, which may influence time-use patterns.

Strengths of this study are that it was conducted in two different countries and used standardised data collection tools at three different time points. Study participants were population based rather than from hospitals which increases the generalisability of the findings. We included matched controls without vision impairment and in general their outcomes remained relatively stable or worsened over time. This provides support to the changes among operated cases being due to cataract surgery and not to other events.

Conclusion

The six year follow up of the Cataract Impact Study is the first study to explore the long term impacts of cataract surgery on people's lives in low income settings. This study has indicated that there are sustained benefits of cataract surgery to a population of older adults in low-income countries in terms of health related quality of life, daily activities and household economics and highlights the importance of cataract surgery in improving the lives of people in the long term.

Acknowledgments

We are very grateful to all the study participants for giving their time so generously. We would also like to thank the field workers, doctors, office managers, data entry staff and drivers who made this study possible.

Author Contributions

Conceived and designed the experiments: HK SP AF CE MR. Performed the experiments: LD LB SP CE MR. Analyzed the data: LD SP HK. Wrote the paper: SP. Revised the article critically for important intellectual content: LD HK LB AF CE MR. Gave final approval of the version to be published: SP LD HK LB AF CE MR.

References

1. Resnikoff S, Pascolini D, Mariotti SP, Pokharel GP (2008) Global magnitude of visual impairment caused by uncorrected refractive errors in 2004. Bull World Health Organ 86: 63–70.
2. Polack S, Kuper H, Eusebio C, Mathenge W, Wadud Z, et al. (2008) The impact of cataract on time-use: results from a population based case-control study in Kenya, the Philippines and Bangladesh. Ophthalmic Epidemiol 15: 372–382.
3. Dandona L, Dandona R, Srinivas M, Giridhar P, Vilas K, et al. (2001) Blindness in the Indian state of Andhra Pradesh. Invest Ophthalmol Vis Sci 42: 908–916.
4. Wadud Z, Kuper H, Polack S, Lindfield R, Rashid Akm M, et al. (2006) Rapid Assessment of Avoidable Blindness and Needs Assessment of Cataract Surgical Services in Satkhira District, Bangladesh. Br J Ophthalmol 90:1225–1229.
5. Mathenge W, Kuper H, Polack S, Onyango O, Nyaga G, et al. (2007) Rapid Assessment of Avoidable Blindness in Nakuru District, Kenya. Ophthalmology 114: 599–605.
6. Eusebio C, Kuper H, Polack S, Enconado J, Tongson N, et al. (2007) Rapid assessment of avoidable blindness in Negros Island and Antique District, Philippines. Br J Ophthalmol 91: 1588–1592.
7. Polack S, Eusebio C, Mathenge W, Wadud Z, Mamun R, et al. (2010) The Impact of Cataract Surgery on Activities and Time-Use: Results from a Longitudinal Study In Kenya, Bangladesh and The Philippines PLoS ONE 5: e10913.
8. Polack S, Eusebio C, Mathenge W, Wadud Z, Mamun R, et al. (2010) The Impact of Cataract Surgery on health related quality of life in Kenya, Bangladesh and The Philippines. Submitted to Ophthalmic Epidemiology. Ophthalmic Epidemiol 17: 387–399.
9. Kuper H, Polack S, Mathenge W, Eusebio C, Wadud Z, et al. (2010) Does cataract surgery alleviate poverty? Evidence from a multi-centre intervention study conducted in Kenya, the Philippines and Bangladesh. PloS One 5: e15431.
10. Polack S, Eusebio C, Fletcher A, Foster A, Kuper H (2010) Visual impairment from cataract and health related quality of life: results from a case-control study in the Philippines. Ophthalmic Epidemiol 17: 152–159.
11. Polack S, Kuper H, Mathenge W, Fletcher A, Foster A (2007) Cataract visual impairment and quality of life in a Kenyan population. Br J Ophthalmol 91: 927–932.
12. Polack S, Kuper H, Wadud Z, Fletcher A, Foster A (2008) Quality of life and visual impairment from cataract in Satkhira district, Bangladesh. Br J Ophthalmol 92: 1026–1030.
13. Kuper H, Polack S, Eusebio C, Mathenge W, Wadud Z, et al. (2008) A case-control study to assess the relationship between poverty and visual impairment from cataract in Kenya, the Philippines, and Bangladesh. PLoS Med 5: e244.
14. Lundqvist B, Monestam E (2006) Longitudinal changes in subjective and objective visual function 5 years after cataract surgery Prospective population-based study. J Cataract Refract Surg 32: 1944–1950.
15. Chandrasekaran S, Wang JJ, Rochtchina E, Mitchell P (2007) Change in health-related quality of life after cataract surgery in a population-based sample. Eye.
16. Turner AG, Magnani RJ, Shuaib M (1996) A not quite as quick but much cleaner alternative to the Expanded Programme on Immunization (EPI) Cluster Survey design. Int J Epidemiol 25: 198–203.
17. Jelsma J, Hansen K, De Weerdt W, De Cock P, Kind P (2003) How do Zimbabweans value health states? Popul Health Metr 1: 11.
18. Shaheen R, Lindholm L (2005) Quality of life among pregnant women with chronic energy deficiency in rural Bangladesh. Health Policy.
19. Tidermark J, Bergstrom G, Svensson O, Tornkvist H, Ponzer S (2003) Responsiveness of the EuroQol (EQ 5-D) and the SF-36 in elderly patients with displaced femoral neck fractures. Qual Life Res 12: 1069–1079.
20. Rabin R, de Charro F (2001) EQ-5D: a measure of health status from the EuroQol Group. Ann Med 33: 337–343.
21. Harvey AS, Taylor ME (2000) Time Use. In: Grosh M, Glewwe P, editors. Designing household survey questionnaires for developing countries Lessons from 15 years of the Living Standards Measurement Study. Washington: The World Bank. pp. 249–275.
22. Grosh M, Glewwe P, editors (2000) Designing household survey questionnaires for developing countries. Lessons from 15 years of the living standards measurement study. Washington, D.C.: World Bank.
23. Filmer D, Pritchett L (2001) Estimating wealth effects without expenditure data - or tears. An application to educational enrollment in states of India. Demography 38: 115–132.
24. UNDP (1995) Human Development Report. Chapter 4: Valuing women's work. UNDP. 87–98 p.

25. Finger RP, Kupitz DG, Fenwick E, Balasubramaniam B, Ramani RV, et al. (2012) The impact of successful cataract surgery on quality of life, household income and social status in South India. PLoS One 7: e44268.
26. Javitt J, Venkataswamy G, Sommer A (1983) The economic and social aspect of restoring sight. In: Henkind P, editor. ACTA: 24th International Congress of Ophthalmology. New York: JP Lippincott. pp. 1308–1312.
27. Fletcher A, Vijaykumar V, Selvaraj S, Thulasiraj RD, Ellwein LB (1998) The Madurai Intraocular Lens Study. III: Visual functioning and quality of life outcomes. Am J Ophthalmol 125: 26–35.
28. Desai P, Reidy A, Minassian DC, Vafidis G, Bolger J (1996) Gains from cataract surgery: visual function and quality of life. Br J Ophthalmol 80: 868–873.
29. Jayamanne DGR, Allen ED, Wood CM, Currie S (1999) Correlation between early, measurable improvment in quality of life and speed of visual rehabilitation after phacoemulsification. J Cataract Refract Surg 25: 1135–1139.
30. Owsley C, McGwin G Jr, Scilley K, Meek GC, Seker D, et al. (2007) Impact of cataract surgery on health-related quality of life in nursing home residents. Br J Ophthalmol 91: 1359–1363.
31. Rasanen P, Krootila K, Sintonen H, Leivo T, Koivisto AM, et al. (2006) Cost-utility of routine cataract surgery. Health Qual Life Outcomes 4: 74.

Alcohol Intake and the Risk of Age-Related Cataracts: A Meta-Analysis of Prospective Cohort Studies

Wei Wang, Xiulan Zhang*

Zhongshan Ophthalmic Center, State Key Laboratory of Ophthalmology, Sun Yat-Sen University, Guangzhou, People's Republic of China

Abstract

Purpose: Epidemiologic studies assessing the relationship between alcohol consumption and the risk of age-related cataracts (ARCs) led to inconsistent results. This meta-analysis was performed to fill this gap.

Methods: Eligible studies were identified via computer searches and reviewing the reference lists of these obtained articles. Pooled estimates of the relative risks (RR) and the corresponding 95% confidence Intervals (CI) were calculated using random effects models.

Results: Seven prospective cohort studies involving a total of 119,706 participants were ultimately included in this meta-analysis. Pooled results showed that there is no substantial overall increased risk of ARC due to heavy alcohol consumption. The estimated RRs comparing heavy drinkers versus non-drinkers were 1.25 (95% CI: 1.00, 1.56) for cataract sugery, 1.06 (95% CI: 0.63, 1.81) for cortical cataracts, 1.26 (95% CI: 0.93, 1.73) for nuclear cataracts, and 0.91 (95% CI: 0.32, 2.61) for posterior subcapsular cataracts (PSCs), respectively. No significant associations between moderate alcohol consumption and cataracts were observed. The pooled RRs comparing moderate drinkers versus non-drinkers were 0.90 (95% CI: 0.64, 1.26) for cataract surgery, 0.97 (95% CI: 0.75, 1.25) for cortical cataracts, 0.91 (95% CI: 0.76, 1.08) for nuclear cataracts, and 0.97 (95% CI: 0.49, 1.91) for PSCs, respectively.

Conclusions: This meta-analysis suggests that there is no substantial overall increased risk of ARC due to alcohol intake. Because of the limited number of studies, the findings from our study must be confirmed in future research via well-designed cohort or intervention studies.

Editor: K. Krishna Sharma, University of Missouri-Columbia, United States of America

Funding: This research was supported by the National Natural Science Foundation of China (81371008). The funders had no role in study design, data collection and analysis, decision to publish, or preparation of the manuscript.

Competing Interests: The authors have declared that no competing interests exist.

* Email: zhangxl2@mail.sysu.edu.cn

Introduction

Age-Related Cataracts (ARCs) remain the leading cause of blindness in developed and developing countries [1–3]. As the world's population ages, visual impairment due to cataracts is on the increase [4]. This is a significant global problem. Although surgical techniques and subsequent outcomes have greatly improved in recent years, the economic cost of cataract surgery remains substantial. Therefore, apart from the surgical extraction of the lens, other primary prevention efforts regarding cataracts should be explored [5].

Alcohol intake may have both harmful and protective effects in terms of ARCs [6–9]. An extensive body of data shows concordant J-shaped associations between alcohol intake and a variety of adverse health outcomes [10]. This may be true regarding ARCs. Epidemiologic studies that have assessed this relationship, however, have not consistently shown that heavy alcohol consumption is associated with a higher risk of ARCs or that moderate alcohol consumption is protective [11–38]. To address this uncertainty, this meta-analysis of the literature was performed to evaluate the associations between alcohol consumption and ARCs. Only prospective cohort studies were included in this study because of the limitations of retrospective studies in terms of assessing the associations of alcohol consumption due to the significance of recall bias in such studies.

Methods

The Preferred Reporting Items for Systematic Reviews and Meta-Analyses (PRISMA) statement was used as a guide to conduct the study, including the strategies for searching, analysis, and the presentation of results, potential bias, interpretation, and writing (Checklist S1).

1. Literature Search

Two authors independently performed literature searches by using the PubMed and Embase databases through December of 2013. The keywords were as follows: (drinking OR alcohol OR ethanol OR wine OR beer OR liquor OR "life stye") AND (cataract OR cataracts OR "lens opacity" OR "lens opacities" OR "lens opacification") AND (cohort OR longitudinal OR inciden* OR follow-up). There were no limits placed on the year or language of publication. References identified from the bibliographies of pertinent articles were also retrieved.

2. Exposure Assessment

There are currently no universally accepted definitions of heavy or moderate alcohol use. Low-risk recommendations vary between less than 10 to 60 g/day among developed nations. In this study, heavy alcohol consumption was defined as ≥20 g/day (equivalent to 2 Australian standard drinks) in accordance with the Australian alcohol guidelines average for male and females [39]. Moderate alcohol consumption was defined as being less than heavy alcohol consumption but more than no alcohol consumption. When possible, nondrinkers were chosed as the reference category; however, in several studies, occasional drinkers were included in the reference category. When more than one estimate in a study fell within the range considered for moderate or heavy alcohol consumption, the corresponding estimates were pooled using the Hamling et al. [40] method, thus taking into account their correlation.

3. Study Selection

Studies were included for analysis if they met the following criteria: (1) had a prospective cohort study design; (2) clearly reported measurements of alcohol consumption; (3) clearly defined ARC as the outcome; and (4) reported the relative risk (RR) and the corresponding 95% Confidence Interval (95%CI) (or the data to calculate them). In studies of the same population, only the latest or the most complete studies were included. Reviews or letters to the editor without original data, editorials, case reports, case-control studies, and cross-sectional studies were excluded.

4. Data Extraction and Study Quality Evaluation

Data extraction and study quality evaluation were performed independently by two reviewers (W.W. and X.Z). Data were extracted using a standardized extraction form, and the assessment of methodological quality was determined by using the Newcastle-Ottawa Scale (NOS) [41]. The NOS consists of three parameters of quality: selection, comparability, and outcome. The NOS assigns a maximum of four points for selection, two points for comparability, and three points for exposure/outcome. A score of nine points on the NOS reflects the highest study quality. Any disagreement was resolved via discussion.

5. Statistical Analysis

RR was used as the common measure of association across studies. The data from individual studies were pooled by using the random-effect model with the DerSimonian-Laird method, which considers within-study and between-study variation [42]. Heterogeneity was assessed using the Cochran Q and I^2 statistics. For the Q statistic, a P value<0.10 was considered statistically significant for heterogeneity; for the I^2 statistic, values of 25%, 50%, and 75% represented mild, moderate, and severe heterogeneity, respectively. To assess the influence of individual studies on the pooled result, sensitivity analyses were performed by excluding each study one by one and recalculating the combined estimates based on the remaining studies. Subgroup analyses were also performed by gender. Publication bias was evaluated via funnel figures, Egger's test (linear regression method), and Begg's test (rank correlation method) [43]. All analyses were performed by using STATA Version 12.0 (StataCorp). A P value less than 0.05 was considered significant, except where otherwise specified. Additionally, data from this meta-analysis are presented in accordance with the checklist proposed by the Meta-Analysis of Observational Studies in Epidemiology (MOOSE) group.

Results

1. Literature Search

The detailed steps of the study selection process are shown in Figure 1. Briefly, we initially identified 425 potentially eligible studies. Thirty-one were considered as potentially relevant studies. Of these, 24 studies were excluded because they did not meet the inclusion criteria or were duplicate publications. Finally, seven cohort studies that met all inclusion criteria were inclued for meta-analysis [29–35]. There was complete agreement between reviewers regarding study eligibility.

2. Study Characteristics and Qualities

The design features and participant characteristics of the studies are presented in Table 1. The seven prospective cohort studies selected provided a total sample size of 119,706 people. Of these studies, four studies were conducted in North America, one in Sweden, one in Australia, and one in China. The mean length of follow-up ranged from 2 to 12 years, with a median of 8 years. One cohort study included only men, and one study included only women. In most studies, participants were 40 years or older, with the exception of one that also included participants in their 30 s. Five studies were population-based studies, whereas two studies consisted of volunteers (the Physicians' Health Study [35] and the

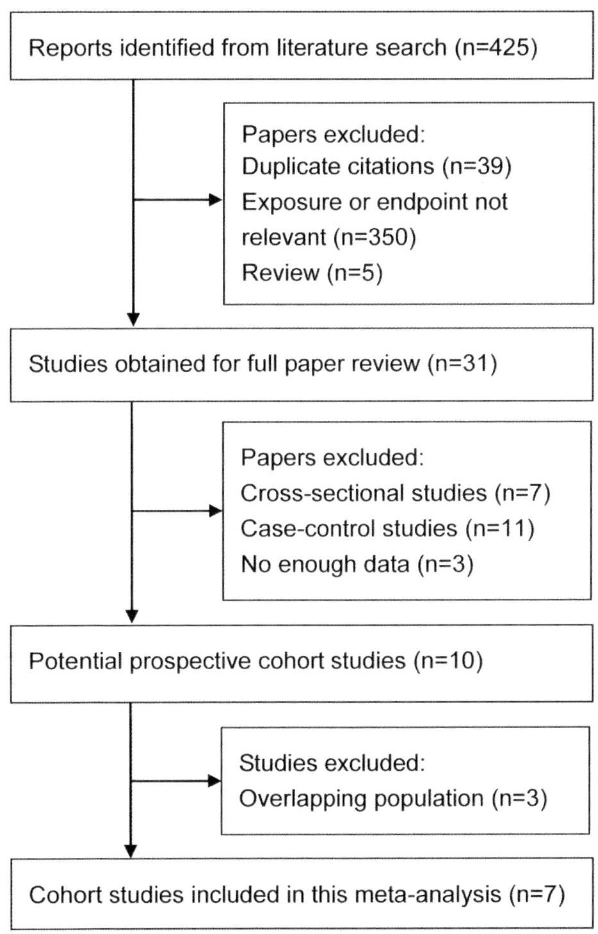

Figure 1. Flow chart of study selection.

Table 1. Characteristic of prospective cohort studies evaluating alcohol consumption and its association with age-related cataract.

First author, year	Study Follow-up	Population (Sample Size, age [years])	ARC Definition and Grading	Adjust variables	Alcohol intake	RR(95%CI) (highest vs lowest)
Storey, 2013	The Salisbury Eye Evaluation Study (SEE), 2 years	Population based, United States (2520, 65 to 84)	The Wisconsin Cataract Grading system	Age, sex, race, education, past steroid use, smoking status, alcohol status, history of hypertension, diabetes, average annual ultraviolet-B exposure	Not clear	Any vs non-drink: Nuclear: 0.87(0.63,1.20); Cortical: 1.39 (0.87,2.20); Any: 1.01 (0.78,1.32)
Kuang, 2013	The Shihpai Fye Study (SPES), 7 years	Population based, China (1361, ≥65)	Lens Opacification Classification System III	Age, sex, education, marital status, waist-to-hip ratio, systolic blood pressure, history of hypertension, diabetes, cardiovascular disease, stroke, smoking history, alcohol drinking, and history of hormone use among women	Not clear	Any vs non-drink: Surgery: 1.12(0.64,1.98); PSC: 1.37(0.67,2.82); Any:1.31(0.95,1.81)
Kanthan, 2010	The Blue Mountains Eye Study (BMES), 10 years	Population based, Australia (3654,49 to 97)	The Wisconsin Cataract Grading system	Age, gender, smoking, diabetes, socioeconomic status, steroid use, and myopia.	0 >0 to ≤1 >1 to ≤2 >2 drinks/day	Heavy vs non-drink: Surgery:2.10(1.16, 3.81); Cortical:0.76 (0.53, 1.10); Nuclear:1.13(0.73.1.76); PSC: 0.65(0.36, 1.19)
Lindblad, 2007	The Swedish Mammography Cohort (SMC), 8 years	Population based, Sweden, female only (34 713, 49 to 83)	The Swedish National Cataract Register	Age, smoking, alcohol consumption, steroid medication use, vitamin supplement use, educational level	<6 6–13 >13–20 >20–30 >30 g/day	Heavy vs non-drink: Surgery:0.84(0.53, 1.33);
Klein, 2003	The Beaver Dam Eye Study (BDES), 10 years	Population based, USA (4926, 43–86)	The Wisconsin Cataract Grading system	Age and Sex	0 >0–5.7 >5.7–14.2 >14.2–48 >48 g/day	Heavy vs non-drink: Cortical:1.13 (0.60,2.31); Nuclear:1.93 (1.08,3.46); PSC:0.37 (0.09,1.56)
Chasan-Taber, 2000	The Nurses' Health Study (NHS), 12 years	Nurse, United States (50461, 30 to 55)	Ophthalmologic records	Age, time period, smoking, body mass index, area of residence, number of physician visits, aspirin use, calories, physical activity, parental history of myocardial infarction, history of diagnosis of elevated cholesterol, hypertension, or diabetes	0 >0–4.9 5.0–14.9 15.0–24.9 ≥25 g/day	Heavy vs non-drink: Cataract: 1.10(0.90, 1.35); Cortical: 2.07 (0.82, 5.24); Nuclear: 1.10(0.74, 1.62); PSC: 2.46(1.09, 5.55)
Manson, 1994	The Physicians' Health Study (PHS), 5 years	Physician, USA, male only (22071, 40 to 84)	Self-report confirmed by medical record review	Age	Not clear	Daily drinkers vs non: Surgery:1.12 (0.64, 1.98); PSC:1.37 (0.67, 2.82); Any:1.31 (0.95, 1.81)

ARC = age-related cataract; CI = confidential interval; PSC = posterior subcapsular cataract.

Nurses Health Study [33], which were conducted as part of other studies consisting of healthcare workers). Alcohol consumption was ascertained via self-report at baseline in each study by using self-administered questionnaires that estimated consumption over the past year. The assessment of ARC varied across studies. Standardized criteria for the diagnosis of cataracts were used in some studies, while in others, cases were diagnosed medically via an ophthalmologist or medical record review. Likewise, the outcome measure of cataracts was not consistent. Many studies used the incidence of cataracts, but some studies used cataract extraction as the measure of outcome. All studies adjusted for age in their analyses. The NOS results showed that the average score was 8.5 (range 8 to 9), indicating that the methodological quality was generally good.

3. Alcohol Intake and ARC Risks

The pooled RR of any drinkers versus non-drinkers forARC risk was summarized in Figure 2, and no significant association were noted. There was moderate heterogeneity among studies ($P = 0.048$; $I^2 = 52.8\%$). In order to analyse the influence of the sample and age, a sensitivity analysis was performed. When The Nurses' Health Study (NHS) (largest number of population and aged 30–55) was excluded from this study, the random-effect pooled estimate of any drinker vs non-drinker for any cataract was

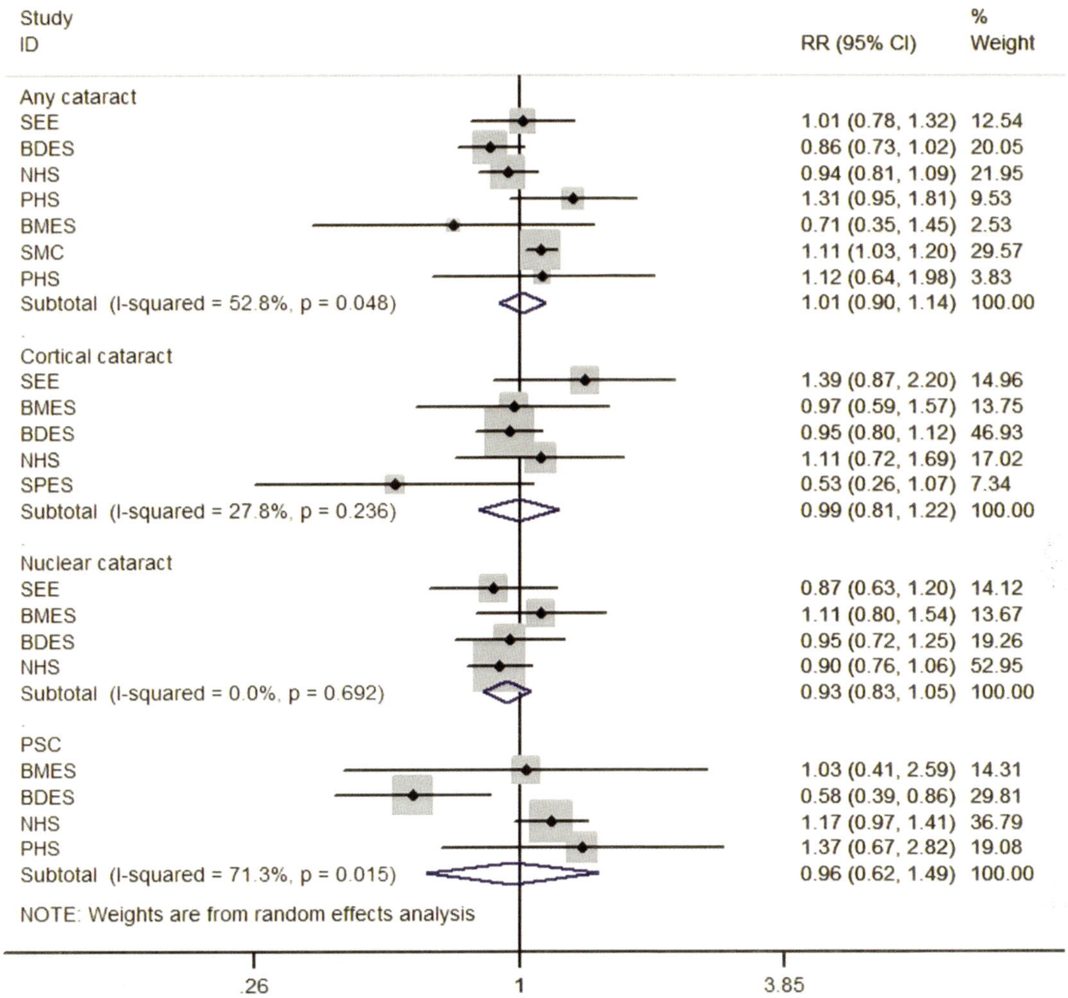

Figure 2. Forest plot for study-specific and pooled relative risk (RR) estimates (Any drinkers versus Non-drinkers) of cataract risk associated with alcohol consumption. SEE = The Salisbury Eye Evaluation Study; BMES = The Blue Mountains Eye Study; BDES = The Beaver Dam Eye Study; NHS = The Nurses' Health Study; SMC = The Swedish Mammography Cohort; SPES = The Shihpai Eye Study; PHS = The Physicians' Health Study; PSC = posterior subcapsular cataract.

1.030 (0.893,1.187), similar to that of all 7 studies. Heterogeneity between studies was not significantly reduced by the sensitivity analysis ($P = 0.064$, $I^2 = 52.0\%$). In addition, subgroup analyses were performed to evaluate whether the pooled estimates of any drink vs non-drink for any cataract were different according to gender. When NHS study and SMC study were excluded individually from this study, the random-effect pooled RR comparing any drinkers to non-drinkers for any cataract was 0.990 (0.825, 1.188), with moderate levels of heterogeneity ($P = 0.174$, $I^2 = 37.0\%$). For the subgroup including studies with only female, the association between alcohol intake and any cataract was also not statistically significant [RR = 1.035 (0.881,1.215)]. However, this should also be interprete with cautions because only two of the seven studies included. These subgroup analyses did not alter the results obtained in cumulative analyses. Hence, the original result was robust.

The RR estimates of moderate drinkers versus non-drinkers were showed in Figure 3. There was also no statistical association. As for heavy drinking versus no drinking, there was a borderline positive association between the risk of cataract surgery and the consumption of ≥20 g/day of alcohol (RR = 1.25, 95% CI: 1.00, 1.56), with moderate heterogeneity ($P = 0.121$; $I^2 = 52.60\%$). With respect to cortical, nuclear, and PS cataracts, the associations were statistically non-significant, with pooled RRs of 1.06 (95% CI: 0.63, 1.81), 1.26 (95% CI: 0.93, 1.73), and 0.91 (95% CI: 0.32, 2.61), respectively (Figure 4). In sensitivity analyses, the results were similar and without great fluctuation (data not shown).

4. Publication Bias

Visual inspection of the funnel plot for the studies evaluating alcohol consumption and its associations with ARC did not identify substantial asymmetry (Figure 5, Figure 6). The Begg rank correlation test and Egger linear regression test also indicated little

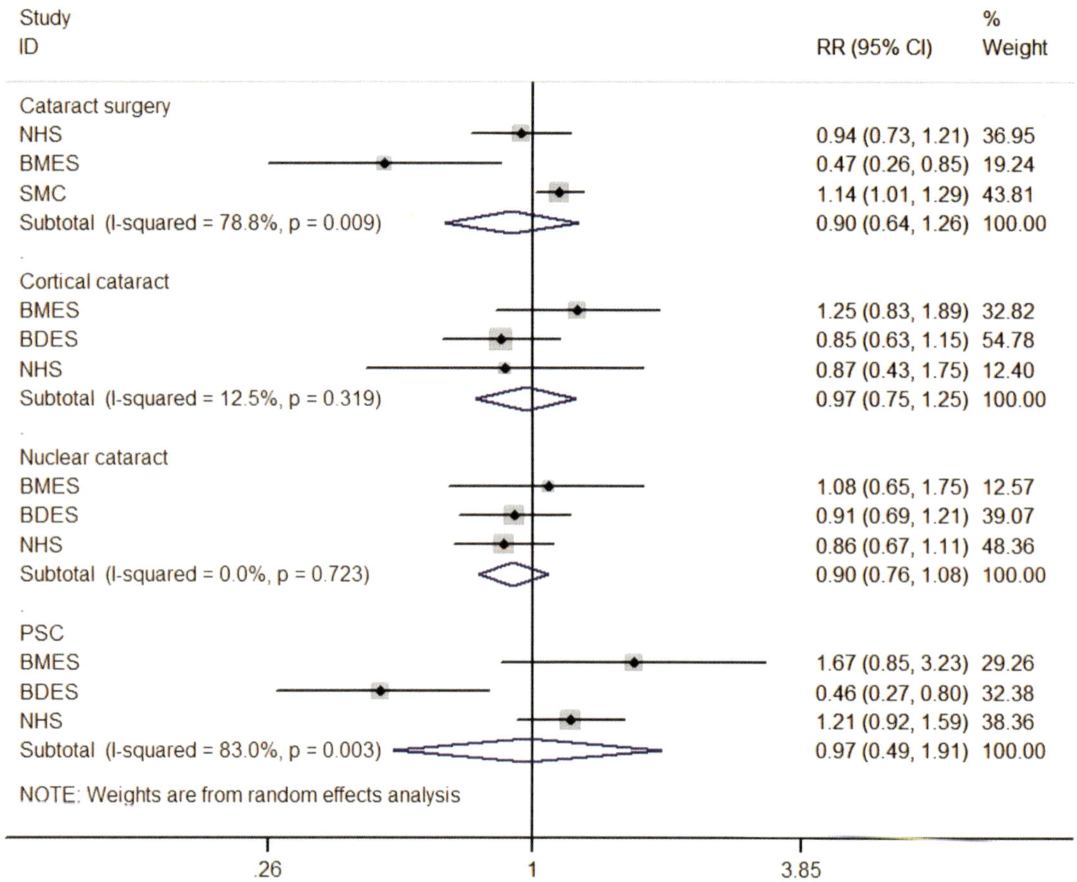

Figure 3. Forest plot for study-specific and pooled relative risk (RR) estimates (Moderate drinkers versus Non-drinkers) of cataract risk associated with alcohol consumption. SEE = The Salisbury Eye Evaluation Study; BMES = The Blue Mountains Eye Study; BDES = The Beaver Dam Eye Study; NHS = The Nurses' Health Study; SMC = The Swedish Mammography Cohort; SPES = The Shihpai Eye Study; PHS = The Physicians' Health Study; PSC = posterior subcapsular cataract.

evidence of publication bias among studies of alcohol intake and ARC risk (Begg's Test P = 1.000 and 0.806; Egger's test P = 0.487 and 0.988).

Discussion

To our knowledge, this is the first meta-analysis to report an association between alcohol consumption and ARC risk. Findings from the current study suggest that there is no substantial increase in the risk of cataract requiring extraction with alcohol intake overall. Similar associations were observed for specific cataract subtypes, however those who reported consuming heavy alcohol had a borderline association with cataract surgery. This combined estimate was robust across sensitivity analyses and had no observed publication bias. However, because of the limited number of studies included, further efforts should be made to confirm these findings.

Alcohol has many metabolic effects and modifies the absorption of drugs and dietary components. These effects may be important in the alcohol-cataract relationship [6]. The lens consists of structural proteins, arranged in a way that allows high transparency. Damaged proteins are eliminated by proteolytic enzymes [44]. With increasing age, the amount of proteolytic enzymes are reduced, thus promoting the formation of protein aggregates, which leads to cataract and loss of visual acuity. Oxidative stress generates free radicals which impair lens proteins, which will aggregate and form opacities [45]. Heavy alcohol consumption induces the microsomal enzyme cytochrome CYP2E1 in the liver. The metabolism of ethanol via this enzyme results in the production of several free radicals. These pro-oxidant molecules generated by the metabolism of alcohol could lead to the aggregation of lens proteins and subsequent cataract formation [46]. In addition, alcohol may augment processes such as membrane damage, alter protein-protein interactions, and disrupt calcium homeostasis [47], all of which contribute to cataract development. However, no substantial association between alcohol consumption and cataract risk was detected in this meta-analysis.

In this study, all RRs were non-significant. With respect to heavy alcohol consumption, the association was borderline significant with RR being 1.25 (1.00 to 1.56). However within the 95% confidence interval is 1.00, hence there may not be significance technically. Furthermore, for studies with small numbers, this study could thus have lacked adequate power to

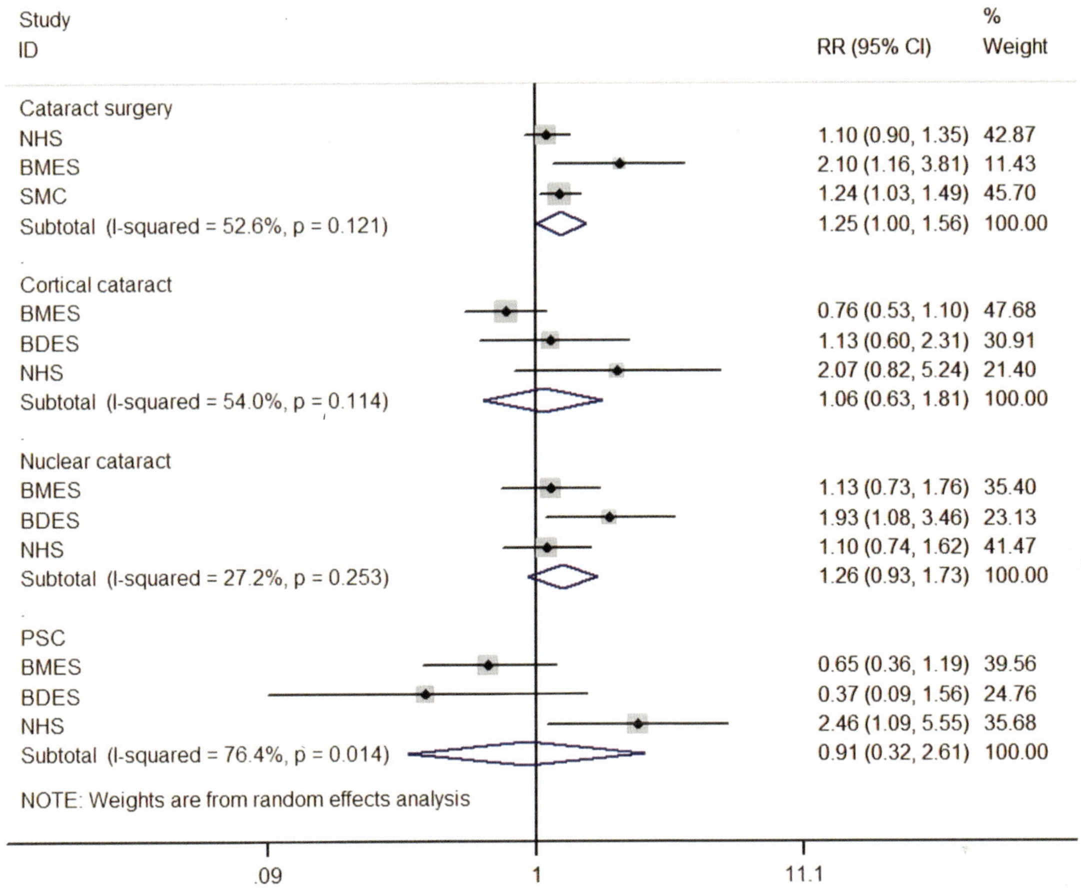

Figure 4. Forest plot for study-specific and pooled relative risk (RR) estimates (Heavy drinkers versus Non-drinkers) of cataract risk associated with alcohol consumption. SEE = The Salisbury Eye Evaluation Study; BMES = The Blue Mountains Eye Study; BDES = The Beaver Dam Eye Study; NHS = The Nurses' Health Study; SMC = The Swedish Mammography Cohort; SPES = The Shihpai Eye Study; PHS = The Physicians' Health Study; PSC = posterior subcapsular cataract.

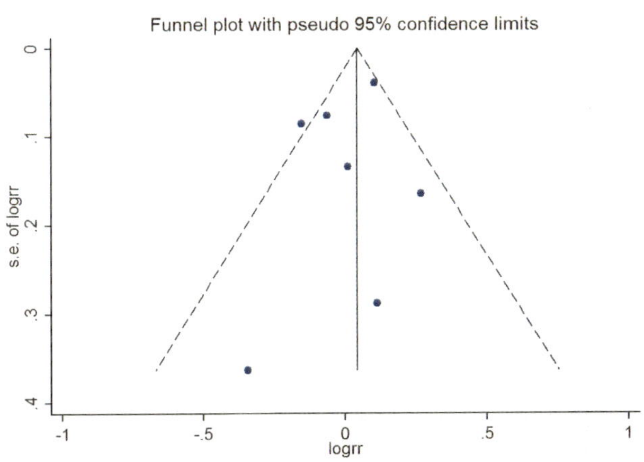

Figure 5. Funnel plot of the association between alcohol intake and risk of any cataract (Any drinkers versus Non-drinkers-Any).

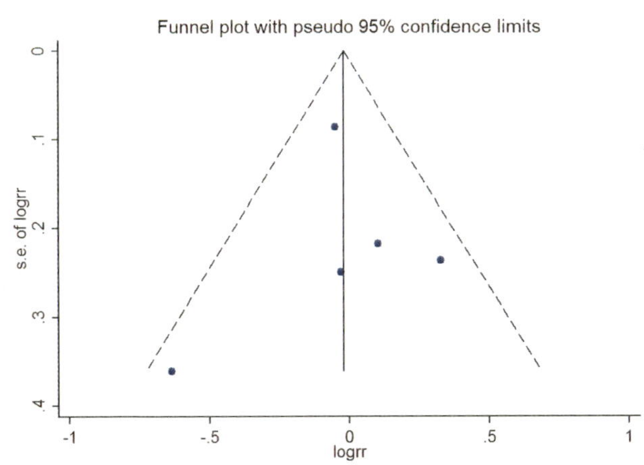

Figure 6. Funnel plot of the association between alcohol intake and risk of cortical cataract (Any drinkers versus Non-drinkers).

detect possible weak associations between alcohol consumption and the development of individual cataract subtypes. The results indicated that if there is an association between cataracts and alcohol, it is relatively weak. In addition, as individuals vary in their ability to detoxify alcohol in the blood, self-reported consumption of alcohol may not accurately reflect alcohol levels in the body or eye [31,32]. Therefore, the findings should be interpreted with caution and require confirmation via future studies. In contrast to heavy alcohol consumption, moderate alcohol consumption has been suggested to have a protective effect regarding ARCs. However, we could not confirm this relationship in this study. We were unable to evaluate the shape of the dose-response curve between alcohol consumption and ARCs because of the small number of studies included. Further prospective cohort studies are needed to determine the shape of the dose-response curve. Despite being an attractive factor, our meta-analysis results do not support alcohol intake to have a major effect to ARC susceptibility.

This meta-analysis has several strengths. First, all the original studies used a prospective cohort study design with good study quality, which greatly reduced the likelihood of recall and selection biases. Second, the use of the random-effects model to derive summary estimates allowed the researchers to account for heterogeneity among studies. Moreover, sensitivity analyses were consistent with primary analysis, providing further indication of the robustness of our results.

This study also has a number of limitations. First, although extensive searches with no limitations in terms of language or year of publication were performed, only seven prospective cohort studies evaluating alcohol consumption and ARC were found. Second, because of the inability to fully adjust for various confounders, the adverse effects of alcohol intake on ARCs could be attributed to other confounders related to alcohol consumption, such as poor nutrition, lack of exercise, and high levels of cigarette smoking [29,30,35]. However, most included studies have adjusted for a wide range of potential confounders. Third, alcohol consumption measured via self-reporting may be misclassified by study participants due to the social stigma attached to heavy consumption and alcoholism [31–34]. In addition, it is possible that heavy drinkers are less likely to participate in studies, which could result in selection biases and also limit the power to detect significant associations with heavy alcohol consumption. Finally, substantial heterogeneity was shown across the component studies. This heterogeneity was not surprising because of variations in the methods of ARC assessment, study designs, and study populations, as well as adjustments across studies.

In conclusion, the present comprehensive meta-analysis provides evidence of a lack of any appreciable association between heavy or moderate alcohol consumption and ARC risk. Because of the limited number of studies, the findings must be confirmed via future research in the form of well-designed cohort or intervention studies. In addition, the underlying mechanisms involved remain to be further elucidated.

Author Contributions

Conceived and designed the experiments: WW XZ. Performed the experiments: WW XZ. Analyzed the data: WW XZ. Contributed reagents/materials/analysis tools: WW XZ. Wrote the paper: WW XZ.

References

1. Prokofyeva E, Wegener A, Zrenner E (2013) Cataract prevalence and prevention in Europe: A literature review. Acta Ophthalmologica 91: 395–405.
2. Huang W, Zheng Y, Wang L, Huang S, Liu B, et al. (2012) Five-year incidence and postoperative visual outcome of cataract surgery in urban southern China: the Liwan Eye Study. Invest Ophthalmol Vis Sci 53: 7936–7942.
3. Richter GM, Choudhury F, Torres M, Azen SP, Varma R (2012) Risk factors for incident cortical, nuclear, posterior subcapsular, and mixed lens opacities: the Los Angeles Latino eye study. Ophthalmology 119: 2040–2047.
4. Fong CS, Mitchell P, Rochtchina E, Teber ET, Hong T, et al. (2013) Correction of Visual Impairment by Cataract Surgery and Improved Survival in Older Persons: The Blue Mountains Eye Study Cohort. Ophthalmology 120: 1720–1727.
5. Agte V, Tarwadi K (2010) The importance of nutrition in the prevention of ocular disease with special reference to cataract. Ophthalmic Res 44: 166–172.
6. Hiratsuka Y, Ono K, Murakami A (2009) Alcohol use and cataract. Curr Drug Abuse Rev 2: 226–229.
7. Hiratsuka Y, Li G (2001) Alcohol and eye diseases: a review of epidemiologic studies. J Stud Alcohol 62: 397–402.
8. West SK, Valmadrid CT (1995) Epidemiology of risk factors for age-related cataract. Surv Ophthalmol 39: 323–334.
9. Hodge WG, Whitcher JP, Satariano W (1995) Risk factors for age-related cataracts. Epidemiologic Reviews 17: 336–346.
10. Wang S, Wang JJ, Wong TY (2008) Alcohol and eye diseases. Surv Ophthalmol 53: 512–525.
11. Theodoropoulou S, Theodossiadis P, Samoli E, Vergados I, Lagiou P, et al. (2011) The epidemiology of cataract: A study in Greece. Acta Ophthalmologica 89: e167–e173.
12. Echebiri SI, Odeigah PG, Myers SN (2010) Case-control studies and risk factors for cataract in two population studies in Nigeria. Middle East Afr J Ophthalmol 17: 303–309.
13. Durant JS, Frost NA, Trivella M, Sparrow JM (2006) Risk factors for cataract subtypes waterclefts and retrodots: two case-control studies. Eye (Lond) 20: 1254–1267.
14. Ughade SN, Zodpey SP, Khanolkar VA (1998) Risk factors for cataract: a case control study. Indian J Ophthalmol 46: 221–227.
15. Phillips CI, Clayton RM, Cuthbert J, Qian W, Donnelly CA, et al. (1996) Human cataract risk factors: significance of abstention from, and high consumption of, ethanol (U-curve) and non-significance of smoking. Ophthalmic Res 28: 237–247.
16. Tavani A, Negri E, La Vecchia C (1996) Food and nutrient intake and risk of cataract. Ann Epidemiol 6: 41–46.
17. Munoz B, Tajchman U, Bochow T, West S (1993) Alcohol use and risk of posterior subcapsular opacities. Arch Ophthalmol 111: 110–112.
18. The Italian-American Cataract Study Group (1991) Risk factors for age-related cortical, nuclear, and posterior subcapsular cataracts. The Italian-American Cataract Study Group. Am J Epidemiol 133: 541–553.
19. Leske MC, Chylack LJ, Wu SY (1991) The Lens Opacities Case-Control Study. Risk factors for cataract. Arch Ophthalmol 109: 244–251.
20. Mohan M, Sperduto RD, Angra SK, Milton RC, Mathur RL, et al. (1989) India-US case-control study of age-related cataracts. India-US Case-Control Study Group. Arch Ophthalmol 107: 670–676.
21. Harding JJ, van Heyningen R (1988) Drugs, including alcohol, that act as risk factors for cataract, and possible protection against cataract by aspirin-like analgesics and cyclopenthiazide. Br J Ophthalmol 72: 809–814.
22. Park S, Kim T, Cho SI, Lee EH (2013) Association between cataract and the degree of obesity. Optom Vis Sci 90: 1019–1027.
23. Xu L, You QS, Jonas JB (2009) Prevalence of alcohol consumption and risk of ocular diseases in a general population: the Beijing Eye Study. Ophthalmology 116: 1872–1879.
24. Tsai SY, Hsu WM, Cheng CY, Liu JH, Chou P (2003) Epidemiologic study of age-related cataracts among an elderly Chinese population in Shih-Pai, Taiwan. Ophthalmology 110: 1089–1095.
25. McCarty CA, Nanjan MB, Taylor HR (2000) Attributable risk estimates for cataract to prioritize medical and public health action. Invest Ophthalmol Vis Sci 41: 3720–3725.
26. Cumming RG, Mitchell P (1997) Alcohol, smoking, and cataracts: the Blue Mountains Eye Study. Arch Ophthalmol 115: 1296–1303.
27. Ritter LL, Klein BE, Klein R, Mares-Perlman JA (1993) Alcohol use and lens opacities in the Beaver Dam Eye Study. Arch Ophthalmol 111: 113–117.
28. Clayton RM, Cuthbert J, Duffy J, Seth J, Phillips CI, et al. (1982) Some risk factors associated with cataract in S.E. Scotland: a pilot study. Trans Ophthalmol Soc U K 102 Pt 3: 331–336.
29. Storey P, Munoz B, Friedman D, West S (2013) Racial differences in lens opacity incidence and progression: the Salisbury Eye Evaluation (SEE) study. Invest Ophthalmol Vis Sci 54: 3010–3018.
30. Kuang TM, Tsai SY, Liu CJ, Ko YC, Lee SM, et al. (2013) Seven-Year Incidence of Age-related Cataracts Among an Elderly Chinese Population in

Shihpai, Taiwan: The Shihpai Eye Study. Invest Ophthalmol Vis Sci 54(9): 6409–6415.
31. Kanthan GL, Mitchell P, Burlutsky G, Wang JJ (2010) Alcohol consumption and the long-term incidence of cataract and cataract surgery: the Blue Mountains Eye Study. Am J Ophthalmol 150: 434–440.
32. Lindblad BE, Hakansson N, Philipson B, Wolk A (2007) Alcohol consumption and risk of cataract extraction: a prospective cohort study of women. Ophthalmology 114: 680–685.
33. Morris MS, Jacques PF, Hankinson SE, Chylack LJ, Willett WC, et al. (2004) Moderate alcoholic beverage intake and early nuclear and cortical lens opacities. Ophthalmic Epidemiol 11: 53–65.
34. Klein BE, Klein R, Lee KE, Meuer SM (2003) Socioeconomic and lifestyle factors and the 10-year incidence of age-related cataracts. Am J Ophthalmol 136: 506–512.
35. Manson JE, Christen WG, Seddon JM, Glynn RJ, Hennekens CH (1994) A prospective study of alcohol consumption and risk of cataract. Am J Prev Med 10: 156–161.
36. Kanthan GL, Wang JJ, Rochtchina E, Tan AG, Lee A, et al. (2008) Ten-year incidence of age-related cataract and cataract surgery in an older Australian population. The Blue Mountains Eye Study. Ophthalmology 115: 808–814.
37. Chasan-Taber L, Willett WC, Seddon JM, Stampfer MJ, Rosner B, et al. (2000) A prospective study of alcohol consumption and cataract extraction among U.S. women. Ann Epidemiol 10: 347–353.
38. Klein BE, Klein RE, Lee KE (1999) Incident cataract after a five-year interval and lifestyle factors: the Beaver Dam eye study. Ophthalmic Epidemiol 6: 247–255.
39. Adams MK, Chong EW, Williamson E, Aung KZ, Makeyeva GA, et al. (2012) 20/20—Alcohol and age-related macular degeneration: the Melbourne Collaborative Cohort Study. Am J Epidemiol 176: 289–298.
40. Hamling J, Lee P, Weitkunat R, Ambuhl M (2008) Facilitating meta-analyses by deriving relative effect and precision estimates for alternative comparisons from a set of estimates presented by exposure level or disease category. Stat Med 27: 954–970.
41. Wells G, Shea B, O'Connell D, Peterson J, Welch V, et al. (2014) The Newcastle-Ottawa Scale (NOS) for assessing the quality of nonrandomised studies in meta-analyses. http://www.ohri.ca/programs/clinical_epidemiology/oxford.asp. Accessed 2014 Aug 29.
42. DerSimonian R, Laird N (1986) Meta-analysis in clinical trials. Control Clin Trials 7: 177–188.
43. Egger M, Davey SG, Schneider M, Minder C (1997) Bias in meta-analysis detected by a simple, graphical test. BMJ 315: 629–634.
44. Werten PJ, Vos E, De Jong WW (1999) Truncation of betaA3/A1-crystallin during aging of the bovine lens; possible implications for lens optical quality. Exp Eye Res 68: 99–103.
45. Nahomi RB, Wang B, Raghavan CT, Voss O, Doseff AI, et al. (2013) Chaperone peptides of alpha-crystallin inhibit epithelial cell apoptosis, protein insolubilization, and opacification in experimental cataracts. J Biol Chem 288: 13022–13035.
46. Balog Z, Sikic J, Vojnikovic B, Balog S (2001) Senile cataract and the absorption activity of cytochrome C oxidase. Coll Antropol 25 Suppl: 33–36.
47. Zeng J, Borchman D, Paterson CA (1998) Acute effect of ethanol on lens cation homeostasis. Alcohol 16: 189–193.

In-the-Bag Intraocular Lens Placement via Secondary Capsulorhexis with Radiofrequency Diathermy in Pediatric Aphakic Eyes

Lixia Luo[❡], Haotian Lin[❡], Weirong Chen[❡], Chunxiao Wang, Xinyu Zhang, Xiangchen Tang, Jianping Liu, Nathan Congdon, Jingjing Chen, Zhuoling Lin, Yizhi Liu*

State Key Laboratory of Ophthalmology, Zhongshan Ophthalmic Center, Sun Yat-sen University, Guangzhou, China

Abstract

Pediatric ophthalmologists increasingly recognize that the ideal site for intraocular lens (IOL) implantation is in the bag for aphakic eyes, but it is always very difficult via conventional technique. We conducted a prospective case series study to investigate the success rate and clinical outcomes of capsular bag reestablishment and in-the-bag IOL implantation via secondary capsulorhexis with radiofrequency diathermy (RFD) in pediatric aphakic eyes, in which twenty-two consecutive aphakic pediatric patients (43 aphakic eyes) enrolled in the Childhood Cataract Program of the Chinese Ministry of Health were included. The included children underwent either our novel technique for secondary IOL implantation (with RFD) or the conventional technique (with a bent needle or forceps), depending on the type of preoperative proliferative capsular bag present. In total, secondary capsulorhexis with RFD was successfully applied in 32 eyes (32/43, 74.4%, age 5.6±2.3 years), of which capsular bag reestablishment and in-the-bag IOL implantation were both achieved in 30 eyes (30/43, 70.0%), but in the remaining 2 eyes (2/32, 6.2%) the IOLs were implanted in the sulcus with a capsular bag that was too small. Secondary capsulorhexis with conventional technique was applied in the other 11 eyes (11/43, 25.6%, age 6.9±2.3 years), of which capsular bag reestablishment and in-the-bag IOL implantation were both achieved only in 3 eyes(3/43, 7.0%), and the IOLs were implanted in the sulcus in the remaining 8 eyes. A doughnut-like proliferative capsular bag with an extensive Soemmering ring (32/43, 74.4%) was the main success factor for secondary capsulorhexis with RFD, and a sufficient capsular bag size (33/43, 76.7%) was an additional factor in successful in-the-bag IOL implantation. In conclusion, RFD secondary capsulorhexis technique has 70% success rate in the capsular bag reestablishment and in-the-bag IOL implantation in pediatric aphakic eyes, particularly effective in cases with a doughnut-like, extensively proliferative Soemmering ring.

Editor: Roy A. Quinlan, University of Durham, United Kingdom

Funding: This study was funded by the Key Projects for Hospital Clinical Disciplines of the Ministry of Health of China in 2010–2012 (Project No.175 in Document 439 of the Planning and Finance Secretary of Ministry of Health). The funders had no role in study design, data collection and analysis, decision to publish, or preparation of the manuscript.

Competing Interests: The authors have declared that no competing interests exist.

* E-mail: yizhi_liu@yahoo.cn

❡ These authors contributed equally to this work.

Introduction

Pediatric cataract patients are commonly left aphakic after lens removal in early childhood, particularly when surgery is performed in the first year of life.[1–3] Secondary intraocular lens (IOL) implantation is considered when an aphakic child is unable to tolerate contact lenses or glasses or when more functional vision without additional correction is desired. [4] Although the ciliary sulcus was the common site of implantation for many years, pediatric ophthalmologists increasingly recognize that the ideal site for IOL implantation is in the bag. In-the-bag implantation sequesters the IOL from the highly reactive uveal tissue and maintains better IOL centration. [5,6].

In many parts of China, pediatric cataract patients do not receive standardized treatment and regular follow-up, possibly because health resources are limited and patient compliance is poor. [7] Clinically, we have encountered serious challenges attempting secondary IOL implantation via conventional techniques in pediatric aphakic eyes, which are commonly characterized by severely fibrotic, fused anterior-posterior-capsulotomy edges and a doughnut-like Soemmering ring after many years without follow-up. In some cases, this ring of intracapsular lens material can become quite bulky, leaving less space in the ciliary sulcus for IOL placement and causing inevitable iris chafing and secondary glaucoma. [8,9] In the past, we most often used a bent needle or forceps for secondary capsulorhexis and reopened the fibrotic, closed capsular bag in an attempt to achieve in-the-bag IOL placement. [10] However, it was not always easy to control the direction of the tear or to complete a continuous curvilinear capsulorhexis. Under these circumstances, when the IOL was placed into the bag, the anterior capsule was likely to tear.

The surgical treatment of pediatric cataracts is constantly changing as a result of advances in the armamentarium of surgeons and microsurgical techniques. Capsular surgery using radiofrequency diathermy (RFD) was originally described by Kloti in 1984 [11] and further examined by Gassmann and colleagues in 1988. [12] Although the RFD technique has been commercially available and in current clinical use for a number of years, we are unaware of any studies that have used RFD for secondary capsulorhexis in pediatric aphakic eyes. [2,3].

In this paper, we present a valuable new procedural addition to RFD that allows the removal of a fibrotic capsule and the reopening of the capsular bag for in-the-bag IOL implantation using RFD. Then, we investigated the success rate and success factors of our novel surgical technique associated with capsular bag reestablishment and in-the-bag IOL implantation in pediatric aphakic eyes with proliferative capsular bags and report the preliminary clinical outcomes of the procedure.

Materials and Methods

Patients

Pediatric patients were selected from the Childhood Cataract Program of the Chinese Ministry of Health (CCPMOH), which initiated a series of ongoing studies on the influence of early interventions on the long-term outcomes of pediatric cataract treatment. [7] The study was approved by the institutional review board of Zhongshan Ophthalmic Center (ZOC), Guangzhou, China. Informed written consent was obtained from at least one parent of each participating child, and the tenets of the Declaration of Helsinki were followed throughout this study.

Pediatric patients were included in this study if they had aphakic eyes after previous cataract surgery and were scheduled to undergo secondary IOL implantation. There was some variation in the surgical technique used for the previous cataract surgery, which was a function of the patient's age, the year of surgery and the degree of posterior capsule opacity. In the previous surgeries, a limbal or scleral tunnel incision was employed, and an anterior capsulotomy was made in a continuous curvilinear manner. The nucleus and cortex were removed using an irrigation/aspiration (I/A) device or an automated vitrectomy instrument, the latter of which was used to create a central posterior capsulotomy and perform a limited anterior vitrectomy in select cases. Peripheral iridectomy was rarely performed.

However, all of the aphakic eyes included in the study were required to have adequate residual capsular support (the diameter of previous posterior capsulotomy≤5 mm) and a capsular bag that was completely closed with anterior-posterior synechia and filled with proliferative cortical material and/or an opaque membrane, which were evaluated with a BX 900® Photo Slit Lamp (Haag-Streit AG, Switzerland) and a Pentacam Scheimpflug Imaging System (Oculus, Germany) before surgery. [13] Furthermore, all of the included children were required to attend all of the follow-up appointments specified in our protocol. Children who were noncompliant with our follow-up protocol were excluded before data collection began.

Surgical Technique (Video S1)

The patients underwent general anesthesia for the surgeries, which were all performed by the same surgeon (Y.L.). The included eyes underwent secondary IOL implantation using either our novel technique (secondary capsulorhexis with RFD) or the conventional technique (secondary capsulorhexis with bent needle or forceps). Our novel surgical technique would be first tried to be applied in the included eyes. However, the conventional technique would be chosen if there was a high risk of unexpected thermal burns of posterior capsule by the RF tip during anterior capsulorhexis. In-the-bag IOL implantation was attempted in all included eyes after the cortical material was removed if the size of peripheral capsular bag was large enough (diameter >8 mm) without capsular tear during anterior capsulorhexis.

Briefly, our novel surgical technique was as follows (Figure 1). After a conjunctival peritomy was made, a 3.2-mm superior scleral tunnel incision was created. We then used sodium hyaluronate to maintain the anterior chamber, and the RF tip (Oertli Instrumente, AG, Switzerland) was inserted into the anterior chamber through the incision. The applied coagulation energy (setting: high energy mode, 500 kHz) easily cut the anterior fibrotic capsule without resistance or complications, but the energy could also burn the posterior capsule if there was not enough cortical material between anterior and posterior capsule. The appearance of a visible bubble line indicated the cutting site. After the cortical material was removed with the I/A device, we implanted an IOL in the peripheral capsular bag. Our IOL of choice for secondary in-the-bag IOL placement is a 3-piece (Sensar AR40e, AMO, Inc. CA, USA) or 1-piece (Acrysof SA60AT, Alcon Laboratories, Inc. Texas, USA) acrylic IOL with a 6.5-mm optic at random, but only 1-piece (Acrysof SA60AT, Alcon Laboratories, Inc. Texas, USA) acrylic IOL was used for sulcus IOL placement, each of which was inserted with an appropriate specialized injector. The subsequent steps included (secondary) capsulorhexis of the posterior capsule with RFD, anterior vitrectomy, irrigation and aspiration. The tunnel incision was sutured with 10-0 nylon sutures. All of the patients received subconjunctival dexamethasone (2 mg) before the surgery was completed.

The conventional technique followed the method described above, with the important exception that a bent needle or forceps was used for the secondary capsulorhexis, which is the standard step recommended in the literature. [10].

Postoperative Medicine Administration Regimen

The standard postoperative regimen consisted of tobradex eye drops (tobramycin 0.3%, dexamethasone 0.1%, Alcon) 4 times per day and tobradex eye ointment (tobramycin 0.3%, dexamethasone 0.1%, Alcon) once per night for 1 month. Subsequently, anti-inflammatory steroid drugs were replaced with a steroid-free drug for another month (pranoprofen eye drops, 4 times per day, Senju Pharmaceutical Co., Ltd. JP). If the intraocular pressure (IOP) was ≥21 mmHg, additional antiglaucoma drugs were administered according to the regimen followed in our previous study. [14].

Follow-up Protocol and Assessment Methods

The follow-up appointments were scheduled according to our previous protocol. [7] Specifically, in this study, follow-up appointments consisted of orthoptic assessment, IOP measurement using a Tono-Pen tonometer (Reichert Inc., Seefeld, Germany), and fundoscopy, which included an optic disc assessment. Concurrently, the degree of anterior segment inflammation and the stability of the IOL were examined with a BX 900® Photo Slit Lamp (Haag-Streit AG, Switzerland) and a Pentacam Scheimpflug Imaging System (Oculus, Germany) at every follow-up visit and documented. The slit lamp photographic images were subjectively evaluated for inflammation and IOL stability, and the software included on the Pentacam device automatically and quantitatively graded the Pentacam images with respect to corneal edema and the stability of the IOL. [15,16] Because young children have poor compliance with examination, we have developed techniques and equipment specific for pediatric ophthalmic examinations. [14] We performed examinations after administering a sedative drug (i.e., chloral hydrate as a sleep aid) or under general anesthesia (if chloral hydrate was contraindicated or unacceptable) for children who were too uncooperative to allow for regular examinations in the clinic.

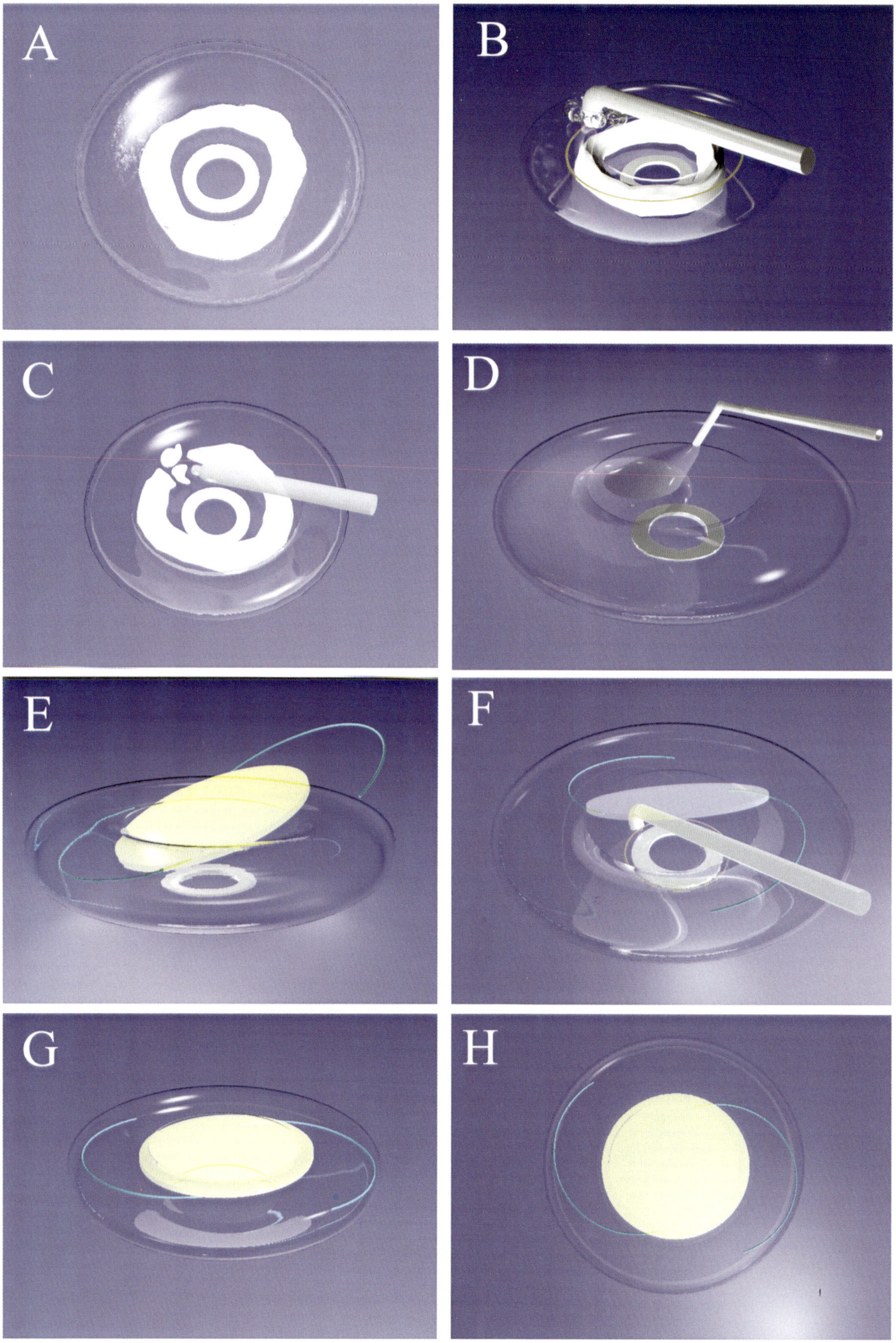
A
B
C
D
E
F
G
H

Figure 1. Schematic diagrams of the surgical techniques of capsular bag reestablishment and in-the-bag IOL implantation via secondary capsulorhexis with RFD. A, We used sodium hyaluronate to maintain the anterior chamber of an aphakic eye with a doughnut-like, extensive Soemmering ring. B, The RF tip was inserted into the anterior chamber to cut the anterior fibrotic capsule with coagulation energy, and the appearance of a visible bubble line indicates the cutting site. C, The cortical material was removed via I/A or a phaco tip using a divide-and-conquer approach. D, The capsular bag was reestablished with sodium hyaluronate. E, An IOL was implanted into the peripheral capsular bag. F, The RF tip was inserted into the anterior chamber again through the tilted IOL to cut the posterior fibrotic capsule. G, The IOL was dialed centrally after secondary capsulorhexis of the posterior capsule. H, The IOL was well-centered and implanted in the bag after the sodium hyaluronate was cleared. Notes: RFD = radiofrequency diathermy, IOL = intraocular lens, I/A = irrigation/aspiration.

Main Outcome Measures

The success rate of secondary capsulorhexis with RFD/in-the-bag IOL placement was defined as the proportion of successful secondary capsulorhexis with RFD/in-the-bag IOL placement among the included cases. Intraoperative complications can include capsular tear, iris or corneal thermal burns by the RF tip, and the presence of residual proliferative material in the vitreous cavity. Postoperative complications can include ocular hypertension (IOP≥21 mmHg), corneal edema, delayed healing of the corneal incision, increased postoperative inflammation, iris synechia, pigmentation dispersion, macular edema, retinal detachment, recurrence of severe tissue reactivity and shrinkage of the capsule. The axial stability of in-the-bag IOL was evaluated with the Pentacam Scheimpflug Imaging System. IOL decentration was recorded using slit lamp photographic images if the edge of the IOL optic could be visualized through the undilated pupil or if the IOL/capsular bag complex appeared decentered. However, the in-the-bag IOL placement and rotation stability were evaluated by comparing slit lamp photographic images after pupil dilation at different follow-up appointments. [16].

Statistical Analysis

Continuous variables were expressed as means ± standard deviations (SD), whereas categorical data were expressed as numbers (n) and percentages (%). Because of the small sample size, Mann-Whitney tests were used to identify differences between our novel technique and the conventional technique. Categorical variables were compared using Fisher's exact test. To look at the factors influencing on surgical success of capsular bag reestablishment and in-the-bag IOL implantation, the type of Soemmering ring, capsular bag size, and age were statistical analyzed between the cases via our novel technique and conventional technique. All statistical tests were two-sided, and the 0.05 level was considered statistically significant. Data were analyzed using SPSS 17.0 (SPSS Inc., Chicago, IL) for Windows.

Results

A total of 43 aphakic eyes of 22 children (age: 6.0±2.3 years), including 17 males (17/22, 77.3%) and 21 children (21/22, 95.5%) with bilateral cataracts, were consecutively recruited from CCPMOH from December 2010 to March 2012. However, 2 children (4 eyes via our novel technique, 4/43, 9.3%) were excluded from analysis of postoperative complications for noncompliance with our follow-up protocol. Altogether (Figure 2), secondary capsulorhexis with RFD was successfully applied in 32 aphakic eyes (32/43, 74.4%, age 5.6±2.3 years), of which capsular bag reestablishment and in-the-bag IOL implantation were also achieved in 30 eyes (30/32, 93.8%), and the IOLs were implanted in the sulcus with a capsular bag that was too small in the remaining 2 eyes (2/32, 6.2%). Secondary capsulorhexis with conventional technique was applied in the other 11 aphakic eyes (11/43, 25.6%, age 6.9±2.3 years), of which capsular bag reestablishment and in-the-bag IOL implantation were both achieved only in 3 eyes (3/11, 27.3%, $p<0.05$ compared with cases via our novel technique), and the IOLs were implanted in the sulcus in the remaining 8 eyes (1 eye with unexpected tear in posterior capsule, 3 eyes with small capsular bag size and failure of capsular bag reestablishment in the other 4 eyes because of close adhesion of residual anterior-posterior-capsule). It is necessary to mention that one of the 11 aphakic eyes via conventional technique was initially applied with our novel RFD technique, but the RFD technique was replaced by the conventional technique because of timely detection of the unexpected thermal burns of posterior capsule by the RF tip during anterior capsulorhexis, resulting in sulcus IOL implantation.

There was a significant correlation between the types of preoperative proliferative capsular bag present and the successful application of secondary capsulorhexis with RFD. If the proliferative capsular bag had an extensive/continuous Soemmering ring (Figure 3A), this type of capsular bag could be successfully applied with our novel surgical technique, although in-the-bag IOL placement in this type of closed, fibrotic capsular bag is difficult to accomplish with the traditional armamentarium and methods. If the aphakic eyes were with a proliferative capsular bag, a sparse/focal Soemmering ring or synechia and an undilatable pupil (Figure 3B), our novel surgical technique was unsuitable because of easily unexpected thermal burn of posterior capsule and should be instead with the conventional technique. The reestablishment of this type of proliferative capsular bag is always difficult. In all, we found that a doughnut-like proliferative capsular bag with an extensive Soemmering ring (32/43, 74.4%) was the main success factor for secondary capsulorhexis with RFD. A sufficient capsular bag size (33/43, 76.7%) was an additional factor in successful in-the-bag IOL implantation. However, age was found not to be a factor influencing on surgical success of capsular bag reestablishment and in-the-bag IOL implantation.

All Soemmering ring material and proliferative membranes in the visual axis were intraoperatively removed without capsular tear in all included eyes, except the stated case of unexpected thermal burns of posterior capsule during anterior capsulorhexis initially by the RF tip. No iris or corneal thermal burns from the RF tip occurred and no residual proliferative material was present in the vitreous cavity during the operation. One week after surgery, the in-the-bag IOL was centered in the peripheral capsular bag with a clear and relatively smooth-edged secondary capsulorhexis in eyes via our novel technique. In eyes via conventional technique, however, the IOL implantation was accompanied by epithelium proliferation scattered in the visual axis and a relatively rough posterior edge after secondary capsulorhexis (Figure 4).

Throughout the postoperative follow-up period (13.3±4.6 months), no corneal edema, delayed corneal incision healing, or inflammatory reaction was found to have been triggered by residual material or the surgical intervention. Furthermore, no iris synechia, pigmentation dispersion, macular edema, retinal detachment, recurrence of severe tissue reactivity or capsule shrinkage were identified. However, ocular hypertension (IOP≥21 mmHg) occurred in 5 eyes (5/28, 17.9%) via our novel technique and 2 eyes (2/11, 18.2%) via conventional technique. Lens epithelium proliferation in the visual axis was identified in 4

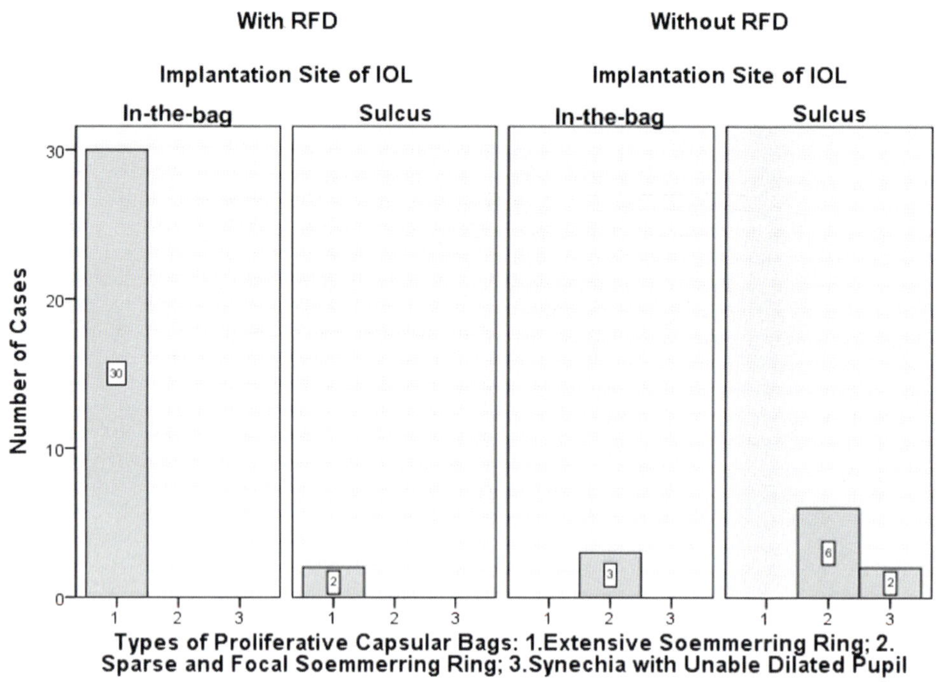

Figure 2. The relationships between different types of proliferative capsular bags, secondary capsulorhexis with/without RFD and the IOL implantation site in two groups. The number of cases is shown in different columns. Proliferative capsular bag Type 1 was included in Group A, and proliferative capsular bag Types 2 and 3 were included in Group B. Notes: RFD = radiofrequency diathermy, IOL = intraocular lenses.

eyes via conventional technique but no eyes via our novel technique (Figure 5). No IOL displacement (decentration, rotation or tilt) was discovered in any of the included eyes upon analysis with the Pentacam Scheimpflug Imaging System or upon comparing the slit lamp photographic images after pupil dilation at different follow-up appointments.

Discussion

In this paper, we presented a new procedural addition to RFD that will be valuable to any clinician responsible for the care of pediatric cataract patients with challenging cases. The procedure involves the removal of a fibrotic capsule and reopening of the capsular bag with RFD for in-the-bag IOL implantation in pediatric aphakic eyes. We recruited 22 consecutive aphakic pediatric patients (43 aphakic eyes) from CCPMOH and conducted this prospective case series study to investigate the success rate and clinical outcomes of novel technique. We found that a high success rate (70%) of capsular bag reestablishment and in-the-bag IOL implantation could be easily achieved with RFD secondary capsulorhexis in pediatric aphakic eyes, particularly those with a doughnut-like, extensively proliferative Soemmering ring. Furthermore, we found significantly decreased lens epithelium proliferation after secondary IOL implantation with RFD secondary capsulorhexis than the conventional technique in pediatric aphakic eyes.

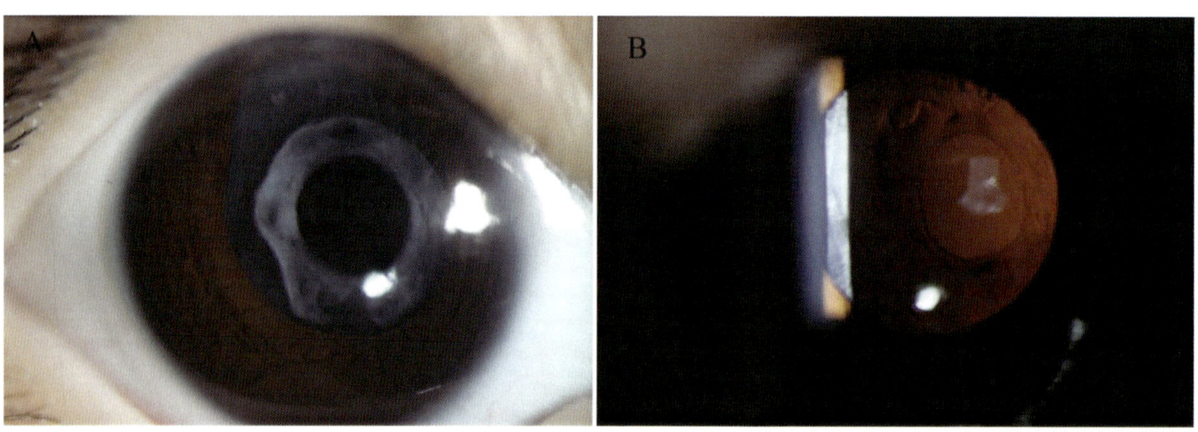

Figure 3. Photograph of an aphakic eye with a proliferative capsular bag. A, The capsular bag was completely closed with anterior-posterior synechia, was filled with proliferative cortical material and had an extensive Soemmering ring. B, The capsular bag was completely closed with anterior-posterior synechia, but it had little cortical material and a sparse and focal Soemmering ring.

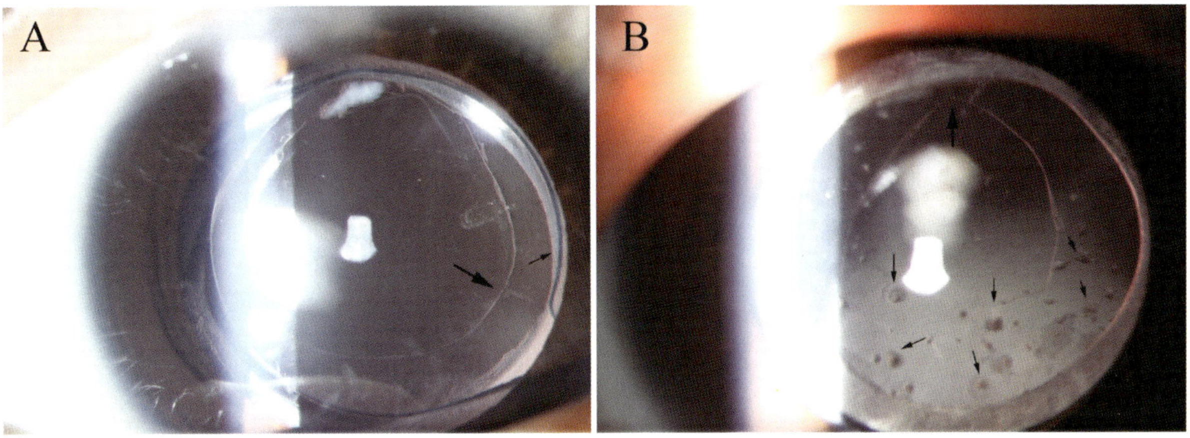

Figure 4. Postoperative photographs of secondary IOL implantation 1 week after surgery. A, The in-the-bag IOL was centered in the peripheral capsular bag with clear anterior (small arrow) and posterior (large arrow) secondary capsulorhexis relative to the smooth edge in one of the eyes underwent our novel surgical technique. B, In-the-bag IOL was accompanied by epithelium proliferation (small arrow) scattered in the visual axis and a relatively rough posterior edge (large arrow) after secondary capsulorhexis in one of the eyes underwent the traditional surgical technique. Notes: IOL = intraocular lenses.

It is well known that the technical ease and success of secondary IOL implantation depends on the capsular support that remains after primary cataract surgery. [13] However, secondary IOL insertions in aphakic pediatric patients present considerable challenges, especially in the presence of severe tissue reactivity, capsular shrinkage and Soemmering ring formation. [17] These complications increase the risk of capsular tear and may lead to the inadvertent sulcus placement of the IOL, which can lead to such additional complications as IOL displacement, pigmentation dispersion and iris damage. [8].

An increasing number of pediatric ophthalmologists have recognized that the ideal site for IOL implantation is in the bag. This placement sequesters the IOL from the highly reactive uveal tissue and maintains better IOL centration. However, in-the-bag secondary IOL implantation presents a challenge in pediatric aphakic eyes with a closed fibrotic capsule bag. [2] In the past, when we performed secondary capsulorhexis to reestablish the fibrotic capsular bag in aphakic patients, we typically used a bent needle and/or forceps. Using this technique, it was always difficult to control the tear direction, and it was difficult to complete a continuous curvilinear capsulorhexis. Early in 1999, Wilson et al. [18] first described a technique for achieving in-the-bag secondary implantation in children. The authors used a vitrector probe to circumferentially cut close to the point of fusion of the anterior and posterior capsules, and they then used a vitrector to remove the Soemmering ring material. In 2008, Gimbel and Venkataraman [19] described an adult patient in whom they performed secondary IOL placement. An anterior capsulotomy was performed using a cystotome, and the Soemmering ring was aspirated using a manual Simcoe cannula, after which the IOL was inserted in the bag. Recently, Dilraj et al. [20] reported a modified technique that was built on previous techniques for Soemmering ring removal in aphakic eyes, followed by the in-the-bag placement of a secondary IOL. Unique to their technique is the use of 20-gauge MST scissors to cut the anterior capsule to complete the anterior capsulotomy, as well as a 2-handed technique to manually fragment and debulk the Soemmering ring, followed by the viscoexpression of large fragments in Dilraj's

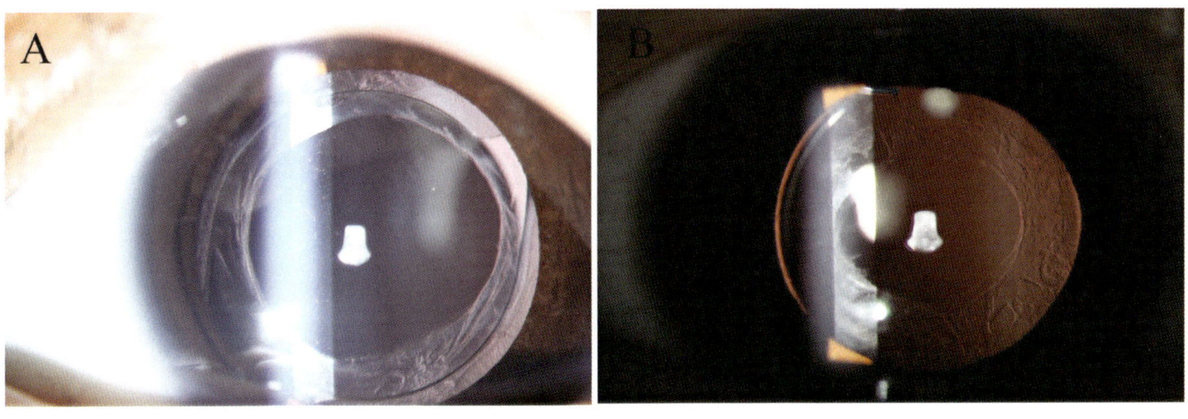

Figure 5. Postoperative photograph of secondary IOL implantation 3 months after surgery. A, The in-the-bag IOL was well-centered in the peripheral capsular bag without any epithelium proliferation in the visual axis in one of the eyes underwent our novel surgical technique. B, Apparent epithelium proliferation and shrinkage of the residual capsular bag was identified in one of the eyes underwent the traditional surgical technique. Notes: IOL = intraocular lenses.

study [20]. However, all of the described techniques in the previous studies are somewhat complex, and their effectiveness and safety profiles were not reported because of the lack of a well-conducted prospective case series study. Furthermore, we are not aware of any studies that have used the RFD technique for secondary capsulorhexis to achieve secondary IOL in-the-bag implantation in pediatric aphakic eyes, despite the fact that the RFD technique has been commercially available and in current clinical use for many years.

Capsulorhexis using RFD was originally reported by Kloti [11] and further researched by Gassmann [12]. With RFD, the capsule is cut and coagulated using a platinum-alloy-tipped probe heated to approximately 160°C by a modulated, high-frequency current of 500 kHz. Although diathermy capsulorhexis techniques have achieved good results in particular clinical situations, [21–23] these techniques are not popular in cataract cases because they offer less elasticity and resistance. [24] The negative reports of decreased capsular elasticity and the lack of an obvious advantage in adult primary capsulorhexis using RFD compared with using traditional forceps may explain why research on the RFD technique has stalled. It is well known that the pediatric capsule is highly elastic, making it difficult to perform capsulorhexis with a bent needle or forceps. Moreover, in secondary IOL implantation cases, it is difficult to distinguish the anterior opening even with capsule staining because of the white proliferative cortical material between the anterior and posterior capsular leafs. However, RFD is easy to perform in this situation, regardless of the proliferative anterior capsular visibility and resistance. In our study, we found that the RF tip could be especially easily controlled to create a highly predictable secondary capsulorhexis in severely proliferative aphakic eyes with a doughnut-like residual capsule. Interestingly, the challenging condition of a doughnut-like proliferative capsular bag with extensive Soemmering ring formation for secondary IOL implantation, either in the bag or in the sulcus, happened to be a critical success factor for the application of our new RFD procedure (reduced risk of unexpected thermal burns of posterior capsule by the RF tip during anterior capsulorhexis); however, studies with a larger sample size are still warranted to further explore the application of our novel technique.

Most patients who present for secondary IOL insertion have a central posterior capsulotomy. In these eyes, inadvertent partial or complete loss of the Soemmering ring into the vitreous cavity is possible when the Soemmering ring is removed using the techniques described in previous studies. Dilraj et al. [20] believed that performing all of the maneuvers for Soemmering ring removal in an ophthalmic viscoelastic-filled eye minimized the risk of Soemmering ring loss. Although Dilraj's technique had the advantage of avoiding the active infusion of the anterior chamber with balanced salt solution if necessary as a vitrector, the use of a Simcoe cannula or phacoemulsification probe to remove Soemmering ring material presented no advantages over the techniques described by Wilson et al. [18] and Gimbel and Venkataraman [19], and there were no reports of the intraoperative complications resulting from the technique in Dilraj's report. In the present study, we performed secondary capsulorhexis of the anterior proliferative capsular bag (Figure 1A) and then immediately cleared all doughnut-like, extensively proliferative material and the Soemmering ring (Figure 1C), which was still separated from the vitreous cavity before we performed the secondary capsulorhexis of the posterior proliferative capsular (Figure1F). In all of the 32 eyes in which RFD was successfully applied, no loss of residual proliferative material into the vitreous cavity occurred during the operation, which showed that our procedure had great effectiveness and excellent safety. Furthermore, no iris or corneal thermal burns due to the RF tip occurred during surgery, which contributed to the excellent safety of our technique.

It is a widely recognized fact that active lens epithelial cells remain after cataract surgery in almost all pediatric cataract patients, despite improvements in surgical techniques, such as hydrodissection and vacuuming of the capsular bag. [2] In our study, we noted that congenital or infantile cataracts in the first year of life have a much more exuberant cortex deposition within the capsular bag than those in children operated on at a later age, which was similar to the findings of Wilson et al. [18] This lens material always forms the extensive Soemmering ring (constituting 74.4% of the eyes in our study). If the ring is sparse, in focal areas and enclosed between the anterior and posterior capsules (constituting 25.6% of the eyes in our study), it may be reasonable to leave it unopened at the time of secondary IOL implantation. However, if the Soemmering ring is extensive, sulcus placement of the IOL risks future IOL tilt and uveitis-glaucoma-hyphema syndrome with subsequent enlargement of the Soemmering ring. [25] Although in-the-bag IOL implantation was not achieved in 2 eyes via our novel technique in this study (while sulcus IOL implantation was achieved) because of the small size of the capsular bag, the extensive proliferative material and Soemmering ring were completely cleared after RFD secondary capsulorhexis, with no signs of IOL tilt or uveitis-glaucoma-hyphema syndrome during our postoperative follow-up. Additionally, the other eyes in our study demonstrated good clinical outcomes without the above mentioned posterior complications.

Most pediatric ophthalmologists suggest that if the anterior capsule overlying the Soemmering ring material is opened, it is best not to leave any Soemmering ring material, as residual material may trigger an inflammatory reaction. [19] In our study, all Soemmering ring material was completely removed intraoperatively in all included eyes, which was indirectly proven by the fact that no secondary inflammation reaction was identified during our follow-up. Although ocular hypertension (IOP≥21 mmHg) occurred in 5 eyes (5/28, 17.9%) via our novel technique and 2 eyes (2/11, 18.2%) via conventional technique, all of the cases of ocular hypertension were self-limiting and presented with steroid-induced characteristics, which are discussed in another study. [14].

Unique to our technique is the use of an RF tip to complete the secondary capsulorhexis of the anterior and posterior capsules separately, which not only exposes the proliferative Soemmering ring material for clearing but also prevents the loss of residual fragments into the vitreous cavity. At the same time, both the anterior and posterior capsular fibrosis at the rhexis edge can be circumferentially cut, and continuous secondary capsulorhexis can be precisely achieved without the risk of a radial capsule tear, which can help maintain IOL stability in the bag. Moreover, swollen capsular edges have been reported after diathermy capsulotomy, such that the lens epithelium was less proliferative and less capsule shrinkage occurred [26]. Interestingly, we found in the current study that lens epithelium proliferation in the visual axis was identified in 4 eyes (4/11, 36.4%) via conventional technique, but in no eyes via our novel technique. We believe that the diathermy used during capsulorhexis, which is unique to our technique, could help to decrease the number of residual active lens epithelial cells and thus prevent long-term epithelium proliferation. A randomized controlled study with a larger sample size is needed to investigate whether there is a significant difference between the occurrence rates of post-operative residual lens epithelium proliferation and the incidence of secondary IOL tilt and decentration due to extensive proliferation.

The results and interpretation of the present study must be understood within the context of the study's strengths and limitations. The study's strengths include its strict, consistent follow-up protocol; the use of reasonably accurate measurements within a national research program (CCPMOH); the first presentation of a valuable new addition to RFD; the first classification of an extensive/continuous Soemmering ring, sparse/focal Soemmering ring, and synechia with and undilatable pupil as three types of proliferative capsular bags; the first clinical outcomes report of this new technique compared with the conventional bent needle or forceps technique; and the first report of the success rate and the first discussion of the success factors for the RFD technique. The study weaknesses must also be acknowledged. Although this study was included in a national program, all of the subjects underwent surgery and were followed at a single center without a randomized and controlled design. Therefore, the results should be confirmed and the indications for the application of RFD secondary capsulorhexis in pediatric aphakic eyes should be further defined in future studies that include large sample sizes with a randomized and controlled design and long-term follow-up.

Despite these limitations, the current study remains one of the first to report that a high success rate of capsular bag reestablishment and in-the-bag IOL implantation could be easily achieved with RFD secondary capsulorhexis in pediatric aphakic eyes with a doughnut-like, extensively proliferative Soemmering ring.\The simplicity, effectiveness, and excellent safety profiles of this procedure make it a valuable addition to the armamentarium of any clinician responsible for these challenging patient cases.

Acknowledgments

Disclaimer: This paper was included in a film presentation at the 2012 ASCRS·ASOA (F49) in Chicago, which was nominated as one of the best films (Video S1). The research protocol was approved by the Institutional Review Board/Ethics Committee of Sun Yat-sen University. Informed consent was obtained from each participant, and the tenets of the Declaration of Helsinki were followed throughout.

Author Contributions

Conducted the study and collected the data: CXW JPL XCT JJC ZLL. Reviewed the manuscript: NC YZL. Conceived and designed the experiments: LXL HTL WRC YZL. Performed the experiments: LXL HTL WRC YZL. Analyzed the data: LXL HTL WRC XYZ NC YZL. Contributed reagents/materials/analysis tools: XCT. Wrote the paper: LXL HTL WRC.

References

1. Chee KY, Lam GC. (2009) Management of congenital cataract in children younger than 1 year using a 25-gauge vitrectomy system. J Cataract Refract Surg 35: 720–724.
2. Lin AA, Buckley EG. (2010) Update on pediatric cataract surgery and intraocular lens implantation. Curr Opin Ophthalmol. 21: 55–9.
3. Forbes BJ, Guo S. (2006) Update on the surgical management of pediatric cataracts. J Pediatr Ophthalmol Strabismus. 43: 143–51; quiz 165–6.
4. Magli A, Forte R, Rombetto L. (2012) Long-term outcome of primary versus secondary intraocular lens implantation after simultaneous removal of bilateral congenital cataract. Graefes Arch Clin Exp Ophthalmol. 14. [Epub ahead of print].
5. Mura JJ, Pavlin CJ, Condon GP, Belovay GW, Kranemann CF, et al. (2010) Ultrasound biomicroscopic analysis of iris-sutured foldable posterior chamber intraocular lenses. Am J Ophthalmol. 149: 245–252.
6. Vasavada AR, Raj SM, Karve S, Vasavada V, Vasavada V, et al. (2010) Retrospective ultrasound biomicroscopic analysis of single-piece sulcus-fixated acrylic intraocular lenses. J Cataract Refract Surg.36: 771–7.
7. Lin H, Chen W, Luo L, Congdon N, Zhang X, et al. (2012) Effectiveness of a short message reminder in increasing compliance with pediatric cataract treatment: a randomized trial. Ophthalmology. 119: 2463–70.
8. Kobayashi H, Hirose M, Kobayashi K. (2000) Ultrasound biomicroscopic analysis of pseudophakic pupillary block glaucoma induced by Soemmering's ring. Br J Ophthalmol 84: 1142–1146.
9. Chen P-F, Lin C-P, Lin S-Y. (2009) Lens material-induced glaucoma 25 years after cataract extraction surgery [letter]. Jpn J Ophthalmol 53: 275–277.
10. Basti S, Greenwald MJ. (1995) Principles and paradigms of pediatric cataract management. Indian J Ophthalmol. 43: 159–76.
11. Kloti R. (1984) Bipolar-Nassfeld-Diathermie in der Mikrochirugie. Klin Monatsbl Augenheilkd 442: 184.6.
12. Gassmann F, Schimmelpfennig B, Kloti R. (1988) Anterior capsulotomy by means of bipolar radio-frequency endodiathermy. J Cataract Refract Surg 14: 673.
13. Wagoner MD, Cox TA, Ariyasu RG, Jacobs DS, Karp CL; American Academy of Ophthalmology. (2003) Intraocular lens implantation in the absence of capsular support: a report by the American Academy of Ophthalmology. Ophthalmology.110: 840–59.
14. Lin HT, Luo LX, Chen WR. (2013) Assessment of the incidence of early-onset ocular hypertension in children receiving topical steroids after cataract surgery. Ophthalmology. In press.
15. Kim KH, Kim WS. (2010) Intraocular lens stability and refractive outcomes after cataract surgery using primary posterior continuous curvilinear capsulorhexis. Ophthalmology. 117: 2278–86.
16. Wang YL, Liu YZ, Wang YQ, He MG, Zhou Q, et al. (2011) [Comparison of stability of acrylic intraocular lens and transparency of lens capsule using Pentacam Scheimpflug System]. Zhonghua Yan Ke Za Zhi. 47: 298–302. Chinese.
17. DeVaro JM, Buckley EG, Awner S, Seaber J. (1997) Secondary posterior chamber intraocular lens implantation in pediatric patients. Am J Ophthalmol.123: 24–30.
18. Wilson ME Jr, Englert JA, Greenwald MJ. (1999) In-the-bag secondary intraocular lens implantation in children. J AAPOS 3: 350–355.
19. Gimbel HV, Venkataraman A. (2008) Secondary in-the-bag intraocular lens implantation following removal of Soemmering ring contents. J Cataract Refract Surg 34: 1246–1249.
20. Grewal DS, Basti S. (2012) Modified technique for removal of Soemmerring ring and in-the-bag secondary intraocular lens placement in aphakic eyes. J Cataract Refract Surg. 38: 739–42.
21. Comer RM, Abdulla N, O'Keefe M. (1997) Radiofrequency diathermy capsulorhexis of the anterior and posterior capsules in pediatric cataract surgery: preliminary results. J Cataract Refract Surg. 23 Suppl 1: 641–644.
22. Findl O, Amon M. (1998) Anterior capsulotomy created by radiofrequency endodiathermy and continuous curvilinear posterior capsulorhexis in a patient with intumescent cataract and primary capsular fibrosis. J Cataract Refract Surg. 24: 870–871.
23. Hausman N, Richard CT. (1991) Investigations on diathermy for anterior capsulotomy. Invest Ophthalmol Vis Sci 32: 2155–2159.
24. Luck J, Brahma AK, Noble BA. (1994) A comparative study of the elastic properties of continuous tear curvilinear capsulorhexis versus capsulorhexis produced by radiofrequency endodiathermy. British Journal of Ophthalmology 78: 392–396.
25. Aonuma H, Matsushita H, Nakajima K, Watase M, Tsushima K, et al. (1997) Uveitis-glaucoma-hyphema syndrome after posterior chamber intraocular lens implantation. Jpn J Ophthalmol 41: 98–100.
26. Butcher JM, Bonshek RD, Raines MF. (1994) Surgical capsulorhexis and diathermy capsulotomy: an ultrastructural comparison. Eur J Implant Refract Surg 6: 344–347.

Prevalence and Risk Factors of Idiopathic Epiretinal Membranes in Beixinjing Blocks, Shanghai, China

Xiao-feng Zhu[1], Jin-juan Peng[1], Hai-dong Zou[1]*, Jiong Fu[2], Wei-wei Wang[2], Xun Xu[1], Xi Zhang[1]

1 Department of Ophthalmology, Shanghai First People's Hospital, Affiliated Shanghai Jiaotong University, Shanghai, China, **2** Beixinjing Community Health Service Center, Shanghai, China

Abstract

Background: To determine the prevalence and risk factors associated with idiopathic epiretinal membranes (iERM) in a Chinese population aged 60 years or older in Beixinjing Blocks, Shanghai.

Methods: This population-based study consisted of 3727 participants (89.7% of the eligible). It was performed to describe the prevalence of iERM and possible demographic, systemic, and ocular factors associated with iERM. Each participant underwent a standardized interview and comprehensive ophthalmic examination. iERM was identified and graded from retinal photographs. Then, a case-control study comparing the participants with vs. without iERM was performed to further study the associations between iERM and blood biochemical test results (including fasting plasma glucose, serum creatinine, total cholesterol, and triglyceride), ocular biological parameters (including the axial length, corneal curvature, refractive diopter, intraocular press, and anterior chamber depth), and the data of optical coherence tomography.

Results: The prevalence of iERM was 1.02%. iERM was significantly associated with diabetes (OR: 2.457; 95% CI: 1.137, 5.309) and a higher level of education (OR: 1.48; 95% CI: 1.123, 1.952). Blood biochemical test results and ocular biological parameters showed no significant differences between the iERM and control groups, whereas the incidence of posterior vitreous detachment in the iERM group was much higher than in the control group (26.5% vs. 8.8%), but this difference was not statistically significant. Moreover, the eyes with iERM had poorer visual acuity than the eyes without iERM ($P<0.05$).

Conclusions: In Beixinjing Blocks, Shanghai, iERM was relatively rare, was associated with diabetes and a higher level of education, and caused a substantial decrease in visual acuity.

Editor: Yingfeng Zheng, Zhongshan Ophthalmic Center, China

Funding: Funding was provided by a key grant from the Shanghai Health Bureau (20114007) and a grant from the Shanghai Leading Talent Reserve Program (40311). No conflicting relationship exists for any author. The funders had no role in study design, data collection and analysis, decision to publish, or preparation of the manuscript.

Competing Interests: The authors have declared that no competing interests exist.

* E-mail: zouhaidong@hotmail.com

These authors contributed equally to this work.

Introduction

Epiretinal membrane (ERM) is a retinal disease resulting in a disturbance of macular vision and predisposing to rhegmatogenous retinal detachment [1], which significantly impair quality of life [2,3]. ERM is characterized by wrinkling or distortion of the macular surface caused by retinal cell migration and proliferation [4–6], and it has been associated with a variety of ocular diseases, such as diabetic retinopathy (DR) [7,8], retinal vein occlusion [4,9], retinal detachment [9–11], and cataract surgery [4,5,7–9,12]. Most cases, however, are termed idiopathic ERM (iERM): they have no antecedent ocular pathology other than posterior vitreous detachment (PVD) or separation [13,14]. While the pathogenesis of iERM is not fully clear, there is growing evidence that PVD plays a critical role in the pathogenesis of iERM through at least two possible mechanisms [15]. First, transient vitreoretinal traction during the development of PVD may cause dehiscences in the internal limiting membrane (ILM) through which glial cells can migrate and proliferate on the inner retinal surface [16–18]. Second, and perhaps more frequently, iERM may result from the proliferation and transdifferentiation of hyalocytes contained within vitreous cortical remnants left on the retinal surface following PVD [19–21].

Epidemiological studies contribute to clarify the pathogenesis and risk factors of iERM. Population-based studies [4,5,7,8,22–28] have reported a great discrepancy (2.2% to 18.5%) in the prevalence of ERM among different ethnic groups. It has been suggested that Asians have a lower prevalence of ERM compared with Caucasians [22,24–26]. Similarly, studies [8,23,25–28] documenting the prevalence of iERM in various populations also shown substantial ethnic variations. The lowest prevalence (3.0%) was reported in the Handan Eye Study [25], and the highest (17.5%) in the Los Angeles Latino eye study (LALES) [23]. Although there have been two population-based studies [24,25] of the ERM prevalence in China, the differences in study design and methodology resulted in a large discrepancy. The Beijing Eye Study [24], including both rural and urban subjects aged 40 years or older, relied solely on retinal photographs, while the Handan

Eye Study [25], including rural subjects aged 30 years or older, relied on retinal photographs and/or optical coherence tomography (OCT). Therefore, further study of ERM in a Chinese urban population is necessary. Moreover, according to population-based studies, in addition to old age [4,7,8,22–25,26,28], which is a recognized risk factor for iERM, other possible risk factors, such as female gender [26], refractive error [4,24,25,28], diabetes [4,8,27], and serum cholesterol [22], are inconsistently associated with iERM. Therefore, in Part I of our study (a population-based study), we aimed to describe the prevalence of iERM in a random sample of the resident population aged 60 years or older in Beixinjing Blocks, Shanghai, China, relied on retinal photographs. Meanwhile we examined risk factors associated with iERM, including ocular, systemic and socio-demographic characteristics.

Previous clinical studies [29–31] concerning the risk factors associated with iERM have been susceptible to selection bias because the cases usually came from hospital patients, who were generally at the second or higher stage of iERM and had subjective symptoms. Thus, in Part II of our study (a case-control study), comparing the participants with vs. without iERM from Part I was performed to further study the differences between the two groups. We have studied some possible iERM risk factors in Part I, such as old age, gender and diabetes, so we carried out a blood biochemical test for the cases and controls as a supplementary evaluation. Partial or complete PVD has been found in 80% to 95% of eyes with iERM in large clinical studies [32–34], and it is likely that the association between iERM and PVD is universal. Therefore, B-mode ultrasound and OCT examinations were conducted to analyze the existence of PVD in eyes with or without iERM. Furthermore, there is some controversy about the association between refractive error and iERM [8,23–26], so we further examined the axial length, corneal curvature, refractive diopter, anterior chamber depth (ACD), and intraocular press (IOP) in cases and controls.

Materials and Methods

Study Design and Population

Beixinjing Blocks, located in the northwest of Shanghai, was selected for the study because of its relatively stable population (43,253 in the 2000 census, and 8,153 aged 60 years or older) and representative demographic and socioeconomic characteristics. Beixinjing Blocks has mostly urban residents whose economic conditions could be classified as middle class in China: average per capita annual incomes among urban households are 36,230 yuan ($5728 US) [35]. Moreover, Beixinjing Blocks has fairly complete health archives for residents and its coverage rate had reached 97.52% in 2001.

This study protocol was approved by the Human Research and Ethics Committee of the Shanghai First People's Hospital, affiliated Shanghai Jiaotong University, and adhered to the tenets of the Declaration of Helsinki.

Part I: Population-based study. Between November 2010 and April 2011, a population-based study of the prevalence of iERM was designed and performed in Beixinjing Blocks. Random cluster sampling was used to select the study sample. Clusters were defined geographically using Residence Administrative Committees (RACs) of approximately 1,000 persons (all ages). By using 2000 census information, the residents of RAC that had total populations larger than 1,500 were subdivided, and the residents of RAC smaller than 500 were grouped in defining clusters for sampling. Forty-two clusters were defined for random sampling. With an estimated 18.9% of the Beixinjing Blocks population aged 60 years or older, the typical cluster was estimated to contain approximately 190 study participants.

The required sample size was calculated based on estimating with 95% confidence the prevalence of ERM in the Handan Eye Study (3.4%) [25]. The required sample size with simple random sampling can be calculated as $n \approx Z^2(p)(1-p)/B^2$ where $p = 0.034$; $B = 0.034(0.25) = 0.0085$ with a 25% error bound; and $Z = 1.96$ for a 95% confidence interval (CI). It was assumed that a cluster design effect as high as 1.5 might be present, which would increase the calculated sample size from 1,746 to 2,619. With an estimated response rate of 90%, the required sample size became 2,910. Accordingly, 16 clusters (with an expected study population of 3,040) were chosen by simple random sampling from the list of 42 clusters.

Two days before the examinations, RACs telephoned the eligible residents, informing them of the examination date and the purpose of the study. The field examinations were mainly carried out in the nearest community meeting room, while home inspections were used to collect data of physically disabled residents. Near the end of this study, the eligible residents who had not participated in the field examination on the previously scheduled day were notified by phone about another examination date.

The research group included one lead ophthalmic doctor who had prior experience organizing large-scale epidemiologic studies, four trained ophthalmologists from Shanghai First People's Hospital, affiliated Shanghai Jiaotong University, and two trained physicians from Bingxinjing Community Hospital. Before formal investigation, the members of the research group had trained for two weeks to understand the purpose of the study, methods, and detailed steps for each variable (such as familiar with correct filling sheets, standard operating procedures of inspection equipment, and diagnosis, classification and grading criteria of iERM). Written informed consent was first obtained from all study participants. A detailed interview was conducted to collect information regarding demographics (including age, gender, employment status, years of formal education after kindergarten, height, and weight), histories of diagnosis and treatment relating to systemic comorbidities (such as hypertension, diabetes, and cardio-cerebrovascular diseases) and ocular diseases (such as DR, cataract, and glaucoma). After that, all eligible participants underwent a comprehensive ophthalmic examination. Visual acuity of each eye was measured using the log of the minimum angle of resolution (LogMAR) Early Treatment Diabetic Retinopathy Study (ETDRS) chart at a distance of 4 m, with illumination ≥300 lux. In participants who were wearing glasses in their daily lives, visual acuity was measured with their spectacles. Both types of visual acuity mentioned above are known as the presenting visual acuity [36]. In addition, pinhole-corrected visual acuity was measured in participants with a presenting visual acuity worse than 0.7 in either eye. Anterior segment examinations with a slit-lamp biomicroscope, refractive media and fundus examinations with a direct ophthalmoscope were conducted by the ophthalmologists. If participants' pinhole-correction visual acuity worse than 0.7 and the vision loss could not be attributed to corneal disease, the examinations were performed after pupil dilatation with 0.5% tropicamide and 0.5% phenylephrine (Mydrin-P; Santen Pharmaceuticals; Japan) except in case of a shallow anterior chamber. A digital 45° non-mydriatic retinal camera (CR-DGi Non-mydriatic Retinal Camera; Canon Inc., Tokyo, Japan) was used to obtain color retinal photographs of ETDRS standard field 1 [37] (centered on the optic disc) and field 2 (centered on the macula) for each eye.

The retinal photographs were assessed respectively by two ophthalmologists with retinal subspecialty training for the presence of ERM and its grading. The prevalence-adjusted bias-adjusted kappa statistic was 0.82 for the presence of ERM, and the kappa statistic was 0.70 for its grading. In case of doubt, the lead ophthalmic doctor reassessed the retinal photographs to make the final diagnosis and grading. In our study, ERM was subdivided as idiopathic or secondary. iERM was defined as ERM occurring in eyes without a secondary cause, such as DR (at least a history of diabetes associated with retinal microaneurysms), retinal vascular disease, retinal detachment, or history of cataract surgery. Moreover, iERM was graded using the method described by Klein et al. [7], which divides iERM into two types, cellophane macular reflex (CMR) and premacular fibrosis (PMF). CMR was defined as a patch or irregular, increased reflection from the inner retinal surface. PMF, a more severe type, was defined as a grayish and opaque appearance of the inner retinal surface combined with superficial retinal folds or traction lines. Participants with both CMR and PMF were allocated to the PMF group. Thus, iERM was detected in 34 participants (1.02%), who were all later confirmed by OCT.

Part II: Case-control study. In November 2011, the 34 participants with iERM as the case group and 34 healthy participants randomly selected (using a computer-generated random number table) as the control group from the participants without ERM were further examined in the Beixinjing community health service center. Cases and controls were well matched in age, sex, body mass index (BMI), and the iERM-associated risk factors (diabetes and higher level of education) obtained from Part I. After explaining the purpose of this study, we obtained the written informed consent from all participants.

Two ophthalmologists, two optometrists and one retinal specialist performed the following examinations. Blood samples were collected for testing plasma glucose, serum total cholesterol, creatinine, and triglyceride after an overnight fast. The uncorrected distance visual acuity (UCDVA) was measured using the ETDRS chart as described in Part I, and near visual acuity was measured using the LogMAR word reading cards at the participant's preferred reading distance. The best-corrected distance visual acuity (BCDVA) was measured after objective refraction by an autorefractor (Nidek ARK900; Nidek Inc., Aichi, Japan). For each eye, IOP by a non-contact tonometry, axial length, K1 (keratometry for flat meridian), K2 (keratometry for steep meridian), and ACD by an IOL-master (Carl Zeiss Meditec, Jena, Germany) were examined at least three times, then the average readings were recorded.

The B-mode ultrasound (10 MHz or 20 MHz, Cine-Scan, Quantel, France) and OCT (Spectralis OCT, Heidelberg Engineering, Heidelberg, Germany) examinations (after 20 minutes' dark adaptation with the pupil naturally dilated or adequate pupil dilatation with Mydrin-P) were conducted on all 68 participants by two ophthalmologists, respectively, who were trained and certified by retinal specialists. Posterior staphyloma and the kinetic movements of both the posterior vitreous and the vitreoretinal traction were observed under biomicroscopy, ophthalmoscopy and B-mode ultrasonography. The PVD before the macular region was confirmed when a complete separation of the posterior hyaloid membrane (a floating continuous thin membrane-like echo in the vitreous cavity under ultrasonography) and an optically or acoustically empty subhyaloid space were both present under ultrasonography, and no vitreoretinal adhesion at the macular region was present under OCT examination.

OCT examinations, including detected iERM in OCT images, were performed in both groups [38]. The retinal thickness of the central fovea, the thickness of iERM, and the distance between the membrane and central fovea were measured. Most of the OCT scans of the macula were centered on the participant's fixation point. When visual acuity in the participant's eye to be scanned was too poor to provide stable fixation, manual positioning of the macula by moving the fixation LED or using external fixation was used. Part of the optic disc was included at the edge of the images to help orient the images.

Data Management and Analysis

Statistical analyses were performed with SPSS statistical software version 13.0 (SPSS Inc., Chicago, IL, USA). An alpha level of $P<0.05$ was chosen as the criterion for significance.

Descriptive statistical analyses were performed to characterize demographic data, visual acuity, and clinical characteristics. Age-standardized prevalence was calculated by direct methods using 2000 Chinese national census population. Logistic regression was employed to determine the independence of potential risk factors for iERM, including continuous (age and BMI) and dichotomous variables (gender, level of education, hypertension, diabetes, cardio-cerebrovascular diseases, and high myopia). Odds ratios (ORs) and 95% CIs were reported. Moreover, the independent-samples t-test and Mantel-Haenszel chi-square test were used to determine the significant differences between the case and control groups.

Results

A total of 4,153 residents were determined as eligible, and 3727 residents underwent interviews and clinic examinations, corresponding to a response rate of 89.7%. Of these, gradable retinal photographs for epiretinal membranes were available for 3571 participants (95.8%, 7,142 eyes; 1,989 women). The mean age was 71.08±7.36 years (median, 71 years; range, 60–98 years). The other 156 participants (4.2%) had un-gradable retinal photographs due to refractive media opacity, such as cataract and vitreous opacity. 245 of 3571 participants (6.9%) were excluded because of a known secondary cause of the development of ERM. DR was present in 32 participants, retinal vascular disease in 50, a history or signs of retinal detachment in 19, and a history of cataract surgery in 162.

Of the resulting 3,326 participants, iERM was detected in 39 eyes of 34 participants according to retinal photographs, for a prevalence of 1.02%. CMR was present in 0.63% (21 eyes of 21 participants) and PMF in 0.39% (14 eyes of 13 participants). The age-specific, gender-specific, and age-standardized (according to the 2000 Chinese national census population aged 60 years or older) prevalence of CMR, PMF and any iERM are listed in Table 1. Participants' demographic and clinical characteristics are shown in Table 2. There were significant differences between the participants with and without iERM in level of education and prevalence of diabetes ($P<0.05$). Compared with the participants without iERM, those with iERM had decreased presenting visual acuity, which was assessed in the worst eye, and a significant difference was observed ($P<0.05$). Moreover, presenting visual acuity was significantly worse in eyes of the participants with PMF than without iERM ($P<0.01$), but the participants with CMR had similar presenting visual acuity to those without iERM (Figure 1). After excluding participants with any known secondary cause for the development of ERM (n = 245), the prevalence of iERM was significantly associated with diabetes (OR: 2.457; 95% CI: 1.137, 5.309) and higher level of education (OR: 1.48; 95% CI: 1.123, 1.952). iERM was not associated with age, gender, BMI, hypertension, cardio-cerebrovascular diseases, or high myopia.

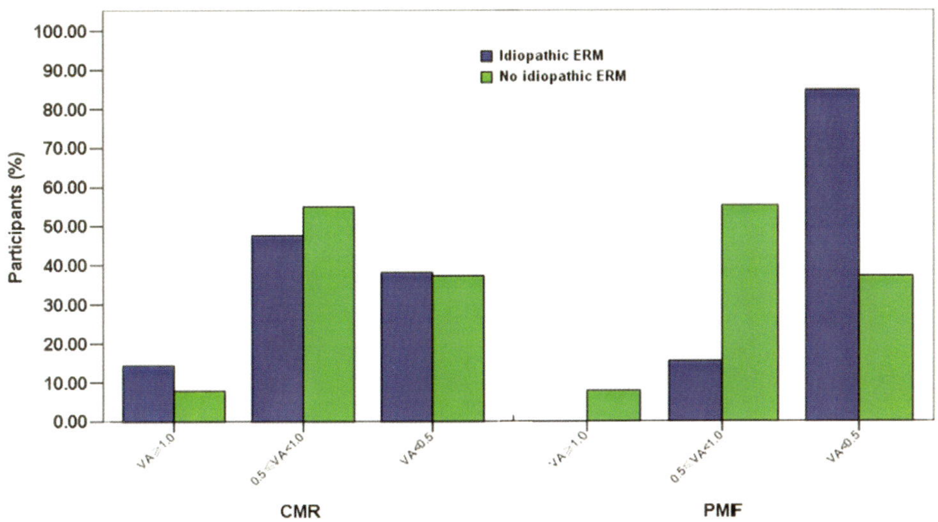

Figure 1. LogMAR presenting visual acuity of idiopathic epiretinal membranes (iERM) and no iERM.

In the case-control study, the demographic characteristics of the 34 participants with iERM and the 34 healthy participants were compared in Table 3. The difference between the two groups was not statistically significant in age, gender, BMI, diabetes history, or level of education. In contrast to serum total cholesterol ($t = 2.47$, $p = 0.02$), the difference between the two groups was not statistically significant in fasting plasma glucose, serum creatinine, or triglyceride ($P > 0.05$). The fasting plasma glucose levels of the iERM group(mean 6.25 mmol/L, SD 1.79) and control group (mean 6.12 mmol/L, SD1.8) were both slightly higher than the normal range (3.9–6.10 mmol/L), and serum total cholesterol was higher in the control group (mean 5.53 mmol/L, SD 1.17; normal range <5.20 mmol/L). In contrast to distance visual acuity ($t = -2.25$, $P = 0.03$) and near visual acuity ($t = -2.32$, $P = 0.02$), the differences in ocular biological parameters, including refractive error, axial length, K1, K2, ACD and IOP, between the two groups were not statistically significant ($P > 0.05$). When we compared the distance visual acuity of the participants with CMR or PMF, respectively, with the controls, the distance visual acuity was significantly lower in the eyes with PMF ($p < 0.01$), while it was similar between CMR and the controls. Twelve eyes of 9 participants (26.5%) with iERM were associated with PVD before the macular region, while 3 participants (8.8%) were associated with PVD in the control group, but the differences between the two groups were not statistically significant ($P = 0.056$). None of the eyes had posterior staphyloma. According to OCT images, there was a significant difference in the mean retinal thickness of the central fovea ($P < 0.01$) between the iERM group (390.78 μm, SD 128.60) and control group (243.55 μm, SD 25.33). Moreover, the mean thickness of iERM was 20.03 μm (SD 13.04), and the mean distance between the membrane and central fovea was 65.76 μm (SD 225.99).

Table 1. Prevalence of idiopathic epiretinal membranes by age and gender.

Variable		Total (n)	CMR (n, %)	PMF (n, %)	Any iERM (n, %)
Sex*	Male	1481	12 (0.8)	5 (0.3)	17 (1.1)
	Female	1845	9 (0.5)	8 (0.4)	17 (0.9)
Age (y)	60–69	1409	8 (0.6)	6 (0.4)	14 (1.0)
	70–79	1507	11 (0.7)	7 (0.5)	18 (1.2)
	80+	410	2 (0.5)	0 (0)	2 (0.5)
Total*		3326	21 (0.6)	13 (0.6)	34 (1.0)

CMR, cellophane macular reflex; PMF, preretinal macular fibrosis; iERM, idiopathic epiretinal membrane.
*Age-standardized prevalence using the 2000 Chinese national census.

Discussion

In this population-based study, we observed an overall iERM prevalence of 1.02% in Beixinjing Blocks, Shanghai, China, which included 0.63% for CMR and 0.39% for PMF. Our study suggests that iERM is less frequent in urban Chinese than reported in samples of Asians from the Handan Eye Study (3.0%) [25] and Singapore Malay Eye Study (9.5%) [2], Caucasians from the Melbourne Visual Impairment Project Study (5.4%) [23] and Latinos from the LALES (17.5%) [8]. Therefore, the prevalence of iERM differs among population-based studies, for reasons unknown. One possible reason may be ethnic differences, as mentioned by some previous studies [22,24]. Interestingly, not just the prevalence of iERM but the prevalence of DR and age-related macular degeneration in our previous studies [39,40] were lower than in Western countries. Another possible reason is different inclusion criteria for eligible participants. In the present study, urban residents aged 60 years or older were randomly selected, while most of the other studies used an inclusion criterion of 40 years or older [8,23,26]. The prevalence of diabetes [4,8,27], a risk factor for iERM, was 20.4% among persons who were aged≥60 years in China [41], and Shanghai, as the largest city and one of the most economically developed areas, has a higher prevalence (aged 60–69 years: 22.4%/male, 22.3%/female; aged 70–74 years: 25.6%/male, 27.2%/female) [42], which was close to the results from the Singapore Malay Eye Study (21.8%) [43], but much lower than the LALES (34.5%) [44]. Therefore, we cannot rule out the possible association between the prevalence of diabetes and the lower prevalence of iERM in Beixinjing Blocks. In addition, cataract surgical rate (CSR) in Beixinjing Blocks (aged≥60 years) was 7,790/million in 2007 [45]. Approximately 8000 cataract surgeries (an exclusion criteria for iERM) per year

Table 2. Demographic and clinical characteristics among the participants (n = 3326) with or without idiopathic epiretinal membrane.*

Characteristic	iERM	No iERM	Statistic value †	P value
Participants [No. (%)]	34 (1.02)	3292 (98.98)		
Mean age (SD, 95% CI), years	71.53 (6.11, 95% CI, 69.40 to 73.66)	70.84 (7.34, 95% CI, 70.59 to 71.09)	t = 0.568	0.57
60–69 [No. (%)]	14 (41.2)	1395 (42.4)	χ2 = 1.356	0.544
70–79 [No. (%)]	18 (52.9)	1489 (45.2)		
80+ [No. (%)]	2 (5.9)	408 (12.4)		
Male [No. (%)]	17 (50.0)	1464 (44.5)	χ2 = 0.416	0.519
Mean BMI (SD, 95%CI)	24.15 (3.02, 95% CI, 23.10 to 25.20)	23.90 (3.27, 95% CI, 23.79 to 24.02)	t = 0.436	0.663
Mean education (SD, 95%CI) years	9.38 (5.38, 95% CI, 7.51 to 11.26)	7.42 (4.47, 95% CI, 7.27 to 7.58)	t = 2.54	0.011 †
Illiterate [No. (%)]	4 (11.8)	468 (14.2)	χ2 = 10.725	0.023 †
Primary school [No. (%)]	6 (17.6)	1143 (34.7)		
Junior high school [No. (%)]	9 (26.5)	814 (24.7)		
Senior high school [No. (%)]	6 (17.6)	551 (16.7)		
College or higher [No. (%)]	9 (26.5)	361 (9.6)		
Systemic comorbidities suffered				
Hypertension [No. (%)]	18 (52.9)	1310 (39.8)	χ2 = 2.425	0.119
Diabetes [No. (%)]	9 (26.5)	435 (13.2)		0.038 ‡
Cardio-cerebrovascular diseases [No. (%)]	6 (17.6)	292 (8.9)		0.118
Hypermyopia [No. (%)]	0 (0)	163 (5.0)		0.411
Mean logMAR presenting VA (SD, 95%CI)	0.44 (0.29, 95% CI, 0.34 to 0.55)	0.54 (0.25, 95% CI, 0.53 to 0.55)	t = −2.263	0.024 ‡
Mean logMAR UCDVA (SD, 95%CI)	0.39 (0.29, 95% CI, 0.29 to 0.50)	0.45 (0.27, 95% CI, 0.44 to 0.46)	t = −1.205	0.228

iERM, idiopathic epiretinal membrane; SD, standard deviation; CI, confidence interval; BMI, body mass index; VA, visual acuity; UCDVA, uncorrected distance visual acuity.
*Idiopathic epiretinal membrane was considered present in participants without a secondary cause (diabetic retinopathy, retinal vascular disease, retinal detachment, or history of cataract surgery) of ERM.
†t: Independent samples t-test; χ2: Pearson chi-square.
‡P<0.05.

have been closer to the western developed countries, which might cause lower prevalence of iERM in Beixinjing Blocks. Nevertheless, some methodological issues should be mentioned. This study used non-stereoscopic 45° retinal photographs to identify and grade iERM, whereas some other studies used 30° stereoscopic retinal photographs and/or OCT [8,23–25]. Even though we

Table 3. Demographic characteristics in the 34 participants with iERM and the 34 healthy participants (control group).

	iERM group	Control group	Statistic value*	P value
No. of participants	34	34		
Mean age (SD) years	72.53 (6.11)	70.44 (7.90)	t = 1.219	0.227
Male [No. (%)]	17 (50.0)	15 (44.1)	χ2 = 0.236	0.627
Mean BMI (SD)	24.15 (3.02)	23.02 (3.54)	t = 1.412	0.163
Levels of education				
Illiterate [No. (%)]	4 (11.8)	4 (12.5)	χ2 = 1.59	0.87
Primary school [No. (%)]	6 (17.6)	3 (9.4)		
Junior high school [No. (%)]	9 (26.5)	10 (31.3)		
Senior high school [No. (%)]	6 (17.6)	7 (21.9)		
College or higher [No. (%)]	9 (26.5)	8 (25)		
Diabetes suffered [No. (%)]	9 (26.5)	4 (11.8)	χ2 = 2.378	0.123

iERM, idiopathic epiretinal membrane; SD, standard deviation.
*χ2: Mantel-Haenszel chi-square; t: independent-samples t-test.

trained ophthalmologists to evaluate the participants for iERM, non-stereoscopic retinal photographs might have resulted in an underestimation of the prevalence of iERM by missing subtle early macular changes, especially CMR.

Consistent with previous studies [4,8,27], our study found that diabetes was positively associated with the prevalence of iERM. Samantha and associates [8] speculated that the high prevalence of iERM (17.5%) in their population-based study was because of its high prevalence of diabetes. These findings suggest diabetes might promote the occurrence and development of iERM. A conceivable pathological mechanism is that synchysis contributes to the precocious and exaggerated PVD in diabetics, and therefore, PVD is significantly more common in diabetics, even in the absence of retinopathy [46].

In addition to diabetes, we found that a higher level of education was associated with iERM, which was consistent with the Beijing Eye Study [24]. In contrast to previous studies, we failed to find a significant association between the prevalence of iERM and other potential risk factors, including older age [4,7,8,22–25,26,28], gender [26], and high myopia [4,8]. It was likely that the number of participants with iERM was too small in our study to detect associations with these factors. Not surprisingly, we found that presenting visual acuity was significantly worse in eyes of participants with iERM or PMF, but not in those with CMR, compared with participants without iERM. These findings are consistent with previous studies [4,7,25]. The presence of PMF alone can cause decreased visual acuity if it involves the center of the fovea [4,7,8]. It was conceivable that most iERM cases detected from retinal photographs or OCT were early-stage iERM, so most patients with iERM had no obvious visual impairment.

In the subsequent case-control study, we unexpectedly found that serum total cholesterol was negatively associated with iERM. However, hypercholesterolemia has been reported as a possible risk factor for iERM in the Hisayama Study [22] and the Multi-Ethnic Study of Atherosclerosis [47]. Although the pathophysiological mechanisms of the formation of iERM are not clear, experimental studies demonstrate that chemoattractants from the serum or vascular endothelial cells may mediate cell migration and proliferation, which might promote the development of iERMs in patients with hyperlipidemia [48,49]. Therefore, we speculated that the cholesterol association was a spurious finding in our study, due to the small sample and possible sampling error.

There is controversy [8,23–26] about the relationship between refractive error and iERM, especially myopia [23,25,28], which might have a positive association with iERM. However, in addition to distance visual acuity and near visual acuity, no ocular biological parameters were significantly different between the two groups in our study. It was notable that the incidence of PVD in the case group was much higher than in the control group, although this difference was not statistically significant. Large clinical studies [32–34,50] have implicated PVD as a factor involved in the genesis of iERM [15]. Therefore, we cannot rule out the possibility that PVD has clinical significance in iERM.

The limitations of our study should be stated. First, blood biochemical parameters, such as serum total cholesterol [22] and fasting plasma glucose [4], that were previously reported as risk factors for iERM were not examined in our population-based study due to the limited resources. Second, it is difficult to complete B-mode ultrasound, OCT, and IOL-master examinations for all participants in large-scale population-based studies, such as the Handan Eye Study [25], in which only 85.3% participants had OCT images from at least one eye that were considered gradable for ERM. Although we performed a further case-control study, residual confounding was also possible. In addition, the diagnosis and grading of iERM could be affected by non-stereoscopic retinal photographs and refractive media opacity, such as cataract and vitreous opacity, which may have led to an underestimation of the prevalence of iERM.

In conclusion, iERM occurs at a relatively low frequency in a population-based sample of Beixinjing Blocks aged 60 years or older. Its prevalence was lower than in Western countries and in Chinese subjects in Handan, and it was associated with diabetes and higher level of education. Furthermore, iERM causes a substantial decrease in visual acuity.

Acknowledgments

The authors thank the staff and participants in Beixinjing study for their valuable skill and support.

Author Contributions

Conceived and designed the experiments: HDZ XX XZ. Performed the experiments: HDZ JJP XFZ JF WWW. Analyzed the data: XFZ JJP HDZ. Contributed reagents/materials/analysis tools: HDZ XFZ. Wrote the paper: XFZ HDZ JJP.

References

1. Snead DR, James S, Snead MP (2008) Pathological changes in the vitreoretinal junction 1: epiretinal membrane formation. Eye 22: 1310–1317.
2. Okamoto F, Okamoto Y, Hiraoka T, Oshika T (2009) Effect of vitrectomy for epiretinal membrane on visual function and vision-related quality of life. Am J Ophthalmol 147: 869–874.
3. Ghazi-Nouri SM, Tranos PG, Rubin GS, Adams ZC, Charteris DG (2006) Visual function and quality of life following vitrectomy and epiretinal membrane peel surgery. Br J Ophthalmol 90: 559–562.
4. Mitchell P, Smith W, Chey T, Wang JJ, Chang A (1997) Prevalence and associations of epiretinal membranes. The Blue Mountains Eye Study, Australia. Ophthalmology 104: 1033–1040.
5. Fraser-Bell S, Guzowski M, Rochtchina E, Wang JJ, Mitchell P (2003) Five-year cumulative incidence and progression of epiretinal membranes: the Blue Mountains Eye Study. Ophthalmology 110: 34–40.
6. Bouwens MD, de Jong F, Mulder P, van Meurs JC (2008) Results of macular pucker surgery: 1- and 5-year follow-up. Graefes Arch Clin Exp Ophthalmol 246: 1693.
7. Klein R, Klein BE, Wang Q, Moss SE (1994) The epidemiology of epiretinal membranes. Trans Am Ophthalmol Soc 92: 403–430.
8. Fraser-Bell S, Ying-Lai M, Klein R, Varma R; The Los Angeles Latino Eye Study Group (2004) Prevalence and associations of epiretinal membranes in latinos: the Los Angeles Latino Eye Study. Invest Ophthalmol Vis Sci 45: 1732–1736.
9. Appiah AP, Hirose T (1989) Secondary causes of premacular fibrosis. Ophthalmology 96: 389–392.
10. Kraushar MF, Morse PH (1988) The relationship between retina surgery and preretinal macular fibrosis. Ophthalmic Surg 19: 843–848.
11. Council MD, Shah GK, Lee HC, Sharma S (2005) Visual outcomes and complications of epiretinal membrane removal secondary to rhegmatogenous retinal detachment. Ophthalmology 112: 1218–1221.
12. Jahn CE, Minich V, Moldaschel S, Stahl B, Jedelhauser P, et al. (2001) Epiretinal membranes after extracapsular cataract surgery(1). J Cataract Refract Surg 27: 753–760.
13. Foos RY (1977) Vitreoretinal juncture; epiretinal membranes and vitreous. Invest Ophthalmol Vis Sci 16: 416–422.
14. Johnson MW (2010) Posterior vitreous detachment: evolution and complications of its early stages. Am J Ophthalmol 149: 371–382.
15. Kishi S, Hagimura N, Shimizu K (1996) The role of the premacular liquefied pocket and premacular vitreous cortex in idiopathic macular hole development. Am J Ophthalmol 122: 622–628.
16. Clarkson JG, Green WR, Massof D (1977) A histopathologic review of 168 cases of preretinal membrane. Am J Ophthalmol 84: 1–17.
17. Smiddy WE, Maguire AM, Green WR, Michels RG, de la Cruz Z, et al. (1989) Idiopathic epiretinal membranes. Ultrastructural characteristics and clinicopathologic correlation. Ophthalmology 96: 811–820.

18. Hiscott PS, Grierson I, Trombetta CJ, Rahi AH, Marshall J, et al. (1984) Retinal and epiretinal glia: an immunohistochemical study. Br J Ophthalmol 68: 698–707.
19. Gandorfer A, Rohleder M, Kampik A (2002) Epiretinal pathology of vitreomacular traction syndrome. Br J Ophthalmol 86: 902–909.
20. Kita T, Hata Y, Kano K, Miura M, Nakao S, et al. (2007) Transforming growth factor-beta2 and connective tissue growth factor in proliferative vitreoretinal diseases: possible involvement of hyalocytes and therapeutic potential of Rho kinase inhibitor. Diabetes 56: 231–238.
21. Yamashita T, Uemura A, Sakamoto T (2008) Intraoperative characteristics of the posterior vitreous cortex in patients with epiretinal membrane. Graefes Arch Clin Exp Ophthalmol 246: 333–337.
22. Miyazaki M, Nakamura H, Kubo M, Kiyohara Y, Iida M, et al. (2003) Prevalence and risk factors for epiretinal membranes in a Japanese population: the Hisayama study. Graefes Arch Clin Exp Ophthalmol 241: 642–646.
23. McCarty DJ, Mukesh BN, Chikani V, Wang JJ, Mitchell P, et al. (2005) Prevalence and associations of epiretinal membranes in the visual impairment project. Am J Ophthalmol 140: 288–294.
24. You Q, Xu L, Jonas JB (2008) Prevalence and associations of epiretinal membranes in adult Chinese: the Beijing eye study. Eye 22: 874–879.
25. Duan XR, Liang YB, Friedman DS, Sun LP, Wei WB, et al. (2009) Prevalence and associations of epiretinal membranes in a rural Chinese adult population: the Handan Eye Study. Invest Ophthalmol Vis Sci 50 : 2018–2023.
26. Kawasaki R, Wang JJ, Mitchell P, Aung T, Saw SM, et al. (2008) Racial difference in the prevalence of epiretinal membrane between Caucasians and Asians. Br J Ophthalmol 92: 1320–1324.
27. Kawasaki R, Wang JJ, Sato H, Mitchell P, Kato T, et al. (2009) Prevalence and associations of epiretinal membranes in an adult Japanese population: the Funagata study. Eye (Lond) 23: 1045–1051.
28. Koh V, Cheung CY, Wong WL, Cheung CM, Wang JJ, et al. (2012) Prevalence and risk factors of epiretinal membrane in Asian Indians. Invest Ophthalmol Vis Sci 53: 1018–1022.
29. Khaja HA, McCannel CA, Diehl NN, Mohney BG (2008) Incidence and clinical characteristics of epiretinal membranes in children. Arch Ophthalmol 126: 632–636.
30. Yazici AT, Alagöz N, Celik HU, Bozkurt E, Alagöz C, et al. (2011) Idiopathic and secondary epiretinal membranes: do they differ in terms of morphology? An optical coherence tomography-based study. Retina 31: 779–784.
31. Arichika S, Hangai M, Yoshimura N (2010) Correlation between thickening of the inner and outer retina and visual acuity in patients with epiretinal membrane. Retina 30: 503–508.
32. Kishi S, Shimizu K (1994) Oval defect in detached posterior hyaloid membrane in idiopathic preretinal macular fibrosis. Am J Ophthalmol 118: 451–456.
33. Appiah AP, Hirose T, Kado M (1988) A review of 324 cases of idiopathic premacular gliosis. Am J Ophthalmol 106: 533–535.
34. Sidd RJ, Fine SL, Owens SL, Patz A (1982) Idiopathic preretinal gliosis. Am J Ophthalmol 94: 44–48.
35. Shanghai Bureau of Statistics (2011) Statistics bulletin for the national economy and social development in Shanghai [in Chinese]. Available at http://www.stats-sh.gov.cn/sjfb/201202/239488.html. Accessed February 24, 2012.
36. Liang YB, Friedman DS, Wong TY, Zhan SY, Sun LP, et al. (2008) Prevalence and causes of low vision and blindness in a rural chinese adult population: the Handan Eye Study. Ophthalmology 115: 1965–1972.
37. Moss SE, Meuer SM, Klein R, Hubbard LD, Brothers RJ, et al. (1989) Are seven standard photographic fields necessary for classification of diabetic retinopathy? Invest Ophthalmol Vis Sci 30: 823–828.
38. Wilkins JR, Puliafito CA, Hee MR, Duker JS, Reichel E, et al. (1996) Characterization of epiretinal membranes using optical coherence tomography. Ophthalmology 103: 2142–2151.
39. Huang XB, Zou HD, Wang N, Wang WW, Fu J, et al. (2009) A prevalence survey of blindness and visual impairment in adults aged equal or more than 60 years in Beixinjing blocks of Shanghai, China. Zhonghua Yan KeZa Zhi 45: 786–792.
40. Peng J, Zou H, Wang W, Fu J, Shen B, et al. (2011) Implementation and first-year screening results of an ocular telehealth system for diabetic retinopathy in China. BMC Health Serv Res 11: 250.
41. Yang W, Lu J, Weng J, Jia W, Ji L, et al. (2010) Prevalence of diabetes among men and women in China. N Engl J Med 362: 1090–1101.
42. Li R, Lu W, Jiang QW, Li YY, Zhao GM, et al. (2012) Increasing prevalence of type 2 diabetes in Chinese adults in Shanghai. Diabetes Care 35: 1028–1030.
43. Sabanayagam C, Wang JJ, Mitchell P, Tan AG, Tai ES, et al. (2011) Metabolic syndrome components and age-related cataract: the Singapore Malay eye study. Invest Ophthalmol Vis Sci 52: 2397–2404.
44. Gatto NM, Varma R, Torres M, Wong TY, Johnson PL, et al. (2012) Retinal microvascular abnormalities and cognitive function in Latino adults in Los Angeles. Ophthalmic Epidemiol 19: 127–136.
45. Huang XB, Zou HD, Wang N, Wang WW, Fu J, et al.(2009) Epidemiological survey of cataract among the elder in Beixinjing Blocks,Shanghai.Int J Ophthalmol 9: 1321–1324. [in Chinese]
46. Foos RY, Kreiger AE, Forsythe AB, Zakka KA (1980) Posterior vitreous detachment in diabetic subjects. Ophthalmology 87: 122–128.
47. Ng CH, Cheung N, Wang JJ, Islam AF, Kawasaki R, et al. (2011) Prevalence and risk factors for epiretinal membranes in a multi-ethnic United States population. Ophthalmology 118: 694–699.
48. Zauberman H, Livni N (1981) Experimental vascular occlusion in hypercholesterolemic rabbits. Invest Ophthalmol Vis Sci 21: 248–255.
49. Smiddy WE, Maguire AM, Green WR, Michels RG, de la Cruz Z, et al. (1989) Idiopathic epiretinal membranes. Ultrastructural characteristics and clinicopathologic correlation. Ophthalmology 96: 811–820.
50. Johnson MW (2005) Perifoveal vitreous detachment and its macular complications. Trans Am Ophthalmol Soc 103: 537–567.

Discrepant Expression of Cytokines in Inflammation- and Age-Related Cataract Patients

Wan Chen[9], **Haotian Lin**[9], **Xiaojian Zhong, Zhaochuan Liu, Yu Geng, Chufang Xie, Weirong Chen***

State Key Laboratory of Ophthalmology, Zhongshan Ophthalmic Center, Sun Yat-sen University, Guangzhou, Guangdong, China

Abstract

Purpose: Inflammatory cataracts secondary to Behcet's disease (BD) or Vogt-Koyanagi-Harada disease (VKH) are thought to result from a pathological dysregulation of cytokines that is different from that of age-related (AR) cataracts. However, little is known about the function of cytokines in the development of inflammatory cataracts. The purpose of this study was to identify possible differences in cytokine expression in inflammation- and age-related cataract patients.

Methods: Analysis techniques involving the concomitant use of a cocktail of antibody-coated non-magnetic beads were used to determine the cytokine expression profiles of BD, VKH and AR cataract patients. Furthermore, anterior chamber aqueous flares and inflammatory cells were quantitatively measured with a laser flare cell meter (LFCM).

Results: The expressions of interleukin-2 (IL-2), IL-4, IL-6, IL-10, IL-17A, and interferon-γ (IFN-γ) were analyzed in aqueous humor (AqH), phytohemagglutinin (PHA)-stimulated and non-PHA-stimulated cultures of peripheral blood mononuclear cells (PBMCs) from the three types of cataract patients. IL-6 and IFN-γ were identified above the detection limits, but, among the BD and VKH cataract patients, only the levels of IL-6 were significantly higher in both the AqH and PBMC non-PHA cultures compared with the levels observed in the AR cataract patients. In contrast, IFN-γ was significantly elevated in the AqH of the BD cataract patients compared with the VKH and AR cataract patients. In the PHA-stimulated PBMC cultures, IL-2, IFN-γ, IL-6, and IL-17A were significantly increased, and the IL-6 level was significantly higher in the VKH patients than in the BD and AR cataract patients. The correlation analyses of the cytokines and inflammation indexes of the AqH obtained with the LFCM revealed that only IL-6 was significantly correlated with the inflammation index.

Conclusion: Distinct expression profiles of cytokines and the correlations of these profiles with in vivo inflammatory indexes for inflammatory and AR cataract patients were identified.

Editor: Matthaios Speletas, University of Thessaly, Faculty of Medicine, Greece

Funding: This study was supported by the National Natural Science Foundation of China (No. 81270980), the Guangdong Technology Programs (No. 2009B080701017) and the Pearl River Science and Technology New Star Project of Guangzhou City (2014J2200060). The funders had no role in study design, data collection and analysis, decision to publish, or preparation of the manuscript.

Competing Interests: The authors have declared that no competing interests exist.

* Email: chenwr_q@aliyun.com

[9] These authors contributed equally to this work.

Introduction

Cataracts secondary to uveitis, such as those that occur in Behcet's disease (BD) and Vogt-Koyanagi-Harada disease (VKH), challenge ophthalmologists in many aspects, including a miotic pupil, iris atrophy, posterior synechiae, pupillary membrane, operation time, perioperative medication, macular edema, severe postoperative inflammation and band keratopathy. The pathogenesis of this type of cataract is thought to be inflammation-related, in contrast to the pathogenesis of age-related (AR) cataracts. However, the expression patterns and function of cytokines during the development of inflammatory cataracts remain unknown.

Cytokines are crucially involved in the regulation of the normal human immune response. Dysregulated cytokine expression participates in the pathogenesis of autoimmune diseases, including BD and VKH. [1–3] Investigations of cytokine expression have advanced our understanding of the pathogeneses of various diseases. Previous studies have provided increasing support for the hypothesis that specific CD4^{+}T helper (Th) cell-mediated immune responses play a central role in the pathogenesis of uveitis. [4] CD4^{+} T cells are crucial for immunoregulation because they orchestrate the function of other immune cell types. CD4^{+} T cells can be sub-classified into groups, which include Th1, Th2, and Th17 cells. Th1 cells, which predominantly secrete IFN-γ, may play a pathogenic role in organ-specific autoimmune and other chronic inflammatory disorders. [5,6] Th2 cells, which primarily produce IL-4, IL-5, and IL-13, exert a strong inhibitory effect on Th1 differentiation and are responsible for the pathogenesis of allergic diseases. [7] Previous studies have suggested that both BD and VKH are predominantly related to the Th1 immune response, and patients with these diseases have increased levels of Th1-associated cytokines, such as interferon-gamma (IFN-γ), interleukin-12 (IL-12), and TNF-a. [8–11] Recently, several investigators have detected increased levels of IL-17 in active BD and VKH patients relative to patients in inactive stages and control healthy subjects. [11–14] Based on these findings, Th17 cells, in addition to Th1 cells, might be involved in the pathogeneses of these two subtypes of uveitis. Therefore, we inferred that there might be differences in the expression levels of IL-2, IL-4, IL-6, IL-10, IL-17A, and IFN-γ between inflammatory cataracts that are secondary to BD and VKH and AR cataracts. Long-standing ocular inflammation is a characteristic of uveitis. Previous studies have shown that aqueous flare can be detected in uveitis patients with long-standing inflammation even when that inflammation has been quiet for 3 months or longer. [15] Therefore, there is also likely to be differences in the aqueous flares and inflammatory cells of patients with BD and VKH cataracts relative to those with AR cataracts.

In this study, we concomitantly used a cocktail of antibody-coated non-magnetic beads to determine the cytokine expression profiles of BD, VKH and AR cataract patients, and we used a laser flare cell photometer (LFCM) to quantitatively measure the anterior chamber aqueous flares and inflammatory cells of these patients.

Methods

Patients

Nine patients (8 males and 1 female) with cortical cataracts secondary to BD (age 41.11±7.22 years) and ten VKH cortical cataract patients (4 males and 6 females, age 47.10±9.78 years) who required cataract surgery between January, 2010 and June, 2011 at the Cataract Treatment Department of Zhongshan Ophthalmic Center were included in the study. BD and VKH were diagnosed based on the International Study Group for Behcet's Disease Criteria [16] and the Revised International Diagnostic Criteria for VKH [17], respectively. There was no significant difference in the duration of disease between the VKH and BD patients ($P = 0.895$). All patients had received low dose prednisone (<20 mg/d) for at least 3 months to ensure that their uveitis was inactive prior to inclusion in this study. Ten age-matched AR cortical cataract patients (4 males and 6 females, age 49.90±10.59 years) with no prior history of uveitis, glaucoma, ocular trauma, rheumatoid arthritis, diabetes or other eye or systematic diseases were also included at the same time period. The three types of cortical cataract patients were matched for age and sex ($P > 0.05$). This study was performed in accordance with the Declaration of Helsinki and with the approval of the Sun Yat-sen University-Zhongshan Ophthalmic Center-Institutional Review Board (SYSU-ZOC-IRB). Written informed consent was obtained from all patients.

Measurement of Preoperative Anterior Chamber Inflammation

Quantitative measurements of anterior chamber aqueous flare and inflammatory cells were obtained preoperatively for the BD, VKH and AR cataract patients with a FC-2000 LFCM (Kowa, Tokyo, Japan) as described in a previous study [18]. Three individual measurements from each eye were averaged, and measurements that were affected by artifacts were discarded. Flare and cell readings are expressed as photon counts per millisecond (pc/ms) and cells/0.5 mm^3, respectively.

Analyses of the Cytokine Expression Profiles

All 29 included patients agreed to provide samples of peripheral blood (10 ml) and aqueous humor (100–200 μl) prior to their cataract surgeries. Peripheral blood mononuclear cells (PBMCs) were prepared from 10 ml of fresh heparinized blood via Ficoll-Hypaque density-gradient centrifugation. To study the production of the related cytokines, the PBMCs were cultured either with or without phytohemagglutinin (PHA) stimulation at a density of 2×10^6 cells/ml for 72 hours. Then, the supernatants were harvested and stored at −70°C until the cytokine analyses. Aqueous humor (100–200 μl) was aspirated from each patient via limbic paracentesis using a 27-gauge needle attached to a tuberculin syringe following the topical application of a local anesthetic, oxybuprocaine hydro-chloride (0.4%, Benoxinate, Chauvin Pharmaceuticals Ltd., Kingston, United Kingdom). The procedure was performed under a surgical microscope before phacoemulsification began. The samples were snap frozen and maintained at −70°C until use. Aqueous humor samples were obtained from all patients with uveitis at the beginning of the surgeries.

The cytokine expression profiles in the supernatants of the PBMC cultures and the aqueous humor samples were determined using a cocktail of antibody-coated non-magnetic beads that enabled concomitant measurements of the levels of IFN-γ, IL-2, IL-4, IL-6, IL-10, and IL-17A (Bio-plex pro-cytokine assay, BIORAD, Hercules, CA, USA). This technology allowed multiple analyses to be conducted on a single 50-μl sample. The analysis was performed following the manufacturer's instructions, and the results were generated using the Bio-Plex 200 system and software.

Statistical Analyses

The data were analyzed using the Statistical Package for Social Sciences (SPSS Version 16.0 for Windows). All data are expressed as the mean ± SD. One-way ANOVA and post-ANOVA pairwise comparisons of the means were conducted using the Kruskal-Wallis test to analyze the differences among the groups. The Mann-Whitney test was also used where indicated by the results of tests of the assumptions of normality and the homogeneity of the variance. Linear regression was used to assess correlations between pairs of variables. For all tests, $P \leq 0.05$ was considered statistically significant.

Results

Anterior Chamber Inflammation

The preoperative flare values of the VKH and BD groups were 18.21±4.80 and 21.72±3.24 pc/ms, respectively, and both of these values were significantly greater than those of the AR group ($P = 0.001$ and $P < 0.001$, respectively). However, no significant difference was found between the two uveitis groups ($P = 0.123$, Table 1). The inflammatory cell counts in the VKH, BD, and AR groups were 6.53±3.54, 5.80±3.21, and 4.03±2.73 cells/0.5 mm^3, respectively. No significant differences were found among these groups ($F = 1.837$, $P = 0.179$, Table 1).

Cytokine Concentrations in the Supernatants of the PBMC Cultures

The IL-2, IL-4, IL-10 and IL-17A contents were below the detection levels in the non-PHA-stimulated PBMC samples of the patients and the AR group. IFN-γ was detected, but no significant differences were found among the three groups ($P = 0.583$, Figure 1). However, we observed that IL-6 was significantly elevated in both the BD and VKH patients compared with the AR cataract patients ($P = 0.017$ and $P = 0.004$, respectively, Figure 1-A).

Table 1. Anterior chamber aqueous flare and inflammatory cells counts of the three groups.

Inflammation parameters	VKH Group	BD Group	AR Group	F	P
Flare values (pc/ms)	18.21±4.80*	21.72±3.24*	5.80±3.17	54.883	0.000
Cell count (cells/0.5 mm^3)	6.53±3.54	5.80±3.21	4.03±2.73	1.837	0.179

Footnotes: *P<0.05 versus the AR samples.

IL-2, IL-6, IL-17A, and IFN-γ were significantly increased in all of the PBMC samples following PHA stimulation, while IL-4 and IL-10 remained at relatively low levels (Figure 1-B). However, no significant differences in the mean levels of the above-mentioned cytokines were observed among the groups (Figure 1). Moreover, IL-6 was significantly increased in the VKH patients compared with the BD patients and the AR cataract patients (P = 0.000 and P = 0.013, respectively, Figure 1-B).

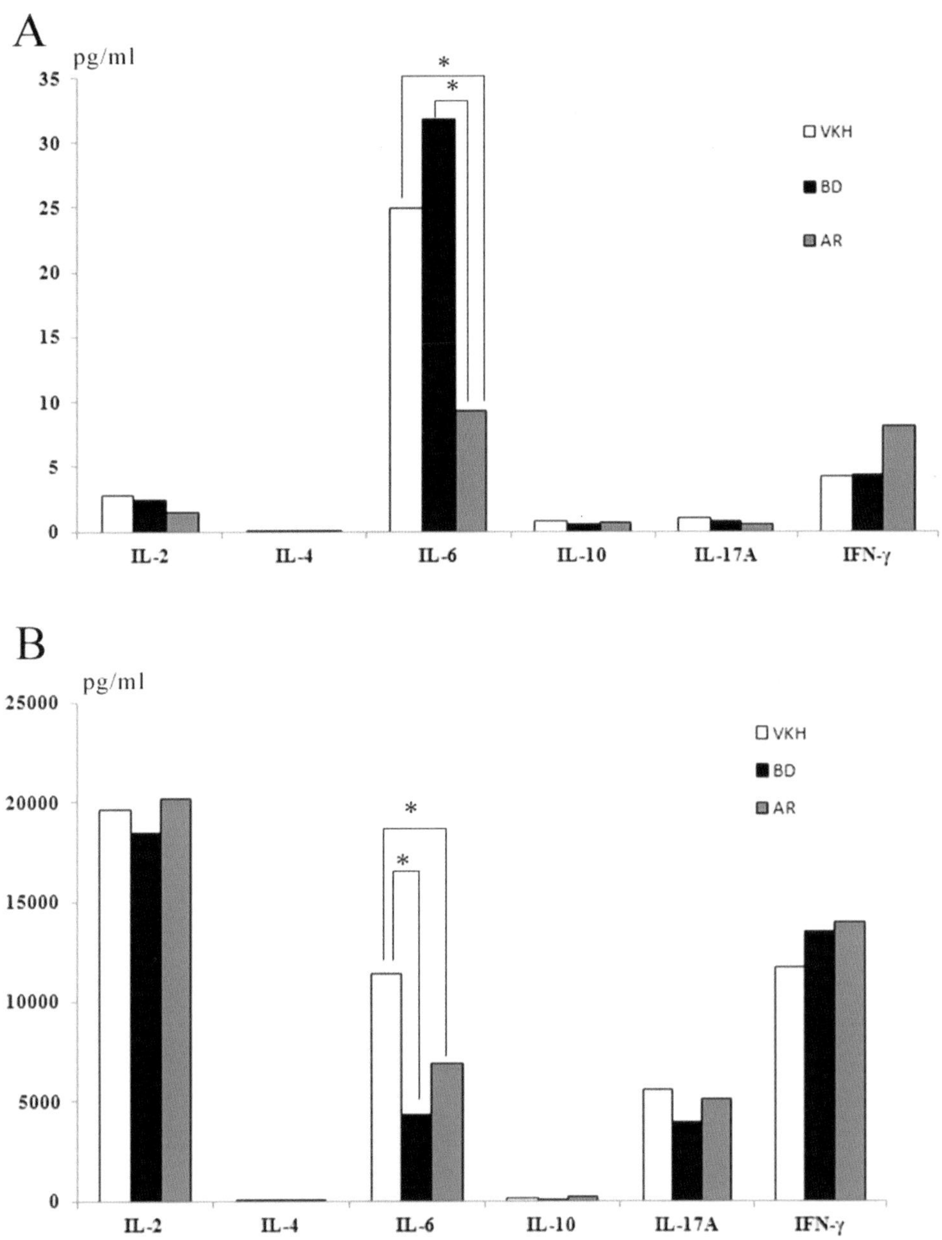

Figure 1. Mean IL-2, IL-4, IL-6, IL-10, IL-17A and IFN-γ levels in the PBMC samples from the VKH and BD patients and the ARs (pg/ml). Panel A, without PHA stimulation; Panel B, with PHA stimulation. *Statistically significant at the 5% level.

Table 2. Comparisons of the mean cytokine levels in the aqueous humor samples among the three groups via ANOVA.

Cytokine	Inflammatory Groups		AR Group	F	P
	VKH	BD			
IL-2	<1.16	<1.16	<1.16		
IL-4	<0.05	<0.05	<0.05		
IL-6	22.96±6.68*	28.34±17.8*	9.31±6.10	7.373	0.003
IL-10	<0.16	<0.16	<0.16		
IL-17A	<0.46	<0.46	<0.46		
IFN-γ	2.21±0.73	10.57±4.90*	1.83±1.29	53.940	0.000

Footnotes: *P <0.05 versus the AR samples.

Cytokine Levels in the Aqueous Humor

The mean cytokine levels among the three groups were compared using the Kruskal-Wallis test, and the results are shown in Table 2. IL-6 and IFN-γ were detected in all aqueous humor samples from the patients with uveitis and the AR group, but the other cytokines were below the detection levels. The IL-6 cytokine levels were significantly higher in the aqueous humors of the VKH and BD patients compared with the AR cataract patients ($P = 0.034$ and $P = 0.003$, respectively), and the difference between the two disease groups was not significant ($P = 0.921$). Moreover, the IFN-γ levels in the aqueous humor samples of the BD patients were significantly higher than those of both the VKH and AR groups ($P = 0.001$ and $P = 0.014$, respectively).

Correlations Between Cytokines Levels and Anterior Chamber Inflammation

The IL-6 levels in the AqH samples of the VKH and BD patients were positively correlated with the preoperative flare

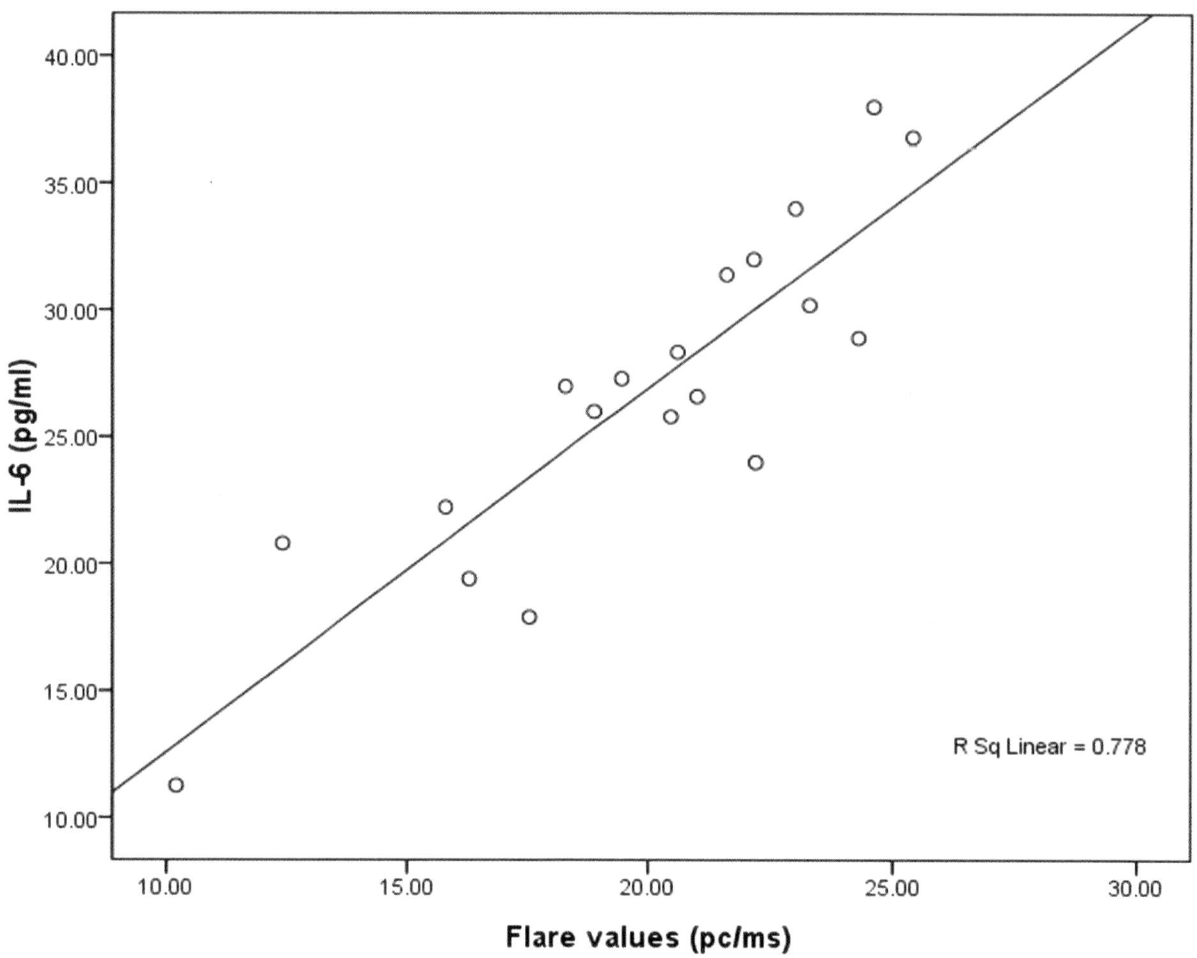

Figure 2. Correlation between the IL-6 levels in the AqH and the preoperative flare values in the VKH and BD patients.

Table 3. The expression levels of cytokines in the peripheral blood and AqH samples of patients with VKH or BD, as reported in previous studies.

Study (Year)	Patients (n)	Origin	Studied cytokines	Stage of disease	Samples	Main results
Sunao Sugita [19] (2012)	BD (10)	Japan	IL-2, IL-4, IL-6, IL-10, TNF-a, IFN-γ	active (6), inactive (4)	AqH	IFN-γ*, IL-2*, TNF-a*, IL-6*, IL-17*
					supernatants of T-cell cultures	IFN-γ*, TNF-a*, IL- 6*, IL-17*
Ahmed M. Abu El-Asrar [20] (2011)	BD (16), VKH (16)	Saudi Arabia	IL-15, IL-17, IFN-γ, TNF-α and IL-10	≥3 cells in the AC	AqH of BD patients	IFN-γ*, IL-15*, IL-17*, TNF-α*, IL-10*
					AqH of VKH patients	IFN-γ*, IL-10*, IL-17*, TNF-α*, IL-15*
A. G. Commodaro [21] (2010)	VKH (21)	Brazil	IFN-γ, IL-10, TGF-β	active (13), inactive (8)	supernatants of PBMC cultures with PHA stimulation	IFN-γ*, IL-10†, TGF-β†
B Li [10] (2005)	VKH (16)	China	IFN-γ, IL-2, IL-4	active (16), inactive (16)	supernatants of PBMC cultures with PHA stimulation and	IFN-γ*, IFN-γ†
					spontaneous secretion of PBMCs	
N AKdeniz [22] (2004)	BD (27)	Turkey	IL-2, IL-6, TNF-a	Active stage	Serum	IL-2*, IL-6*, TNF-a*
Midori Misumi [23] (2003)	BD (18)	Japan	TN F-a, IFN-γ, IL-12, IL-4	active (6), inactive (4)	supernatants of PBMC cultures with PHA stimulation	IFN-γ*, IL-4*, IFN-γ†
					spontaneous secretion of PBMCs	TNF-a*, IL-12*, IFN-γ*,IFN-γ†
Cem Evereklioglu [24] (2002)	BD (37)	Turkey	TNF-a, IL-1β, sIL-2R, IL-6, IL-8	active (17), inactive (20)	Serum	TNF-a*, sIL-2R*, IL-6*, IL-8*, IL-6†

Footnotes: *Cytokines elevated in the active stage of the disease; †cytokines elevated in the inactive stage of the disease.

values ($r = 0.778$ and $P = 0.000$, respectively, Figure 2). However, we found no correlation between the IL-6 level in the PBMCs and the flare values in the uveitis patients ($P = 0.297$ and $P = 0.599$, respectively). Furthermore, there were no correlations between IL-6 levels and cell counts ($P = 0.250$ and $P = 0.385$, respectively). Although the IFN-γ levels in the AqH samples from the BD patients were significantly higher than the levels observed in the samples from both the VKH and AR groups, we found no correlations between the IFN-γ levels in the AqH and the anterior chamber Flare values ($r = 0.481$, $P = 0.190$) and cell counts ($r = 0.065$, $P = 0.790$) of the BD patients.

Discussion

Until now, little was known about the function of cytokines in the development of inflammatory cataracts. Cytokines are crucial in the regulation of normal human immune responses and related diseases. Based on a systematic review of previous studies, we have summarized the expressions of cytokines in patients with VKH and BD in Table 3. We inferred that the expressions of IL-2, IL-4, IL-6, IL-10, IL-17A, and IFN-γ were the most likely to differ between inflammatory cataracts that are secondary to BD and VKH and AR cataracts. Therefore, we concomitantly used a cocktail of antibody-coated non-magnetic beads to determine the expression profiles of these cytokines in BD, VKH and AR cataract patients. The expression levels of IL-2, IL-4, IL-6, IL-10, IL-17A, and IFN-γ were analyzed in the AqH, and PHA-stimulation and non-PHA-stimulated cultures of PBMCs from these three types of cataract patients. In addition, we used LFCM to quantitatively measure the anterior chamber aqueous flares and inflammatory cell levels of these patients to identify any possible differences among the groups of patients and any relationships between the cytokine levels and the clinical inflammation indexes.

In our study, IL-6 was significantly increased in the AqH and the secretions of the PBMCs of both the BD and VKH patients compared with the AR cataract patients, whereas no statistically significant difference was observed between the BD and VKH patients. Previous studies have reported increased levels of IL-6 in the AqH, supernatants of PBMC cultures, the sera of active BD patients, and the AqH and vitreous humor of active VKH patients. [19,22,24,25] Similar to the result of our study, Cem Evereklioglu et al. [24] reported that even inactive patients with BD exhibit significantly higher IL-6 levels compared with AR subjects. IL-6 is a critical mediator of the induction of inflammation and is an essential factor in the differentiation of Th17s. However, there were no signs of acute inflammation in the BD or VKH cataract patients; the inflammatory cells counts of these patients were similar to those of the AR group ($F = 1.837$, $P = 0.179$). Therefore, the presence of IL-6 in the AqH samples of these patients could not have merely been the consequence of an acute inflammatory process. Interestingly, we found that the preoperative aqueous flare values were positively correlated with the IL-6 levels in the AqH of the VKH and BD patients but not with the levels in the secretions of the PBMCs; these findings indicate that the elevated IL-6 level in the AqH, rather than some systemic effect, was correlated with a long-term impairment of the blood-aqueous barrier function.

The role of IFN-γ, which is the main signature cytokine of the Th1 lineage, was intensively studied in EAU models in the 1990s. [26] Moreover, the Th1 subset has been thought of as a major pathogenic effector T cell subset since those studies. Most of the previous studies reported increased levels of IFN-γ in the ocular fluids, supernatants of PBMC cultures and sera of active VKH and BD patients. [10,19–21,23] In the present study, the aqueous IFN-γ level was significantly higher in the patients with BD than in the patients with VKH. This result is consistent with those of Abu El-Asrar et al., [20] who reported that the levels of IFN-γ in the aqueous humor are significantly higher in patients with BD than in patients with VKH and patients with HLA-B27-associated uveitis. Therefore, it is tempting to speculate that the Th1-type immune responses are more potent in patients with BD than in patients with VKH. In this study, we found no significant correlation between IFN-γ levels in the AqH and the flare values in BD patients ($r = 0.481$, $P = 0.190$), and this finding is indicative of a weak correlation between the IFN-γ level and the impairment of the blood-aqueous barrier function. However, this finding may be due to the limited number of patients recruited for our study. Another interesting finding is that the IL-17A expression levels were below the detection level in the AqH and PBMC samples from the uveitis patients and AR cataract patients who were not subjected to PHA stimulation. With PHA stimulation, the IL-17A levels were significantly elevated in all of the PBMC samples, and no significant differences among the groups were found. Previous studies have reported high IL17 levels in the peripheral blood and even in the AqH of patients with active VKH or BD but not in these fluids from patients in the inactive phase. [12,19,20,27] These results indicate that IL-17 contributes to the active proinflammatory pattern that is characteristic of inflammatory diseases of patients with active VKH or BD.

The IL-10 expression patterns of VKH and BD patients vary across different studies. Abu El-Asrar [20] reported increased levels of IL-10 in the AqH of active VKH and BD patients. However, Sunao Sugita [19] failed to detect IL-10 in the AqH of active VKH or BD patients. Notably, A. G. Commodaro [21]found high expression levels of IL-10 in the supernatants of PBMC cultures that were stimulated with PHA from inactive VKH patients. The main biological functions of IL-10 seem to be the limitation and termination of inflammatory responses and the regulation of the differentiation and proliferation of several immune cells, such as T cells, B cells, natural killer cells, antigen-presenting cells, and granulocytes. Immunoregulatory responses involve the upregulation of IL-10 in an attempt to control the inflammation. Therefore, the level of IL-10 might be related to the prognosis of, rather than the activity of, the disease.

Finally, in our study, the expression level of IL-4 was below the detection threshold in both the peripheral blood and the AqH, which is consistent with previous studies [10,19]. The weak correlation between VKH/BD and Th2 might be one of the mechanisms that are responsible. However, the subjects in our study were all in the inactive period, which also may have contributed to these results. In terms of IL-2, there were no significant differences among the three groups in either the AqH or the peripheral blood; this result was most likely due to the subjects being in the inactive period because previous studies have found notably increased levels of IL-2 in active VKH/BD patients.

The results and interpretation of the current study must be understood within the context of its strengths and limitations. Strengths of the study include the combination of clinical and basic research, with ideal prospective and controlled design. Translational medicine is an important direction of current medical research, which will enhance the understanding of the pathogeneses and improve the prognosis of clinical treatment of different diseases. Weaknesses of the study must also be acknowledged: though this was a controlled study, the patients could not be randomized and the number of participants is limited. Further, BD and VKH may be at different stages of disease activity and any comparison between these two diseases may be inaccurate. Last, because of ethical reason, the samples of peripheral blood and aqueous humor could only be obtained at a time point prior to their cataract surgeries and the dynamic changes of cytokines of an individual patient could not be studied in vivo. Despite these limitations, this remains one of first studies to demonstrate distinct expression profiles of cytokines and the correlations of those expression profiles with the in vivo inflammation indexes of the inflammatory and AR cataract patients. Further studies are required to identify the functions of these discrepantly-expressed cytokines (such as IL-6) and to clarify their possible roles in the formation of inflammatory cataracts.

Author Contributions

Conceived and designed the experiments: WC HTL WRC. Performed the experiments: WC WRC. Analyzed the data: WC HTL. Contributed reagents/materials/analysis tools: XJZ ZCL YG CFX. Wrote the paper: HTL WC.

References

1. O'Shea JJ, Ma A, Lipsky P (2002) Cytokines and autoimmunity. Nat Rev Immunol 2: 37–45.
2. Zhou ZY, Chen SL, Shen N, Lu Y (2012) Cytokines and Behcet's disease. Autoimmunity reviews 11: 699–704.
3. Damico FM, Bezerra FT, Silva GC, Gasparin F, Yamamoto JH (2009) New insights into Vogt-Koyanagi-Harada disease. Arq Bras Oftalmol 72: 413–420.
4. Imai Y, Ohno S (2002) Helper T-cell subsets in uveitis. Int Ophthalmol Clin 42: 25–32.
5. Lohmann T, Laue S, Nietzschmann U, Kapellen TM, Lehmann I, et al. (2002) Reduced expression of Th1-associated chemokine receptors on peripheral blood lymphocytes at diagnosis of type 1 diabetes. Diabetes 51: 2474–2480.
6. Jager A, Kuchroo VK (2010) Effector and regulatory T-cell subsets in autoimmunity and tissue inflammation. Scand J Immunol 72: 173–184.
7. Romagnani S (1995) Biology of human TH1 and TH2 cells. J Clin Immunol 15: 121–129.
8. Raziuddin S, Al-Dalaan A, Bahabri S, Siraj AK, Al-Sedairy S (1998) Divergent cytokine production profile in Behcet's disease. Altered Th1/Th2 cell cytokine pattern. J Rheumatol 25: 329–333.
9. Hamzaoui K, Hamzaoui A, Guemira F, Bessioud M, Hamza M, et al. (2002) Cytokine profile in Behçet's disease patients. Scandinavian journal of rheumatology 31: 205–210.
10. Li B, Yang P, Zhou H, Huang X, Jin H, et al. (2005) Upregulation of T-bet expression in peripheral blood mononuclear cells during Vogt-Koyanagi-Harada disease. Br J Ophthalmol 89: 1410–1412.
11. Liu X, Yang P, Lin X, Ren X, Zhou H, et al. (2009) Inhibitory effect of Cyclosporin A and corticosteroids on the production of IFN-gamma and IL-17 by T cells in Vogt-Koyanagi-Harada syndrome. Clin Immunol 131: 333–342.
12. Hamzaoui K, Bouali E, Ghorbel I, Khanfir M, Houman H, et al. (2011) Expression of Th-17 and RORγt mRNA in behçet's disease. Medical science monitor: international medical journal of experimental and clinical research 17: R227.
13. Wang C, Tian Y, Lei B, Xiao X, Ye Z, et al. (2012) Decreased IL-27 expression in association with an increased Th17 response in Vogt-Koyanagi-Harada disease. Invest Ophthalmol Vis Sci 53: 4668–4675.
14. Chi W, Zhu X, Yang P, Liu X, Lin X, et al. (2008) Upregulated IL-23 and IL-17 in Behcet patients with active uveitis. Invest Ophthalmol Vis Sci 49: 3058–3064.
15. Oshika T, Nishi M, Mochizuki M, Nakamura M, Kawashima H, et al. (1989) [Quantitative assessment of aqueous flare intensity and cell count in uveitis]. Nihon Ganka Gakkai Zasshi 93: 1032–1037.
16. Weichsler B, Davatchi F, Mizushima Y, Hamza M, Dilsen N, et al. (1990) Criteria for diagnosis of Behçet's disease. Lancet 335: 1078–1080.
17. Read RW, Holland GN, Rao NA, Tabbara KF, Ohno S, et al. (2001) Revised diagnostic criteria for Vogt-Koyanagi-Harada disease: report of an international committee on nomenclature. Am J Ophthalmol 131: 647–652.
18. Fang W, Zhou H, Yang P, Huang X, Wang L, et al. (2008) Longitudinal quantification of aqueous flare and cells in Vogt-Koyanagi-Harada disease. Br J Ophthalmol 92: 182–185.

19. Sugita S, Kawazoe Y, Imai A, Yamada Y, Horie S, et al. (2012) Inhibition of Th17 differentiation by anti-TNF-alpha therapy in uveitis patients with Behcet's disease. Arthritis Res Ther 14: R99.
20. El-Asrar AM, Struyf S, Kangave D, Al-Obeidan SS, Opdenakker G, et al. (2011) Cytokine profiles in aqueous humor of patients with different clinical entities of endogenous uveitis. Clin Immunol 139: 177–184.
21. Commodaro AG, Peron J, Genre J, Arslanian C, Sanches L, et al. (2010) IL-10 and TGF-β Immunoregulatory Cytokines rather than Natural Regulatory T Cells are Associated with the Resolution Phase of Vogt-Koyanagi-Harada (VKH) Syndrome. Scandinavian journal of immunology 72: 31–37.
22. Akdeniz N, Esrefoglu M, Keles MS, Karakuzu A, Atasoy M (2004) Serum interleukin-2, interleukin-6, tumour necrosis factor-alpha and nitric oxide levels in patients with Behcet's disease. ANNALS-ACADEMY OF MEDICINE SINGAPORE 33: 596–599.
23. Misumi M, Hagiwara E, Takeno M, Takeda Y, Inoue Y, et al. (2003) Cytokine production profile in patients with Behcet's disease treated with infliximab. Cytokine 24: 210–218.
24. Evereklioglu C, Er H, Turkoz Y, Cekmen M (2002) Serum levels of TNF-alpha, sIL-2R, IL-6, and IL-8 are increased and associated with elevated lipid peroxidation in patients with Behcet's disease. Mediators Inflamm 11: 87–93.
25. de Boer JH, Van Haren M, de Vries-Knoppert W, Baarsma GS, De Jong P, et al. (1992) Analysis of IL-6 levels in human vitreous fluid obtained from uveitis patients, patients with proliferative intraocular disorders and eye bank eyes. Current eye research 11: 181–186.
26. Caspi RR, Chan CC, Grubbs BG, Silver PB, Wiggert B, et al. (1994) Endogenous systemic IFN-gamma has a protective role against ocular autoimmunity in mice. J Immunol 152: 890–899.
27. Matsuoka K, Inoue N, Sato T, Okamoto S, Hisamatsu T, et al. (2004) T-bet upregulation and subsequent interleukin 12 stimulation are essential for induction of Th1 mediated immunopathology in Crohn's disease. Gut 53: 1303–1308.

Gender Difference in the Association of Metabolic Syndrome and Its Components with Age-Related Cataract: The Korea National Health and Nutrition Examination Survey 2008-2010

Young-Hoon Park[1], Jeong Ah Shin[1], Kyungdo Han[2,3], Hyeon Woo Yim[3], Won-Chul Lee[3], Yong-Moon Park[3,4]*

1 Department of Ophthalmology and Visual Science, College of Medicine, The Catholic University of Korea, Seoul, Korea, **2** Department of Biostatistics, College of Medicine, The Catholic University of Korea, Seoul, Korea, **3** Department of Preventive Medicine, College of Medicine, The Catholic University of Korea, Seoul, Korea, **4** Department of Epidemiology and Biostatistics, Arnold School of Public Health, University of South Carolina, Columbia, South Carolina, United States of America

Abstract

Purpose: To explore the relationship of the metabolic syndrome (MetS) and its components with age-related cataract in a representative Korean population.

Methods: We analyzed the data from the Korea National Health and Nutrition Examination Surveys (2008–2010). A total of 11,076 adults (4,811 men and 6,265 women) aged 40 and over who completed ophthalmologic examination were evaluated. Cataract was defined as the presence of cortical, nuclear, anterior (sub)capsular or posterior subcapsular cataract, from slit-lamp examination or previous cataract surgery. MetS was defined according to the Joint Interim Statement proposed in 2009 from the International Diabetes Federation and the American Heart Association/National Heart, Lung, and Blood Institute.

Results: The prevalence of cataract and MetS in this population was 39.4% (37.1% for men and 41.6% for women) and 38.5% (37.6% for men and 39.4% for women), respectively. Cataract prevalence tended to increase with the number of MetS components in both genders (both $P < 0.001$). After being controlled for confounders, however, MetS was significantly associated with cataract only in women (adjusted odds ratio (aOR), 1.24; 95% confidence interval (CI), 1.02–1.50]. Reduced HDL cholesterol, elevated fasting glucose, and elevated triglycerides were also significantly associated with cataract in women (aOR, 95% CI; 1.27 (1.07–1.50), 1.23 (1.01–1.50), and 1.26 (1.04–1.52), respectively). In the subgroup analysis for cataract subtype, MetS and reduced HDL cholesterol were significantly associated with nuclear cataract in women (aOR, 95% CI; 1.25 (1.07–1.55) and 1.25 (1.03–1.52), respectively). However, such associations were not found in men.

Conclusions: Our results suggest that MetS and its components appear to be associated with age-related cataract only among Korean women, especially in nuclear cataract.

Editor: Yingfeng Zheng, Zhongshan Ophthalmic Center, China

Funding: This work was financially supported by research grants from the Catholic Medical Center Research Foundation made in the program year of 2011. The funders had no role in study design, data collection and analysis, decision to publish, or preparation of the manuscript.

Competing Interests: The authors have declared that no competing interests exist.

* E-mail: markYMpark@gmail.com

Introduction

Cataract is the most common age-related eye disease and a leading cause of blindness and poor vision. The World Health Organization (WHO) reports that cataract is responsible of nearly 50% of blindness in the world (37 million blind people) [1].

In general, the risk factors of cataract are aging, smoking, ultraviolet radiation exposure, and genetic factors [2,3], whereas the epidemiological evidence is still controversial for antioxidants, alcohol consumption, and supplement use [3–6]. Some epidemiological studies have shown positive associations between the risk of cataract and various metabolic abnormalities. Diabetes and hyperglycemia have long been recognized as risk factors for cataract in several studies [7–10]. Obesity or central obesity [11–15], and serum lipid levels [15–17] have also been found to increase the risk of cataract, whereas the relationship between cataract with systolic and diastolic blood pressure is controversial [15,18,19].

Recent studies have documented that MetS is associated with ocular disorders such as glaucoma, diabetic and nondiabetic retinopathy [20–23]. Although a few previous studies have suggested that MetS is associated with cataract [24–28], the association between MetS and its components with cataract has not been properly evaluated in Asian populations because a standardized definition for MetS has not been used in these populations [28].

The present study investigated the association of MetS and its components with age-related cataract and its subtype in a representative Korean population.

Methods

Study population

The Korea National Health and Nutrition Examination Survey (KNHANES) is an ongoing cross-sectional survey for the non-institutionalized civilian population of South Korea. A complex, stratified, multistage probability sampling design based on age, sex, and region was used in this survey to represent the Korean population. Since KNHANES IV, a rolling sampling design also has been used so that the samples from each year are independent and homogeneous. KNHANES, coordinated by the Korean Ministry of Health and Welfare, included a health interview survey, a health examination survey, and a nutrition survey. Since 2008, ophthalmologic interviews and examinations have also been conducted. This survey was reviewed and approved by the Institutional Review Board of the Korea Centers for Disease Control and Prevention, and all participants provided written informed consent.

In the present analysis, we limited the study population to adults aged 40 years or older who participated in all three parts of the survey in addition to ophthalmologic interviews and examinations. Therefore, our final study population for the analysis included 11,076 participants (4,811 men and 6,265 women).

Assessment of cataract

Ophthalmologic examinations were conducted by ophthalmologists from the Korean Ophthalmologic Society in cooperation with the Korea Centers for Disease Control and Prevention (KCDC). Participants underwent a comprehensive eye slit-lamp examination (Haag-Streit BQ-900; Haag-Streit AG, Koeniz, Switzerland) by ophthalmologists. Cataracts were graded according to the Lens Opacities Classification System III (LOCS) standard photographs, regarding nuclear, cortical, anterior (sub) capsular, posterior subcapsular, and mixed type cataract [29,30]. Pseudophakic and aphakic eyes were included as operated cataracts for the purpose of the statistical analysis. Pseudophakic and aphakic eyes were included as operated cataracts for the purpose of the statistical analysis. However, these phenotypes were not assigned to any subgroup of cataract. In addition, any exclusion criteria for the pseudophakic patients were not applied.

Measurements

The health interview survey was performed by trained interviewers. All participants were asked about their demographic and socioeconomic characteristics including residential area, education, income, and occupation. The ophthalmologic surveys were also conducted. The subjects were categorized in the group with outdoor activity if they participated in regular outdoor activity for the past ten years. Respondents who were exposed to sunlight more than five hours per day were categorized as the sun exposure group. Family history of eye disease was designated if the subject's family members in a direct line had any cataract, glaucoma, strabismus, blepharoptosis, retinopathy, or other eye diseases. Respondents were categorized into two groups: ever-smokers (current smokers and ex-smokers) and non-smokers. Alcohol consumption was determined by questioning the participants about their drinking behavior during the month before the health interview. Alcohol consumption status was classified into two groups as non- to moderate drinkers (< 30.0 g alcohol/day) and heavy drinkers (≥ 30.0 g alcohol/day) [31], after converting the average frequency and amount of alcoholic beverages into the amount of pure alcohol (in grams) consumed per day. The subjects who engaged in moderate or vigorous exercise on a regular basis were designated as those who exercised regularly.

Anthropometric measurements of the participants were performed by specially trained examiners. Waist circumference was measured to the nearest 0.1 cm in a horizontal plane at the level of the midpoint between the iliac crest and the costal margin at the end of a normal expiration. The body mass index (BMI) was calculated as the individual's weight in kilograms divided by the square of the individual's height in meters. Blood pressure was measured three times on the right arm while the individual was in a seated position after at least 5 minutes of rest using a mercury sphygmomanometer (Baumanometer; Baum, Copiague, NY). The final blood pressure value was obtained by averaging the values of the second and third blood pressure measurements.

Blood samples were obtained after a minimum fasting time of 8 hours. The serum levels of glucose, total cholesterol (TC), high-density lipoprotein (HDL) cholesterol, triglycerides, creatinine, asparate aminotransferase (AST), and alanine aminotransferase (ALT) were measured enzymatically using a Hitachi automatic analyser 7600 (Tokyo, Japan). Hemoglobin (Hb) was measured by the SLS hemoglobin (NoCyanide) method using a XE-2100D (Sysmex/Japan). Insulin resistance was calculated using the homeostasis model assessment (HOMA) estimate of insulin resistance (HOMA-IR = fasting insulin [uU/ml] X fasting glucose [mmol/l]/22.5) [32].

Definition of Metabolic Syndrome

MetS was defined using the criteria proposed by the American Heart Association (AHA) and the National Heart, Lung, and Blood Institute (NHLBI) together with the International Diabetes Federation (IDF) in 2009 [33]. MetS was defined as (1) a waist circumference ≥ 90 cm in men and ≥ 80 cm in women, according to the IDF criteria for Asian countries; (2) a fasting glucose ≥ 100 mg/dl or being on medication use for elevated glucose; (3) fasting triglycerides ≥ 150 mg/dl or cholesterol-lowering medication use; (4) HDL- cholesterol < 40 mg/dL in men and < 50 mg/dL in women or cholesterol-lowering medication use; and (5) systolic blood pressure ≥ 130mmHg and/or diastolic blood pressure ≥ 85 mm Hg or being on an antihypertensive drug treatment for patients with a history of hypertension. MetS diagnosis requires at least three of the five components to be present.

Statistical analysis

All data are presented as means ± SE for continuous variables or proportions (SE) for categorical variables. Statistical analyses were conducted using the SAS (version 9.2; SAS Institute, Inc., Cary, NC, USA) survey procedure to take into account the complex sampling design with sampling weights of KNHANES and to provide nationally representative prevalence estimates. In order to minimize the effect of variations among the survey years, all the analyses performed in this study were adjusted for survey year. In addition, we conducted stratified analyses to assess the effect modification by gender in the association of MetS and its components with age-related cataract and cataract subtype. Multiple logistic regression analyses were performed to estimate the magnitude of the association of cataract with MetS and its components, and two statistical models based on the characteristics of the variables were used. One model included age and survey year. Subsequently, socioeconomic and lifestyle-related characteristics including income, education, residential area, smoking status, drinking alcohol, exercise, occupation (farmer or fisher), family history of eye disease, and sun exposure were included based on the results from the univariate analysis. The effect modification by gender was also tested by entering the interaction term (gender*MetS) in the full model. A $P < 0.05$ was considered statistically significant.

Results

1. The prevalence and related characteristics of metabolic syndrome

The prevalence of MetS in this population was 38.5% (95% confidence interval (CI), 37.4–39.7%; 37.6% for men and 39.4% for women). The prevalence of individual components of MetS was 40.4% for abdominal obesity, 37.7% for elevated triglycerides, 49.6% for low HDL cholesterol, 45.8% for high BP, and 36.2% for elevated glucose. Table 1 shows the characteristics of the participants by MetS status. Subjects with MetS were more likely to be older in both genders. Urban residence, higher education, and family history of eye disease were lower, whereas low income, occupation of farmer or fisher, sun exposure, and regular exercise were higher in women with MetS. Occupation of farmer or fisher and regular exercise were lower, whereas heavy drinker was higher in men with MetS.

2. The prevalence and related characteristics of cataract

The prevalence of cataract in participants aged 40 years or older was 39.4% (95% CI, 37.2–41.6%; 37.1% for men and 41.6% for women) and that in participants aged 60 years or older over was 79.8% (95% CI, 77.5 – 82.1%; 77.2% for men and 81.8% for women). The prevalence was 22.8% (95% CI, 20.3 – 25.3%) for nuclear type, 9.1% (95% CI, 7.8 – 10.4%) for cortical type, 4.2% (95% CI, 2.9 – 8.7%) for mixed type, 0.7% (95% CI, 0.3 – 1.3%) for anterior(sub)capsular type, and 0.3% (95% CI, 0.0 – 0.7%) for posterior subcapsular type in participants aged 40 years or older (figure 1). Table 2 shows characteristics of the participants by age-related cataract. These results indicate that prevalence of cataract tended to increase with age in both genders ($P< 0.001$). The prevalence of cataract was higher in women than men ($P<0.001$). Urban residence, higher education, family history of eye disease, and heavy drinker were lower, whereas low income, occupation of farmer or fisher, and sun exposure were higher in both genders with cataract. Ever-smoker was higher in men, and regular exercise was lower in women.

3. The associations of metabolic syndrome with age-related cataract

Figure 2 shows that the prevalence of cataract rose with an increase in the number of metabolic syndrome components in both genders (both $P <0.0001$), although the increasing trend was larger in women. Figure 3 shows the gender difference in the relationship between prevalence of cataract and metabolic syndrome components. The prevalence of cataract was higher in all MetS components for women (all $P <0.0001$), but it was higher only in low HDL ($P= 0.031$), high glucose ($P <0.0001$), and high BP ($P <0.0001$) for men.

Table 3 shows the results of multiple logistic regression analyses. There were significant effect modifications of gender on age ($P = 0.023$) in the full model, which supported the rationale for stratified analyses by gender. After being controlled for confounders, MetS was significantly associated with cataract in women

Table 1. Characteristics of the participants according to the presence or absence of metabolic syndrome by gender.

	Overall proportion	Total		P	Men		P	Women		P
		absence	presence		absence	presence		absence	presence	
Sex (%)				0.134						
male	48.5(0.4)	49.8(0.7)	47.9(0.9)							
female	51.5(0.4)	50.2(0.7)	52.1(0.9)							
Age (years)				<.001			<.001			<.001
40–49	38.4(0.8)	56.8(1.1)	10.0(0.9)		45.0(1.3)	34.5(1.5)		49.9(1.2)	17.8(1.1)	
50–59	29.2(0.7)	32.4(0.9)	24.4(1.0)		30.0(1.1)	33.0(1.4)		28.5(0.9)	29.0(1.2)	
60–69	17.5(0.5)	8.9(0.5)	30.6(0.8)		14.8(0.7)	20.8(1.0)		12.5(0.7)	27.0(1.0)	
≥70	14.9(0.5)	1.8(0.2)	35.0(1.2)		10.2(0.6)	11.7(0.8)		9.0(0.6)	26.2(1.2)	
Residence (urban)	74.9(2.1)	76.2(2.0)	73.7(2.2)	0.013	74.6(2.3)	76.1(2.3)	0.348	77.8(2.0)	71.5(2.4)	<.001
Education (>6yrs)	67.0(0.8)	74.6(0.9)	58.4(1.2)	<.001	78.9(1.0)	79.5(1.2)	0.699	70.2(1.1)	39.1(1.4)	<.001
Income (lowest quartile)	21.6(0.7)	17.2(0.8)	26.4(1.0)	<.001	16.8(0.9)	18.1(1.0)	0.289	17.7(0.9)	34.0(1.3)	<.001
Occupation (farmer/fisher)	10.2(1.1)	10.3(1.2)	10.1(1.1)	0.833	13.3(1.6)	10.2(1.3)	0.010	7.3(0.9)	10.0(1.2)	0.003
Outdoor activities (yes)	98.3(0.4)	98.4(0.4)	98.3(0.5)	0.794	98.8(0.3)	98.1(0.6)	0.084	97.9(0.6)	98.5(0.6)	0.295
Sun exposure (yes)	25.7(1.0)	25.1(1.1)	26.6(1.3)	0.179	33.6(1.4)	32.8(1.5)	0.660	16.7(1.1)	20.8(1.6)	<.001
Family history of eye disease (yes)	18.1(0.5)	20.6(0.7)	15.6(0.7)	<.001	18.2(0.9)	17.1(1.2)	0.471	22.9(0.9)	14.2(0.9)	<.001
Ever-smoker (yes)	44.1(0.5)	44.1(0.8)	44.6(1.0)	<.001	81.1(0.9)	83.7(1.1)	0.074	7.3(0.6)	8.7(0.7)	0.136
Heavy drinker (yes)	18.0(0.6)	16.2(0.7)	20.7(1.0)	<.001	24.1(1.1)	30.8(1.5)	<.001	6.1(0.7)	5.4(0.8)	0.505
Regular exercise (yes)	25.5(0.7)	27.4(0.8)	24.0(0.8)	<.001	29.1(1.1)	25.4(1.3)	0.017	74.3(1.0)	77.3(1.2)	0.025

Data are presented as the means±SE or % (SE).

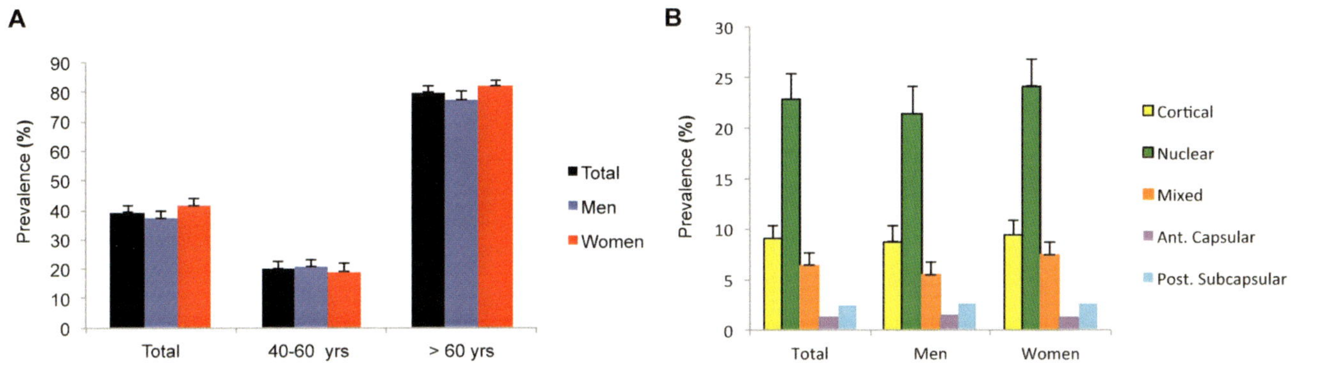

Figure 1. Prevalence of age-related cataract according to gender: by age group (A) and by the subtype of cataract (B). The error bars represent the upper 95% confidence intervals.

(adjusted odds ratio (aOR), 1.24; 95% confidence interval (CI), 1.03–1.49). Cataract prevalence increased with the number of MetS components in women (P = 0.007). Especially, the odds of cataract in subjects with 4 to 5 MetS components were significantly higher compared with subjects with none to one MetS component (aOR, 1.47; 95% CI, 1.12–1.93). Reduced HDL cholesterol, elevated fasting glucose, and elevated triglycerides were also significantly associated with cataract in women (aOR, 95% CI; 1.26 (1.07–1.49), 1.23 (1.02–1.49), and 1.26 (1.04–1.52), respectively). In the subgroup analysis for cataract subtype, MetS and reduced HDL cholesterol were significantly associated with nuclear subtype in women (aOR, 1.24; 95% CI, 1.01–1.54 and 1.24 (1.02–1.50), respectively). Also, the prevalence of the nuclear subtype of cataract increased with the number of MetS components in women (*P* = 0.037).

However, no significant association between MetS and cataract was found in men. In addition, there was no association between MetS and other subtypes of cataract including anterior (sub)capsular, posterior subcapsular, and mixed type cataract.

Discussion

To the best of our knowledge, this is the first large population based study to examine the association of age-related cataract with MetS and its components among a representative Korean population stratified by gender. In this cross-sectional study, conducted as part of KNHANES 2008–2010, MetS and its

Table 2. Characteristics of the participants according to the presence or absence of age-related cataract by gender.

	Overall proportion	Total		*P*	Men		*P*	Women		*P*
		absence	presence		absence	presence		absence	presence	
Sex (%)				<.001						
male	48.5(0.4)	50.4(0.7)	45.7(0.7)							
female	51.5(0.4)	49.6(0.7)	54.3(0.7)							
Age (yrs)				<.001			<.001			<.001
40–49	38.4(0.8)	56.8(1.1)	10.0(0.9)		57.9(1.3)	11.6(1.1)		55.8(1.3)	8.7(1.0)	
50–59	29.2(0.7)	32.4(0.9)	24.4(1.0)		31.7(1.1)	28.4(1.5)		33.1(1.1)	20.9(1.0)	
60–69	17.5(0.5)	8.9(0.5)	30.6(0.8)		8.7(0.6)	31.6(1.3)		9.2(0.6)	29.8(1,0)	
≥70	14.9(0.5)	1.8(0.2)	35.0(1.2)		1.8(0.3)	28.4(1.3)		1.9(0.3)	40.6(1.4)	
Residence (urban)	74.9(2.1)	79.2(2.0)	68.3(2.8)	<.001	78.4(2.1)	69.7(2.9)	<.001	80.1(2,0)	67.1(2.8)	<.001
Education (> 6 yrs)	67.0(0.8)	81.5(0.8)	44.5(1.2)	<.001	87.0(0.9)	63.1(1.5)	<.001	75.8(1.0)	28.8(1.4)	<.001
Income (Lowest quartile)	21.6(0.7)	12.5(0.7)	35.8(1.2)	<.001	10.9(0.7)	30.0(1.3)	<.001	14.1(0.8)	40.8(1.4)	<.001
Occupation (farmer/fisher)	10.0(1.1)	6.9(0.8)	14.8(1.8)	<.001	8.5(1.0)	17.2(2.2)	<.001	5.2(0.7)	12.7(1.6)	<.001
Outdoor activities (yes)	98.3(0.4)	98.6(0.4)	97.9(0.7)	0.207	99.0(0.4)	98.0(0.7)	0.194	98.3(0.4)	97.9(0.7)	0.405
Sun exposure (yes)	25.7(1.0)	21.7(0.9)	32.0(1.7)	<.001	29.9(1.2)	39.0(1.8)	<.001	13.3(0.9)	26.1(1.9)	<.001
Family history of eye disease (yes)	18.1(0.5)	21.5(0.7)	12.9(0.7)	<.001	20.5(1.0)	12.5(0.9)	<.001	22.5(0.9)	13.2(0.8)	<.001
Ever-smoker (yes)	44.1(0.5)	44.9(0.7)	42.8(0.8)	0.048	81.7(0.8)	82.7(1.0)	<.001	7.5(0.6)	9.2(0.7)	0.078
Heavy drinker (yes)	18.0(0.6)	19.6(0.7)	14.8(0.9)	<.001	28.9(1.1)	22.8(1.3)	<.001	7.4(0.7)	3.4(0.6)	<.001
Regular exercise (yes)	25.5(0.7)	27.0(0.8)	23.3(1.0)	0.002	28.1(1.1)	25.7(1.4)	0.161	25.8(0.9)	21.3(1.1)	<.001

Data are presented as the means±SE or % (SE).

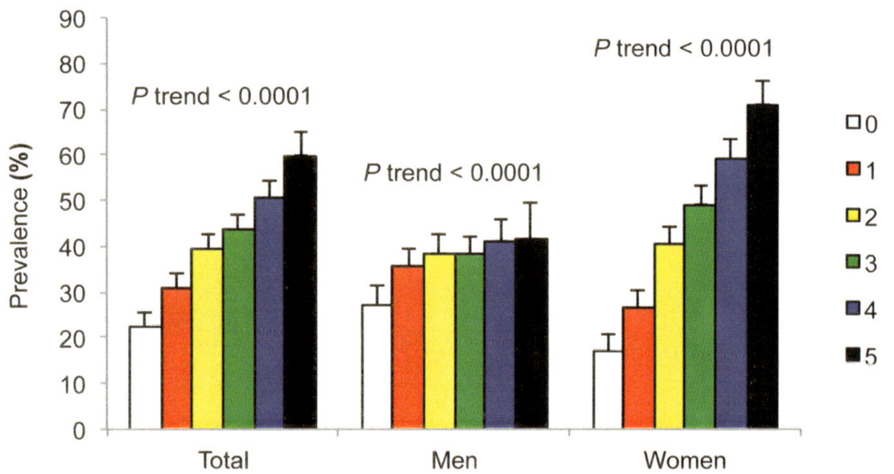

Figure 2. Prevalence of age-related cataract according to the increasing number of MetS components by gender. The error bars represent the upper 95% confidence intervals. All P for trend were < 0.0001.

components including reduced HDL cholesterol, elevated fasting glucose, and elevated triglycerides were positively associated with the risk of age-related cataract only in women. In addition, the prevalence of age-related cataract increased with the number of MetS components in women. These phenomena were also observed in the nuclear subtype of cataract.

Gender difference in the association between MetS and age-related cataract was consistent with the data from some existing studies [16,17,24,25,27]. In the present study, there was no significant relation between MetS and cataract in Korean men. The reason is not clear but a few studies have reported strong associations of some components of MetS with cataract among women [15,17,24]. This gender specific association might be explained by differences of hormonal [34] and life-style related characteristics [35] of MetS between men and women. In addition, there has been some evidence that gender difference in MetS contributes to the gender-related differential risk of cardiovascular disease [36].

MetS components could be potential risk factors of cataract, especially as all of them are associated with age. The data about the relationship between cataract and all five MetS components are controversial in many studies [10,13,16,18,20,37]. Galeone et al. [27] and Sabanayagam C et al. [28] reported that cataract prevalence increased with increasing number of metabolic syndrome components in both men and women. However, Lindblad BE et al. [25] suggested that MetS and its components, abdominal adiposity, diabetes, and hypertension, seem to be associated with an increased risk for cataract extraction, especially among women aged less than 65 years.

Our study found a tendency for an increase in the percent rate of cataract among women with reduced HDL cholesterol. Similar data were found in the Beaver Dam Eye Study: higher serum HDL cholesterol was associated with a decreased risk of cataract [17]. A strong association was found between low levels of HDL cholesterol and the development of lens opacities of adults of both genders from South Africa [38]. Animal studies have shown

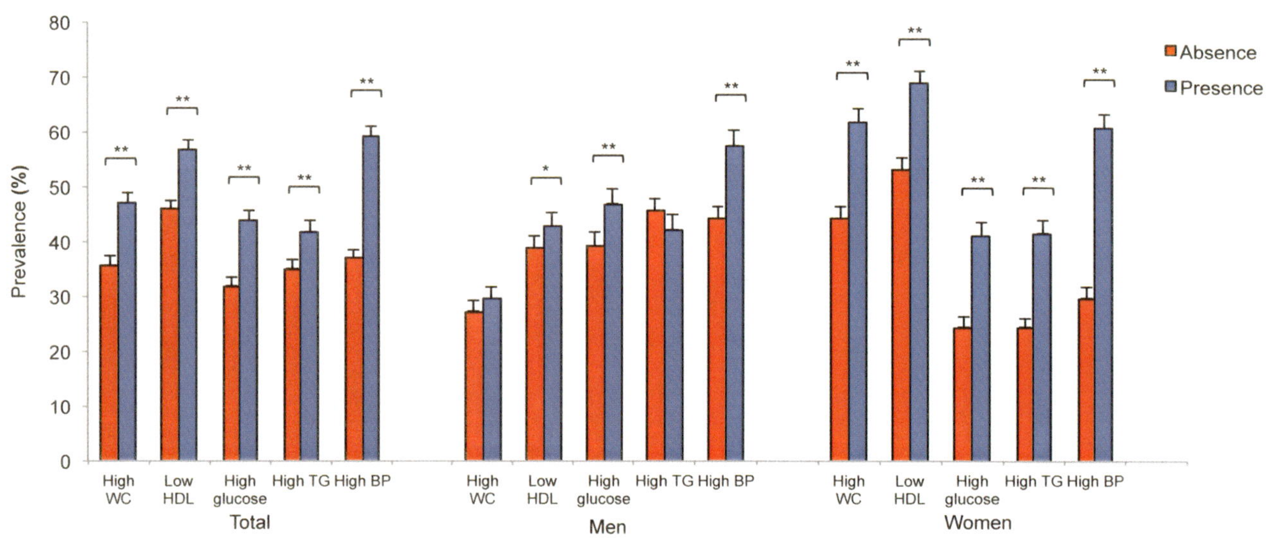

Figure 3. Prevalence of age-related cataract according to the absence or presence of MetS components by gender. The error bars represent the upper 95% confidence intervals (*$P<0.05$, **$P<0.0001$).

Table 3. Association of metabolic syndrome and its components with age-related cataract by gender.

Variables	Total cataract				Cortical subtype				Nuclear subtype			
	Model1		Model2		Model1		Model2		Model1		Model2	
	OR(95% CI)	*P*	OR(95% CI)	*P*	OR(95% CI)	*P*	OR(95% CI)	*P*	OR(95% CI)	*P*	OR(95% CI)	*P*
Male												
MetS (presence vs. absence)	1.00(0.83,1.20)	0.973	0.95(0.79,1.14)	0.548	0.93(0.67,1.29)	0.646	0.90(0.63,1.26)	0.543	1.13(0.89,1.43)	0.331	1.07(0.85,1.34)	0.572
Number of MetS components												
0–1	1		1		1		1		1		1	
2	1.15(0.90,1.46)		1.11(0.87,1.43)		1.19(0.84,1.70)		1.16(0.82,1.63)		1.08(0.78,1.48)		1.04(0.74,1.44)	
3	1.11(0.87,1.40)		1.05(0.82,1.34)		0.89(0.58,1.36)		0.86(0.55,1.34)		1.25(0.92,1.70)		1.17(0.86,1.60)	
4–5	1.00(0.77,1.30)		0.92(0.71,1.20)		1.10(0.71,1.72)		1.06(0.67,1.67)		1.06(0.74,1.52)		0.99(0.71,1.39)	
P for trend	0.885		0.634		0.93		0.907		0.463		0.767	
MetS component												
High waist circumference	1.02(0.85,1.23)	0.830	0.95(0.80,1.15)	0.615	0.83(0.58,1.18)	0.288	0.84(0.59,1.21)	0.323	1.23(0.97,1.55)	0.082	1.14(0.91,1.42)	0.264
Low HDL	0.99(0.83,1.19)	0.944	0.01(0.84,1.22)	0.888	0.90(0.66,1.22)	0.485	0.93(0.68,1.27)	0.791	1.06(0.83,1.34)	0.659	1.09(0.85,1.39)	0.519
High glucose	1.03(0.86,1.22)	0.757	1.01(0.85,1.20)	0.949	0.94(0.69,1.28)	0.685	0.90(0.66,1.24)	0.521	1.14(0.91,1.43)	0.245	1.14(0.92,1.41)	0.248
High triglycerides	1.00(0.83,1.19)	0.963	0.95(0.80,1.14)	0.611	1.19(0.87,1.62)	0.278	1.11(0.82,1.52)	0.543	0.97(0.78,1.22)	0.817	0.95(0.76,1.18)	0.637
High blood pressure	1.04(0.86,1.26)	0.692	1.00(0.82,1.22)	0.990	1.27(0.93,1.72)	0.133	1.24(0.92,1.69)	0.180	0.92(0.71,1.18)	0.511	0.87(0.68,1.12)	0.278
Female												
MetS (presence vs. absence)	1.21(1.01,1.46)	0.036	1.24(1.03,1.49)	0.030	0.84(0.62,1.14)	0.274	0.89(0.66,1.19)	0.430	1.23(1.01,1.50)	0.048	1.24(1.01,1.54)	0.046
Number of MetS components												
0–1	1		1		1		1		1		1	
2	1.19(0.93,1.53)		1.23(0.94,1.61)		0.85(0.56,1.30)		0.91(0.59,1.40)		1.17(0.85,1.59)		1.20(0.86,1.68)	
3	1.24(0.99,1.55)		1.25(0.98,1.60)		0.62(0.43,0.91)		0.67(0.46,0.96)		1.33(1.01,1.75)		1.34(1.01,1.80)	
4–5	1.39(1.08,1.80)		1.47(1.12,1.93)		0.94(0.61,1.44)		1.03(0.67,1.58)		1.30(0.96,1.76)		1.37(0.99,1.90)	
P for trend	0.011		0.007		0.503		0.797		0.046		0.037	
MetS component												
High waist circumference	1.09(0.90,1.32)	0.388	1.11(0.91,1.36)	0.297	0.75(0.55,1.00)	0.051	0.78(0.57,1.06)	0.115	1.12(0.88,1.41)	0.364	1.15(0.90,1.48)	0.270
Low HDL	1.27(1.08,1.50)	0.005	1.26(1.07,1.49)	0.006	1.15(0.87,1.52)	0.318	1.14(0.87,1.50)	0.336	1.26(1.04,1.52)	0.018	1.24(1.02,1.50)	0.031
High glucose	1.19(0.98,1.43)	0.065	1.23(1.02,1.49)	0.030	0.98(0.72,1.34)	0.903	1.01(0.74,1.39)	0.952	1.13(0.90,1.41)	0.294	1.20(0.95,1.51)	0.132
High triglycerides	1.20(0.99,1.44)	0.052	1.26(1.04,1.52)	0.020	1.03(0.76,1.39)	0.842	1.12(0.84,1.50)	0.442	1.14(0.92,1.40)	0.236	1.18(0.95,1.46)	0.140
High blood pressure	1.03(0.86,1.24)	0.755	1.08(0.89,1.30)	0.463	0.99(0.74,1.31)	0.932	1.07(0.80,1.42)	0.614	1.00(0.81,1.24)	0.992	1.03(0.83,1.29)	0.772

Data are presented as the odds ratio (95% confidence interval).Abbreviation: MetS, Metabolic syndrome; HDL, high density lipoprotein cholesterol.
Model 1: adjusted by age and survey year; model 2: adjusted by socioeconomic and lifestyle-related characteristics including income, education, residential area, smoking status, drinking alcohol, exercise, occupation (farmer or fisher), family history of eye disease, and sun exposure.

acceleration of the development of diabetic cataracts by hyperlipidemia and low HDL in rats [39]. Inflammation and oxidative stress resulting from reduced HDL cholesterol levels could induce cataract formation [28,40–42]. These findings are in contrast to the results of Sabanayagam C et al. [28]. They reported that there were no significant associations between high-serum triglycerides or low-serum HDL and cataract in a Malay population. However, an association was observed between low HDL levels and cortical cataract in their study. In addition, some studies have reported associations of high-triglyceride of low-HDL levels with cataract among specific subpopulations as in our report [16,24,38]. Especially, Paunksnis A et al. [24] have suggested that the percent rate of cataract was significantly higher among women with higher arterial pressure, central obesity, and elevated triglyceride level than among women without those MetS components. The results of these studies correspond well with the present study.

High glucose has been considered a risk factor for cataract in several epidemiologic studies, both cohort and case-control studies [7,9,15,43]. No significant association was observed in a cohort study [24]. Diabetes may be related to cataract by glycation of the lens proteins [44,45]. Diabetes has been shown to be associated with cataract in several Asian populations [28,46]. Mechanisms proposed to explain increased cataractogenesis from elevated blood glucose and diabetes include non-enzymatic glycosylation of lens proteins, leading to oxidation, cross-linking, aggregation, and precipitation, and polyol accumulation, in which aldose reductase catalyzes the conversion of glucose to sorbitol [26,47]. Sorbitol accumulation generates increased osmotic pressure, causing swelling and eventual rupture of lens fiber cells [48]. Lens proteins are highly susceptible to the advanced glycation events because of their continuous exposure to the elevated environmental glucose levels [49].

Many studies have found a positive association of cataract with high blood pressure, especially systolic hypertension in both genders [18,24,37]. In the Blue Mountains Eye Study, hypertension was associated with a lower prevalence of nuclear cataract [50]. In the POLA Study, hypertension decreased the risk of cataract surgery [43], while in a study from Italy, hypertension was associated with an increased risk of cataract extraction in women [15]. However, conflicting findings on the relationship between blood pressure and cataract exist across other studies [7,18,19,26,37,50,51]. In the present study, there was no association between elevated blood pressure and cataract in both Korean men and women. On balance, current evidence suggests that neither hypertension nor antihypertensive medications are likely to be major cataract risk factors.

In the subgroup analysis for cataract subtype, MetS and reduced HDL cholesterol were significantly associated with nuclear cataract in women (aOR, 95% CI; 1.24 (1.01–1.54) and 1.24 (1.02–1.50), respectively). However, no significant association between MetS and cataract was found in men. These findings are different from the Singapore Malay Eye Study in that MetS showed a modest association with cortical subtypes, although this association might be biased due to not using a standard definition of MetS. [28].

The relationship between cataract subtypes and MetS components is controversial in the previous studies. Klein BE et al. [17] suggested that higher HDL cholesterol was associated with decreased risk of cortical cataract in women. Jacques PF et al. [13] reported that diabetes and measures of adiposity were unrelated to the prevalence of cortical and nuclear cataract. The Framingham Studies findings suggested that fasting hypertriglyceridemia $\geq$ 250 mg/dL was associated with the increased risk of posterior subcapsular cataract in men but no associations were noted between serum lipid/lipoprotein variables and risk of cortical or nuclear cataract [16]. We could not suggest the possible explanation for the association of MetS and its components with nuclear cataract in detail. However, Tan JSL et al. reported that the presence of MetS was associated with an increased risk of incident cortical, posterior capsular cataract and nuclear cataract, and baseline diabetes predicted nuclear cataract after considering age and other factors in The Blue Mountains Eye Study. [26] Although Tan JSL et al's and our findings are generally inconsistent with previous findings for the association of MetS with cortical or posterior subcapsular cataract, the reason for the disparity of findings may also partly be due to racial/ethnic differences in the study population and use of different grading systems for cataract and lens opacities. Further studies are warranted to confirm the relationship between MetS and nuclear cataract.

The prevalence of cataract in adults Koreans aged 40 years or older was 38.5% (37.6% for men and 39.4% for women). The prevalence of cataract was similar to those reported in other Asian populations [28,29], where no statistically significant differences in prevalence were observed in relation to gender. However, women showed a significantly higher prevalence of cataract than men in the present study.

Our study should be interpreted with consideration of the following limitations. First, this study was a cross-sectional analysis; therefore, causal relationships could not be identified, nor were the mechanisms of these associations explored. Second, cataracts were graded according to the Lens Opacities Classification System III (LOCS) standard photographs, regarding only nuclear, cortical, anterior (sub)capsular, posterior subcapsular, and mixed type cataract but the grading of cataract was not measured. Therefore, the relationships cannot be assessed between the severity of cataract and MetS components in this study.

Despite these limitations, this study used a nationally representative sample of adults in Korea, which is a crucial strength of our study. Also, cataract was diagnosed by direct slit-lamp examination. Moreover, to the best of our knowledge this is the first large population-based study in Asia to examine the association between MetS based on the strict definition and age-related cataract.

Taken together, MetS was significantly associated with age-related cataract in women. In addition, reduced HDL cholesterol, elevated fasting glucose, and elevated triglycerides were significantly associated with cataract in women. In the subgroup analysis for cataract subtype, MetS and reduced HDL cholesterol were significantly associated with nuclear cataract in women. However, such associations were not found in men. In conclusion, our results suggest that there may be gender differences in the association between MetS and age-related cataract in Korean adults.

Acknowledgments

We thank Song Ie Kim, a nursing student at the Catholic University of Korea, for her assistance in preparing the manuscript.

Author Contributions

Conceived and designed the experiments: YHP YMP. Analyzed the data: KH HWY WCL YMP. Wrote the paper: YHP JAS YMP.

References

1. Resnikoff S, Pascolini D, Etya'ale D, Kocur I, Pararajasegaram R, et al. (2004) Global data on visual impairment in the year 2002. Bull World Health Organ 82: 844–851.
2. Hodge WG, Whitcher JP, Satariano W (1995) Risk factors for age-related cataracts. Epidemiol Rev17: 336–346.
3. Klein BEK, Klein R (2007) Lifestyle exposures and eye diseases in adults. Am J Ophthalmol 144: 961–969.
4. Abraham AG, Condon NG, West Gower E (2006) The new epidemiology of cataract. Ophthalmol Clin North Am 19: 415–425.
5. Wu SY, Leske MC (2000) Antioxidants and cataract formation: a summary review. Int Ophthalmol Clin 40: 71–81.
6. West S (2007) Epidemiology of cataract: accomplishments over 25 years and future directions. Ophthalmic Epidemiol 14:173–178.
7. Klein BE, Klein R, Lee KE (1998) Diabetes, cardiovascular disease, selected cardiovascular disease risk factors, and the 5-year incidence of age-related cataract and progression of lens opacities: the Beaver Dam Eye Study. Am J Ophthalmol 126: 782–790.
8. Saxena S, Mitchell P, Rochtchina E (2004) Five-year incidence of cataract in older persons with diabetes and pre-diabetes. Ophthalmic Epidemiol 11: 271–277.
9. Rowe NG, Mitchell PG, Cumming RG, Wans JJ (2000) Diabetes, fasting blood glucose and age-related cataract: the Blue Mountains Eye Study. Ophthalmic Epidemiol 7: 103–114.
10. Hennis A, Wu S-Y, Nemesure B, Leske MC, Barbados Eye Studies Group (2004) Risk factors for incident cortical and posterior subcapsular lens opacities in the Barbados Eye Studies. Arch Ophthalmol 122: 525–530.
11. Hiller R, Podgor MJ, Sperduto RD, Nowroozi L, Wilson PW, et al. (1998) A longitudinal study of body mass index and lens opacities. The Framingham Studies. Ophthalmology 105: 1244–1250.
12. Weintraub JM, Willett WC, Rosner B, Colditz GA, Seddon JM, et al. (2002) A prospective study of the relationship between body mass index and cataract extraction among US women and men. Int J Obes Relat Metab Disord 26: 1588–1595.
13. Jacques PF, Moeller SM, Hankinson SE, Chylack LT, Rogers G, et al. (2003) Weight status, abdominal adiposity, diabetes, and early age-related lens opacities. Am J Clin Nutr 78: 400–405.
14. Klein BE, Klein R, Lee KE, Jensen SC (2001) Measures of obesity and age-related eye diseases. Ophthalmic Epidemiol 8: 251–262.
15. Tavani A, Negri E, La Vecchia C (1995) Selected diseases and risk of cataract in women. A case-control study from northern Italy. Ann Epidemiol 5: 234–238.

16. Hiller R, Sperduto RD, Reed GF, D'Agostino RB, Wilson PWF (2003) Serum lipids and age-related lens opacities: a longitudinal investigation: the Framingham Studies. Ophthalmology 110: 578–583.
17. Klein BE, Klein R, Lee KE (1997) Cardiovascular disease, selected cardiovascular disease risk factors, and age-related cataracts: the Beaver Dam Eye Study. Am J Ophthalmol 123: 338–346.
18. Younan C, Mitchell P, Cumming R, Rochtchina E, Panchapakesan J, et al. (2003) Cardiovascular disease, vascular risk factors and the incidence of cataract and cataract surgery: the Blue Mountains Eye Study. Ophthalmic Epidemiol 10: 227–240.
19. Schaumberg DA, Glynn RJ, Christen WG, Ajani UA, Stürmer T, et al. (2001) A prospective study of blood pressure and risk of cataract in men. Ann Epidemiol 11: 104–110.
20. Tan GS, Wong TY, Fong C-W, Aung T, Singapore Malay Eye Study (2009) Diabetes, metabolic abnormalities, and glaucoma. Arch Ophthalmol 127: 1354–1361.
21. Costa LA, Canani LH, Lisbôa HRK, Tres GS, Gross JL (2004) Aggregation of features of the metabolic syndrome is associated with increased prevalence of chronic complications in Type 2 diabetes. Diabet Med 21: 252–255.
22. Kawasaki R, Tielsch JM, Wang JJ, Wong TY, Mitchell P, et al. (2008) The metabolic syndrome and retinal microvascular signs in a Japanese population: the Funagata study. Br J Ophthalmol 92: 161–166.
23. Wong TY, Duncan BB, Golden SH, Klein R, Couper DJ, et al. (2004) Associations between the metabolic syndrome and retinal microvascular signs: the Atherosclerosis Risk In Communities study. Invest Ophthalmol Vis Sci 45: 2949–2954.
24. Paunksnis A, Bojarskiene F, Cimbalas A, Cerniauskiene LR, Luksiene DI, et al. (2007) Relation between cataract and metabolic syndrome and its components. Eur J Ophthalmol 17: 605–614.
25. Lindblad BE, Håkansson N, Philipson B, Wolk A (2008) Metabolic syndrome components in relation to risk of cataract extraction: a prospective cohort study of women. Ophthalmology 115: 1687–1692.
26. Tan JSL, Wang JJ, Mitchell P (2008) Influence of diabetes and cardiovascular disease on the long-term incidence of cataract: the Blue Mountains eye study. Ophthalmic Epidemiol 15: 317–327.
27. Galeone C, Petracci E, Pelucchi C, Zucchetto A, La Vecchia C, et al. (2010) Metabolic syndrome, its components and risk of age-related cataract extraction: a case-control study in Italy. Ann Epidemiol 20: 380–384.
28. Sabanayagam C, Wang J, Mitchell P (2011) Metabolic Syndrome Components and Age-Related Cataract: The Singapore Malay Eye Study. Invest Ophthalmol Vis Sci 52: 2397-2404.
29. Seah SKL, Wong TY, Foster PJ, Ng TP, Johnson GJ (2002) Prevalence of lens opacity in Chinese residents of Singapore: the tanjong pagar survey. Ophthalmology109: 2058–2064.
30. Lim LS, Tai ES, Aung T, Tay WT, Saw SM, et al. (2009) Relation of age-related cataract with obesity and obesity genes in an Asian population. Am J Epidemiol 169: 1267–1274.
31. Agarwal DP (2002) Cardioprotective effects of light-moderate consumption of alcohol: a review of putative mechanisms. Alcohol Alcohol 37: 409–415.
32. Matthews DR, Hosker JP, Rudenski AS, Naylor BA, Treacher DF, et al. (1985) Homeostasis model assessment: insulin resistance and beta-cell function from fasting plasma glucose and insulin concentrations in man. Diabetologia 28: 412–419.
33. Alberti KG, Eckel RH, Grundy SM, Zimmet PZ, Cleeman JI, et al. (2009) Harmonizing the Metabolic Syndrome: a joint interim statement of the International Diabetes Federation Task Force on Epidemiology and Prevention; National Heart, Lung, and Blood Institute; American Heart Association; World Heart Federation; International Atherosclerosis Society; and International Association for the Study of Obesity. Circulation 120: 1640–1645.
34. Banos G, Guarner V, Perez-Torres I (2011) Sex steroid hormones, cardiovascular diseases and the metabolic syndrome. Cardiovasc Hematol Agents Med Chem 9: 137-146.
35. Lee DH, Kim YM, Jekal Y, Park S, Kim KC, et al. (2013) Low levels of physical activity are associated with increased metabolic syndrome risk factors in Korean adults. Diabetes Metab J 37: 132-139.
36. Regitz-Zagrosek V, Lehmkuhl E, Weickert MO (2006) Gender differences in the metabolic syndrome and their role for cardiovascular disease. Clin Res Cardiol 95: 136-147.
37. Klein BE, Klein R, Jensen SC, Linton KL (1995) Hypertension and lens opacities from the Beaver Dam Eye Study. Am J Ophthalmol 119: 640–646.
38. Meyer D, Parkin D, Maritz FJ, Liebenberg PH (2003) Abnormal serum lipoprotein levels as a risk factor for the development of human lenticular opacities. Cardiovasc J S Afr 14: 60–64.
39. Tsutsumi K, Inoue Y, Yoshida C (1999) Acceleration of development of diabetic cataract by hyperlipidemia and low high-density lipoprotein in rats. Biol Pharm Bull 22: 37–41.
40. Klimov AN, Gurevich VS, Nikiforova AA, Shatilina LV, Kuzmin AA, et al. (1993) Antioxidative activity of high density lipoproteins in vivo. Atherosclerosis 100: 13–18.
41. Varma SD, Chand D, Sharma YR, Kuck JF Jr, Richards RD (1984) Oxidative stress on lens and cataract formation: role of light and oxygen. Curr Eye Res 3: 35–57.
42. von Eckardstein A, Hersberger M, Rohrer L (2005) Current understanding of the metabolism and biological actions of HDL. Curr Opin Clin Nutr Metab Care 8: 147–152.
43. Delcourt C, Cristol JP, Tessier F, Léger CL, Michel F, et al. (2000) Risk factors for cortical, nuclear, and posterior subcapsular cataracts: the POLA study. Pathologies Oculaires Liées à l'Age. Am J Epidemiol 151: 497–504.
44. Stevens VJ, Rouzer CA, Monnier VM, Cerami A (1978) Diabetic cataract formation: potential role of glycosylation of lens crystallins. Proc Natl Acad Sci U S A 75: 2918–2922.
45. Kinoshita JH, Fukushi S, Kador P, Merola LO (1979) Aldose reductase in diabetic complications of the eye. Metabolism 28: 462–469.
46. Wong TY, Loon SC, Saw SM (2006) The epidemiology of age related eye diseases in Asia. Br J Ophthalmol 90: 506–511.
47. Stitt AW (2001) Advanced glycation: an important pathological event in diabetic and age related ocular disease. Br J Ophthalmol 85: 746–753.
48. Lee AY, Chung SK, Chung SS (1995) Demonstration that polyol accumulation is responsible for diabetic cataract by the use of transgenic mice expressing the aldose reductase gene in the lens. Proc Natl Acad Sci U S A 92: 2780–2784.
49. Di Benedetto A, Aragona P, Romano G, Romeo G, Di Cesare E, et al. (1999) Age and metabolic control influence lens opacity in type I, insulin-dependent diabetic patients. J Diabetes Complicat 13: 159–162.
50. Goodrich ME, Cumming RG, Mitchell P, Koutts J, Burnett L (1999) Plasma fibrinogen and other cardiovascular disease risk factors and cataract. Ophthalmic Epidemiol 6: 279–290.
51. Leske MC, Wu SY, Hyman L, Li X, Hennis A, et al. (1999) Diabetic retinopathy in a black population: the Barbados Eye Study. Ophthalmology 106: 1893–1899.

Prevalence and Associations of Incomplete Posterior Vitreous Detachment in Adult Chinese: The Beijing Eye Study

Lei Shao[1], Liang Xu[2], Qi Sheng You[2], Ya Xing Wang[2], Chang Xi Chen[2], Hua Yang[2], Jin Qiong Zhou[2], Jost B. Jonas[2,3], Wen Bin Wei[1]*

1 Beijing Tongren Eye Center, Beijing Tongren Hospital, Capital Medical University, Beijing, China, **2** Beijing Institute of Ophthalmology, Beijing Tongren Hospital, Capital Medical University, Beijing, China, **3** Department of Ophthalmology, Medical Faculty Mannheim of the Ruprecht-Karls University, Heidelberg, Germany

Abstract

Purpose: To determine prevalence and associations of incomplete posterior vitreous detachment (PVD).

Methods: The population-based cross-sectional Beijing Eye Study 2011 included 3468 individuals with a mean age of 64.6±9.8 years (range: 50–93 years). A detailed ophthalmic examination was performed including spectral-domain optical coherence tomography (SD-OCT). Incomplete PVD was differentiated into type 1 (shallow PVD with circular perifoveal vitreous attachment), type 2 (PVD reaching fovea but not foveola), type 3 (shallow PVD with pinpoint vitreous attachment at the foveola), and type 4 (PVD completely detached from the macula, attached to the optic disc).

Results: An incomplete PVD was detected in 3948 eyes (prevalence: 60.5±0.6%; 95% Confidence Interval (CI): 59.3%,61.7%) of 2198 subjects (67.1±0.8%;95%CI: 65.6%,68.7%). Type 1 PVD was seen in 3090 (78.3%) eyes, type 2 PVD in 504 (12.8%) eyes, type 3 PVD in 70 (1.8%) eyes, and type 4 PVD in 284 (7.2%) eyes. Prevalence of incomplete PVD was associated with younger age ($P<0.001$;OR:0.91), male gender ($P<0.001$;OR:0.64), rural region of habitation ($P<0.001$;OR:0.49), larger corneal diameter ($P=0.04$;OR:0.91), better best corrected visual acuity ($P=0.02$;OR:0.41), and hyperopic refractive error ($P<0.001$;OR:1.15). The type of incomplete PVD was associated with higher age ($P<0.001$), urban region of habitation ($P<0.001$), myopic refractive error ($P=0.001$), thinner cornea ($P=0.005$), and better best corrected visual acuity ($P=0.056$).

Conclusions: In adult Chinese in Greater Beijing, prevalence of an incomplete PVD (detected in 67.1% subjects) was associated with younger age, male gender, rural region of habitation, larger corneal diameter, better best corrected visual acuity and hyperopic refractive error.

Editor: Andreas Wedrich, Medical University Graz, Austria

Funding: This work was supported by State Natural Sciences Fund (grant #81041018) and Natural Sciences Fund of Beijing government (grant #7092021, 7112031). The funders had no role in study design, data collection and analysis, decision to publish, or preparation of the manuscript.

Competing Interests: The authors have declared that no competing interests exist.

* E-mail: wenbing_wei@yahoo.com.cn

Introduction

The vitreous body fills the inner volume of the posterior segment of the eye and is metabolically more active than previously thought [1,2]. It is connected with the inner wall of the eye at the optic nerve head as Martegiani's ring, with the periphery of the retina and the pars plana as the vitreous basis of Salzmann, and with the posterior surface of the lens as Wiegert's ligamentum hylaoideo-capsulare. Losing its gel-like consistency with increasing age, the vitreous body can eventually detach from the retina and optic disc, an occurrence clinically described as posterior vitreous detachment (PVD). It leads to subjective symptoms such as floaters or "mouches volantes", and can be the reason for increasing vitreoretinal traction resulting in a rhegmatogenous retinal detachment. The condition of the posterior vitreous has been described to be connected also with other diseases such macular holes, macular edema in various retinal diseases such as retinal vein occlusions, and age-related macular degeneration [3–5]. Due to limitations in the three-dimensional optical resolution of ophthalmoscopy and fundus photography, a PVD, in particular an incomplete PVD as precursor of a complete PVD, could not reliably be diagnosed. With the clinical introduction of spectral-domain optic coherence tomography (SD-OCT), however, the posterior surface of the vitreous in the region of a PVD could be imaged [6–9]. In view of the clinical and pathogenic importance of a PVD, we therefore conducted the present study to assess the prevalence of a PVD and its associated factors in population-based investigation.

Methods

Ethics Statement

The Medical Ethics Committee of the Beijing Tongren Hospital approved the study protocol and all participants gave informed written consent, according to the Declaration of Helsinki.

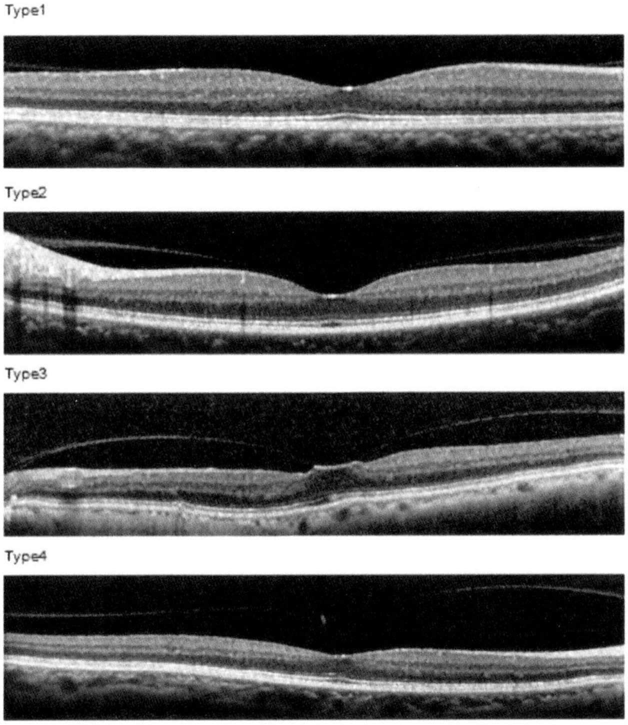

Figure 1. Classification of an incomplete posterior vitreous detachment (PVD). Type 1: shallow PVD which did not reach the foveal region of the macula; type 2: the PVD reached the fovea but did not extend to the foveola as the center of the fovea; type 3: a shallow PVD with pinpoint foveal vitreous traction on the foveola; type 4: the posterior vitreous was completely detached from the macula including the foveola, but was attached to the optic nerve head.

The Beijing Eye Study 2011 is a population-based cross-sectional study in Northern China. It was carried out in 5 communities in the urban district of Haidian in the North of Central Beijing and in 3 communities in the village area of Yufa of the Daxing District south of Beijing. The only eligibility criterion for inclusion into the study was an age of 50+ years. In 2011, the 8 communities had a total population of 4403 individuals aged 50 years or older. In total, 3468 individuals (1963 (56.6%) women) participated in the eye examination, corresponding to an overall response rate of 78.8%. The study was divided into a rural part (1633 (47.1%) subjects; 943 (57.7%) women) and an urban part (1835 (52.9%) subjects; 1020 (55.6%) women). The mean age was 64.6±9.8 years (median, 64 years; range, 50–93 years).

All examinations were carried out in the communities, either in schoolhouses or in community houses. Trained research technicians asked the study participants questions providing information on demographic variables, socioeconomic background, and known major systemic diseases. Fasting blood samples were taken for measurement of blood lipids, glucose and glycosylated hemoglobin HbA1c. Blood pressure was measured. Body height and weight and the circumference of the waist and hip were recorded. The ophthalmic examination included measurement of presenting visual acuity (VA) and uncorrected VA. Best corrected VA was assessed by automatic refractometry (Auto Refractometer AR-610, Nidek Co., Ltd, Tokyo, Japan). If uncorrected VA was lower than 1.0, we additionally performed subjective refractometry. Intraocular pressure was measured by pneumotonometry by an experienced ophthalmologist. A slit lamp examination carried out by an experienced ophthalmologist assessed lid abnormalities, Meibomian gland dysfunction, corneal disorders, and peripheral anterior chamber depth using van Herick's method. Using optical low-coherence reflectometry (Lensstar 900® Optical Biometer, Haag-Streit, 3098 Koeniz, Switzerland), biometry of the right eyes was performed for measurement of the anterior corneal curvature, central corneal thickness, anterior chamber depth, lens thickness and axial length. The pupil was dilated using tropicamide once or twice, until the pupil diameter was at least 6 mm. The anterior segment was measured by slit-lamp adapted optical coherence tomography (OCT) (Heidelberg Engineering Co., Dossenheim, Germany). Digital photographs of the cornea and lens and retro-illuminated photographs of the lens were taken using the Neitz CT-R camera (Neitz Instruments Co., Tokyo, Japan). Monoscopic photographs of the macula and optic disc were taken using a fundus camera (Type CR6-45NM, Canon Inc. U.S.A.). The optic nerve head, peripapillary area, and macula were scanned by two spectral-domain OCTs (iVue SD-OCT; Optovue Inc. Fremont, CA, U.S.A.; Spectralis, Heidelberg Engineering, Heidelberg, Germany). The study has been described in detail recently [10,11].

The macular region was imaged by spectral-domain optical coherence tomography (SD-OCT; Spectralis®, Wavelength: 870 nm; Heidelberg Engineering Co., Heidelberg, Germany). The examination included 31 sections, each of comprised 9 averaged scans and which were obtained in an area of an 8.8 mm×8.8 mm rectangle centered on the fovea. The subfoveal choroidal thickness was measured using the enhanced depth imaging modality. The horizontal and vertical sections running through the foveal center were selected for further analysis. We differentiated between four types of an incomplete PVD. Type 1 was characterized by a shallow PVD which did not reach the foveal region of the macula. In type 2, the PVD reached the fovea but did not extend to the foveola as the center of the fovea. Type 3 showed a shallow PVD with a pinpoint foveal vitreous traction on the foveola. In type 4, the posterior vitreous was completely detached from the macula including the foveola, but was attached to the optic nerve head (Fig. 1). We measured the length of the vitreous attached to the macula in the four quadrants (temporal, nasal, superior, inferior), and the height of the incomplete PVD in the four quadrants at 750 μm distant to the foveola. The measurements were performed using the Heidelberg Eye Explorer software (version 5.3.3.0; Heidelberg Engineering Co., Heidelberg, Germany).

Only those subjects with OCT images of the macula were included into the study. The statistical analysis was performed using a commercially available statistical software package (SPSS for Windows, version 20.0, SPSS, Chicago, IL, USA). In a first step, the prevalence of an incomplete PVD was calculated. In a second step, we performed a univariate logistic regression analysis with the incomplete PVD as dependent parameter and ocular and general parameters as independent parameters. In a third step, we performed a multivariate logistic regression analysis, with an incomplete PVD as dependent parameter and all those parameters as independent parameters which were significantly associated with incomplete PVD in univariate analysis. From this full model, non-significant terms were removed step by step. 95% Confidence intervals (CI) were presented. All *P*-values were 2-sided and were considered statistically significant when the values were less than 0.05.

Results

Out of the 3468 subjects included in the study, OCT images with sufficient quality for examination were available for 6530 eyes of 3276 (94.5%) participants (1844 (56.3%) women). The mean

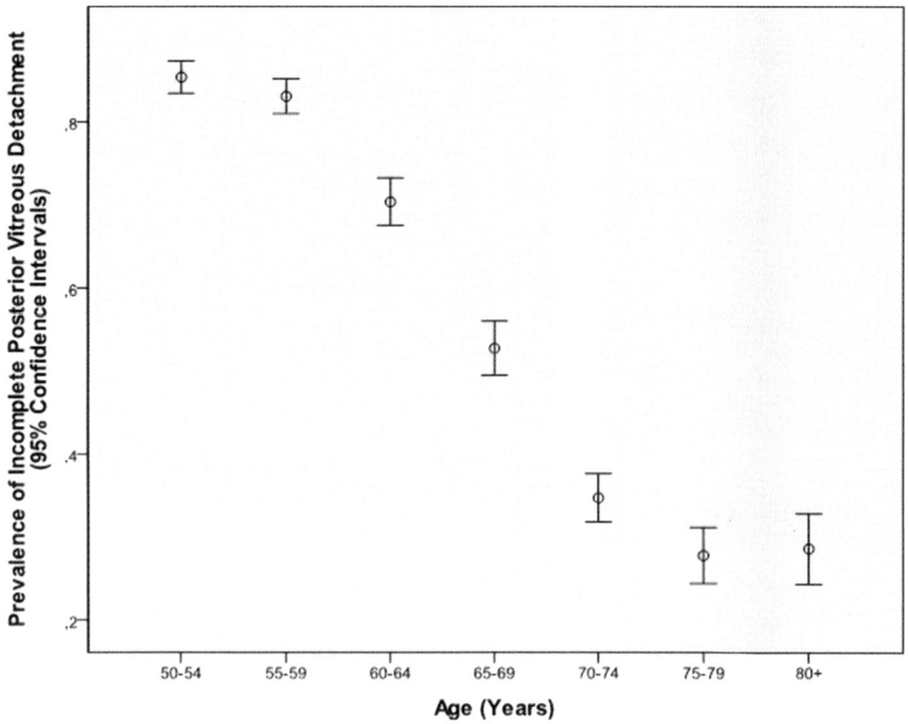

Figure 2. Diagram showing the distribution of the prevalence of incomplete posterior vitreous detachment stratified by age groups in the Beijing Eye Study 2011.

age was 64.3±9.6 years (median: 63 years; range: 50 to 93 years), the mean refractive error (spherical equivalent) was −0.18±2.04 diopters (median: 0.25 diopters; range: −22.0 to +7.50 diopters). For 192 (5.5%) eyes, OCT images could not be examined either because images were not taken or because available images could not be assessed owing to lens opacities or vitreous clouding. The group of subjects without incomplete PVD examinations as compared with the group of subjects with incomplete PVD examinations was significantly older (70.1±11.2 years versus 64.3±9.6 years; P<0.001; 95%CI: 4.15, 7.39) but did not vary significantly in gender (P = 0.12) and refractive error (P = 0.29).

An incomplete PVD was detected in 3948 (60.5%) eyes (prevalence rate (mean ± SE): 60.5±0.6%; 95% CI: 59.3%, 61.7%) of 2198 (67.1%) subjects (prevalence rate: 67.1±0.8%; 95% CI: 65.6%, 68.7%). Mean age of all subjects with incomplete PVD was 61.4±8.7 years (median, 59.0 years; range, 50–91 years), mean refractive error was −0.01±1.64 diopters (median, 0.25 diopter; range, −18.00 to +7.50 diopter). The frequency of an incomplete PVD was significantly (P<0.01; $\chi 2$ test) the highest in the nasal region (3902 (98.8%) eyes), followed by the superior region (3701 (93.7%) eyes), the temporal region (3493 (88.5%) eyes), and finally the inferior region (3083 (78.1%) eyes).

Out of the group of eyes with an incomplete PVD (n = 3948), a type 1 PVD was detected in 3090 (78.3%) eyes, type 2 PVD in 504 (12.8%) eyes, a type 3 PVD in 70 (1.8%) eyes, and a type 4 PVD in 284 (7.2%) eyes. An incomplete PVD affecting one quadrant only was seen in 159 (4.0%) eyes. In 321 (8.1%), the incomplete PVD was present in two quadrants, in 494 (12.5%) eyes in three quadrants, and 2974 (75.3%) eyes showed an incomplete PVD in all four quadrants.

The mean length of the scan with attached vitreous in the eyes with an incomplete PVD was significantly (*P* = 0.001) longer in the temporal macular region (2556±906 μm; range: 751–4819 μm) and in the inferior macular region (2510 ± 829 μm; range: 696–4462 μm) than in the nasal macular region (2277±485 μm; range: 704–4840 μm; *P*<0.001), in which it was significantly (*P*<0.001) longer than in the superior macular region (2073±713 μm; range, 486–4164 μm).

The mean height of the incomplete PVD at 750 μm distant from the foveal center was significantly (*P*<0.001) higher superiorly (239±204 μm; range: 0–1186 μm) than temporally (221±203 μm; range: 0–848 μm), where it was significantly (*P* = 0.04) higher than nasally (215±200 μm; range: 0–854 μm), where finally it was higher (*P* = 0.003) than inferiorly (206±210 μm; range: 0–1297 μm).

In univariate logistic analysis, presence of an incomplete PVD was significantly associated with the systemic parameters of younger age (*P*<0.001) (Fig. 2), male gender (*P* = 0.02), rural region of habitation (*P*<0.001), taller body height (*P*<0.001), higher body weight (*P*<0.001), higher body mass index (*P*<0.001), higher diastolic blood pressure (*P*<0.001), higher serum concentrations of low-density lipoproteins (*P* = 0.002) and creatinine (*P*<0.001), absence of self-reported diabetes mellitus (*P*<0.001) and arterial hypertension (*P*<0.001), smoking (*P*<0.001), higher alcohol consumption (*P*<0.001), and higher frequency of reported snoring (*P* = 0.006), no self-reported diagnosis of cerebral infarction or hemorrhage (*P*<0.001), and of coronary heart disease (*P*<0.001); and with the ocular parameters of shorter axial length (*P*<0.001), hyperopic refractive error (P<0.001), shorter anterior chamber depth (*P* = 0.009), thinner lens (*P*<0.001), thinner central corneal thickness (*P* = 0.045), smaller corneal diameter (*P* = 0.012), better best corrected VA (logMAR) (*P*<0.001), thicker subfoveal retinal thickness (*P* = 0.002) and choroidal thickness(*P*<0.001), higher intraocular pressure (*P*<0.001), and absence of cataract surgery(*P*<0.001) (Table 1). It was not significantly associated with

Table 1. Factors Associated with Incomplete Posterior Vitreous Detachment in the Beijing Eye Study (Univariate Analysis).

Parameter	*P*-Value	Odds Ratio	95% Confidence Interval	
Age	<0.001	0.90	0.89	0.90
Gender	0.02	0.79	0.71	0.87
Region of habitation	<0.001	0.27	0.24	0.30
Body height	<0.001	1.02	1.01	1.03
Body weight	<0.001	1.03	1.02	1.03
Body Mass Index	<0.001	1.07	1.05	1.09
Cognitive level	<0.001	1.04	1.01	1.06
Diastolic Blood pressure	<0.001	1.03	1.02	1.04
Systolic Blood pressure	0.11			
Low-Density Lipoproteins	0.002	1.17	1.06	1.29
Creatinine	<0.001	0.99	0.98	1.00
Self-reported diabetes mellitus	<0.001	0.59	0.47	0.73
Self-reported Arterial hypertension	<0.001	0.65	0.56	0.76
Smoking	<0.001	1.56	1.41	1.73
Alcohol consumption	<0.001	1.22	1.16	1.28
Snoring	0.006	1.17	1.05	1.31
Self-reported Cerebral Infarction	<0.001	0.48	0.36	0.63
Self-reported coronary heart disease	<0.001	0.52	0.43	0.63
Axial length	<0.001	0.70	0.66	0.76
Refractive error	<0.001	1.13	1.09	1.17
Anterior chamber depth	0.009	0.82	0.71	0.95
Lens Thickness	<0.001	0.42	0.33	0.53
Central corneal thickness	0.045	1.00	1.00	1.00
Corneal diameter	0.01	0.90	0.83	0.98
Best corrected visual acuity (logMAR)	<0.001	0.01	0.01	0.02
Focal retinal thickness	0.002	0.82	0.71	0.95
Subfoveal choroidal thickness	<0.001	1.01	1.01	1.01
Intraocular pressure	<0.001	1.07	1.04	1.10
Cataract surgery	<0.001	0.31	0.23	0.43

the systemic parameters of systolic blood pressure ($P = 0.11$), serum concentrations of high-density lipoproteins ($P = 0.52$), cholesterol ($P = 0.09$), triglycerides ($P = 0.07$) and glucose ($P = 0.52$); and with the ocular parameters of pupil diameter ($P = 0.95$) and corneal steepness ($P = 0.10$) (Table 1).

Model building for the multivariate analysis began with all significant factors from the univariate associations (Table 1). From this full model, non-significant terms were removed in a step-wise manner, starting with the parameters with the highest *P*-values. In the final model, presence of incomplete PVD was significantly associated with younger age ($P<0.001$; OR: 0.91), male gender ($P<0.001$; OR: 0.64), rural region of habitation ($P<0.001$; OR: 0.49), shorter corneal diameter ($P = 0.04$; OR: 0.91), better best corrected VA (logMAR) ($P = 0.02$; OR: 0.41), and hyperopic

Table 2. Factors Associated with Incomplete Posterior Vitreous Detachment Using Multivariate Logistic Regression Models in the Beijing Eye Study.

Factor	*P*-value	Odds Ratio	95% Confidence Interval	
Age	<0.001	0.91	0.90	0.92
Gender	<0.001	0.64	0.54	0.77
Region of habitation	<0.001	0.49	0.41	0.59
Corneal diameter	0.04	0.91	0.84	0.99
Best corrected visual acuity (logMAR)	0.02	0.41	0.19	0.87
Refractive Error (Diopters)	<0.001	1.15	1.10	1.20

Table 3. Factors Associated with the Stage of Incomplete Posterior Vitreous Detachment Using Multivariate Regression Models in the Beijing Eye Study.

Parameter	*P*-Value	Standardized Coefficient Beta	Regression Coefficient B	95% Confidence Interval
Age (Years)	<0.001	0.39	0.04	0.04, 0.05
Region of Habitation	<0.001	0.13	0.23	0.16, 0.30
Refractive Error (Diopters)	0.001	−0.07	−0.04	−,0.64, −0.02
Best Corrected Visual Acuity (logMAR)	0,056	0.05	0.40	−0.010, 0.81
Central Corneal Thickness (μm)	0.005	0.06	0.002	0.000, 0.003

refractive error (*P*<0.001; OR: 1.15) (Table 2). The prevalence of incomplete PVD was no longer significantly associated with systemic parameters of body height (P = 0.57) and weight (P = 0.73), diastolic blood pressure (P = 0.17), serum concentrations of low-density lipoproteins (P = 0.91) and creatinine (P = 0.76), the self-reported diagnosis of cerebral infarction or hemorrhage (P = 0.50), known diabetes mellitus (P = 0.50) and arterial hypertension (P = 0.19), alcohol consumption (P = 0.56) and snoring (P = 0.26); and with the ocular parameters of anterior chamber depth (P = 0.14), lens thickness (P = 0.21), central corneal thickness (P = 0.62), subfoveal choroidal thickness (P = 0.51), intraocular pressure (P = 0.20), and cataract surgery (P = 0.93). In an intra-individual inter-eye comparison, side difference in the prevalence of an incomplete PVD was associated with a side difference in refractive error: the eye with the incomplete PVD as compared with the contralateral eye had a significantly more hyperopic refractive error (*P*= 0.01).

The type (or stage) of incomplete PVD was significantly associated with higher age (*P*<0.001), urban region of habitation (*P*<0.001), myopic refractive error (*P*= 0.004), lower best corrected VA (*P*<0.001), longer axial length (*P*<0.001), thicker central corneal thickness (*P*= 0.001), and thicker lens (*P*<0.001). It was not significantly associated with gender (*P*= 0.09), corneal diameter (*P*= 0.77), and anterior chamber depth (*P*= 0.15). In multivariate analysis, stage of incomplete PVD remained to be significantly associated with higher age (*P*<0.001), urban region of habitation (*P*<0.001), myopic refractive error (*P*= 0.001), thinner central corneal thickness (*P*= 0.005), and marginally significantly with better best corrected VA (*P*= 0.056).

Discussion

In our population-based study on adult Chinese in Greater Beijing, the prevalence of an incomplete PVD (60.5±0.6% per eye; 67.1±0.8% per subject) was significantly associated with younger age (*P*<0.001), male gender (*P*<0.001), rural region of habitation (*P*<0.001), larger corneal diameter (*P*= 0.04), better best corrected VA (logMAR) (*P*= 0.02), and hyperopic refractive error (*P*<0.001). Reversely, the type (or stage) of incomplete PVD was significantly associated with older age (*P*<0.001), urban region of habitation (*P*<0.001), myopic refractive error (*P*= 0.001), thinner central corneal thickness (*P*= 0.005), and marginally significantly with better best corrected VA (*P*= 0.056).

These results cannot be compared with other population-based investigations, since only few population-based studies, such as the Sydney Myopia Study on school children, the Handan Study on adult Chinese in China, and the Singapore Chinese Eye Study, have applied OCT technology for imaging of the posterior ocular segment; none of these studies, however, examined the presence of a PVD [12–15]. In a hospital-based study by Hayreh and colleagues, the frequency of a complete PVD was assessed in 1,481 subjects with a mean age of 63.5±15.0 years [16]. The presence of a complete PVD was assessed by indirect and direct ophthalmoscopy, fundus biomicroscopy and by using a Hruby. A complete PVD was observed in 38% of the eyes of men aged 65+ years, and in 57% of the eyes of women aged 65+ years [16]. If one takes into account that an incomplete PVD as assessed in our study is the precursor of a complete PVD as assessed in Hayreh's study, and if one considers that in Hayreh's study due to the limitations of the applied technology not all complete PVDs may have been detected, the figures in Hayrehs study are complementary and thus compatible with the results of our study. In our study, an incomplete PVD was detected in 33% of the eyes of men aged 65+ years, and in 24% of the eyes of women aged 65+ years. Ignoring the different study types (population-based versus hospital-based) and the different study samples (Chinese versus Whites) and summarizing the prevalence figures of Hayrehs study and of our study leads to a figure of 29% (100%–38% (complete PVD) – 33% (incomplete PVD)) of the men and 19% (100%–57% (complete PVD)–24% (incomplete PVD)) of the women aged 65+ years who either had an attached posterior vitreous or in whom a complete PVD was overlooked in Hayrehs study. In a hospital-based study by Schwab and colleagues on emmetropic eyes of 271 Caucasians with a mean age of 76±8 years, an incomplete PVD was detected in 68% of the eyes by OCT or by ultrasound [17]. That figure is also comparable with the result of our study.

In the present study, the prevalence of an incomplete PVD was highest in the nasal sector (98.8%) and the superior region (93.7%), followed by the temporal region (88.5%), and finally the inferior sector (78.1%). A similar sequence of sectors was found in a previous study by Uchino and colleagues in which the superior quadrant was most frequently affected followed by temporal, inferior and nasal quadrant [18]. The reasons for the differences between the four sectors in the frequency of an incomplete PVD have remained unclear, however, regional variations in the liquefaction of the vitreous body and effects of the gravity could have played a role. The sequence of sectors with respect to the frequency of an incomplete PVD was paralleled by the sequence of sectors with respect to the longest line of attached vitreous. The line of attached vitreous was longest in the temporal region and inferior region, followed by the nasal region and the superior region. Correspondingly, the mean height of an incomplete PVD at 750 μm distant from the foveal center was highest in the superior region, followed by the temporal sector, the nasal region, and finally the inferior sector.

Interestingly, Hayreh's study revealed that the occurrence of a complete PVD was significantly correlated with older age (*P*<0.001), myopic refractive error (*P*<0.001), female gender

($P<0.001$), and surgical aphakia ($P<0.001$) [16]. These findings confirm our results, if one considers an incomplete PVD as the precursor of a complete PVD: In our study, the prevalence of an incomplete PVD was associated with younger age, male gender, and hyperopic refractive error (Table 2). In a parallel manner, the stage of an incomplete PVD in our study was associated with older age, female gender, and myopic refractive error (Table 3). An association between PVD and female gender was also reported by Chuo et al. [19], who specifically found a significant association between vitamin B6 intake and PVD amongst premenopausal women but not amongst postmenopausal women. They concluded that high estrogen levels in premenopausal women may be protective against PVD and that hormonal changes associated with menopause may lead to changes in the vitreous, predisposing to PVD. The higher levels of intake of vitamin B6 which were associated with the development of PVD in premenopausal women might have been explained through an anti-estrogen effect. An age-related decline in the prevalence of an incomplete PVD has also been reported by Schwab and colleagues [17]. Parallel to age, hyperopic refractive error (or short axial length) was related with a higher prevalence of an incomplete PVD in our study. This primarily paradox relationship may be explained if one again considers the incomplete PVD as complimentary to and as precursor of a complete PVD, so that hyperopia would be associated with a reduced prevalence of complete PVD. Correspondingly, the stage of an incomplete PVD was significantly associated with myopic refractive error (Table 3). An incomplete PVD was detected significantly more often in men than in women in our study, after adjusting for factors such as age, region of habitation, and refractive error. The reason for the gender differences has remained unclear. In contrast to previous studies [16,17], status after cataract surgery was not correlated with an incomplete PVD in our study. Reason for the differences between the studies may have been that the frequency of cataract surgery in the Beijing Eye Study 2011 was relatively low (5.2%) preventing a statistically significant relationship between cataract surgery and detected incomplete PVD.

The associations between incomplete PVD and focal retinal thickness, subfoveal choroidal thickness, anterior chamber depth and lens thickness as found in univariate analysis were no longer statistically significant in the multivariate analysis after adjusting for age, gender, region of habitation, corneal diameter, best corrected VA and refractive error. It showed that the associations between the prevalence of incomplete PVD and retinal thickness, subfoveal choroidal thickness, anterior chamber depth and lens thickness were merely explained by the confounding effects of the associations between prevalence of incomplete PVD and age, gender, region of habitation, corneal diameter, best corrected VA and refractive error. The reason for the relationship between incomplete PVD and better best corrected VA has remained unclear. One may speculate that the macula may function better if the vitreous is partially (or later on, completely) detached from the macula.

The findings in our study may have clinical importance since the status of the vitreous including its attachment to, detachment from, the posterior pole is or may be associated with other clinical entities. A PVD has been considered to play a role in the pathogenesis of rhegmatogenous retinal detachments the prevalence of which increase with age. In a parallel manner, the prevalence of an incomplete PVD decreased with older age in our study. Population-based studies such as the Beijing Eye study, the Central India Eye and Medical Study and the Singapore Indian Eye Study have shown that age-related macular degeneration is associated with hyperopia or a shorter axial length [10,20.21]. Eyes with shorter axial length, i.e. hyperopic eyes, have a less destructed vitreous body and a lower prevalence of PVD as also shown in our present study. If a compact attached vitreous is a risk factor for the development of age-related macular degeneration, one may infer that the induction of a posterior PVD and partial liquefaction of the vitreous body may potentially be helpful to prevent age-related macular degeneration. If that is the case, one may hypothetically consider the intravitreal use of microplasmin which was shown to induce a posterior PVD and vitreous liquefaction so that macular holes could be closed in some eyes just by the intravitreal microplasmin injection [22]. In a similar manner, diabetic retinopathy, in particular proliferative diabetic retinopathy, is associated with hyperopia, and thus potentially with the attachment or detachment of the posterior vitreous. Other diseases the prevalence of which are related with PVD are macular holes, cystoid macular edema as consequence of a vitreo-macular traction syndrome, and macular edema due to other reasons such as retinal vein occlusions. Future studies may assess whether the results of our current study help in understanding the pathogenesis of these disorders by showing the associations of a PVD with other ocular and general parameters.

Potential limitations of our study should be mentioned. First, the OCT technology could not distinguish between a completely attached vitreous body and a complete PVD. All figures presented in this study therefore relate only to an incomplete PVD, while the frequency of a complete PVD was deduced from the age-related decline of the prevalence of an incomplete PVD (Fig. 2). Second, the OCT method may not have imaged all incomplete PVDs. Third, as in any population-based study, non-participation is of general concern. In our study, however, the response rate was reasonable with 78.8% of the invited subjects participating in the study. Fourth, findings from our study as cross-sectional investigation do not allow to directly drawing conclusions on cause-relationships. Strengths of our study are that it is the first population-based study searching for the prevalence and associations between ocular and systemic parameters and an incomplete PVD.

In conclusion, in adult Chinese in Greater Beijing, an incomplete PVD was detected in 60.5% eyes or 67.1% subjects. While the prevalence of an incomplete PVD was associated with younger age, male gender, rural region of habitation, larger corneal diameter, better best corrected VA and hyperopic refractive error, the progressive stage of incomplete PVD was associated with higher age, urban region of habitation, and myopic refractive error.

Author Contributions

Conceived and designed the experiments: LX QSY YXW JBJ WBW. Performed the experiments: LS LX QSY YXW CXC HY JQZ JBJ WBW. Analyzed the data: LS YXW JBJ. Contributed reagents/materials/analysis tools: LX JBJ WBW. Wrote the paper: LS YXW JBJ.

References

1. Sebag J (1989) The vitreous: structure, function, and pathobiology. New York: Springer-Verlag 80–95.
2. Shui YB, Holekamp NM, Kramer BC, Crowley JR, Wilkins MA, et al. (2009) The gel state of the vitreous and ascorbate-dependent oxygen consumption: relationship to the etiology of nuclear cataracts. Arch Ophthalmol 127:475–482.

3. Krebs I, Brannath W, Glittenberg C, Zeiler F, Sebag J, et al. (2007) Posterior vitreomacular adhesion: a potential risk factor for exudative age-related macular degeneration? Am J Ophthalmol 144: 741–746.
4. Johnson MW (2005) Tractional cystoid macular edema. A subtle variant of the vitreomacular traction syndrome. Am J Ophthalmol 140: 184–192.
5. Panozzo G, Mercanti A (2007) Vitrectomy for myopic traction maculopathy. Arch Ophthalmol 125: 767–772.
6. Hee MR, Puliafito CA, Wong C, Duker JS, Reichel E, et al. (1995) Optical coherence tomography of macular holes. Ophthalmology 102: 748–756.
7. Gallemore RP, Jumper JM, McCune BW, Jaffe GJ, Postel EA, et al. (2000) Diagnosis of vitreoretinal adhesions in macular disease with optical coherence tomography. Retina 20: 115–120.
8. Mirza RA, Johnson MW, Jampol LM (2007) OCT use in evaluation of the vitreoretinal interface: a review. Surv Ophthalmol 52: 397–421.
9. Koizumi H, Spaide RF, Fisher YL, Freund KB, Klancnik JM Jr, et al. (2008) Three-dimensional evaluation of vitreomacular traction and epiretinal membrane using spectral domain optical coherence tomography. Am J Ophthalmol 145: 509–517.
10. Xu L, Li Y, Zheng Y, Jonas JB (2006) Associated factors for age-related maculopathy in the adult population in China. The Beijing Eye Study. Br J Ophthalmol 90(9): 1087–1090.
11. Xu L, Cao WF, Wang YX, CHen CX, Jonas JB (2008) Anterior chamber depth and chamber angle and their associations with ocular and general parameters. The Beijing Eye Study. Am J Ophthalmol 145: 929–936.
12. Huynh SC, Wang XY, Rochtchina E, Mitchell P (2006) Distribution of macular thickness by optical coherence tomography: findings from a population-based study of 6-year-old children. Invest Ophthalmol Vis Sci 47: 2351–2357.
13. Eriksson U, Holmström G, Alm A, Larsson E (2009) A population-based study of macular thickness in full-term children assessed with Stratus OCT: normative data and repeatability. Acta Ophthalmol 87: 741–745.
14. Duan XR, Liang YB, Friedman DS, Sun LP, Wong TY, et al. (2010) Normal macular thickness measurements using optical coherence tomography in healthy eyes of adult Chinese persons: the Handan Eye Study. Ophthalmology 117: 1585–1594.
15. Koh VT, Tham YC, Cheung CY, Wong WL, Baskaran M, et al. (2012) Determinants of ganglion cell-inner plexiform layer thickness measured by high-definition optical coherence tomography. Invest Ophthalmol Vis Sci 53: 5853–5839.
16. Hayreh SS, Jonas JB (2004) Posterior vitreous detachment: clinical correlations. Ophthalmologica 218: 333–343.
17. Schwab C, Ivastinovic D, Borkenstein A, Lackner EM, Wedrich A, et al. (2012) Prevalence of early and late stages of physiologic PVD in emmetropic elderly population. Acta Ophthalmol 90: 179–184.
18. Uchino E, Uemura A, Ohba N (2001) Initial stages of posterior vitreous detachment in healthy eyes of older persons evaluated by optical coherence tomography. Arch Ophthalmol 119: 1475–1479.
19. Chuo JY, Lee TY, Hollands H, Morris AH, Reyes RC, et al. (2006) Risk factors for posterior vitreous detachment: a case-control study. Am J Ophthalmol 142: 931–937.
20. Jonas JB, Nangia V, Kulkarni M, Gupta R, Khare A (2012) Factors associated with early age-related macular degeneration in Central India. The Central India Eye and Medical Study. Acta Ophthalmol 90: e185–191.
21. Cheung CM, L Xi, Cheng CY, Zheng Y, Mitchell P, et al. (2013) Prevalence of and risk factors for age-related macular degeneration among Indian persons living in Singapore and India. Am J Ophthalmol In Press.
22. Stalmans P, Benz MS, Gandorfer A, Kampik A, Girach A, et al. (2012) Enzymatic vitreolysis with ocriplasmin for vitreomacular traction and macular holes. N Engl J Med 367: 606–615.

31

Myo/Nog Cells: Targets for Preventing the Accumulation of Skeletal Muscle-Like Cells in the Human Lens

Jacquelyn Gerhart[1¤a], Marvin Greenbaum[2], Victoria Scheinfeld[1], Paul FitzGerald[3], Mitchell Crawford[1], Arturo Bravo-Nuevo[1], Meghan Pitts[1], Mindy George-Weinstein[1*¤b]

1 Lankenau Institute for Medical Research, Wynnewood, Pennsylvania, United States of America, **2** Lankenau Medical Center, Wynnewood, Pennsylvania, United States of America, **3** Department of Cell Biology and Human Anatomy, School of Medicine, University of California Davis, Davis, California, United States of America

Abstract

Posterior capsule opacification (PCO) is a vision impairing condition that arises in some patients following cataract surgery. The fibrotic form of PCO is caused by myofibroblasts that may emerge in the lens years after surgery. In the chick embryo lens, myofibroblasts are derived from Myo/Nog cells that are identified by their expression of the skeletal muscle specific transcription factor MyoD, the bone morphogenetic protein inhibitor Noggin, and the epitope recognized by the G8 monoclonal antibody. The goal of this study was to test the hypothesis that depletion of Myo/Nog cells will prevent the accumulation of myofibroblasts in human lens tissue. Myo/Nog cells were present in anterior, equatorial and bow regions of the human lens, cornea and ciliary processes. In anterior lens tissue removed by capsulorhexis, Myo/Nog cells had synthesized myofibroblast and skeletal muscle proteins, including vimentin, MyoD and sarcomeric myosin. Alpha smooth muscle actin (α-SMA) was detected in a subpopulation of Myo/Nog cells. Areas of the capsule denuded of epithelial cells were surrounded by Myo/Nog cells. Some of these cell free areas contained a wrinkle in the capsule. Depletion of Myo/Nog cells eliminated cells expressing skeletal muscle proteins in 5-day cultures but did not affect cells immunoreactive for beaded filament proteins that accumulate in differentiating lens epithelial cells. Transforming growth factor-betas 1 and 2 that mediate an epithelial-mesenchymal transition, did not induce the expression of skeletal muscle proteins in lens cells following Myo/Nog cell depletion. This study demonstrates that Myo/Nog cells in anterior lens tissue removed from cataract patients have undergone a partial differentiation to skeletal muscle. Myo/Nog cells appear to be the source of skeletal muscle-like cells in explants of human lens tissue. Targeting Myo/Nog cells with the G8 antibody during cataract surgery may reduce the incidence of PCO.

Editor: Ram Nagaraj, Case Western Reserve University, United States of America

Funding: This study was funded by the Sharp-Strumia Research Foundation (http://www.mainlinehealth.org/sharpe-strumia) and March of Dimes (http://www.marchofdimes.com) awarded to Dr. George-Weinstein and the National Institutes of Health (EY08747) awarded to Dr. FitzGerald. The funders had no role in the study design, data collection and analysis, decision to publish, or preparation of the manuscript.

Competing Interests: Targeting Myo/Nog cells in the lens is described in the patent entitled "Compositions and Methods for the Treatment and Prevention of Lens Fibrotic Diseases", US 13/132,745. The G8 monoclonal antibody is under product development by Genisphere, LLC, Hatfield, PA.

* E-mail: George-weinstein@rowan.edu

These authors contributed equally to this work.

¤a Current address: Genisphere, LLC, Hatfield, Pennsylvania, United States of America
¤b Current address: Department of Biomedical Sciences, Cooper Medical School of Rowan University, Camden, New Jersey, United States of America

Introduction

Posterior capsule opacification (PCO) is a vision impairing condition that arises in some patients following cataract surgery [1,2]. Visual acuity is compromised by the formation of Elschnig pearls that consist of differentiating lens cells (regenerative PCO) and the emergence of myofibroblasts that migrate onto the lens capsule and deposit extracellular matrix (fibrotic PCO) [3]. The fibrotic form of PCO has been attributed to lens epithelial cells that undergo an epithelial to mesenchymal transition (EMT) and a transdifferentiation to myofibroblasts [2,4]. Several families of molecules have been implicated in the emergence of myofibroblasts in lens tissue [43], including transforming growth factor beta (TGF-β) that induces an epithelial to mesenchymal transition (EMT), cell migration, synthesis of alpha smooth muscle actin (α-SMA), contraction and production of extracellular matrix in anterior and posterior lens tissue [4–18]. Contractions of myofibroblasts produce folds and wrinkles in the thick basement membrane surrounding the lens called the capsule [19].

Myofibroblasts in the chick embryo lens originate from Myo/Nog cells that are incorporated into the eye during early stages of development [20–22]. Myo/Nog cells, which exist at low frequency in many tissues, are identified by their expression of mRNA for the skeletal muscle specific transcription factor MyoD, the bone morphogenetic protein (BMP) inhibitor Noggin and the cell surface molecule recognized by the G8 monoclonal antibody (mAb) [20,21,23–27]. Expression of MyoD is the hallmark of Myo/Nog cells' commitment to the skeletal muscle lineage, while their release of Noggin is critical for modulating BMP signaling, morphogenesis and differentiation [20,21,26,28]. Depletion of Myo/Nog cells in the blastocyst results in severe malformations of the body wall, central nervous system and the eyes due to deregulated BMP signaling [20,21,26].

In addition to their role as the primary producer of Noggin, Myo/Nog cells react to a perturbation in homeostasis in multiple tissues [22,26,27]. The propensity of Myo/Nog cells to respond to wounding reflects, in part, their innate capacity for migration and expression of muscle proteins [20–22,24,25,29]. When removed from embryonic and fetal tissues and cultured in serum-free medium, they translate MyoD mRNA and undergo terminal skeletal muscle differentiation [24,25,28,29]. *In vivo*, Myo/Nog cells do not appear to translate MyoD mRNA or synthesize sarcomeric proteins under homeostatic conditions [21,25,30]. However, when activated by apoptotic cells, epidermal abrasion, tumorigenesis, or incisions in embryonic lens tissue, Myo/Nog cells rapidly increase in number and migrate to the wound [22,26,27].

The goals of this study were to determine whether the human lens contains Myo/Nog cells and characterize their behavior in anterior lens tissue removed by capsulorhexis during cataract surgery. The effect of Myo/Nog cell depletion on the accumulation of myofibroblasts in anterior lens tissue was tested *in vitro*.

Materials and Methods

Human Anterior Segments

Human anterior segments from three donors were obtained through the National Disease Research Interchange (Philadelphia, PA, USA). Lens sections from an additional three donors were acquired from Excalibur Pathology, Inc. (Oklahoma City, OK, USA). The age of the donors ranged from 52 to 96 years old. Five eyes were procured 3–8 hours postmortem. The sixth eye was procured 13 hours postmortem. Eyes were immediately placed in fixative and shipped the same day. Lenses from one donor were fixed in 4% paraformaldehyde for approximately 24 hours, cut in quarters and embedded in OCT compound for cryosectioning. Lenses from the other five donors were fixed in a modified Davidson's fixative containing 14% ethyl alcohol, 14% formalin and 6.25% glacial acetic acid (Excalibur Pathology, Inc., USA) and embedded in paraffin. This fixation method produced preservation of lens morphology superior to that of paraformaldehyde. Tissue was sectioned at 10 µm. Some sections were stained with Hematoxylin 7211 and Eosin-Y (Richard-Allan Scientific, Kalamazoo, MI, USA).

Human Anterior Lens Tissue

Anterior lens tissue was removed by capsulorhexis from 283 patients during cataract surgery. The patients ranged from 55 to 91 years old. Approximately 2/3 of the patients were female. The most common cataract subtype was nuclear sclerosis, which in the majority of cases, was accompanied by cortical and less commonly, posterior subcapsular cataracts. The tissue was fixed in 2% paraformaldehyde within 10 minutes of its removal from 66 patients. Each whole piece of anterior lens tissue was cut in half before processing for histological analysis. Other pieces of unfixed anterior lens tissue were cultured by a modification of the methods of Wormstone et al. [31] and Ishizaki et al. [32]. Four edges of the capsule were pressed to a 35 mm tissue culture dish. Lens tissue was cultured in serum and protein-free DMEM/F12 medium (GIBCO/Life Technologies, Grand Island, NY, USA) at 37°C in 5% CO_2 in air.

In Situ Hybridization and Immunofluorescence Localization

Sections of the anterior segment or anterior lens tissue removed during cataract surgery were examined for the expression of the G8 epitope and mRNAs for MyoD and Noggin by incubating with the G8 IgM MAb [25] and goat anti-mouse IgM µ chain antibodies conjugated with DyLight 488 (Invitrogen/Molecular Probes, Eugene, OR, USA), followed by incubation in Cy3 labeled 3DNA™ dendrimer nanoparticles (Genisphere, LLC, Hatfield, PA, USA) [33]. The following anti-sense sequences were conjugated to 3DNA: human MyoD1 (NM_002478.4:5′-CTGTCCGGCCTGATTTGT GGTTAAGGA-3′) and mouse Noggin (NM_008711.2:5′-TCTCGTTCAGATCC TTCTCCTTAGGGTCAAA-3′) [34,35]. The sequence to mouse Noggin was 94% homologous to human Noggin (29 out of 31 bases) [36] and showed the same co-localization pattern with the G8 mAb in murine and human tissues [27].

Sections of the anterior segment and anterior lens tissue were double labeled with the G8 IgM mAb to tag Myo/Nog cells, and IgG mAbs to vimentin (AMF-17b) [37], alpha smooth muscle actin (α-SMA) (directly conjugated with fluorescein; Sigma-Aldrich, St. Louis, MO, USA) (markers of myofibroblasts), MyoD1 protein (NCL-MyoD1; Novocastra Labs Ltd, UK), slow sarcomeric myosin (A4.951) [38], neonatal and adult sarcomeric myosin heavy chain (MF30) [39], the skeletal muscle specific, T-tubule associated 12101 antigen (12101) [40] and cardiac and skeletal muscle troponin T (CT3) [41] (markers of striated muscle) by previously described methods [23,25]. Double labeling was also performed with the G8 mAb and goat polyclonal antibodies to Noggin (AF719; R&D Systems, Minneapolis, MN, USA) and rabbit polyclonal antibodies to filensin [42] and CP49 [43,44]. Controls for non-specific staining included the E12 IgM mAb [29], 2H3 IgG mAb to neurofilament protein [45] and a goat polyclonal antiserum to the homeobox protein LBX1 expressed in the central nervous system and some developing muscles [46] (Santa Cruz Biotechnology, Dallas, TX, USA). Monoclonal antibodies to vimentin, sarcomeric myosins, the 12101 antigen, troponin T and neurofilament protein were obtained from the Developmental Studies Hybridoma Bank (developed under the auspices of the NICHD and maintained by the University of Iowa, Dept. of Biology, Iowa City, IA, USA).

Primary antibodies were visualized with species- and subclass-specific fluorescent secondary antibodies, including goat anti-mouse or anti-rabbit IgG, goat anti-mouse IgM µ chain and donkey anti-goat IgG conjugated with DyLights 488 or 549 (Jackson ImmunoResearch, West Grove, PA, USA). Nuclei were stained with Hoechst dye 33258 (Sigma-Aldrich). Labeling was analyzed with the Nikon Eclipse E800 epifluorescence microscope equipped with the Evolution QE Optronics video camera and Image Pro Plus image analysis software program (Media Cybernetics, Rockville, MD, USA), and Nikon Eclipse Ti Confocal microscope and NIS-Elements software. Figures were annotated and uniformly adjusted for brightness and contrast with Adobe Photoshop 6.0.

The percentage of labeled cells in anterior lens tissue was determined by counting the total numbers of stained and unstained cells in 20 consecutive fields across the entire tissue. The number of cells in 20 fields varied between 1,124 and 2,284. The accuracy of this sampling method was determined by comparing the percentage of labeled cells in 20 fields to the percentage in the entire tissue. The values for each combination of antibodies used for double labeling are the mean ± standard deviation of anterior lens tissue from different patients.

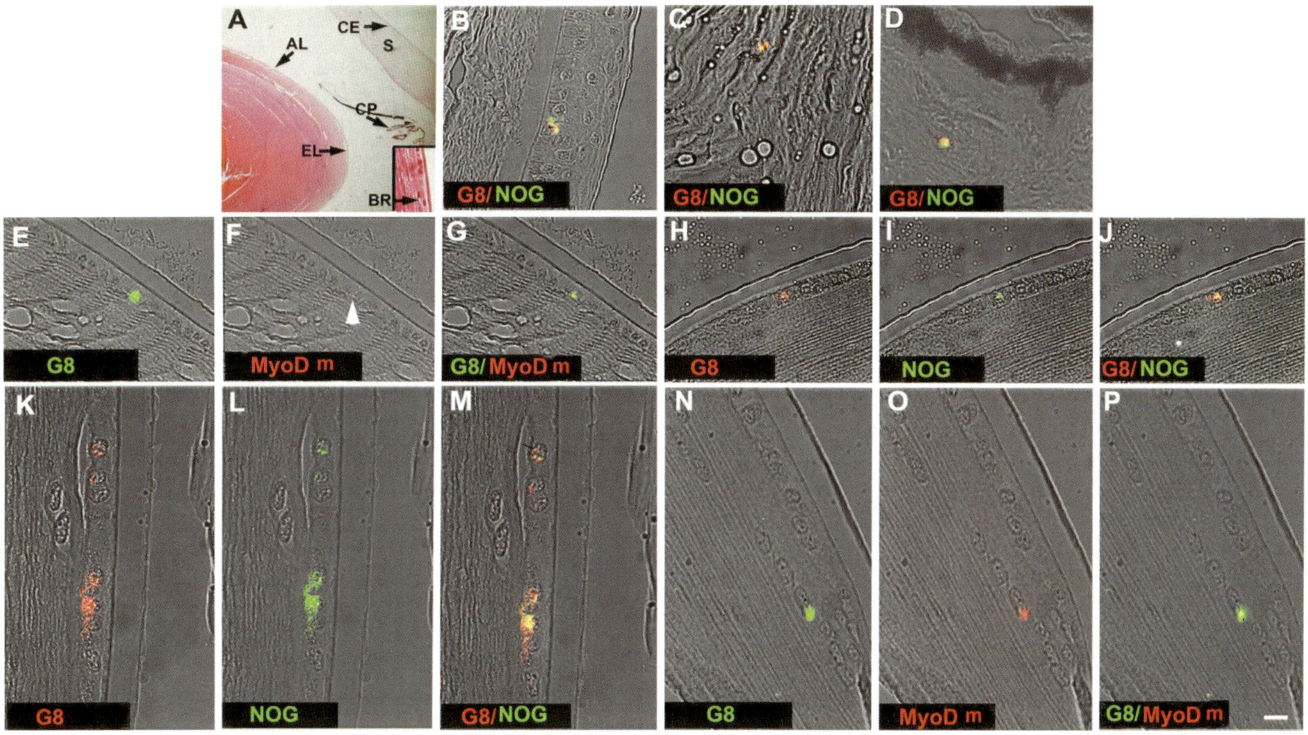

Figure 1. Distribution of Myo/Nog cells in the human anterior segment. Tissue sections through the anterior segment were stained with H&E (A) or double labeled with G8 and dendrimers to MyoD mRNA (MyoD m) or an antibody to Noggin (NOG) (B–P). The primary antibodies and colors of the fluorescent dendrimers and secondary antibodies are indicated in each photograph. Photographs are the merged images of DIC and fluorescence. Overlap of green and red appears yellow in merged images. Myo/Nog cells labeled for G8, MyoD mRNA and Noggin protein were present in the anterior (E–J), equatorial (K–M) and bow regions (N–P) of the lens, corneal epithelium (B), corneal stroma (C) and ciliary processes (D). AL = anterior lens, EL = equatorial lens, BR = bow region of the lens shown in the inset in A, CP = ciliary process, CE = corneal epithelium, S = corneal stroma. Bar = 135 µm in A and 9 µm in B–I.

Depletion of Myo/Nog Cells in Anterior Lens Cultures

Cultures containing anterior lens tissue were incubated in Hanks buffered saline containing 0.1% bovine serum albumen (Sigma-Aldrich) and the G8 mAb or baby rabbit complement (Cedar Lane, Inc., Hornby, Ontario, Canada, USA) alone, or a pre-mixed solution of G8 and complement 20 hours after plating [21]. Explants were stained with a fluorescent secondary antibodies to visualize the G8 mAb, and terminal deoxynucleotidyl transferase dUTP nick end labeling (TUNEL) reagents (Roche Diagnostics, Mannheim, Germany) five hours after treatment [26]. Other treated explants were incubated in culture medium for an additional 4 days and then stained with antibodies to muscle and beaded filament lens proteins.

Treatment of Wounded Anterior Lens Tissue with TGF-β

Whole pieces of anterior lens tissue were cut in half and pressed to a culture dish. In some cultures, tissue was treated with the G8 mAb and complement to deplete Myo/Nog cells immediately after plating. A scratch wound was produced by gently abrading the epithelium with a knife by modification of the method of Wormstone et al. [4,14]. The location of the wound was marked at the edge of the tissue with a dissecting needle. Following wounding, explants were incubated in one ml of DMEM/F12 medium alone or DMEM/F12 containing 10 ηg/ml human recombinant TGF-β2 (Sigma-Aldrich and R&D Systems, Inc., Minneapolis, MN, USA) or human recombinant TGF-β1 (Sigma-Aldrich). Some cultures were treated simultaneously with TGF-β1 or −β2 and 10 ηg/ml human recombinant Noggin (PeproTech, Inc., Rocky Hill, NJ, USA). Media were replenished 48 hours later. Cultures were fixed 48 or 120 hours following the initiation of treatment.

Statistical Analyses

The two-tailed Student's t-test was used to compare the percentages of cells labeled with antibodies to G8, α-SMA, MyoD, myosin, filensin and CP49 in treated and control cultures.

Use of Human Tissue and Ethics Statement

This research followed the tenets of the Declaration of Helsinki. Written informed consent was obtained from the subjects following an explanation of the study. The project was approved by the Institutional Review Board of Main Line Hospitals.

Results

Myo/Nog Cells are Present in the Anterior Segment of the Human Eye

Tissue sections from the anterior segment of six donors were probed for G8, MyoD mRNA and Noggin to determine whether Myo/Nog cells are present in the human lens. None of the donors were reported to have had a history of lens disease. *In situ* hybridization was carried out with Cy3 labeled 3DNA dendrimers that are extremely sensitive and precise reagents for localizing mRNA in single cells in fresh and sectioned tissue [20,21,23,25–27,33]. Double labeling with the G8 mAb and dendrimers to MyoD mRNA or an antibody to Noggin revealed the presence of small numbers of Myo/Nog cells in the lens, epithelial and stromal layers of the cornea, and ciliary processes (Figure 1). Each 10 μm section of the whole lens contained an average of 4±4 (n = 60) Myo/Nog cells among the lens epithelial cells. Of the total cells in the lens labeled with the G8 mAb, 28%, 40% and 31% were present in the anterior, equatorial and bow regions, respectively. Single or clusters of Myo/Nog cells were found in each of these regions, although they were not visible in all three areas in every section (Figure 1E–P). Only one Myo/Nog cell was found between the cortical fibers. These results are consistent with our findings in the chick embryo [20] and adult mice and rabbits (unpublished data) in which the eyes were removed and fixed immediately upon death.

Myo/Nog Cells in Anterior Lens Tissue Removed by Capsulorhexis Express Markers of Myofibroblasts and Skeletal Muscle Cells

Anterior lens tissue, which is more readily available than whole lenses and can be obtained within minutes of surgery, was used to explore the properties of Myo/Nog cells in the human lens. Every piece of anterior lens tissue that was fixed within 10 minutes of capsulorhexis contained a small population of cells labeled with the G8 mAb (3% ±2, number of patients (n = 66) (Figure 2). MyoD mRNA was detected in practically all G8+ cells (98% ±2, n = 4) (Figure 2A–C), and only a few MyoD mRNA+ cells lacked staining for G8 (4% ±4, n = 4). Most Myo/Nog cells had translated MyoD mRNA into protein (Table 1; Figure 2D–F). Noggin was localized in 99% of the G8+ cells (Table 1; Figure 2G–I).

Single or small clusters of 2–4 Myo/Nog cells appeared to be randomly distributed among the lens epithelial cells (Fig. 2A–I). Approximately 35% of the anterior lenses contained clusters ranging from 4–40 Myo/Nog cells lying on the apical surface of the epithelial cells (Figure 2J–L). The presence of apical clusters did not appear to correlate with the age (55–89 years), cataract subtype (nuclear sclerosis with or without cortical and/or posterior subcapsular) or grade (2–4) of the donor. Most lenses lacked G8+ cells along the incision created during the initiation of capsulorhexis (Figure 2M); however, in 15% of the specimens, G8+ cells were intermittently aligned along the incisional edge (Figure 2O). By contrast, all cells along the entire periphery of the tissue were intensely labeled with an antibody to the intermediate filament protein vimentin, (Figure 2N and P). Less intense vimentin staining was observed throughout the epithelium (Figure 2N and P). The specificity of staining with the G8 and vimentin antibodies along the edge of the tissue was demonstrated by the absence of fluorescence when the tissue was incubated with the E12 IgM mAb, 2H3 IgG mAb and their respective secondary antibodies (Figure 2R and S) or secondary antibodies alone (not shown). Thus, in some samples, Myo/Nog cells appear at the incisional border of the tissue.

The state of differentiation of Myo/Nog cells in the lens was determined by screening for markers of myofibroblasts and skeletal muscle cells. Low numbers of cells throughout the lens tissue were labeled with antibodies to muscle proteins (Table 1; Figure 3). Whereas only a small percentage of the G8+ cells contained detectable levels of α-SMA, most or all G8+ cells had synthesized MyoD, sarcomeric myosins, the skeletal muscle specific, T-tubule associated 12101 molecule and troponin T (Table 1), indicating that Myo/Nog cells synthesize proteins characteristic of skeletal muscle.

Approximately 76% of the anterior lenses contained small areas in which the epithelial cells had been denuded from the capsule. These areas were distant from the edges of the tissue pressed against the tissue culture dish. A wrinkle was present in the capsule in at least one of these cell free areas in approximately one third of the samples (Figure 3I, L, U and V). Myo/Nog cells had formed a thickened rim around these cell free areas (Figure 3A–V). Most of

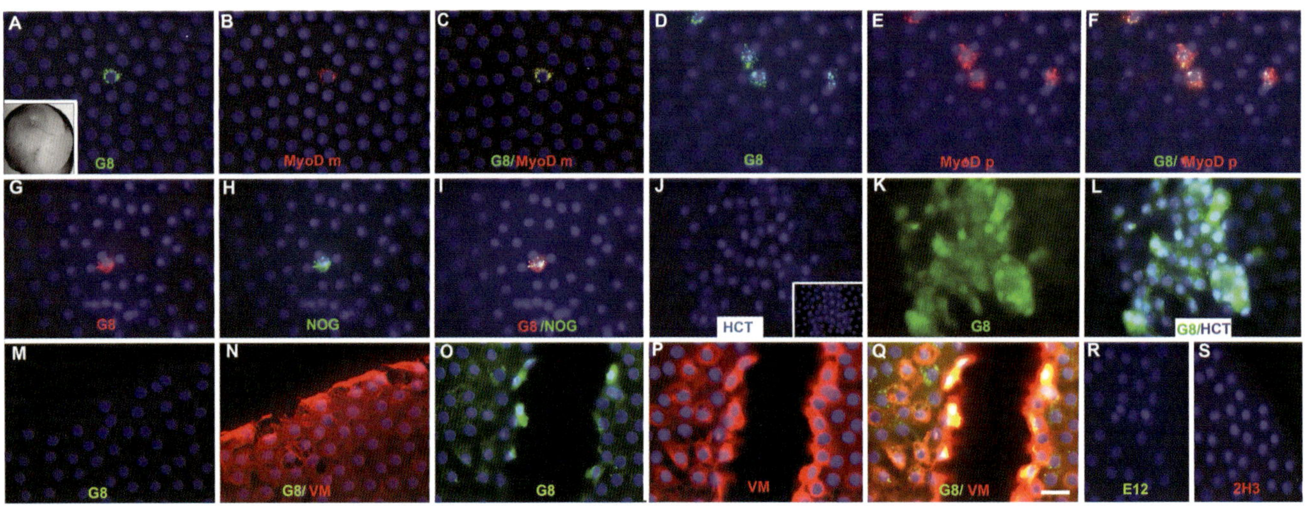

Figure 2. Distribution of Myo/Nog cells in human anterior lens tissue removed during cataract surgery. A low magnification DIC image of anterior lens tissue fixed after capsulorhexis is shown in the inset in A. Tissue was double labeled with the G8 mAb and dendrimers to MyoD mRNA (MyoD m) or antibodies to MyoD protein (MyoD p), Noggin (NOG) or vimentin (VM). The primary antibodies and colors of the fluorescent dendrimers and secondary antibodies are indicated in each photograph. Unmerged images precede the merged images shown in C, F, I, L and Q. Overlap of green and red appears yellow in merged images. Nuclei were stained with Hoechst dye (HCT) (blue). Anterior lens tissue contained single, small groups or large clusters of Myo/Nog cells throughout the epithelium (A–L). Photographs in J-L illustrate a cluster of G8+ cells lying on the apical surface of lens epithelial cells. The underlying layer of nuclei in the same field is shown in the inset in J. G8+ cells were present along the cut edge of some (O) but not all samples (M). Vimentin staining was most intense at the periphery of the tissue (N and P). Tissue incubated with the E12 IgM or 2H3 IgG and their respective secondary antibodies lacked fluorescence (R and S). Bar = 5 mm in the inset in A and 9 μm in the other photomicrographs.

Table 1. Myo/Nog cells in anterior lens tissue are immunoreactive for proteins found in skeletal muscle and lens tissue.

Antibody	% Ab Positive	% Ab Positive with G8	% G8 Positive with other Ab
MyoD	2±2	100	94±12
Noggin	3±2	99±1	99±2
Vimentin	92±10	6±2	100
α-SMA	1±1	30±26	12±11
Sarcomeric Myosin	4±1	93±16	90±19
12101	4±2	81±27	90±12
Troponin T	2±1	100	54±25

Anterior lens tissue was fixed within 10 minutes of capsulorhexis and double labeled with G8 and other antibodies (Ab) and species and subclass specific fluorescent secondary antibodies. % Ab Positive = number of fluorescent cells ÷ total number of cells in 20 fields X 100. % Ab Positive with G8 = number of antibody positive cells co-labeled with G8 ÷ total antibody positive cells X 100. Percent G8 Positive Cells with Other Ab = number of G8 positive cells co-labeled with the other antibody ÷ total number of G8 positive cells X 100. Four cultures were scored for each pair of antibodies except G8+ Noggin (n = 9) and G8+ α-SMA (n = 10).

the G8+ cells surrounding the bare areas of capsule expressed MyoD mRNA and stained with antibodies to MyoD protein, Noggin, α-SMA, vimentin (not shown), sarcomeric myosin, 12101 and troponin T (Figure 3A–V). The specificity of antibody binding in Myo/Nog cells was demonstrated by the lack of staining around the edges of cell free areas following incubation with the E12 and 2H3 mAbs, the LBX1 goat polyclonal antiserum and their respective secondary antibodies (Figure 3W–Y), or secondary antibodies alone (not shown). Although Myo/Nog cells expressed sarcomeric proteins, they did not appear striated. Some Myo/Nog cells were present on the capsule within the cell free areas and had extended processes towards the wrinkle (Figure 3V).

Depletion of Myo/Nog Cells in Cultures of Anterior Lens Tissue Prevents the Accumulation of Cells Expressing Muscle Proteins

The effect of depleting Myo/Nog cells on the accumulation of muscle cells in explants of anterior lens tissue was determined by lysing cells that bound the G8 mAb with complement [21]. Five hours following treatment with G8 and complement, 99% ±1 of the G8+ cells, but only 3% ±3 of the G8- cells (n = 5) were

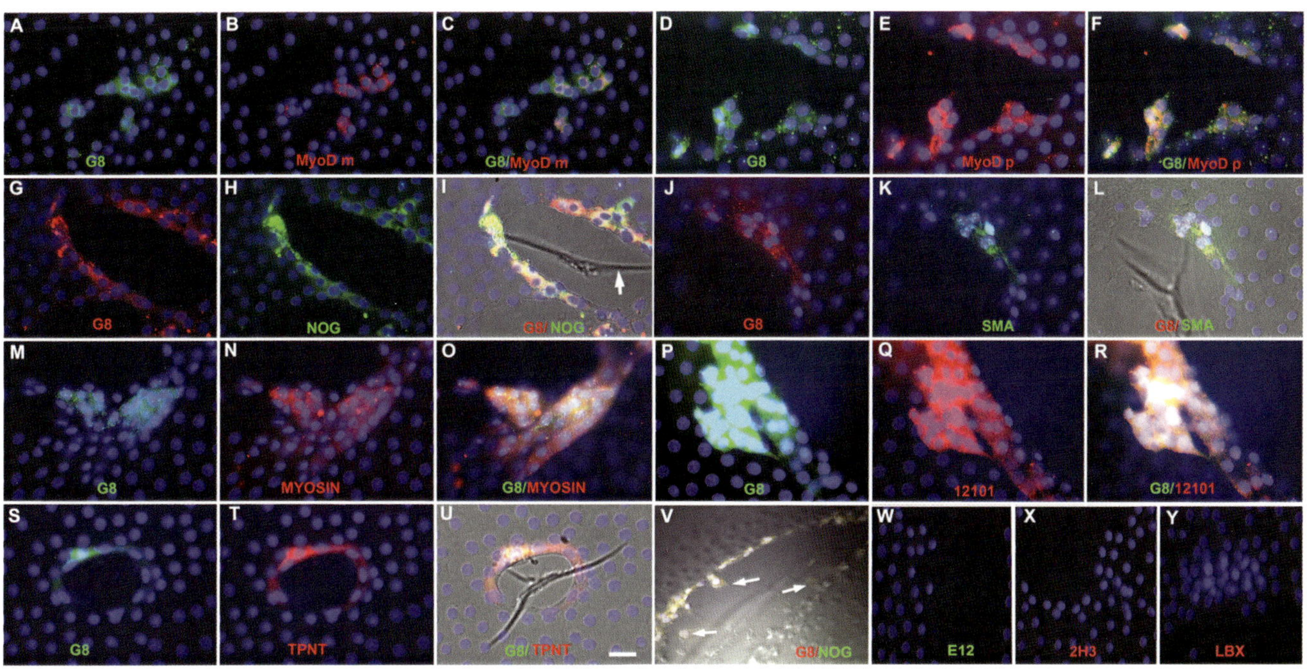

Figure 3. Myo/Nog cells in human anterior lens tissue express muscle proteins. Anterior lens tissue fixed after capsulorhexis was double labeled with the G8 mAb and dendrimers to MyoD mRNA (MyoD m) or antibodies to MyoD protein (MyoD p), Noggin (NOG), α-SMA, sarcomeric myosin heavy chain (MYOSIN), the skeletal muscle specific 12101 antigen (12101) and troponin T (TPNT). The primary antibodies and colors of the fluorescent dendrimers and secondary antibodies are indicated in each photograph. Overlap of green and red appears yellow in merged images. Nuclei were stained with Hoechst dye (blue). Panels I, L, U and V are quadruple merged images of DIC and fluorescence showing wrinkles in the capsule (arrow in I). G8+ cells co-stained for MyoD mRNA, Noggin and muscle proteins surrounded cell free areas of the capsule (A–V). Some Myo/Nog cells had migrated onto the capsule (arrows in V). Tissue incubated with the E12 or 2H3 mAbs, or an antiserum to LBX1 and their respective secondary antibodies, lacked fluorescence (W–Y). Bar = 9 μm.

undergoing apoptosis, as indicated by TUNEL staining (Figure 4A). In cultures treated with the G8 mAb or complement only, 2% ±2 and 5% ±8 of the G8+ and G8- cells, respectively, were TUNEL+ (n = 6) (Figure 4B and C). This experiment demonstrates that Myo/Nog cells are specifically targeted when lens explants are treated with G8 and complement.

Four days following Myo/Nog cell depletion, cultures were labeled with antibodies to G8 and muscle proteins. Treatment with both G8 and complement eliminated G8+ cells in 12 out of 16 cultures and left only a few G8+ cells in the remaining cultures (Table 2, Figure 4D–H). The percentage of α-SMA+ cells was reduced approximately 6-fold following treatment with G8 and complement (Table 2, Figure 4E) and only 1% ±3 of the α-SMA+ cells were co-labeled with the G8 mAb. Complete elimination of G8+ cells in 5-day cultures was accompanied by an absence of MyoD+ and sarcomeric myosin+ cells (Figure 4E and F). By contrast, ablation of Myo/Nog cells did not prevent the accumulation of cells immunoreactive for the beaded filament proteins filensin and CP49 that are synthesized in differentiating lens cells (Table 2, Figure 4G and H). Control cultures treated with G8 (Table 2, Figure 4I–M) or complement alone contained cells with muscle and beaded filament proteins (Table 2). These experiments demonstrate that Myo/Nog cells are not replenished following treatment with the G8 mAb and complement, and the depletion protocol inhibits the accumulation of myogenic cells.

TGF-β Does Not Induce Expression of Skeletal Muscle Proteins in the Absence of Myo/Nog Cells

Anterior lens tissue depleted of Myo/Nog cells was further challenged to produce muscle cells by creating a scratch wound in the epithelium and incubating with TGF-β2 [4,15,47–49]. The wound healing response varied within and between treatment groups. Cells had partially filled in the wound within 48 hours in two out of three untreated explants (Figure 5A). Treatment with TGF-β2 for two days resulted in partial to complete wound closure in four out of 7 explants (Figure 5B). Only one out of five explants displayed partial wound healing following ablation of Myo/Nog cells (Figure 5C). The combination of Myo/Nog cell depletion, wounding and treatment with TGF-β2 resulted in the loss of approximately 50–90% of the cells by 48 hours (Figure 5D). We

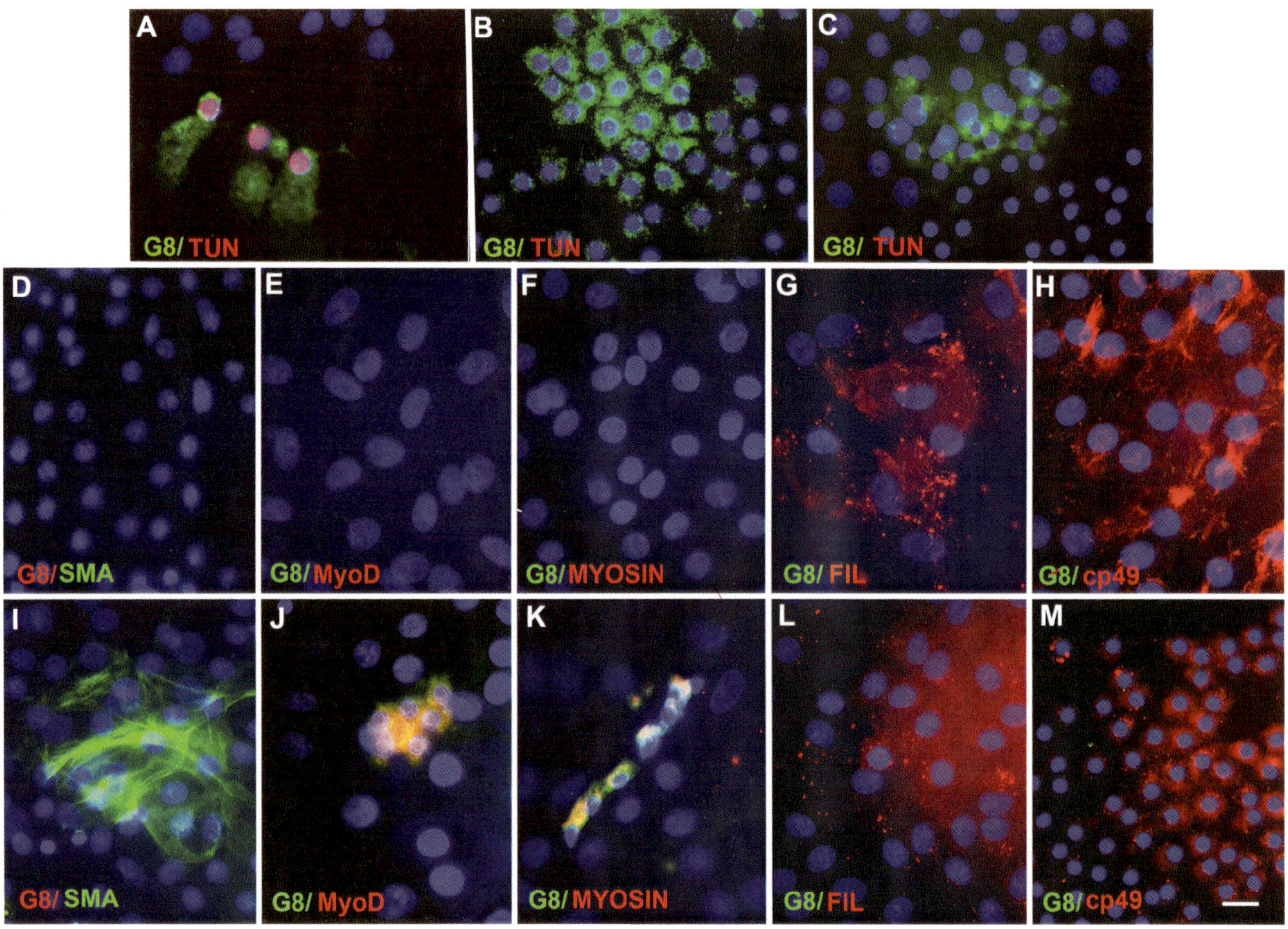

Figure 4. Effects of targeting Myo/Nog cells with the G8 mAb and complement in anterior lens explants. Explants of lens tissue were incubated with the G8 mAb and complement (A, D–H), G8 only (B, I–M) or complement only (C). Five hours later, the tissue was double labeled with the G8 mAb (green) and TUNEL reagents (red). Nuclei were stained with Hoechst dye. G8+, but not G8- cells, were TUNEL+ following treatment with G8 and complement (A). G8+ cells were not TUNEL+ when treated with G8 or complement alone (B and C). Five days following ablation, explants were double labeled with antibodies to G8 and MyoD, α-SMA, sarcomeric myosin heavy chain (MYOSIN), filensin and cp49. The colors of the fluorescent secondary antibodies are indicated in each photograph. Overlap of green and red appears yellow in merged images. Ablation of Myo/Nog cells prevented the accumulation of G8+, MyoD+ and α-SMA+ cells, but not filensin+ and cp49+ cells (D–H). Both muscle and beaded filament proteins were detected in explants treated with the G8 mAb alone (I–M). Bar = 9 μm.

Table 2. Effect of depleting Myo/Nog cells on the accumulation of cells immunoreactive for muscle and beaded filament proteins in anterior lens cultures.

	G8 mAb Tx	Comp Tx	G8 mAb+Comp Tx
% G8+	11±13 (19)	18±12 (4)	0.1±0.1 (16)
% α-SMA+	22±15 (4)	24±14 (4)	4±4 (6)
% MyoD+	5±5 (5)	ND	0 (6)
% Myosin+	5±1 (4)	ND	0 (4)
% Filensin+	18±8 (4)	ND	12±9 (4)
% CP49+	12±5 (4)	ND	24±12 (4)

Anterior lens tissue was incubated with the G8 mAb or complement (Comp) alone, or G8 and complement, 20 hours after plating. Cultures were double labeled with antibodies to G8 and α-SMA, MyoD, sarcomeric myosin, filensin or CP49 on the fifth day in culture. Values are the mean ± standard deviation of the number of antibody-positive cells ÷ total cells X 100. The number of cultures scored is indicated in parentheses. No significant differences were found between the percentages of G8+ or α-SMA+ cells treated with either the G8 mAb or complement alone. Significant differences were found in cultures treated with either the G8 mAb or complement alone and G8+ complement in the percentages of G8+ (0.003 and 0.0001, respectively), α-SMA+ (0.02 and 0.006, respectively), MyoD+ (0.0001) and myosin+ cells (0.0001). No significant differences were found between the percentages of filensin+ and CP49+ cells in cultures treated with G8 or G8+ complement.

reasoned that the detrimental effect of TGF-β2 in explants lacking Myo/Nog cells could reflect the loss of Noggin. Indeed, addition of Noggin at the same time as TGF-β2 prevented cell loss throughout the explant in the absence of Myo/Nog cells, and the wounds were partially or completely filled in all five explants (Figure 5E and F).

By the fifth day after wounding, α-SMA+, MyoD+ and sarcomeric myosin+ cells were abundant in the wounds in untreated and TGF-β2 treated explants (Figure 6A–D). By contrast, no MyoD+ or myosin+ cells were detected within the wounds or throughout the tissue following depletion of Myo/Nog cells in the presence or absence TGF-β2 and Noggin (Figure 6E–H; Table 3). The percentages of α-SMA+ cells varied between explants (Table 3). Five out of six explants treated with TGF-β2 had less than 8% α-SMA+ cells; however in one explant, 60% were α-SMA+. The higher percentage of α-SMA+ cells in this tissue did not appear to correlate with age or the type or grade of cataract (age 70 with nuclear sclerosis (NS), grade 2 compared to those with ≤8% α-SMA+ cells, ages 65–86 with NS, NS with cortical (C) or NS with posterior subcapsular (PS) cataract, grades 2–4). The percentages of α-SMA+ cells remained consistently low following depletion of Myo/Nog cells in the presence or absence of TGF-β2 (Table 3).

Unlike treatment with TGF-β2, cell loss was not observed in response to TGF-β1 following depletion of Myo/Nog cells

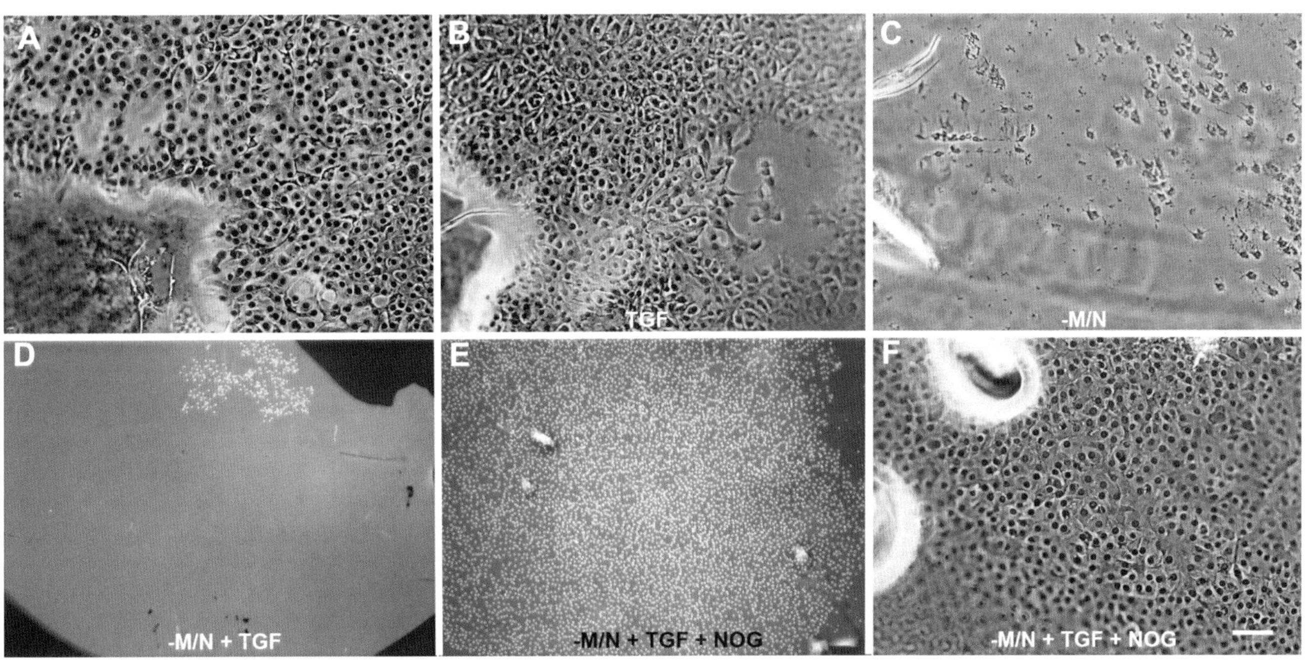

Figure 5. Effects of Myo/Nog cell depletion and TGF-β2 on wound healing in anterior lens explants. A scratch wound was created in explants of anterior lens tissue. Cells had populated the capsule denuded of cells within 48 hours of wounding (A). The wound was also covered with cells following treatment with TGF-β2 (B). Few cells were present in the wound of an explant depleted of Myo/Nog cells (-M/N) (C). The combination of wounding, depletion of Myo/Nog cells and treatment with TGF-β2 resulted in a loss of most cells from the capsule (D). Addition of Noggin (NOG) prevented cell loss resulting from depletion of Myo/Nog cells and treatment with TGF-β2 (E) and promoted wound healing (F). Bar = 27 μm in A-C and F, and 135 μm in D and E.

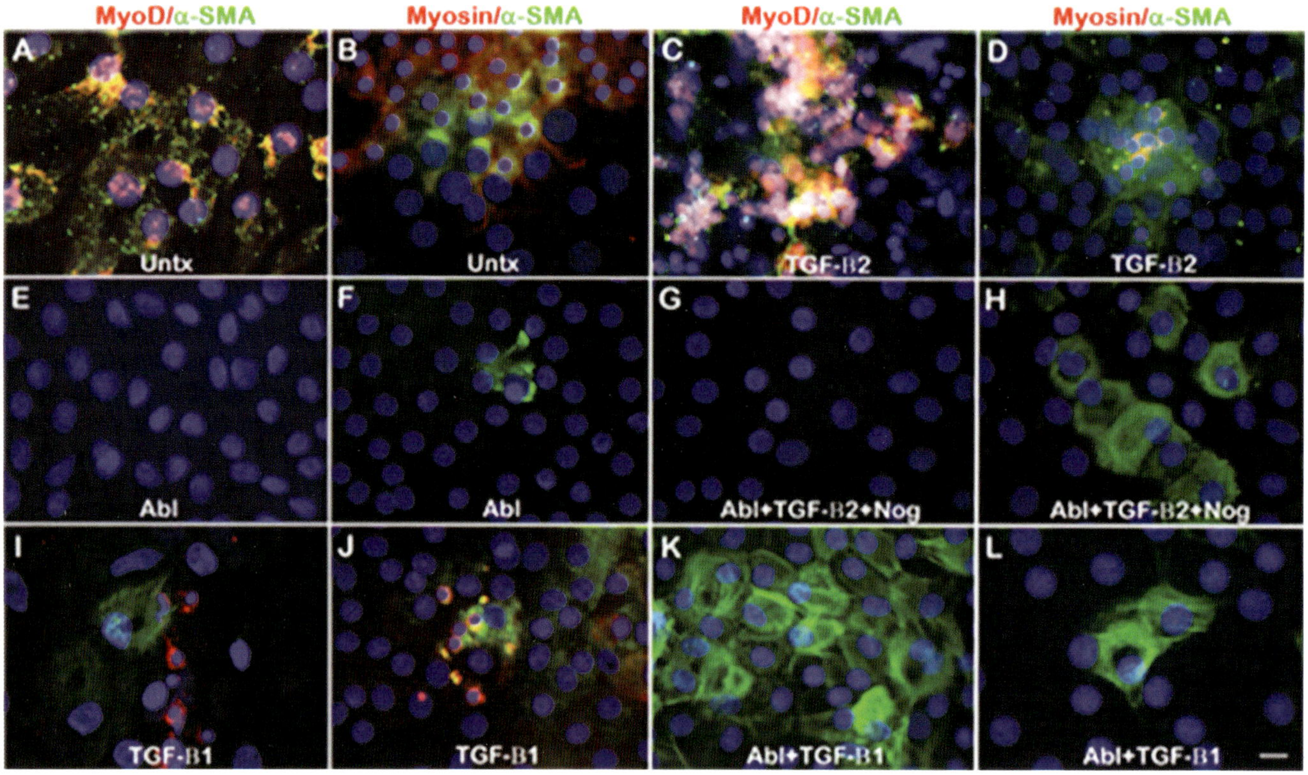

Figure 6. Effect of TGF-β on the accumulation of cells with muscle proteins following wounding and depletion of Myo/Nog cells. Anterior lens explants were wounded and incubated in medium alone (untx) or medium containing TGF-β2 or −β1. Myo/Nog cells were ablated (abl) in some explants prior to wounding. Cells were double labeled with antibodies to α-SMA (green) and MyoD or sarcomeric myosin (red). Nuclei were stained with Hoechst dye. Photographs were taken of the wounded area. Explants incubated in the presence or absence of TGF-β2 or −β1 contained α-SMA+, MyoD+ and myosin+ cells (A–D, I and J). Following depletion of Myo/Nog cells, α-SMA+ cells were less prevalent in the wounds of untreated (E and F) and TGF-β2 treated explants (G and H) than those treated with TGF-β1 (K). No MyoD+ or myosin+ cells were observed in the wounds following Myo/Nog cell depletion and incubation in the presence (G, H, K and L) or absence (E and F) of TGF-β2 or −β1. Bar = 9 μm.

(Figure 6I and J). In the presence of Myo/Nog cells, no significant differences were observed in the percentages of α-SMA+, MyoD+ or sarcomeric myosin+ cells with or without TGF-β1 or −β2, or between the two TGF-βs, with the exception of TGF-β1's effect on increasing the size of the MyoD+ population (0.04). Following Myo/Nog cell depletion, the percentage of α-SMA+ cells was greater in response to TGF-β1 compared to TGF-β2 and Noggin (0.03); however, the results were highly variable (Table 3; Figure 6G, H, K and L). Large numbers of α-SMA+ cells did not appear to correlate with age or the type and grade of cataract (99% α-SMA+: ages 74 and 88, NS/C, grade 2/2 and NS/C/PS, grade 2/2/1, respectively; 22–27% α-SMA+: ages 83 and 74, NS/C, 2/2 and NS, 3, respectively). As was the case with TGF-β2, no MyoD+ or sarcomeric myosin+ cells were detected following

Table 3. Effect of TGF-β on the accumulation of cells with muscle proteins in the presence and absence of Myo/Nog cells.

Treatment	% α-SMA+	% MyoD+	% Myosin+
Wd	6±6 (7)	4±3 (4)	11±9 (3)
Ab+Wd	2±2 (3)	0 (3)	0 (3)
Wd+TGF-β2	12±21 (7)	7±2 (3)	5±3 (4)
Ab+Wd+TGF-β2+Nog	3±4 (4)	0 (3)	0 (4)
Wd+TGF-β1	12±11 (5)	8±2 (4)	4±2 (3)
Ab+Wd+TGF-β1	62±43 (4)	0 (4)	0 (4)
Ab+Wd+TGF-β1+Nog	13±13 (4)	0 (4)	0 (4)

Some explants of anterior lens tissue were treated with the G8 mAb and complement to ablate (Ab) Myo/Nog cells. All explants were wounded (Wd) by scratching the epithelium. Explants were cultured in DMEM/F12 medium alone or medium containing TGF-β2 or −β1 with or without Noggin (Nog). Cells were double labeled with antibodies to α-SMA and MyoD or sarcomeric myosin. Values are the mean ± standard deviation of the number of antibody positive cells ÷ total cells X 100. The number of cultures scored is indicated in parentheses. Neither TGF-β2 nor −β1 stimulated the accumulation of MyoD+ or myosin+ cells following Myo/Nog cell ablation.

depletion of Myo/Nog cells and treatment with TGF-β1 with or without Noggin (Figure 6K and L; Table 3). Combined, these results demonstrate that neither form of TGF-β stimulates the accumulation of cells expressing skeletal muscle proteins in the absence of Myo/Nog cells.

Discussion

PCO occurs in approximately 10–20% in adults and 40–100% in children within two years of cataract surgery [50–53]. The incidence of PCO continues to rise three to six years post-operatively [52]. Although PCO may be ameliorated with Yttrium Aluminum Garnet (Nd:YAG) laser treatment, Nd:YAG:laser is not available worldwide and some patients develop serious complications from the procedure, including corneal edema and retinal detachment [1]. The incidence of PCO has been reduced or delayed by improvements in surgical and drug delivery techniques and intraocular lens composition and design [54,55]; however, prevention of PCO remains an important goal in ophthalmology.

Fibrotic disease of the lens has been attributed to lens epithelial cells that undergo an EMT and a transdifferentiation to myofibroblasts [2,4]. The capacity of epithelial cells in multiple tissues to undergo an EMT has been widely demonstrated in the developing embryo and during the invasion and metastasis of carcinomas [56–58]. However, multiple non-epithelial sources of myofibroblasts have been identified within the tumor stroma, wounds and fibrotic tissues [59–63], indicating that EMT is not necessarily required for the appearance of muscle-like cells in pathological environments.

We propose that a subpopulation of inherently myogenic cells within the lens contributes to the fibrotic form of PCO. In the embryo, these Myo/Nog cells originate in the epiblast, migrate and are integrated into the lens and retina during early stages of development [20,21]. The origin of MyoD+/Noggin+/G8+ cells in the human lens is unknown, but their molecular signature and behaviors resemble those of Myo/Nog cells in avian, rodent and other human tissues [20–22,27]. The premise that Myo/Nog cells in the human lens are a separate population from the lens fiber lineage is supported by the fact that G8+ cells specifically synthesize skeletal muscle proteins and their depletion prevents the emergence of skeletal muscle-like cells over time in culture without affecting the accumulation of cells immunoreactive for beaded filament proteins. These data are consistent with our previous findings demonstrating that Myo/Nog cells are a distinct subpopulation within the embryonic lens and they retain their myogenic properties in a variety of non-muscle tissues [20,21,25,28].

The behavioral repertoire of Myo/Nog cells may be viewed as a continuum that is regulated by the environment. The parent Myo/Nog cell modulates the activities of BMPs in a variety of tissues and has repressed myogenic potential, as evidenced by the expression of MyoD mRNA without detectable levels of translation under homeostatic conditions [20,21,26,28]. When isolated from the embryo and cultured in serum free medium, Myo/Nog cells translate MyoD mRNA, differentiate, fuse and assemble sarcomeres [24,25,29]. In response to a perturbation of homeostasis *in vivo*, Myo/Nog cells expand in number and rapidly appear at the wound [22,26,27]. Both Myo/Nog cells in the cataractous human lens (present study) and myofibroblasts [64–67] express multiple skeletal muscle genes, including MyoD, but they do not fuse or assemble sarcomeres [62,64–67]. Even α-SMA, a commonly used marker for myofibroblasts and smooth muscle, is also expressed in embryonic and neonatal skeletal muscle [68]. Therefore, the development of Myo/Nog cells into myofibroblasts in response to injury appears to represent a partial, yet functional fulfillment of their myogenic potential.

The innate capacity of Myo/Nog cells to synthesize contractile proteins and their distribution around discontinuities in the epithelium are consistent with the interpretation that they were responsible for producing wrinkles in the capsule. Holes in the epithelium, called intercellular vesicles, were observed in sections of cataractous lenses [69,70]. Gaps between human anterior epithelial cells can be produced from contractions induced by saline, acetylcholine or mechanical stimulation [71]. Importantly, expression of α-SMA is not required for contraction in lens cultures [49], suggesting that the expression of other muscle proteins, such as those synthesized by Myo/Nog cells, may be important mediators of capsular wrinkling.

While Myo/Nog cells in the human lens may have surrounded areas of the capsule denuded of epithelial cells and extended lamellipodia towards the wrinkle prior to surgery, their less common appearance at the cut edge of the tissue within 10 minutes of capsulorhexis may reflect a rapid migration to the wound, as observed in the chick embryo lens and murine skin [22,27]. Another relatively rare phenomenon observed in this study was the appearance of Myo/Nog cells on the apical surface of lens epithelial cells. To our knowledge, cells interposed between the anterior epithelium and fibers *in vivo* have not been reported; however, in chick embryo capsular bag cultures, Myo/Nog cells do migrate on the surface of epithelial cells [22]. The occasional accumulation of Myo/Nog cells on the apical surface of lens epithelial cells and at the edge of the tissue may result from mechanical stretching that occurred during capsulorhexis and/or wounding of the epithelial sheet.

Depleting Myo/Nog cells in lens explant cultures significantly reduced the α-SMA+ population and eliminated MyoD+ and sarcomeric myosin+ cells. Addition of TGF-β1 or −β2 had variable effects on the accumulation of α-SMA+ cells that did not correlate with the type or grade of the cataract, and therefore, may reflect subtle differences in the tissue or its handling. Previous reports have documented a more consistent elevation of α-SMA in human lens cells by TGF-β [4,14,15,49]. Differences between the results reported herein and previous studies may be attributed to the source of the tissue (anterior lens tissue, posterior capsular bag model or a lens epithelial cell line), method of measuring α-SMA (Western blot, RT-PCR or qualitative versus quantitative immunofluorescence microscopy), and length of exposure to TGF-βs (2–28 days).

While the effects of TGF-βs on α-SMA expression were variable, neither TGF-β1 nor −β2 stimulated the emergence of MyoD+ or sarcomeric myosin+ cells following depletion of Myo/Nog cells. These experiments further support the conclusion that Myo/Nog cells are a primary source of contractile myofibroblasts that express multiple skeletal muscle proteins following injury to lens tissue. Furthermore, Myo/Nog cells may modulate potential interactions between the BMP and TGF-β signaling pathways in the human lens, as evidenced by the ability of exogenous Noggin to prevent cell loss in response to TGF-β2.

This study provides proof of concept that Myo/Nog cells are potential targets in the human lens for reducing the fibrotic form of PCO and capsular wrinkling. Testing the safety and efficacy of Myo/Nog cell depletion in a preclinical model of cataract surgery may further establish the feasibility of immunotherapy to prevent secondary cataract formation. Depletion of Myo/Nog cells may also prove therapeutic in other tissues prone to fibrosis.

Acknowledgments

The authors thank Drs. Michele Paessler and Gregory Bramblett for their insights and suggestions during the course of this study. Some of the data included in this manuscript was presented in May 2012 at the annual meeting of the Association for Research in Vision and Ophthalmology.

Author Contributions

Conceived and designed the experiments: MG-W JG MG PF. Performed the experiments: JG VS MC AB-N MP. Analyzed the data: MG-W JG VS MG PF MC AB-N. Contributed reagents/materials/analysis tools: MG PF. Wrote the paper: MG-W.

References

1. Awasthi N, Guo S, Wagner BJ (2009) Posterior capsular opacification: a problem reduced but not yet eradicated. Arch Ophthalmol 127: 555–562.
2. Wormstone IM, Wang L, Liu CS (2009) Posterior capsule opacification. Exp Eye Res 88: 257–269.
3. Raj SM, Vasavada AR, Joar K, Vasavada VA, Vasavada VA (2007) Post-operative capsular opacification: A review. Int J Biomed Sci 3: 13.
4. Wormstone IM, Tamiya S, Anderson I, Duncan G (2002) TGF-beta2-induced matrix modification and cell transdifferentiation in the human lens capsular bag. Invest Ophthalmol Vis Sci 43: 2301–2308.
5. Liu J, Hales AM, Chamberlain CG, McAvoy JW (1994) Induction of cataract-like changes in rat lens epithelial explants by transforming growth factor beta. Invest Ophthalmol Vis Sci 35: 388–401.
6. Kurosaka D, Nagamoto T (1994) Inhibitory effect of TGF-beta 2 in human aqueous humor on bovine lens epithelial cell proliferation. Invest Ophthalmol Vis Sci 35: 3408–3412.
7. Gordon-Thomson C, de Iongh RU, Hales AM, Chamberlain CG, McAvoy JW (1998) Differential cataractogenic potency of TGF-beta1, -beta2, and -beta3 and their expression in the postnatal rat eye. Invest Ophthalmol Vis Sci 39: 1399–1409.
8. Saxby L, Rosen E, Boulton M (1998) Lens epithelial cell proliferation, migration, and metaplasia following capsulorhexis. Br J Ophthalmol 82: 945–952.
9. Richiert DM, Ireland ME (1999) TGF-beta elicits fibronectin secretion and proliferation in cultured chick lens epithelial cells. Curr Eye Res 18: 62–71.
10. Lee EH, Joo CK (1999) Role of transforming growth factor-beta in transdifferentiation and fibrosis of lens epithelial cells. Invest Ophthalmol Vis Sci 40: 2025–2032.
11. Marcantonio JM, Rakic JM, Vrensen GF, Duncan G (2000) Lens cell populations studied in human donor capsular bags with implanted intraocular lenses. Invest Ophthalmol Vis Sci 41: 1130–1141.
12. Saika S, Okada Y, Miyamoto T, Ohnishi Y, Ooshima A, et al. (2001) Smad translocation and growth suppression in lens epithelial cells by endogenous TGFbeta2 during wound repair. Exp Eye Res 72: 679–686.
13. Saika S, Miyamoto T, Ishida I, Shirai K, Ohnishi Y, et al. (2002) TGFbeta-Smad signalling in postoperative human lens epithelial cells. Br J Ophthalmol 86: 1428–1433.
14. Wormstone IM, Tamiya S, Eldred JA, Lazaridis K, Chantry A, et al. (2004) Characterisation of TGF-beta2 signalling and function in a human lens cell line. Exp Eye Res 78: 705–714.
15. Wormstone IM, Anderson IK, Eldred JA, Dawes LJ, Duncan G (2006) Short-term exposure to transforming growth factor beta induces long-term fibrotic responses. Exp Eye Res 83: 1238–1245.
16. Lovicu FJ, Schulz MW, Hales AM, Vincent LN, Overbeek PA, et al. (2002) TGFbeta induces morphological and molecular changes similar to human anterior subcapsular cataract. Br J Ophthalmol 86: 220–226.
17. de Iongh RU, Wederell E, Lovicu FJ, McAvoy JW (2005) Transforming growth factor-beta-induced epithelial-mesenchymal transition in the lens: a model for cataract formation. Cells Tissues Organs 179: 43–55.
18. Banh A, Deschamps PA, Gauldie J, Overbeek PA, Sivak JG, et al. (2006) Lens-specific expression of TGF-beta induces anterior subcapsular cataract formation in the absence of Smad3. Invest Ophthalmol Vis Sci 47: 3450–3460.
19. McDonnell PJ, Zarbin MA, Green WR (1983) Posterior capsule opacification in pseudophakic eyes. Ophthalmology 90: 1548–1553.
20. Gerhart J, Pfautz J, Neely C, Elder J, DuPrey K, et al. (2009) Noggin producing, MyoD-positive cells are crucial for eye development. Dev Biol 336: 30–41.
21. Gerhart J, Elder J, Neely C, Schure J, Kvist T, et al. (2006) MyoD-positive epiblast cells regulate skeletal muscle differentiation in the embryo. J Cell Biol 175: 283–292.
22. Walker JL, Zhai N, Zhang L, Bleaken BM, Wolff I, et al. (2010) Unique precursors for the mesenchymal cells involved in injury response and fibrosis. Proc Natl Acad Sci U S A 107: 13730–13735.
23. Gerhart J, Baytion M, DeLuca S, Getts R, Lopez C, et al. (2000) DNA dendrimers localize MyoD mRNA in presomitic tissues of the chick embryo. J Cell Biol 149: 825–834.
24. Gerhart J, Neely C, Stewart B, Perlman J, Beckmann D, et al. (2004) Epiblast cells that express MyoD recruit pluripotent cells to the skeletal muscle lineage. J Cell Biol 164: 739–746.
25. Gerhart J, Bast B, Neely C, Iem S, Amegbe P, et al. (2001) MyoD-positive myoblasts are present in mature fetal organs lacking skeletal muscle. J Cell Biol 155: 381–392.
26. Gerhart J, Scheinfeld VL, Milito T, Pfautz J, Neely C, et al. (2011) Myo/Nog cell regulation of bone morphogenetic protein signaling in the blastocyst is essential for normal morphogenesis and striated muscle lineage specification. Dev Biol 359: 12–25.
27. Gerhart J, Hayes C, Scheinfeld V, Chernick M, Gilmour S, et al. (2012) Myo/Nog cells in normal, wounded and tumor bearing skin. Exp Dermatol 21: 466–468.
28. Gerhart J, Neely C, Elder J, Pfautz J, Perlman J, et al. (2007) Cells that express MyoD mRNA in the epiblast are stably committed to the skeletal muscle lineage. J Cell Biol 178: 649–660.
29. Strony R, Gerhart J, Tornambe D, Perlman J, Neely C, et al. (2005) NeuroM and MyoD are expressed in separate subpopulations of cells in the pregastrulating epiblast. Gene Expr Patterns 5: 387–395.
30. George-Weinstein M, Gerhart J, Reed R, Flynn J, Callihan B, et al. (1996) Skeletal myogenesis: the preferred pathway of chick embryo epiblast cells in vitro. Dev Biol 173: 279–291.
31. Wormstone IM, Liu CS, Rakic JM, Marcantonio JM, Vrensen GF, et al. (1997) Human lens epithelial cell proliferation in a protein-free medium. Invest Ophthalmol Vis Sci 38: 396–404.
32. Ishizaki Y, Voyvodic JT, Burne JF, Raff MC (1993) Control of lens epithelial cell survival. J Cell Biol 121: 899–908.
33. Gerhart J, Baytion M, Perlman J, Neely C, Hearon B, et al. (2004) Visualizing the Needle in the Haystack: In Situ Hybridization With Fluorescent Dendrimers. Biol Proced Online 6: 149–156.
34. Pinney DF, Pearson-White SH, Konieczny SF, Latham KE, Emerson CP Jr (1988) Myogenic lineage determination and differentiation: evidence for a regulatory gene pathway. Cell 53: 781–793.
35. Tonegawa A, Takahashi Y (1998) Somitogenesis controlled by Noggin. Dev Biol 202: 172–182.
36. Valenzuela DM, Economides AN, Rojas E, Lamb TM, Nunez L, et al. (1995) Identification of mammalian noggin and its expression in the adult nervous system. J Neurosci 15: 6077–6084.
37. Isaacs WB, Cook RK, Van Atta JC, Redmond CM, Fulton AB (1989) Assembly of vimentin in cultured cells varies with cell type. J Biol Chem 264: 17953–17960.
38. Webster C, Silberstein L, Hays AP, Blau HM (1988) Fast muscle fibers are preferentially affected in Duchenne muscular dystrophy. Cell 52: 503–513.
39. Bader D, Masaki T, Fischman DA (1982) Immunochemical analysis of myosin heavy chain during avian myogenesis in vivo and in vitro. J Cell Biol 95: 763–770.
40. Kintner CR, Brockes JP (1984) Monoclonal antibodies identify blastemal cells derived from dedifferentiating limb regeneration. Nature 308: 67–69.
41. Jin J, Lin J C, Lin JJ-C (1989) Troponin T isoform switching during heart development. Ann NY Acad Sci 588: 393–396.
42. Alizadeh A, Clark J, Seeberger T, Hess J, Blankenship T, et al. (2003) Targeted deletion of the lens fiber cell-specific intermediate filament protein filensin. Invest Ophthalmol Vis Sci 44: 5252–5258.
43. Alizadeh A, Clark JI, Seeberger T, Hess J, Blankenship T, et al. (2002) Targeted genomic deletion of the lens-specific intermediate filament protein CP49. Invest Ophthalmol Vis Sci 43: 3722–3727.
44. Yoon KH, Blankenship T, Shibata B, Fitzgerald PG (2008) Resisting the effects of aging: a function for the fiber cell beaded filament. Invest Ophthalmol Vis Sci 49: 1030–1036.
45. Dodd J, Morton SB, Karagogeos D, Yamamoto M, Jessell TM (1988) Spatial regulation of axonal glycoprotein expression on subsets of embryonic spinal neurons. Neuron 1: 105–116.
46. Jagla K, Dolle P, Mattei MG, Jagla T, Schuhbaur B, et al. (1995) Mouse Lbx1 and human LBX1 define a novel mammalian homeobox gene family related to the Drosophila lady bird genes. Mech Dev 53: 345–356.
47. Hales AM, Chamberlain CG, McAvoy JW (1995) Cataract induction in lenses cultured with transforming growth factor-beta. Invest Ophthalmol Vis Sci 36: 1709–1713.
48. de Iongh RU, Lovicu FJ, Overbeek PA, Schneider MD, Joya J, et al. (2001) Requirement for TGFbeta receptor signaling during terminal lens fiber differentiation. Development 128: 3995–4010.
49. Dawes LJ, Eldred JA, Anderson IK, Sleeman M, Reddan JR, et al. (2008) TGF beta-induced contraction is not promoted by fibronectin-fibronectin receptor interaction, or alpha SMA expression. Invest Ophthalmol Vis Sci 49: 650–661.
50. Sharma N, Pushker N, Dada T, Vajpayee RB, Dada VK (1999) Complications of pediatric cataract surgery and intraocular lens implantation. J Cataract Refract Surg 25: 1585–1588.
51. Baratz KH, Cook BE, Hodge DO (2001) Probability of Nd:YAG laser capsulotomy after cataract surgery in Olmsted County, Minnesota. Am J Ophthalmol 131: 161–166.
52. Boureau C, Lafuma A, Jeanbat V, Smith AF, Berdeaux G (2009) Cost of cataract surgery after implantation of three intraocular lenses. Clin Ophthalmol 3: 277–285.

53. Apple DJ, Solomon KD, Tetz MR, Assia EI, Holland EY, et al. (1992) Posterior capsule opacification. Surv Ophthalmol 37: 73–116.
54. Findl O, Buehl W, Bauer P, Sycha T (2007) Interventions for preventing posterior capsule opacification. Cochrane Database Syst Rev: CD003738.
55. Bertelmann E, Kojetinsky C (2001) Posterior capsule opacification and anterior capsule opacification. Curr Opin Ophthalmol 12: 35–40.
56. Hay ED (1995) An overview of epithelio-mesenchymal transformation. Acta Anat (Basel) 154: 8–20.
57. Lim J, Thiery JP (2012) Epithelial-mesenchymal transitions: insights from development. Development 139: 3471–3486.
58. Nieto MA (2011) The ins and outs of the epithelial to mesenchymal transition in health and disease. Annu Rev Cell Dev Biol 27: 347–376.
59. Rock JR, Barkauskas CE, Cronce MJ, Xue Y, Harris JR, et al. (2011) Multiple stromal populations contribute to pulmonary fibrosis without evidence for epithelial to mesenchymal transition. Proc Natl Acad Sci U S A 108: E1475–1483.
60. Kriz W, Kaissling B, Le Hir M (2011) Epithelial-mesenchymal transition (EMT) in kidney fibrosis: fact or fantasy? J Clin Invest 121: 468–474.
61. Barth PJ, Westhoff CC (2007) CD34+ fibrocytes: morphology, histogenesis and function. Curr Stem Cell Res Ther 2: 221–227.
62. Gabbiani G (2003) The myofibroblast in wound healing and fibrocontractive diseases. J Pathol 200: 500–503.
63. De Wever O, Demetter P, Mareel M, Bracke M (2008) Stromal myofibroblasts are drivers of invasive cancer growth. Int J Cancer 123: 2229–2238.
64. Sappino AP, Schurch W, Gabbiani G (1990) Differentiation repertoire of fibroblastic cells: expression of cytoskeletal proteins as marker of phenotypic modulations. Lab Invest 63: 144–161.
65. Schaart G, Pieper FR, Kuijpers HJ, Bloemendal H, Ramaekers FC (1991) Baby hamster kidney (BHK-21/C13) cells can express striated muscle type proteins. Differentiation 46: 105–115.
66. Ogata I, Saez CG, Greenwel P, Ponce Mde L, Geerts A, et al. (1993) Rat liver fat-storing cell lines express sarcomeric myosin heavy chain mRNA and protein. Cell Motil Cytoskeleton 26: 125–132.
67. Mayer DC, Leinwand LA (1997) Sarcomeric gene expression and contractility in myofibroblasts. J Cell Biol 139: 1477–1484.
68. Woodcock-Mitchell J, Mitchell JJ, Low RB, Kieny M, Sengel P, et al. (1988) Alpha-smooth muscle actin is transiently expressed in embryonic rat cardiac and skeletal muscles. Differentiation 39: 161–166.
69. Michael R, Vrensen GF, van Marle J, Lofgren S, Soderberg PG (2000) Repair in the rat lens after threshold ultraviolet radiation injury. Invest Ophthalmol Vis Sci 41: 204–212.
70. Maddala R, Deng PF, Costello JM, Wawrousek EF, Zigler JS, et al. (2004) Impaired cytoskeletal organization and membrane integrity in lens fibers of a Rho GTPase functional knockout transgenic mouse. Lab Invest 84: 679–692.
71. Andjelic S, Zupancic G, Perovsek D, Hawlina M (2011) Human anterior lens capsule epithelial cells contraction. Acta Ophthalmol 89: e645–653.

Identification and Functional Analysis of GJA8 Mutation in a Chinese Family with Autosomal Dominant Perinuclear Cataracts

Dongmei Su[1]❡, Zhenfei Yang[2]❡, Qian Li[1], Lina Guan[1], Huiling Zhang[1], Dandan E[1], Lei Zhang[1], Siquan Zhu[2]*, Xu Ma[1]*

1 Department of Genetics, National Research Institute for Family Planning, Beiing, China, **2** Capital Medical University,Beijing Ophthalmology and Visual Sciences Key Lab, Beijing, China

Abstract

Congenital cataract is a clinically and genetically heterogeneous group of eye disorders that causes visual impairment and childhood blindness. The purpose of this study was to identify the genetic defect associated with autosomal dominant congenital perinuclear cataract in a Chinese family. A detailed family history and clinical data of the family were recorded, and candidate gene sequencing was performed to screen for mutation-causing disease in our study. Direct sequencing revealed a c.601G>A (p.E201K) transversion in exon 2 of GJA8. This mutation co-segregated with all affected individuals in the family and was not found in unaffected family members or 100 unrelated controls. The function and mechanism of novel GJA8 point mutation E201K in Chinese patients were then investigated in this study. We found E201K aberrantly located in cytoplasm and prevented its location in the plasma membrane. Induction of E201K expression led to a decrease in cell growth and viability by MTT (3-(4,5-Dimethylthiazol-2-yl)-2,5-diphenyltetrazolium bromide) assay. Our study provides important evidence that GJA8 is a disease-causing gene for congenital cataract and that mutation of GJA8 has a potential causative effect.

Editor: Andreas R. Janecke, Innsbruck Medical University, Austria

Funding: This research was supported by grants from the Central Public-interest Scientific Institution Basal Research Fund (Grant No. 2010GJSSJKA07). The funders had no role in study design, data collection and analysis, decision to publish, or preparation of the manuscript.

Competing Interests: The authors have declared that no competing interests exist.

* E-mail: jswkysgc@126.com (XM); siquanzhu@sina.com (SZ)

❡ These authors contributed equally to this work.

Introduction

Congenital cataract is the most common cause of treatable childhood blindness. More than 1 million blind children in Asia suffer from cataract [1]. Genetically, autosomal dominant inheritance (ADCC) is the most common mode of transmission, and nearly a third of cases show a positive family history [2,3]. The prevalence of congenital cataracts is 1 to 6 per 10,000 live births [4]. Approximately half are inherited, either in isolation or as part of a syndrome of ocular or systemic anomalies [2].The penetrance of congenital cataract is almost complete but expressivity is highly variable. According to morphology, congenital cataracts can be classified into several subtypes: sutural, pulverulent, whole lens, nuclear, lamellar(also referred to as perinuclear), cortical, polar, cerulean, coralliform, and other minor subtypes [5,6]. These cataract subtypes can result from mutations at different genetic loci and can have different inheritance patterns.

To date, more than 30 independent loci and 20 cataract-related genes have been identified as being associated with isolated autosomal dominant congenital cataract (ADCC). Several genes are highly expressed in the lens and have been associated with congenital cataracts that can be considered as candidate genes for hereditary cataracts. And these genes include gap junction protein, alpha 3, *(GJA3)*, and gap junction protein, alpha 8, *(GJA8)*; crystallins such as αA-crystallin (CRYAA), βA1-crystallin (CRYBA1), βB1-crystallin (CRYBB1), βB2-crystallin (CRYBB2), γC-crystallin (CRYGC), γD-crystallin (CRYGD) and γS-crystallin (CRYGS), intrinsic member protein (LIM2), and major intrinsic protein (MIP), cytoskeletal proteins, such as beaded filament structural protein 1 (BFSP1), beaded filament structural protein 2 (BFSP2), transcription factors, such as paired-like homeodomain 3 (PITX3), heat shock transcription factor 4 (HSF4), Maf-like protein gene (MAF), and paired box gene 6 (PAX6), and others, such as chromatin modifying protein 4B (CHMP4B) and Eph-receptor type-A2 (EPHA2) and so on[7–12].

In this study, we applied a functional candidate approach to test the known genes in a Chinese family. A novel missense mutation in GJA8 was identified to be responsible for the cataracts in the family. Functional analysis showed that mutation of GJA8 prevented its location in the plasma membrane and led to a decrease in cell growth and proliferation. These results suggest the novel missense mutation in GJA8 may contribute to the development of nuclear cataract.

Methods

Family Data and Clinical Examination

The three generation Chinese cataract family was recruited from Beijing tongren hospital, capital medical University, Beijing, China. The research was approved by the ethics committee of

Capital Medical University. Informed consent was obtained from all participants of the family, from Guangdong province. The study protocol followed the principles of the Declaration of Helsinki.

Detailed family medical history was recorded by interviewing the family members. All participating members underwent ophthalmic examination including visual acuity, slit lamp examination, intraocular pressure measurement, ultrasonography, fundus examination of the dilated pupil. Slit-lamp photography was performed to document the phenotype of the cataract patients. 100 unrelated subjects without cataracts were recruited from the Ophthalmology Clinic of Beijing Tongren Hospital as normal controls. They were given complete ophthalmologic examinations and did not have eye diseases except mild myopia.

Clinical Examination and Isolation of Genomic DNA

About 2 ml of peripheral blood was collected from the family members who took part in the study. Genomic DNA was extracted from blood using the QIAamp Blood kit (Qiagen, Valencia, CA).

Mutation Screening

We used the functional candidate gene analysis approach, 11 candidate genes, including CRYAA, CRYAB, CRYBA1, CRYBB1, CRYBB2, CRYGC, CRYGD, CRYGS, GJA3, GJA8, MIP, HSF4, and BFSP2 were analyzed. Each exon and intron-exon junction of the genes were amplified by polymerase chain reaction (PCR) with primers listed in Table 1. The PCR products of proband were sequenced using ABI 3730 Automated Sequencer (PE Biosystems, Foster City, CA). The sequencing results were analyzed using Chromas 2.33 (http://www.technelysium.com.au/chromas.html) and compared to the reference sequence in the NCBI (http://www.ncbi.nlm.nih.gov/) database.

Bioinformatics Analysis

The amino acid sequences of GJA8 from several different species were obtained from NCBI GenBank and conservation analysis was performed by CLC Main Workbench Software (Aarhus, Denmark). The function impact of the mutation was predicted by PolyPhen (http://genetics.bwh.harvard.edu/pph2/).

Cell Culture and Transfection

The cell lines Hela were maintained in Iscove's modified Dulbecco's medium supplemented with 10% fetal bovine serum, 100 mg/ml penicillin and 100 mg/ml streptomycin in a humidified atmosphere containing 5% CO_2 at 37°C. Transfection was carried out using Lipofectamine 2000 (Invitrogen Corporation, Carlsbad, CA, USA).

Western Blotting

Total proteins were extracted from Hela cells transfected with GJA8-WT-GFP (wild-type), GJA8-E201K-GFP and GFP vector plasmids. After electrophoresis, a polyvinylidene fluoride membrane was incubated with anti-β-actin antibody (Sigma) and anti-GFP (Abcam). The signals were visualized by using the chemiluminescent substrate method with the SuperSignal West Pico kit provided by Pierce Co.

Subcellular Localization

Hela cells were seeded in six-well tissue culture plates 24 h prior to transfection at approximately 60% confluency. GFP-GJA8 expression constructs containing wild-type or mutants were transfected using Lipofectamine 2000, according to the manufacturer's instructions. Forty-eight hours after transfection, the cells were then analyzed by fluorescence microscopy.

Cell Proliferation and MTT (3-(4,5-Dimethylthiazol-2-yl)-2,5-diphenyltetrazolium bromide) Assay

The protocol is adapted from literature methods [13,14]. Briefly, After transfection, Iscove's modified Dulbecco's medium was supplemented with 5 mg/ml MTT (3-(4,5-Dimethylthiazol-2-yl)-2,5-diphenyltetrazolium bromide) solution for 4 h at 37°C. Thereafter, the medium was aspirated, and the formazan product was solubilized with 100 µl of methyl sulfoxide MTT solution was removed. Viability was assessed by measuring the absorbance at 492 nm with microplatereader.

Results

Clinical Evaluation

Eleven family members of a three-generation cataract Chinese family participated in the study (five affected and six unaffected individuals) (Fig. 1A). All patients in this pedigree had bilateral cataracts. The spectrum of all patients belong to lamellar (perinuclear) cataracts, which is an subtype of congenital cataracts. Most patients experienced decreased visual acuity at 3 years of age, followed by a gradual decrease in visual acuity until surgery was required. The proband, who was a 22-year-old boy, had decreased vision at 3 years of age and was diagnosed with bilateral lamellar (perinuclear) cataract at the age of 22. Slit-lamp examination revealed opacification of perinuclear cataract with opacities involving the nucleus (Fig. 1B). His best corrected visual acuity was 0.3/0.4.

Mutation Analysis

We identified a transversion of G>A at c.601 in exon 2 of *GJA8* in all affected individuals via direct gene sequencing of the coding regions of the candidate genes (Fig .2A). However, we did not find this mutation in any unaffected family members, or in the 100 unrelated control individuals (Fig. 2B). We found no further gene mutations in individuals from the studied family, except for a few nonpathogenic single nucleotidepolymorphisms (SNPs).

Bioinformatics Analysis

The c.601G>A mutation resulted in a substitution of glutamic acid (Glu) with Lysine (Lys) at the 201st amino acid position (E201K). CLC Main Workbench Software revealed that the Glu at the 201st amino acid position is highly conserved among many species (Fig. 3). Furthermore, the structure and function impact of the GJA8 E201K mutation was predicted by PolyPhen (http://genetics.bwh.harvard.edu/pph2/), and the result indicated that E201K could probably be damaging, with a score of 0.999 [15,16].

Functional Analysis

The amount of each of the in-vitro translated wild-type and mutant GJA8 proteins were detected by western blot analysis with anti-GFP antibody (Fig. 4A). The GJA8 WT and GJA8 E201K mutant proteins were expressed at similar levels in western blot analysis of the cell lysates, indicating that mutation did not result in the expression or instability of the protein.

We then examined the subcellular location of GJA8 wild-type and mutant protein. Subcellular localization was determined using C-terminal GFP fusion constructs of mutant and wild-type GJA8, followed by fluorescence microscopy. GFP as a control was located in the nucleus and cytoplasm and GJA8 WT was mainly detected in the plasma membrane (Fig. 4B). GJA8 E201K was aberrantly located in the cytoplasm, indicating that E201K mutation of GJA8 prevented its location in the plasma membrane.

To test directly whether expression of GJA8 mutation had a deleterious effect on cell growth or proliferation, we compared the

Table 1. Primers used for PCR.

Name	Forward (5′–3′)	Reverse (5′–3′)
CRYAA-1	AGCAGCCTTCTTCATGAGC	CAAGACCAGAGTCCATCG
CRYAA-2	GGCAGGTGACCGAAGCATC	GAAGGCATGGTGCAGGTG
CRYAA-3	GCAGCTTCTCTGGCATGG	GGGAAGCAAAGGAAGACAGA
CRYAB-1	AACCCCTGACATCACCATTC	AAGGACTCTCCCGTCCTAGC
CRYAB-2	CCATCCCATTCCCTTACCTT	GCCTCCAAAGCTGATAGCAC
CRYAB-3	TCTCTCTGCCTCTTTCCTCA	CCTTGGAGCCCTCTAAATCA
CRYBA1–1	GGCAGAGGGAGAGCAGAGTG	CACTAGGCAGGAGAACTGGG
CRYBA1–2	AGTGAGCAGCAGAGCCAGAA	GGTCAGTCACTGCCTTATGG
CRYBA1–3	AAGCACAGAGTCAGACTGAAGT	CCCCTGTCTGAAGGGACCTG
CRYBA1–4	GTACAGCTCTACTGGGATTG	ACTGATGATAAATAGCATGAACG
CRYBA1–5	GAATGATAGCCATAGCACTAG	TACCGATACGTATGAAATCTGA
CRYBA1–6	CATCTCATACCATTGTGTTGAG	GCAAGGTCTCATGCTTGAGG
CRYBB1–1	CCCTGGCTGGGGTTGTTGA	TGCCTATCTGCCTGTCTGTTTCTC
CRYBB1–2	TAGCGGGGTAATGGAGGGTG	AGGATAAGAGTCTGGGGAGGTGG
CRYBB1–3	CCTGCACTGCTGGCTTTTATTTA	TCTCCAGAGCCCAGAACCATG
CRYBB1–4	CCAACTCCAAGGAAACAGGCATA	CCTCCCTACCCACCATCATCTC
CRYBB1–5	TAGACAGCAGTGGTCCCTGGAGA	AGCACTGGGAGACTGTGGAAGG
CRYBB1–6	CCTAGAAAAGGAAACCGAGGCC	AGCGAGGAAGTCACATCCCAGTA
CRYBB2–1	GTTTGGGGCCAGAGGGGAGTGGT	TGGGCTGGGGAGGGACTTTCAGTA
CRYBB2–2	CCTTCAGCATCCTTTGGGTTCTCT	GCAGTTCTAAAAGCTTCATCAGTC
CRYBB2–3	GTAGCCAGGATTCTGCCATAGGAA	GTGCCCTCTGGAGCATTTCATAGT
CRYBB2–4	GGCCCCCTCACCCATACTCA	CTTCCCTCCTGCCTCAACCTAATC
CRYBB2–5	CTTACCCTTGGGAAGTGGCAATGG	TCAAAGACCCACAGCAGACAAGTT
CRYGC-1	TGCATAAAATCCCCTTACCG	CCTCCCTGTAACCCACATTG
CRYGC-2	TGGTTGGACAAATTCTGGAAG	CCCACCCCATTCACTTCTTA
CRYGD-1	CAGCAGCCCTCCTGCTAT	GGGTCCTGACTTGAGGATGT
CRYGD-2	GCTTTTCTTCTCTTTTTATTTCTGG	AAGAAAGACACAAGCAAATCAGT
CRYGS-2	GAAACCATCAATAGCGTCTAAATG	TGAAAAGCGGGTAGGCTAAA
CRYGS-3	AATTAAGCCACCCAGCTCCT	GGGAGTACACAGTCCCCAGA
CRYGS-4	GACCTGCTGGTGATTTCCAT	CACTGTGGCGAGCACTGTAT
GJA3–1	CGGTGTTCATGAGCATTTTC	CTCTTCAGCTGCTCCTCCTC
GJA3–2	GAGGAGGAGCAGCTGAAGAG	AGCGGTGTGCGCATAGTAG
GJA3–3	TCGGGTTCCCACCCTACTAT	TATCTGCTGGTGGGAAGTGC
GJA8–1	CCGCGTTAGCAAAAACAGAT	CCTCCATGCGGACGTAGT
GJA8–2	GCAGATCATCTTCGTCTCCA	GGCCACAGACAACATGAACA
GJA8–3	CCACGGAGAAAACCATCTTC	GAGCGTAGGAAGGCAGTGTC
GJA8–4	TCGAGGAGAAGATCAGCACA	GGCTGCTGGCTTTGCTTAG
MIP-1	GTGAAGGGGTTAAGAGGC	GGAGTCAGGGCAATAGAG
MIP-2,3	CGGGGAAGTCTTGAGGAG	CACGCAGAAGGAAAGCAG
MIP-4	CCACTAAGG TGGCTGGAA	CTCATGCCCCAAAACTCA
HSF4–1	CATCCCATCCAGCCAGCCTTTTC	GGGCATGGGTGTTCACTGACGT
HSF4–2	CCTCGACCCATATCCCCGTAAG	GCAGGAGCAAGGCAGGCAGTC
HSF4–3	GCGGGAATGAGCAAAGAGGAGG	GCCAAGGCAGGAGAGAGGAAGG
HSF4–4	TCCCCAGCCTCGCCATTCT	CCCGGTGAAGGAGTTTCCAGAG
HSF4–5	GCTGGGGCCTGAGGGAG	GGCTTCCATCTTCTCTTCCTTTT
BFSP2 (1a)	AATGCACAAACCCAAATGGT	AGGCCCTGSSGACACT
BFSP2 (1b)	GAGAGGCGAGTGGTAGTGGA	GGCCTCAGCCTACTCACAAC
BFSP2 (2)	TGCAGACAGAGCATTTCCAC	GAGGGGTGTGAGCTGGATAA
BFSP2 (3)	GCTGCAATTGCCTTCATTTT	GGGTAACCTGACCCAACTTCA

Table 1. Cont.

Name	Forward (5′–3′)	Reverse (5′–3′)
BFSP2 (4)	TCTGTGAAGCCTGTGTCTGG	CCCGGCCTCAATTATTCTTT
BFSP2 (5)	ACCCAGGAGGAGGAGGTTGT	GGGAATCCCCTGGAAACTAA
BFSP2 (6)	GGGGAATAGTCCAGGCTACC	ATGGGTGCCTATGTGAGAGGG
BFSP2 (7)	TTGTTCCAAAGGCCAGATTC	CACTCAAGGGAATCCTTCCA

effects of induced GJA8 WT and GJA8 E201K expression on cell numbers. As shown in Fig. 4C, a dramatic decrease in cell numbers was observed when comparing GJA8 E201K-transfected cells with GJA8 WT- transfected cells. Quantitation of these results revealed that the number of cells transfected with GJA8 E201K was only about 60% of that observed in cells transfected with GJA8 WT (Fig. 4D). Similarly, induction of GJA8 E201K expression dramatically reduced cell viability compared to GJA8 WT cells by MTT assay (Fig. 4E).

Discussion

In this study we identified a novel G>A mutation of *GJA8* in a three-generation Chinese pedigree, which was associated with perinuclear opacities of the lens involving the nucleus. This mutation co-segregated with the phenotype and was not found in 100 unrelated control individuals.

Perinuclear cataracts affect the regions of the perinucleus, but the nucleus is clear. Perinuclear cataracts may occur in isolation or are associated with opacities involving other lens regions. However, genes associated with perinuclear cataract were not clearly identified. Mutations in *GJA8* have been considered as cataractogenesis in humans. To date, 17 mutations in this gene have been identified to contribute to assorted phenotypic cataracts [29]. In this study, we identified a novel mutation, c.601G>A in *GJA8*, which was associated with perinuclear cataract in a Chinese family.

Our study showed that GJA8WT protein was mainly detected in the plasma membrane, whereas GJA8E201K was aberrantly located in the cytoplasm. GJA8 belong to the connexin gene family [17]. Each connexin includes cytoplasmic amino and carboxyl termini as well as four transmembrane domains linked by a single cytoplasmic loop and two extracellular domains, E1 and E2 [18,19], which are thought to play a role in connexon docking and channel gating. E201K mutation of GJA8 located in the second extracellular domains and the 201st residue is quite near the transmembrane domain. The cytoplasmic location of GJA8E201K mutant protein may be explained by the proximity of the E201K residue to the fourth transmembrane domain of GJA8.

GJA8, an important component of gap junction channels, plays an important role in intercellular communication and transfer of molecules [20]. The lens is an avascular organ dependent on gap junction-mediated transportation of ion gradients and metabolic materials and intercellular communication for organ function and homeostasis [21–24]. In our study, we found that induction of GJA8E201K expression dramatically reduced cell viability and proliferation compared to GJA8WT cells. At the cellular level,

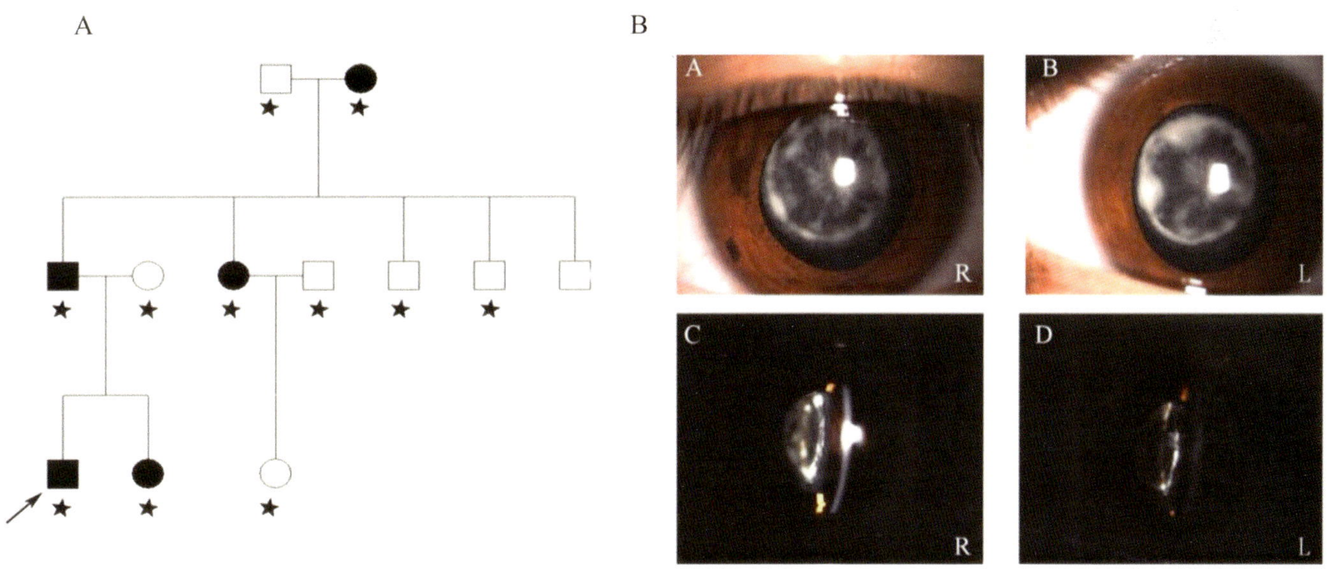

Figure 1. Clinical evaluation of A Chinese family with autosomal dominant cataracts. (A) A Chinese family that has had autosomal dominant cataracts. The arrow indicates the proband. Pedigree of a Chinese three-generation family with autosomal dominant cataract. The black symbols indicate individuals with a diagnosis of congenital cataract performed by genetic analysis. The arrow indicates the proband. The asterisk indicates family members who attended this study. (B) *Slit-lamp photographs of the proband.* A and C in the photograph: Slit-lamp photographs of the proband (III:1) show perinuclear cataract in the right eye. B and D in the photograph: The photographs of the proband (III:1) show perinuclear cataract involving the nucleus of the left eye.

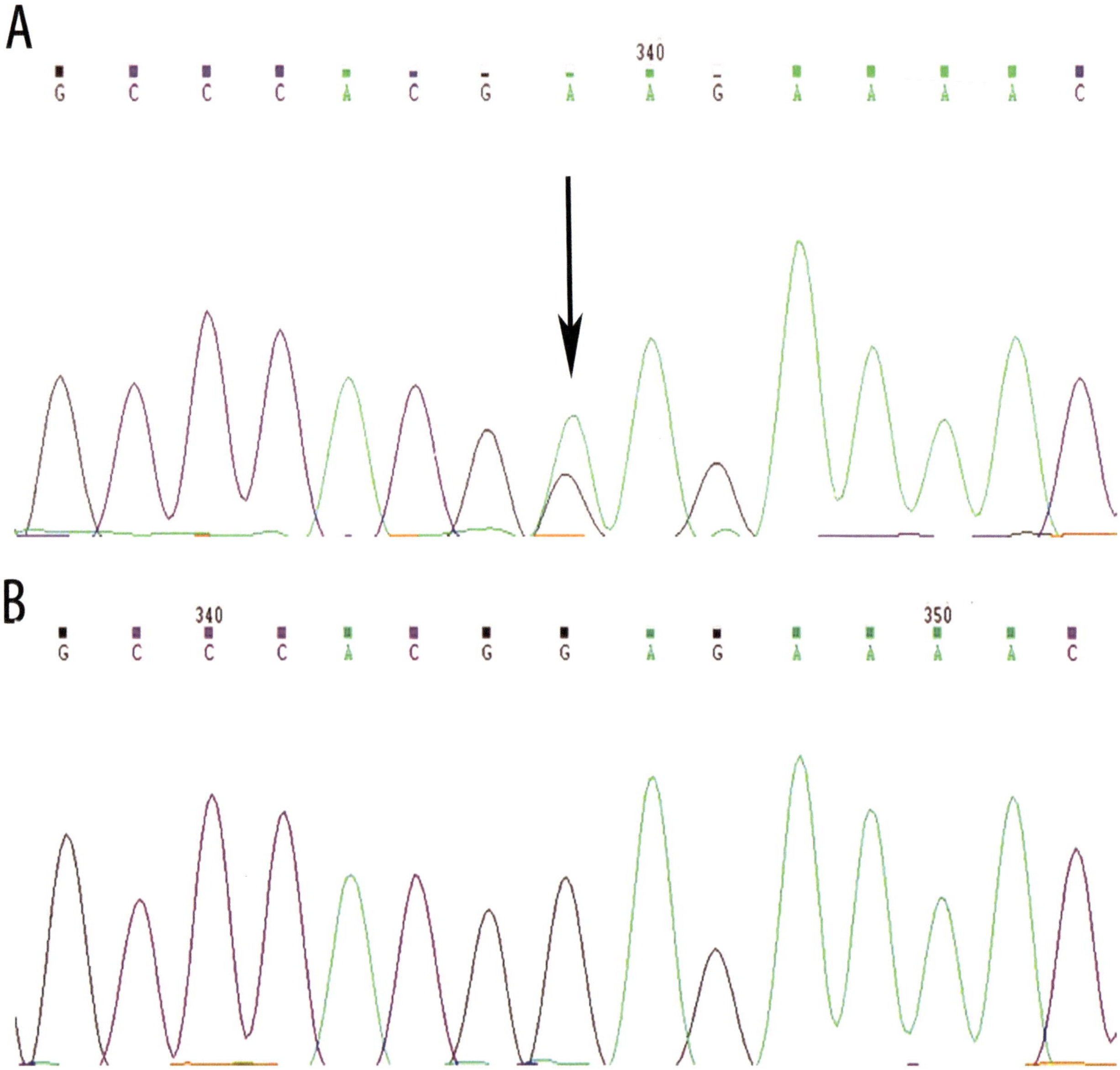

Figure 2. Partial sequence of GJA8 at exon2. A: Sequence of affected individual. In panel A, the heterozygous mutation c.601G>A was identified in all affected participants. B: Sequence of unaffected individual.

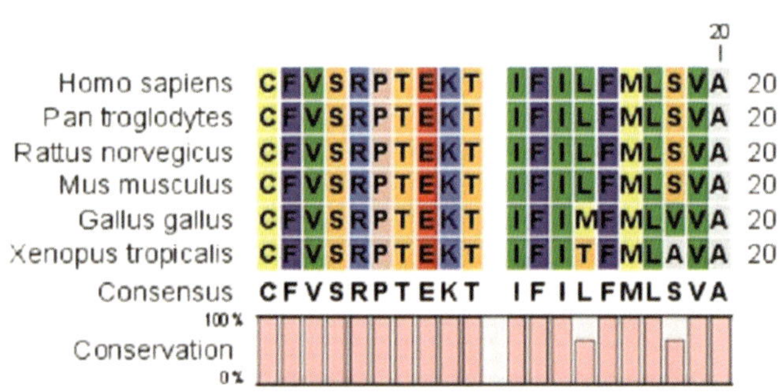

Figure 3. A multiple-sequence alignment of the amino acid sequence in GJA8 from different species. The alignment data indicates that the Glu at the 201st amino acid position is highly conserved among many species (indicated by an arrow).

GJA8E201K aberrant location may lead to capacity deficiency of GJA8E201K to form functional hemichannels, and trigger a complex sequence of events including loss of membrane potential, disruption of transmembrane ion gradients, and subsequent decreased metabolic activity, and finally decreased cell growth.

Our data showed that induction of GJA8 E201K expression for 72 hours led to a decrease in the number of cells and reduction of cell viability. Recent studies have shown that gap junctional coupling provided through wild-type GJA8 had been implicated in cell proliferation. Peter et al had showed that G46V mutation of GJA8 decreased the viability of cells obtaining GJA8 G46V protein. Our in-vitro over-expression of the GJA8 E201K mutation has a similar toxic effect on cell growth as reported for other GJA8 mutations [25–29], however we cannot exclude that in-vivo, the effect of the p.E201K mutation might be mediated by its mislocalization in the cytoplasm, being unable to contribute to the cell metabolism in the lens.

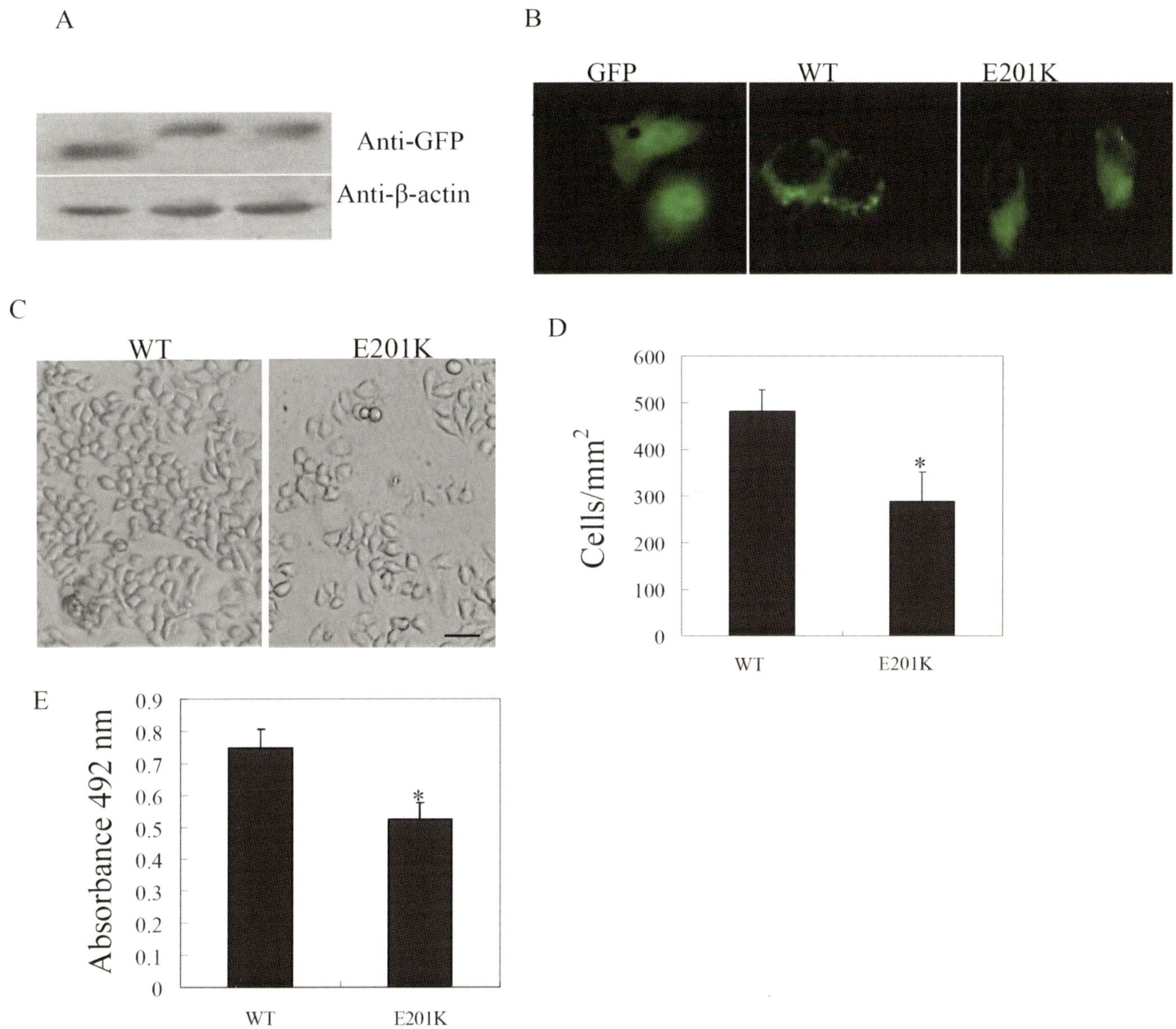

Figure 4. Functional analysis of GJA8 mutation. (A) Western blotting of wild-type and mutant GJA8. Hela cells were transfected with GJA8WT and GJA8E201K expression plasmids, respectively and western blotting was performed with GFP antibody. (B) Subcellular localization of GJA8. GFP-GJA8 expression constructs containing wild-type or mutant were transfected into Hela cells using Lipofectamine 2000. Localization of wild-type and mutant GJA8 GFP-fusion protein in transfected Hela cells was viewed using a fluorescent microscope. (C) Induction of GJA8E201K protein expression decreased the number of cells. Phase contrast photomicrographs from cells containing wild-type or mutant GJA8. GJA8WT (left panel) and GJA8E201K (right panel) cells were observed using a phase contrast microscope after transfection for wild-type and mutant GJA8 expression plasmids for 72 hours. Bar, 100 μm. (D) Graph shows the quantitation of these data as mean ± S.E.M. of the number of cells containing wild-type or mutant GJA8, respectively. *, $p<0.05$; **, $p<0.01$ ($n=3$). (E) Induction of GJA8E201K protein expression decreased the viability of cells by MTT assay. Cells were transfected with wild-type and mutant GJA8 vectors for 3 days and cell viability was tested using MTT assay.

Acknowledgments

We thank the patients and their families for participation in this study. We are grateful to all the people who helped us successfully complete the research.

Author Contributions

Conceived and designed the experiments: DS XM. Performed the experiments: ZY LG HZ DE LZ. Analyzed the data: QL. Contributed reagents/materials/analysis tools: ZY SZ. Wrote the paper: DS.

References

1. Francis PJ, Berry V, Bhattacharya SS, Moore AT (2000) The genetics of childhood cataract. J Med Genet 37: 481–8.
2. Francis PJ, Moore AT (2004) Genetics of childhood cataract. Curr Opin Ophthalmol15: 10–5.
3. Reddy MA, Francis PJ, Berry V, Bhattacharya SS, Moore AT(2004) Molecular genetic basis of inherited cataract and associated phenotypes. Surv Ophthalmol 49: 300–15.
4. Holmes JM, Leske DA, Burke JP, Hodge DO (2003) Birth prevalence of visually significant infantile cataract in a defined U.S. population. Ophthalmic Epidemiol. Apr;10(2): 67–74.

5. Zhang LY, Yam GH, Tam PO, Lai RY, Lam DS, et al. (2009) An αA-crystallin gene mutation, Arg12Cys, causing inherited cataract-microcornea exhibits an altered heat-shock response. Mol Vis 15: 1127–1138.
6. Zhang Q, Guo X, Xiao X, Yi J, Jia X, et al. (2004) Clinical description and genome wide linkage study of Y-sutural cataract and myopia in a Chinese family. Mol Vis10: 890–900.
7. de Figueirêdo ES, de Vasconcellos JP, Arieta CE, de Melo MB (2011) Novel human CRYGD rare variant in a Brazilian family with congenital cataract. Mol Vis 17: p. 2207–11.
8. Hejtmancik JF (2008) Congenital cataracts and their molecular genetics. Semin Cell Dev Biol; 19: 134–49.
9. Burdon KP, Wirth MG, Mackey DA, Russell-Eggitt IM, Craig JE, et al (2004) Investigation of crystallin genes in familial cataract, and report of two disease associated mutations. Br J Ophthalmol; 88: 79–83.
10. Vanita V, Hennies HC, Singh D, Nürnberg P, Sperling K, et al (2006) A novel mutation in GJA8 associated with autosomal dominant congenital cataract in a family of Indian origin. Mol Vis; 12: 1217–22.
11. Boyadjiev SA, Justice CM, Eyaid W, McKusick VA, Lachman RS, et al (2003) A novel dysmorphic syndrome with open calvarial sutures and sutural cataracts maps to chromosome 14q13-q21. Hum Genet; 113: 1–9.
12. Zhu Y, Shentu X, Wang W, Li J, Jin C, et al (2010) Chinese family with progressive childhood cataracts and IVS3+1G>A CRYBA3/A1 mutations. Mol Vis16: 2347–53.
13. Buch K, Peters T, Nawroth T, Sänger M, Schmidberger H, et al (2012) Determination of cell survival after irradiation via clonogenic assay versus multiple MTT Assay–a comparative study. Radiat Oncol. Jan 3; 7: 1.
14. Price P, McMillan TJ (1990) Use of the tetrazolium assay in measuring the response of human tumor cells to ionizing radiation. Cancer Res. Mar 1;50(5): 1392–6.
15. Bennett TM, Shiels A (2011) A recurrent missense mutation in GJA3 associated with autosomal dominant cataract linked to chromosome 13q. Mol Vis.;17: 2255–62.
16. Need AC, Shashi V, Hitomi Y, Schoch K, Shianna KV, et al (2012) Clinical application of exome sequencing in undiagnosed genetic conditions. J Med Genet. Jun;49(6): 353–61.
17. Gerido DA, White TW (2004) Connexin disorders of the ear, skin, and lens. Biochim Biophys Acta 1662: 159–170.
18. Bruzzone R, White TW, Paul DL (1996) Connections with connexins: the molecular basis of direct intercellular signaling. Eur J Biochem 238: 1–27.
19. Harris AL (2001) Emerging issues of connexin channels: biophysics fills the gap. Q Rev Biophys 34: 325–472.
20. White TW, Bruzzone R, Goodenough DA, Paul DL (1992) Mouse Cx50, a functional member of the connexin family of gap junction proteins, is the lens fiber protein MP70. Mol Biol Cell 3: 711–720.
21. Francis P, Berry V, Bhattacharya S, Moore A (2000) Congenital progressive polymorphic cataract caused by a mutation in the major intrinsic protein of the lens, MIP (AQP0). Br J Ophthalmol 84(12): p.1376–9.
22. Willecke K, Eiberger J, Degen J, Eckardt D, Romualdi A, et al (2002) Structural and functional diversity of connexin genes in the mouse and human genome. Biol Chem 383: 725–737.
23. Beahm DL, Hall JE (2002) Hemichannel and junctional properties of connexin 50. Biophys J 82: 2016–2031.
24. Klein BE, Howard KP, Sivakumaran TA, Klein R (2012) The relationship of cataract and cataract extraction to age-related macular degeneration: the Beaver Dam Eye Study. Ophthalmology 119(8): 1628–33.
25. Minogue PJ, Tong JJ, Arora A, Russell-Eggitt I, Hunt DM, et al (2009) A mutant connexin50 with enhanced hemichannel function leads to cell death. Invest Ophthalmol Vis Sci. Dec;50(12): 5837–45.
26. Tong JJ, Minogue PJ, Guo W, Chen TL, Beyer EC, et al (2011) Different consequences of cataract-associated mutations at adjacent positions in the first extracellular boundary of connexin50. Am J Physiol Cell Physiol. May;300(5): C1055–64.
27. Breitman ML, Clapoff S, Rossant J, Tsui LC, Glode LM, et al (1987) Genetic ablation: targeted expression of a toxin gene causes microphthalmia in transgenic mice. Science 238: 1563–1565.
28. Landel CP, Zhao J, Bok D, Evans GA (1988) Lens-specific expression of recombinant ricin induces developmental defects in the eyes of transgenic mice. Genes Dev 2: 1168–1178.
29. Hu S, Wang B, Zhou Z, Zhou G, Wang J, et al (2010) A novel mutation in GJA8 causing congenital cataract-microcornea syndrome in a Chinese pedigree. Mol Vis 16: 1585–1592.

Age-Related Cataract, Cataract Surgery and Subsequent Mortality: A Systematic Review and Meta-Analysis

E Song[1¶], Hongpeng Sun[2¶], Yong Xu[2], Yana Ma[2], Hong Zhu[2], Chen-Wei Pan[2*]

1 Lixiang Eye Hospital of Soochow University, Suzhou, China, **2** School of Public Health, Medical College of Soochow University, Suzhou, China

Abstract

Purpose: Changes in lens may reflect the status of systemic health of human beings but the supporting evidences are not well summarized yet. We aimed to determine the relationship of age-related cataract, cataract surgery and long-term mortality by pooling the results of published population-based studies.

Methods: We searched PubMed and Embase from their inception till March, 2014 for population-based studies reporting the associations of any subtypes of age-related cataract, cataract surgery with all-cause mortality. We pooled the effect estimates (hazards ratios [HRs]) under a random effects model.

Results: Totally, we identified 10 unique population-based studies including 39,659 individuals at baseline reporting the associations of any subtypes of cataract with all-cause mortality from 6 countries. The presence of any cataract including cataract surgery was significantly associated with a higher risk of death (pooled HR: 1.43, 95% CI, 1.21, 2.02; $P<0.001$; $I^2=64.2\%$). In the meta-analysis of 9 study findings, adults with nuclear cataract were at higher risks of mortality (pooled HR: 1.55, 95% CI, 1.17, 2.05; $P=0.002$; $I^2=89.2\%$). In the meta-analysis of 8 study findings, cortical cataract was associated with higher risks of mortality (pooled HR: 1.26, 95% CI, 1.12, 1.42; $P<0.001$, $I^2=29.7\%$). In the meta-analysis of 6 study findings, PSC cataract was associated with higher risks of mortality (pooled HR: 1.37, 95% CI, 1.04, 1.80; $P=0.03$; $I^2=67.3\%$). The association between cataract surgery and mortality was marginally non-significant by pooling 8 study findings (pooled HR: 1.27, 95% CI, 0.97, 1.66; $P=0.08$; $I^2=76.6\%$).

Conclusions: All subtypes of age-related cataract were associated with an increased mortality with nuclear cataract having the strongest association among the 3 cataract subtypes. However, cataract surgery was not significantly related to mortality. These findings indicated that changes in lens may serve as markers for ageing and systemic health in general population.

Editor: Yingfeng Zheng, Zhongshan Ophthalmic Center, China

Funding: The authors have no support or funding to report.

* Email: pcwonly@gmail.com

These authors also contributed equally to this work.

Introduction

Visual impairment (VI) is a global health burden, associated with increased mortality in different ethnic groups [1–5]. Age-related cataract, including nuclear, cortical and posterior subcapsular (PSC) cataract, is a leading cause of visual impairment worldwide [6–13]. Although age-related cataract seems to increase the risk of death, the relationship of different cataract subtypes and mortality remains unclear. It is important for clinicians and ophthalmologists to understand the associations between different cataract subtypes and mortality as the pathophysiology, treatment and impact on visual functioning of the 3 subtypes are different [14]. A clearer understanding of the relationship between cataract subtypes and mortality may provide further insights into the pathogenesis of these conditions. In addition, if a specific subtype of cataract is associated with increased mortality, lens imaging targeting this subtype may be a useful tool for the assessment of systemic health and ageing of the whole body. This research question is also of great importance from public health perspectives regarding the increasing burden of cataract throughout the world. The question of whether age-related cataracts are associated with an increased risk of death or whether the association between increased mortality and the occurrence of the cataract is caused simply by the relationship with higher age is unclear.

To address this gap, we conducted a systematic review and meta-analysis to examine the association between different subtypes of age-related cataract, cataract surgery and long term mortality from available population-based studies.

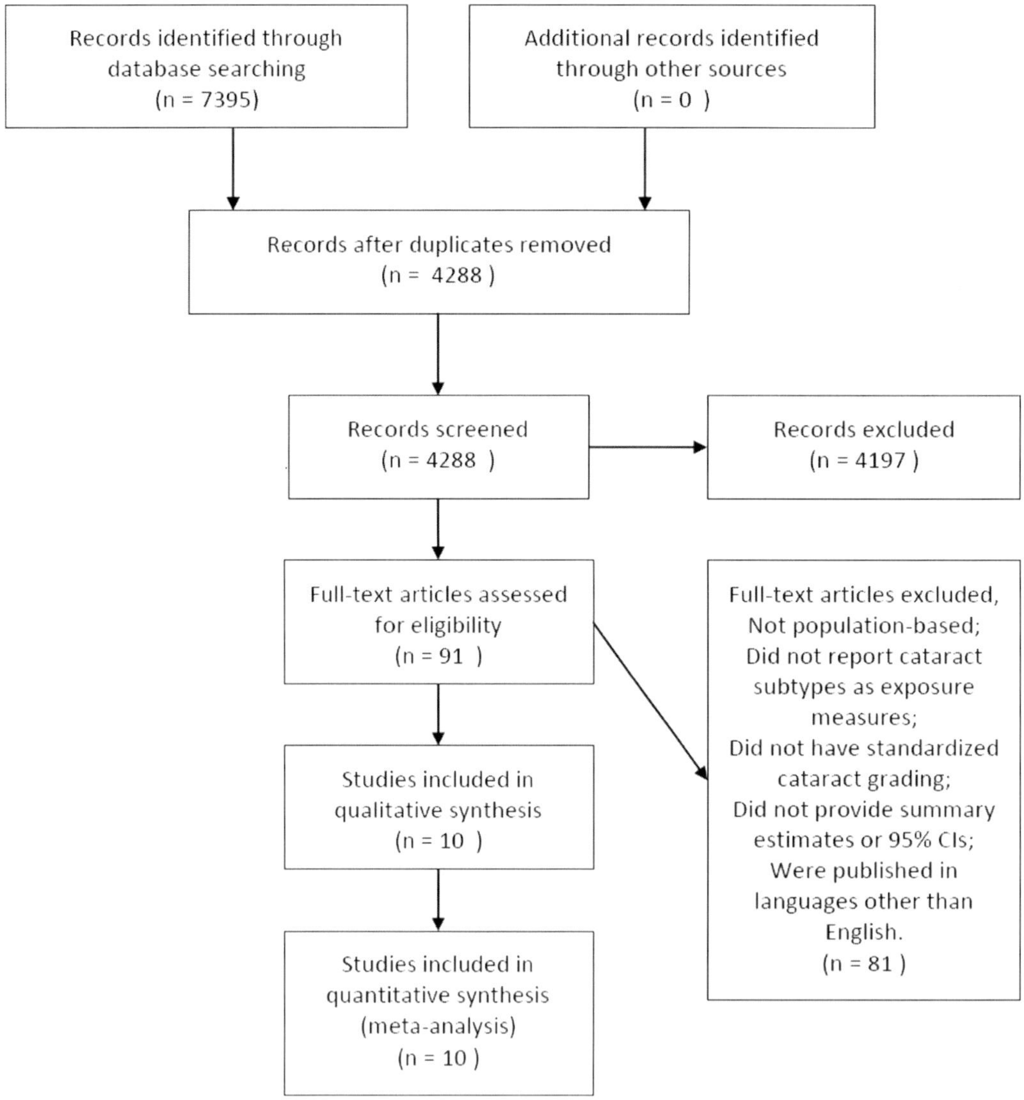

Figure 1. Flow diagram showing the selection process for inclusion of studies.

Methods

Ethnics Statement

The study was approved by the Ethics Committee, Medical College of Soochow University and followed the tenets of the Declaration of Helsinki.

Search Strategy and Inclusion Criteria

The method for performing this meta-analysis is similar with our previously work on overweight/obesity and cataract [15]. We performed this systematic review and meta-analysis to examine the association of different subtypes of age-related cataract, cataract surgery and mortality based on the Meta-analysis of Observational Studies in Epidemiology guidelines [16]. We searched the electronic databases of PubMed and Embase for relevant papers reporting the longitudinal association of age-related cataract, cataract surgery with all-cause mortality published up to March, 2014 with the following search terms (formatted for PubMed search): ((“vision, low”[MeSH Terms] OR (“vision”[All Fields] AND “low”[All Fields]) OR “low vision”[All Fields] OR (“visual”[All Fields] AND “impairment”[All Fields]) OR “visual impairment”[All Fields] OR “vision disorders”[MeSH Terms] OR (“vision”[All Fields] AND “disorders”[All Fields]) OR “vision disorders”[All Fields] OR (“visual”[All Fields] AND “impairment”[All Fields])) OR (“cataract”[MeSH Terms] OR “cataract”[All Fields]) OR (“cataract”[MeSH Terms] OR “cataract”[All Fields] OR (“lens”[All Fields] AND “opacity”[All Fields]) OR “lens opacity”[All Fields]) OR (“cataract extraction”[MeSH Terms] OR (“cataract”[All Fields] AND “extraction”[All Fields]) OR “cataract extraction”[All Fields]) OR (“cataract extraction”[MeSH Terms] OR (“cataract”[All Fields] AND “extraction”[All Fields]) OR “cataract extraction”[All Fields] OR (“cataract”[All Fields] AND “surgery”[All Fields]) OR “cataract surgery”[All Fields])) AND ((“mortality”[Subheading] OR “mortality”[All Fields] OR “mortality”[MeSH Terms]) OR (“mortality”[Subheading] OR “mortality”[All Fields] OR “survival”[All Fields] OR “survival”[MeSH Terms]) OR (“death”[MeSH Terms] OR “death”[All Fields])). Titles and abstracts of the studies were independently reviewed by 2 authors (ES and HPS). All duplicate articles were removed. Inconsistencies during the literature search

Table 1. Characteristics of the included studies.

Author (year)	Study Name	Location	Ethnicity	Sample Size at baseline	Age at baseline (years)	Follow up period (yrs)	Incidence of mortality: N (%)
Knudtson et al (2006)	The Beaver Dam Eye Study	United States	Whites	4926	43–84	14	1576 (32)
Nucci et al (2004)	The Priverno Eye Study	Italy	Italians	860	45–69	7	44 (5.1)
Clemons et al (2004)	The Age-Related Eye Disease Study	United States	Whites	4753	55–81	9	534 (11)
Cugati et al (2007)	The Blue Mountains Eye Study	Australia	Whites	3654	≥49	11	1051 (28.9)
Hennis et al (2000)	The Barbados Eye Study	United States	Blacks	4709	40–84	4	306 (6.8)
Borger et al (2003)	The Rotterdam Study	Netherlands	Whites	6339	≥55	7	1359 (21.4)
West et al (2004)	The Salisbury Eye Project	United States	Whites and Blacks	2520	65–84	2	147 (5.8
Xu et al (2009)	The Beijing Eye Study	China	Chinese	4439	≥40	5	143 (3.2)
McCarty et al (2001)	Melbourne Visual Impairment Project	Australia	White	3271	40–98	5	231 (7.1)
Khanna et al (2013)	The Andhra Pradesh Eye Diseases Study	India	Indians	4188	≥30	11	799 (19.1)

were resolved by consensus and the reference lists of all identified studies were screened.

We included studies if they were population-based, reported any subtypes of age-related cataract or cataract surgery as an independent variable and all-cause mortality as the outcome measure. The Age-Related Eye Disease Study [1] is a multi-center intervention trial rather than a population-based observational study, which has reported the association between major age-related eye diseases and mortality. As the study participants covered a wide geographical areas and the sample size was large, we feel the results should be included in the meta-analysis. We only included studies in which age-related cataract was assessed based on standardized protocols. Furthermore, we included studies only if the summary estimates such as the relative risk (RR) or hazards ratios (HR) with 95% confidence interval (CI) were reported in the paper, or allowed for calculation based on the data presented in the paper. We summarized the measures of association as HR for all the studies. We excluded studies if they were not population-based, did not have standardized cataract grading, or were published in languages other than English. If one study reported two results at different follow-up periods, the result with a longer follow-up period was included in the analysis.

Data Extraction and Assessment of Study Quality

For each study in the analyses, information on first author, publication year, study name, study location, ethnic group, sample size at baseline, age range of the study participants at baseline, follow-up periods, definitions of age-related cataract and mortality, summary estimates and corresponding 95% CI, and confounding factors adjusted for were extracted and recorded in a form designed previously.

The study quality were assessed using the tool described by Sanderson et al [17]. The variables examined included the methods for selecting study participants, methods for measuring exposure (age-related cataract or cataract surgery) and outcome variable (all-cause mortality), design-specific sources of bias, methods for controlling confounding, statistical methods and conflict of interest.

Statistical Methods for the Meta-analysis

The meta-analysis was performed using Stata version 12.0 (StataCorp, College Station, TX). We meta-analyzed the fully-adjusted study-specific risk estimates under random effects model, accounting for both within and between study variability. All-cause mortality was treated as the outcome measure while nuclear, cortical, PSC cataract or cataract surgery were analyzed as the independent variable. Statistical heterogeneity among studies was evaluated using I^2 Statistic [18]. Values of 0 to 24%, 25% to 49%, 50% to 74%, and more than 75% denote no, low, moderate, and high heterogeneity, respectively [19]. Publication bias was assessed using the Egger regression asymmetry test and the Begg's test.

Results

Literature Search and Characteristics of Included Studies

The literature search yielded 4288 unique titles from the two electronic databases. In total, 91 articles were retrieved for full-text review, 12 of which met all the predefined inclusion criteria. However, two studies reported 2 results at different follow-up periods [2,5,20–21] and only the result with a longer follow-up period were included. Finally, 10 unique population-based studies [1–2,21–28] were included in this meta-analysis. (**Figure 1**)

Characteristics of the 10 studies included in the meta-analysis are summarized in **Table 1**. Among the 10 studies, 2 were

Table 2. Assessment of methodological quality of included studies.

Study	Methods for selecting study participants	Methods for measuring exposure (cataract)	Methods for measuring outcome (mortality)	Design-specific sources of bias	Methods for controlling confounding, and statistical methods	Conflict of Interest
Knudtson et al (2006)	4926 persons aged from 43 to 84 years in the period from September 15, 1987, to May 4, 1988, participated in the baseline examination of the population-based Beaver Dam Eye Study and were followed by about 10 years.	Wisconsin Grading System	National Death Index was used for matching against national death data.	Lost to follow up bias; survival bias; chance finding; residual confounding	Adjustments for age, sex, proteinuria, history of cancer, BMI, ratio of total to high-density lipoprotein cholesterol level, smoking, pulse rate,diabetes status, cardiovascular disease history, sedentary lifestyle, education, and systolic blood pressure were made using Cox proportional hazards models	None reported
Nucci et al (2004)	860 legal residents of Priverno represented 70% of a random sample selected to participate in the Di.S.Co. Project—a population-based study on cardiovascular risk factors carried out by the Italian National Institute of Health.	Slit-lamp examination	Review of municipality records	Lack of statistical power; lost to follow up bias; survival bias; chance finding; residual confounding	Adjusting for age, gender, diabetes, serum cholesterol, high-density lipoprotein cholesterol, and cardiovascular diseases using Cox proportional-hazards regression model.	None reported
Clemons et al (2004)	A total of 4757 persons aged 55 to 81 years at enrollment were entered into the study at 11 clinical centers between 1992 and 1998 and were followed up by 9 years	The Age-Related Eye Disease Study (AREDS) system	Hospital records and death certificates.	Lost to follow up bias; chance finding; residual confounding	Cox proportional-hazards regression model adjusting for age, sex, race, education, smoking status, body mass index, diabetes mellitus, angina, cancer, and hypertension	None reported
Cugati et al (2007)	Australian adults aged 49 years and older at baseline in the Blue Mountains area were followed up for about 11 years	Wisconsin Grading System	The Australian National Death Index data	Lost to follow up bias; survival bias; chance finding; residual confounding	Cox regression models assessed associations between cataract and mortality risk during 11 years after adjusting for age, sex, BMI, hypertension, diabetes mellitus, current smoking, and history of stroke, angina, or myocardial infarction	None reported
Hennis et al (2000)	The studies were based on a simple random sample of Barbados African Americans, 40 to 84 years old. 4631 persons completed baseline examinations at the study site. Surviving members of the cohort were invited to return for a 4-year follow-up visit.	Lens Opacities Classification System II	Ministry of Health records	Lost to follow up bias; survival bias; chance finding; residual confounding	Cox proportional-hazards regression. age; gender; self-reported history of diabetes, cardiac disease, and stroke, or combination of these major illnesses; family history of diabetes and hypertension; body mass index; waist-to-hip ratio; alcohol use; and cigarette smoking.	None reported
Borger et al (2003)	A prospective cohort study of all residents aged 55 years and older from a suburb of Rotterdam	Lens Opacities Classification System II	Municipal registry and medical records.	Lost to follow up bias; chance finding; residual confounding	Cox proportional hazard regression analysis, adjusted for appropriate confounders (age, gender, smoking status, body mass index, cholesterol level, atherosclerosis, hypertension, history of cardiovascular disease, and diabetes mellitus)	None reported
West et al (2004)	A random sample of 2520 residents of Salisbury aged 65 to 84 years was recruited for a home interview and an examination at the SEE clinic. Two-year follow-up was conducted.	Wilmer grading scheme.	Hospital records and the National Death Index	Lost to follow up bias; survival bias; chance finding; residual confounding	Logistic regression model adjusting for age, sex, smoking, diabetes, cormorbid conditions and body mass index.	None reported
Xu et al (2009)	At baseline in 2001, the Beijing Eye Study examined 4439 subjects with an age of 40 years or more. In 2006, all study participants were invited for a follow-up examination.	The Age-Related Eye Disease Study (AREDS) system	Death certificate, hospital medical records	Lost to follow up bias; survival bias; chance finding; residual confounding	Logistic regression was used to investigate the associations of the binary dependent variable mortality with the continuous or categorical independent variables.	None reported

Table 2. Cont.

Study	Methods for selecting study participants	Methods for measuring exposure (cataract)	Methods for measuring outcome (mortality)	Design-specific sources of bias	Methods for controlling confounding, and statistical methods	Conflict of Interest
McCarty et al(2001)	Cluster random sampling was employed to identify nine pairs of census collector districts in the Melbourne statistical division from which to recruit eligible residents. Baseline examinations were conducted between 1992 and 1994. In 1997, 5 year follow up examinations of the original cohort commenced.	Wilmer grading scheme.	National Death Index	Lack of statistical power, lost to follow up bias; survival bias; chance finding; residual confounding	Multivariate logistic regression adjusting for age, sex, country of birth, smoking, hypertension, arthritis, best corrected visual acuity, age related maculopathy, glaucoma, uncorrected refractive error,diabetes,gout and cardiovascular disease.	None reported
Khanna et al (2013)	A large-scale prevalence survey of blindness and visual impairment was conducted between 1996–2000 on 10,293 individuals of all ages in three rural and one urban clusters in Andhra Pradesh, Southern India. More than a decade later, participants in rural clusters were traced to determine ocular risk factors for mortality.	Wilmer grading scheme.	Questionnaire	Lack of statistical power, lost to follow up bias; survival bias; chance finding; residual confounding	Cox-proportional hazard model after adjusting for age, gender, diabetes, hypertension, body mass index, smoking and education status	None reported

conducted in Asia [22–23], 2 were in Australia [21,24], 2 were in Europe [25–26] and the remaining 4 were in the United States [1–2,27–28]. The 10 cohort studies comprised a total of 39,659 individuals at baseline. The sample sizes at baseline ranged from 860 to 6,339. The follow-up periods ranged from 2 to 14 years. The range of mortality rates in all identified studies was very wide (from 3.2% to 32%), which may be due to methodological issues including various ages of enrollment at baseline, follow-up periods and ethnic groups.

Quality Assessment of the Included Studies

All studies graded cataract based on standardized protocols such as the Wisconsin grading system, the Wilmer grading system or the Lens Opacity Classification System [29–31]. In most of the included studies, mortality data were reviewed and retrieved from official records or hospital medical records. All studies adjusted for age in the multivariate analysis; however, diabetes, the most important confounding factor was not adjusted for in one study. All studies gave loss to follow-up rates and described sampling methods in the baseline examinations, albeit in varying degrees. However, only 6 studies outlined specific exclusion criteria and provided information on non-responders. Conflicts of interest were not reported in all included studies. The detailed assessment of study quality of the included study is described in **Table 2**.

Age-related cataract and mortality

Adults with any cataract or cataract surgery previously were more like to die (pooled HR: 1.43, 95% CI, 1.21, 2.02; $P<0.001$; $I^2=64.2\%$). In the meta-analysis of 9 study findings, adults with nuclear cataract were at higher risks of mortality (pooled HR: 1.55, 95% CI, 1.17, 2.05; $P=0.002$; $I^2=89.2\%$) (**Figure 2**). In the meta-analysis of 8 study findings, cortical cataract was associated with higher risks of mortality (pooled HR: 1.26, 95% CI, 1.12, 1.42; $P<0.001$, $I^2=29.7\%$) (**Figure 3**). In the meta-analysis of 6 study findings, PSC cataract was associated with higher risks of mortality (pooled HR: 1.37, 95% CI, 1.04, 1.80; $P=0.03$; $I^2=67.3\%$) (**Figure 4**). The association between cataract surgery and mortality was marginally non-significant by pooling 8 study findings (pooled HR: 1.27, 95% CI, 0.97, 1.66; $P=0.08$; $I^2=76.6\%$)(**Figure 5**). After excluding the Salisbury Eye Project with a follow-up period of only 2 years, all cataract subtypes were still associated with mortality (data not shown).

Table 3 shows the association between cataract and mortality by follow-up years of the identified studies and cataract diagnosis. The estimates were more robust in studies with longer follow-up periods or more standardized grading systems (graded by lens photographs).

There was no evidence of publication bias as indicated by a non-significant Egger test (all $P>0.05$) and Begg's test (all $P>0.05$) in all analyses.

Discussion

In this systematic review and meta-analysis of population-based studies, all subtypes of age-related cataract were associated with increased mortality with nuclear cataract having the strongest association among the 3 cataract subtypes. However, cataract surgery was not significantly related to mortality. These findings indicated that changes in lens may serve as markers for ageing and systemic health in the general population.

Our meta-analysis confirmed the longitudinal association between nuclear cataract (nuclear sclerosis of the lens) and increased mortality reported in previous studies. In addition, we found that the association of nuclear cataract with increased

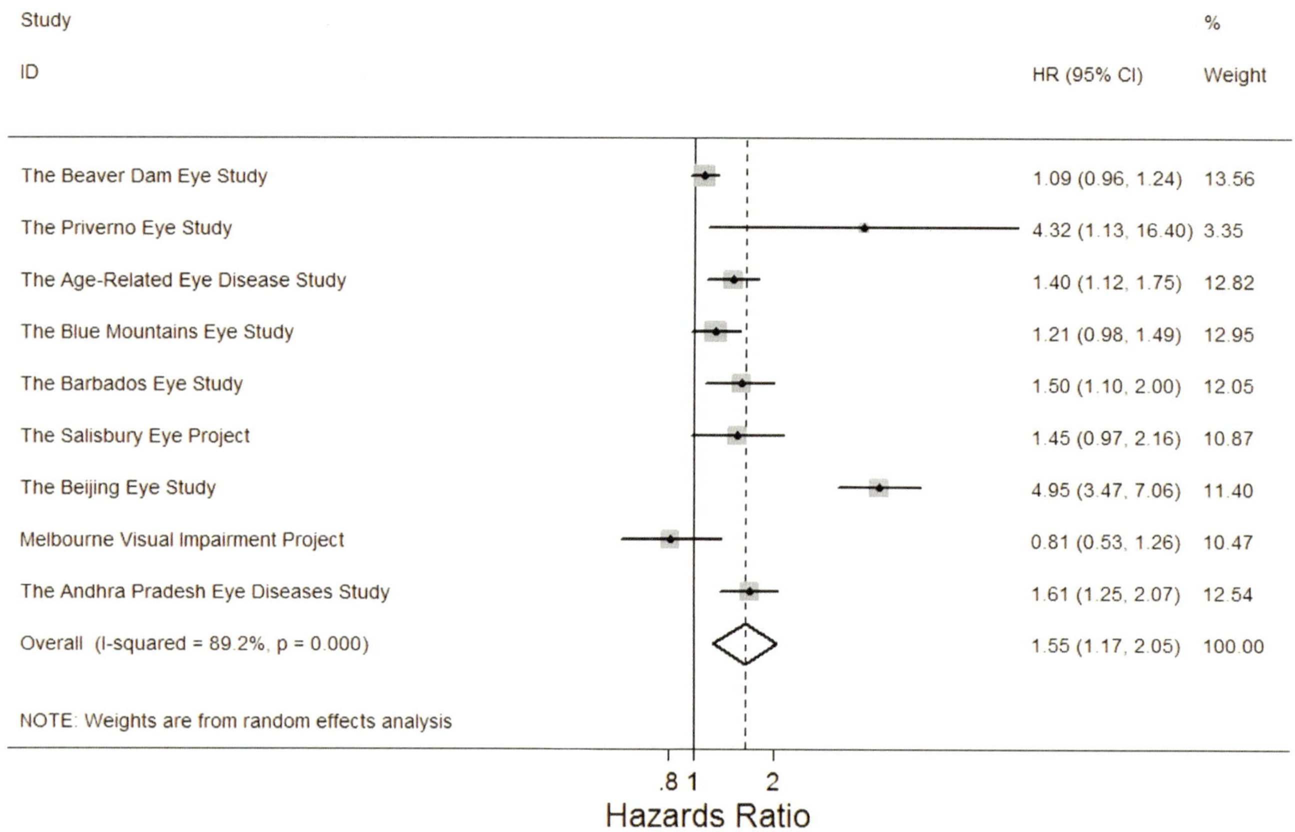

Figure 2. Random effects meta-analysis investigating the association between nuclear cataract and all-cause mortality. HR = hazards ratio; CI = confidence interval.

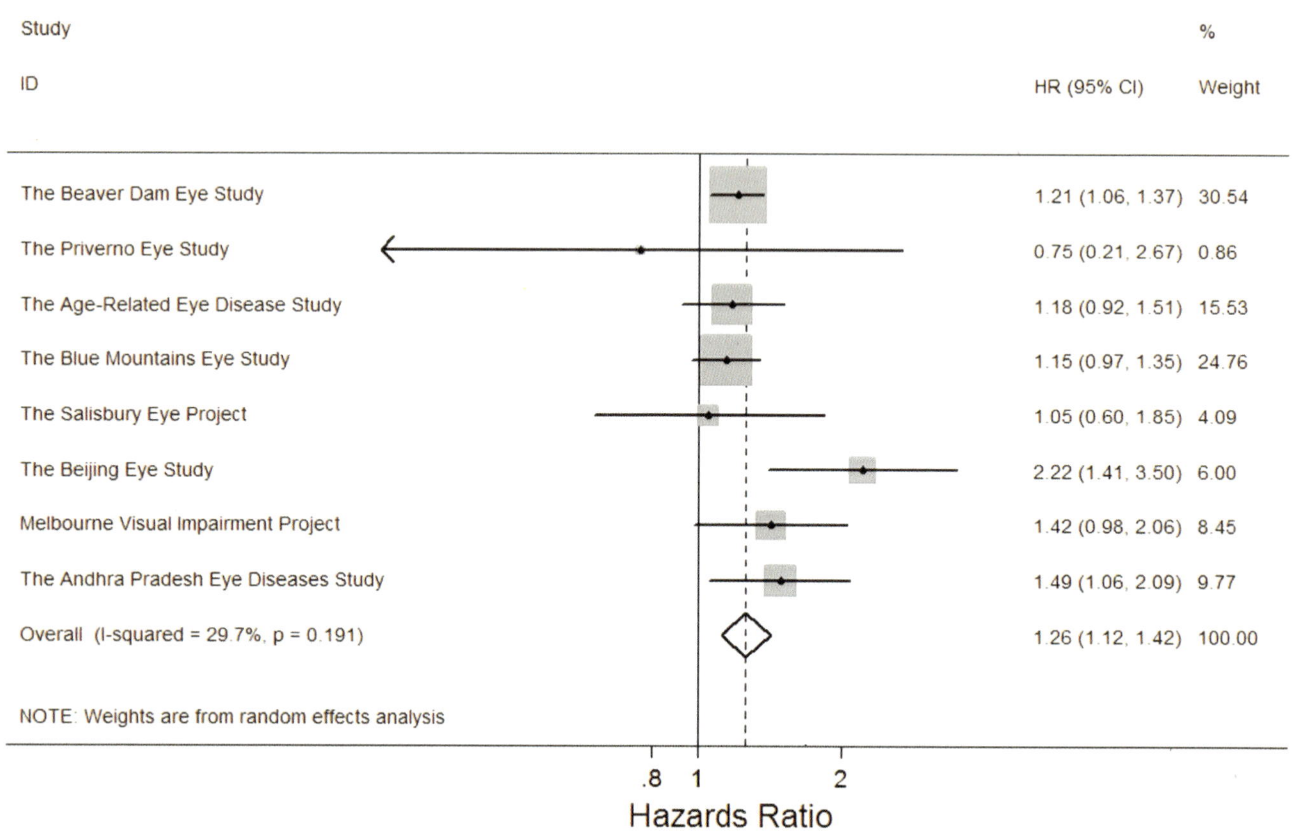

Figure 3. Random effects meta-analysis investigating the association between cortical cataract and all-cause mortality. HR = hazards ratio; CI = confidence interval.

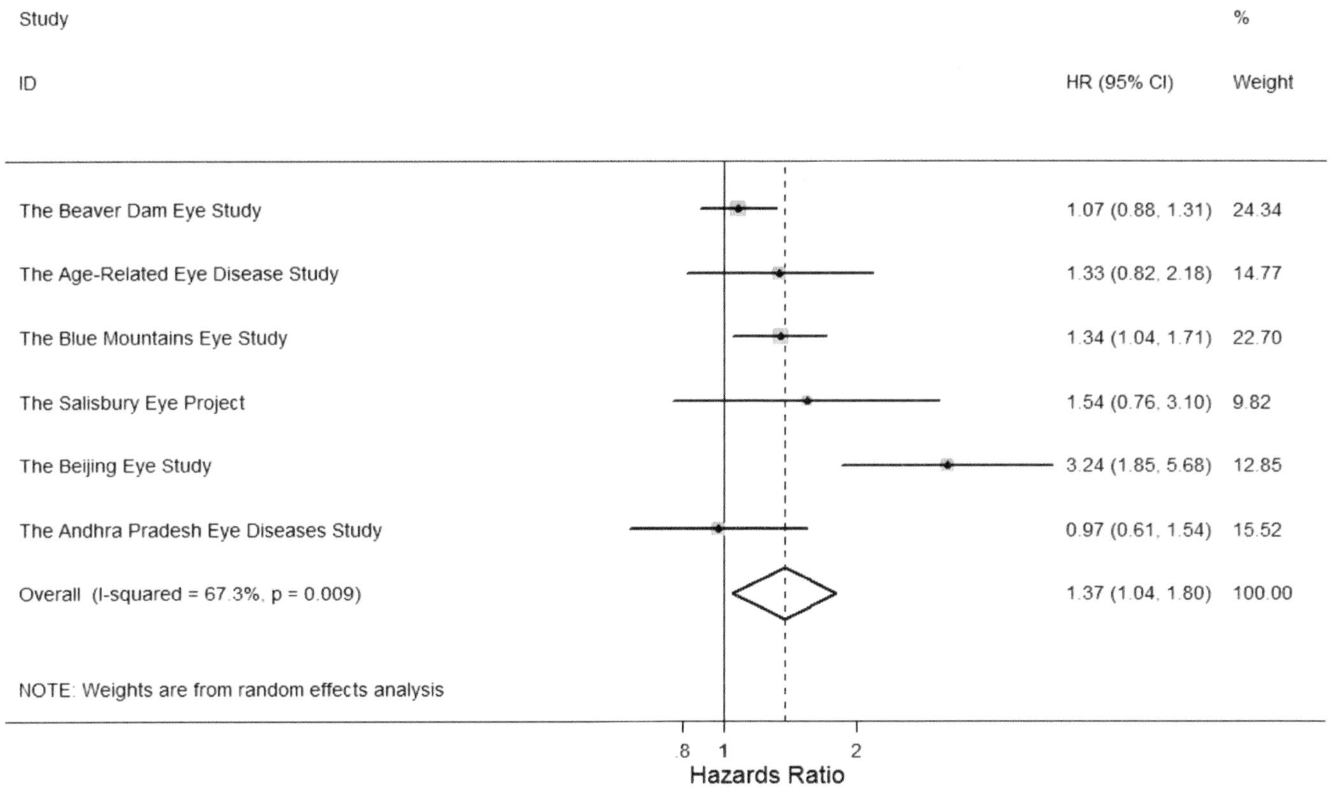

Figure 4. Random effects meta-analysis investigating the association between posterior subcapsular cataract and all-cause mortality. HR = hazards ratio; CI = confidence interval.

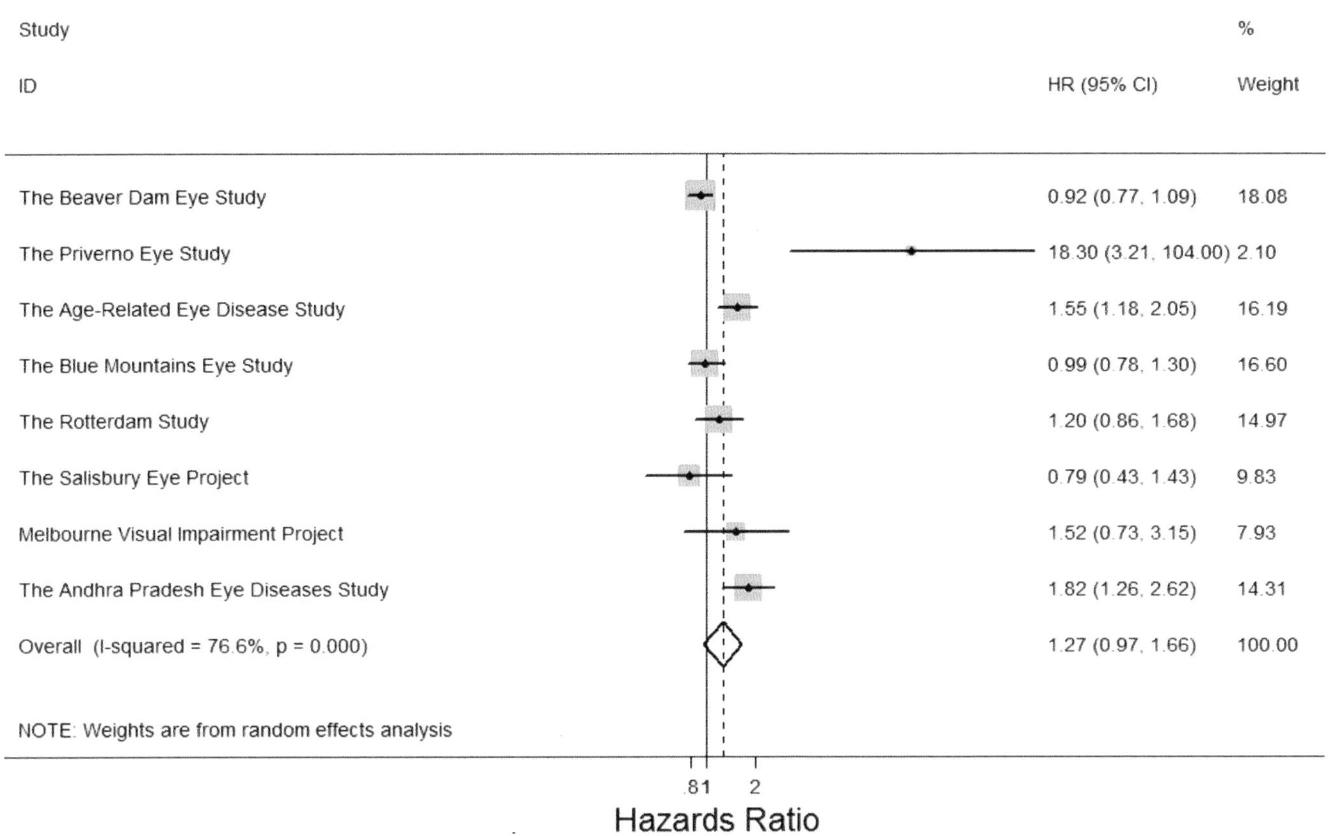

Figure 5. Random effects meta-analysis investigating the association between cataract surgery and all-cause mortality. HR = hazards ratio; CI = confidence interval.

Table 3. Association between cataract and mortality by follow-up years and cataract diagnosis.

	Nuclear cataract				Cortical Cataract				Posterior Subcapsular Cataract				Cataract Surgery			
	N	HR	95% CI	I2 (%)	N	HR	95% CI	I2 (%)	N	HR	95% CI	I2 (%)	N	HR	95% CI	I2 (%)
Follow-up years																
More than 5 years	5	1.32	1.09, 1.60	68.0	5	1.2	1.10, 1.32	0	4	1.16	1.01, 1.33	0	6	1.33	0.98,1.80	82.1
No more than 5 years	4	1.73	0.84, 3.56	93.6	3	1.52	1.03,2.25	55	2	2.31	1.12, 4.77	61.9	2	1.06	0.56,2.00	45.6
Cataract diagnosis																
By photographs	7	1.50	1.09, 2.06	91.5	7	1.27	1.13, 1.44	36	6	1.37	1.04, 1.80	67.3	6	1.2	0.92, 1.56	74.8
By Ophthalmologist clinically	2	2.07	0.80, 5.35	56.3	1	0.75	0.21, 2.67	-	0	-	-	-	2	4.08	0.29, 58.07	89

N = number of studies RR = hazards ratio CI = confidence interval.

mortality was strongest among all of the three cataract subtypes. Nuclear sclerosis of the lens may be a marker for changes in structural proteins of the whole body, mainly resulting from oxidation that cause diminished function [32]. For example, the levels of glutathione (GSH), one of the most important antioxidant agents of the lens, are found to be much higher in the outer cortex fiber cells where GSH is synthesized [33]. Reduced GSH reaches the lens nucleus by diffusion from the surface fiber cells through an abundant network of gap junctions [34]. With increasing age, a greater percentage of GSH is oxidized in the nucleus, making it more susceptible to oxidation [35]. Chronic oxidative stress, especially in brain and immune cells, could accelerate the rate of ageing, leading to an increased mortality in adults with nuclear cataract.

Compared with nuclear cataract, we found a weaker but significant association between cortical cataract and less survival. In the Blue Mountains Eye Study, the association between cortical cataract and increased mortality was no longer significant in persons without diabetes, indicating that the observed association may be confounded by the presence of diabetes [5]. Diabetes is one of the most consistent determinants for cortical cataract [36–38]. In this systematic review, most of the included studies have adjusted for the effect of diabetes in the multivariate analysis (**Table 2**), indicating that the association between cortical cataract and mortality may be, at least partially, independent. UV light exposure could increase the risk of cortical cataract [39]. Exposure to UV light, a known risk factor for cortical cataract, can lead to oxidative stress in the lens, which is a main cause for cortical cataract. This process is similar with other systemic causes of oxidative stress, which may increase the risk of systemic morbidity [40].

The association of PSC cataract and mortality was also positively significant in this meta-analysis although there were fewer studies reporting this association compared with other subtypes. At current stage, we were unable to provide a reasonable biological explanation for this observed association. Animal studies have demonstrated that injection of peroxidative substances into the vitreous resulted in the formation of PSC cataract [41], which may be mediated by peroxidative damage of the whole body.

We found a marginally non-significant association between cataract surgery and mortality, which may be a balanced effect of aged-related cataract and good knowledge of health. Adults who have undergone cataract surgery certainly had cataract previously, which may increase the risk of long term mortality. On the other hand, they tend to have better knowledge of health and healthier lifestyle compared with those who did not. For example, in the Beaver Dam Eye Study, adults with cataract surgery were more likely to take vitamin supplements [2]. Also, adults with previous cataract surgery may have better access to health care services. A clinical trial investigating the effect of cataract surgery on survival in cataract patients may be useful to confirm this finding.

Our meta-analysis may have some important clinical implications. Previous studies have shown that age-related cataract is associated with systemic comorbidities [42] and general functional decline [43] in older adults. We confirmed that these systemic comorbidities and functional decline are sufficient to cause death in the general population. Therefore, we propose that lens imaging may be a necessary clinical examination for normal heath screening of older adults and should not be limited only in eye clinics. Currently, there are various technologies [44–45] for lens imaging and it remains controversial which one is the best to quantify lens opacity in elderly adults.

There are several strengths of the meta-analysis. The qualities of the included studies were relatively high with population-based samples achieving reasonable follow-up rates and the use of standardized grading systems for age-related cataract. Limitations of this meta-analysis should also be acknowledged. First, the potential biases in the original studies, methodological issues and different strategies for adjusting for confounders could affect the results from this meta-analysis. The longitudinal association of age-related cataract and mortality may have been confounded by other unadjusted factors or selection bias. Second, different studies used different cataract grading system, sampling strategies, follow-up period, and ways of mortality measures, which would affect the estimates of mortality. These differences could have also contributed to the observed high heterogeneity across studies. Thirdly, most included studies only reported the association between cataract and all-cause mortality and therefore we were unable to summarize the association between cataract and the cause of mortality. Fourthly, the number of the contributing prospective studies was small and therefore, detailed subgroups analysis may not be feasible. Finally, although there was no evidence of publication bias as indicated by a non-significant Egger test and Begg's test, publication bias could still be of concern because studies that report statistically significant results are more likely to get published than studies that report non-significant results, and this could have distorted the findings of our meta-analyses.

In conclusion, this systematic review and meta-analysis confirmed a longitudinal associations of all age-related cataract subtypes but not cataract surgery with increased mortality. The association was strongest for nuclear cataract. Clinically, ophthalmologists and clinicians should be aware that lens imaging may be a useful tool for the assessment of ageing of the whole body.

Author Contributions

Conceived and designed the experiments: ES HS CWP. Performed the experiments: ES HS. Analyzed the data: HS YX YM. Contributed reagents/materials/analysis tools: CWP. Wrote the paper: ES HS YX YM HZ CWP.

References

1. Clemons TE, Kurinij N, Sperduto RD (2004) Associations of mortality with ocular disorders and an intervention of high-dose antioxidants and zinc in the Age-Related Eye Disease Study: AREDS Report No. 13. Arch Ophthalmol 122: 716–726.
2. Knudtson MD, Klein BE, Klein R (2006) Age-related eye disease, visual impairment, and survival: the Beaver Dam Eye Study. Arch Ophthalmol 124: 243–249.
3. Foong AW, Fong CW, Wong TY, Saw SM, Heng D, et al. (2008) Visual acuity and mortality in a chinese population. The Tanjong Pagar Study. Ophthalmology 115: 802–807.
4. Li Z, Sun D, Liu P, Zhang L, Bai J, et al. (2011) Visual impairment and mortality in a rural adult population (the Southern Harbin eye study). Ophthalmic Epidemiol 18: 54–60.
5. Wang JJ, Mitchell P, Simpson JM, Cumming RG, Smith W (2001) Visual impairment, age-related cataract, and mortality. Arch Ophthalmol 119: 1186–1190.
6. Duerksen R, Limburg H, Carron JE, Foster A (2003) Cataract blindness in Paraguay–results of a national survey. Ophthalmic Epidemiol 10: 349–357.
7. Dunzhu S, Wang FS, Courtright P, Liu L, Tenzing C, et al. (2003) Blindness and eye diseases in Tibet: findings from a randomised, population based survey. Br J Ophthalmol 87: 1443–1448.
8. Zheng Y, Lavanya R, Wu R, Wong WL, Wang JJ, et al. (2011) Prevalence and causes of visual impairment and blindness in an urban Indian population: the singapore Indian eye study. Ophthalmology 118: 1798–1804.
9. Thulasiraj RD, Nirmalan PK, Ramakrishnan R, Krishnadas R, Manimekalai TK, et al. (2003) Blindness and vision impairment in a rural south Indian population: The aravind comprehensive eye survey. Ophthalmology 110: 1491–1498.
10. Murthy GV, Gupta S, Ellwein LB, Munoz SR, Bachani D, et al. (2001) A population-based eye survey of older adults in a rural district of Rajasthan: I. Central vision impairment, blindness, and cataract surgery. Ophthalmology 108: 679–685.
11. Zhao J, Ellwein LB, Cui H, Ge J, Guan H, et al. (2010) Prevalence of vision impairment in older adults in rural China: the China Nine-Province Survey. Ophthalmology 117: 409–416, 416 e401.
12. Hyman L, Wu SY, Connell AM, Schachat A, Nemesure B, et al. (2001) Prevalence and causes of visual impairment in The Barbados Eye Study. Ophthalmology 108: 1751–1756.
13. Varma R, Ying-Lai M, Klein R, Azen SP (2004) Prevalence and risk indicators of visual impairment and blindness in Latinos: the Los Angeles Latino Eye Study. Ophthalmology 111: 1132–1140.
14. Chew M, Chiang PP, Zheng Y, Lavanya R, Wu R, et al. (2012) The impact of cataract, cataract types, and cataract grades on vision-specific functioning using Rasch analysis. Am J Ophthalmol 154: 29–38 e22.
15. Pan CW, Lin Y (2014) Overweight, Obesity, and Age-Related Cataract: A Meta-analysis. Optom Vis Sci 91: 478–483.
16. Stroup DF, Berlin JA, Morton SC, Olkin I, Williamson GD, et al. (2000) Meta-analysis of observational studies in epidemiology: a proposal for reporting. Meta-analysis Of Observational Studies in Epidemiology (MOOSE) group. JAMA 283: 2008–2012.
17. Sanderson S, Tatt ID, Higgins JP (2007) Tools for assessing quality and susceptibility to bias in observational studies in epidemiology: a systematic review and annotated bibliography. Int J Epidemiol 36: 666–676.
18. Higgins JP, Thompson SG, Deeks JJ, Altman DG (2003) Measuring inconsistency in meta-analyses. BMJ 327: 557–560.
19. Higgins JP, Thompson SG (2002) Quantifying heterogeneity in a meta-analysis. Stat Med 21: 1539–1558.
20. Klein R, Klein BE, Moss SE (1995) Age-related eye disease and survival. The Beaver Dam Eye Study. Arch Ophthalmol 113: 333–339.
21. Cugati S, Cumming RG, Smith W, Burlutsky G, Mitchell P, et al. (2007) Visual impairment, age-related macular degeneration, cataract, and long-term mortality: the Blue Mountains Eye Study. Arch Ophthalmol 125: 917–924.
22. Xu L, Wang YX, Wang J, Jonas JJ (2009) Mortality and ocular diseases: the Beijing Eye Study. Ophthalmology 116: 732–738.
23. Khanna RC, Murthy GV, Giridhar P, Krishnaiah S, Pant HB, et al. (2013) Cataract, visual impairment and long-term mortality in a rural cohort in India: the Andhra Pradesh Eye Disease Study. PLoS One 8: e78002.
24. McCarty CA, Nanjan MB, Taylor HR (2001) Vision impairment predicts 5 year mortality. Br J Ophthalmol 85: 322–326.
25. Borger PH, van Leeuwen R, Hulsman CA, Wolfs RC, van der Kuip DA, et al. (2003) Is there a direct association between age-related eye diseases and mortality? The Rotterdam Study. Ophthalmology 110: 1292–1296.
26. Nucci C, Cedrone C, Culasso F, Cesareo M, Regine F, et al. (2004) Association between lens opacities and mortality in the Priverno Eye Study. Graefes Arch Clin Exp Ophthalmol 242: 289–294.
27. West SK, Munoz B, Istre J, Rubin GS, Friedman SM, et al. (2000) Mixed lens opacities and subsequent mortality. Arch Ophthalmol 118: 393–397.
28. Hennis A, Wu SY, Li X, Nemesure B, Leske MC (2001) Lens opacities and mortality: the Barbados Eye Studies. Ophthalmology 108: 498–504.
29. Klein BE, Klein R, Linton KL, Magli YL, Neider MW (1990) Assessment of cataracts from photographs in the Beaver Dam Eye Study. Ophthalmology 97: 1428–1433.
30. Chylack LT, Jr., Wolfe JK, Singer DM, Leske MC, Bullimore MA, et al. (1993) The Lens Opacities Classification System III. The Longitudinal Study of Cataract Study Group. Arch Ophthalmol 111: 831–836.
31. Chylack LT, Jr., Leske MC, McCarthy D, Khu P, Kashiwagi T, et al. (1989) Lens opacities classification system II (LOCS II). Arch Ophthalmol 107: 991–997.
32. Li L, Duker JS, Yoshida Y, Niki E, Rasmussen H, et al. (2009) Oxidative stress and antioxidant status in older adults with early cataract. Eye (Lond) 23: 1464–1468.
33. Giblin FJ (2000) Glutathione: a vital lens antioxidant. J Ocul Pharmacol Ther 16: 121–135.
34. Sweeney MH, Garland DL, Truscott RJ (2003) Movement of cysteine in intact monkey lenses: the major site of entry is the germinative region. Exp Eye Res 77: 245–251.
35. Ye L, Li Q, Cai X, Deng P (2005) Expression of TGF-beta2 mRNA and PCNA, FN protein in lens epithelial cells in age-related nuclear and cortex cataract. J Huazhong Univ Sci Technolog Med Sci 25: 578–581.
36. Machan CM, Hrynchak PK, Irving EL (2012) Age-related cataract is associated with type 2 diabetes and statin use. Optom Vis Sci 89: 1165–1171.
37. Rowe NG, Mitchell PG, Cumming RG, Wans JJ (2000) Diabetes, fasting blood glucose and age-related cataract: the Blue Mountains Eye Study. Ophthalmic Epidemiol 7: 103–114.
38. Klein BE, Klein R, Lee KE (1998) Diabetes, cardiovascular disease, selected cardiovascular disease risk factors, and the 5-year incidence of age-related

cataract and progression of lens opacities: the Beaver Dam Eye Study. Am J Ophthalmol 126: 782–790.
39. Taylor HR, West SK, Rosenthal FS, Munoz B, Newland HS, et al. (1988) Effect of ultraviolet radiation on cataract formation. N Engl J Med 319: 1429–1433.
40. Witztum JL (1994) The oxidation hypothesis of atherosclerosis. Lancet 344: 793–795.
41. Goosey JD, Tuan WM, Garcia CA (1984) A lipid peroxidative mechanism for posterior subcapsular cataract formation in the rabbit: a possible model for cataract formation in tapetoretinal diseases. Invest Ophthalmol Vis Sci 25: 608–612.
42. Nemet AY, Vinker S, Levartovsky S, Kaiserman I (2010) Is cataract associated with cardiovascular morbidity? Eye 24: 1352–1358.
43. Klein BEK, Klein R, Knudtson MD (2006) Frailty and age-related cataract. Ophthalmology 113: 2209–2212.
44. Belikova J, Synek S (2013) Correlation of age-related cataract density graded by the Scheimpflug Imaging System with visual function and phacoemulsification energy. Coll Antropol 37 Suppl 1: 25–30.
45. Grewal DS, Grewal SP (2012) Clinical applications of Scheimpflug imaging in cataract surgery. Saudi J Ophthalmol 26: 25–32.

Permissions

All chapters in this book were first published in PLOS ONE, by The Public Library of Science; hereby published with permission under the Creative Commons Attribution License or equivalent. Every chapter published in this book has been scrutinized by our experts. Their significance has been extensively debated. The topics covered herein carry significant findings which will fuel the growth of the discipline. They may even be implemented as practical applications or may be referred to as a beginning point for another development.

The contributors of this book come from diverse backgrounds, making this book a truly international effort. This book will bring forth new frontiers with its revolutionizing research information and detailed analysis of the nascent developments around the world.

We would like to thank all the contributing authors for lending their expertise to make the book truly unique. They have played a crucial role in the development of this book. Without their invaluable contributions this book wouldn't have been possible. They have made vital efforts to compile up to date information on the varied aspects of this subject to make this book a valuable addition to the collection of many professionals and students.

This book was conceptualized with the vision of imparting up-to-date information and advanced data in this field. To ensure the same, a matchless editorial board was set up. Every individual on the board went through rigorous rounds of assessment to prove their worth. After which they invested a large part of their time researching and compiling the most relevant data for our readers.

The editorial board has been involved in producing this book since its inception. They have spent rigorous hours researching and exploring the diverse topics which have resulted in the successful publishing of this book. They have passed on their knowledge of decades through this book. To expedite this challenging task, the publisher supported the team at every step. A small team of assistant editors was also appointed to further simplify the editing procedure and attain best results for the readers.

Apart from the editorial board, the designing team has also invested a significant amount of their time in understanding the subject and creating the most relevant covers. They scrutinized every image to scout for the most suitable representation of the subject and create an appropriate cover for the book.

The publishing team has been an ardent support to the editorial, designing and production team. Their endless efforts to recruit the best for this project, has resulted in the accomplishment of this book. They are a veteran in the field of academics and their pool of knowledge is as vast as their experience in printing. Their expertise and guidance has proved useful at every step. Their uncompromising quality standards have made this book an exceptional effort. Their encouragement from time to time has been an inspiration for everyone.

The publisher and the editorial board hope that this book will prove to be a valuable piece of knowledge for researchers, students, practitioners and scholars across the globe.

List of Contributors

Kyung-Sun Na and Choun-Ki Joo
Department of Ophthalmology and Visual Science, Seoul St. Mary's Hospital, College of Medicine, The Catholic University of Korea, Seoul, Korea

Yong-Gyu Park and Kyungdo Han
Department of Biostatistics, The Catholic University of Korea, Seoul, Korea

Kyung-Sun Na and Jee Won Mok
Catholic Institutes of Visual Science, The Catholic University of Korea, Seoul, Korea

Kyung-Sun Na
Department of Health Promotion Center, Seoul St. Mary's Hospital, College of Medicine, The Catholic University of Korea, Seoul, Korea

Peng Zhou, Hong-Fei Ye, Yong-Xiang Jiang, Jin Yang, Xiang-Jia Zhu, Xing-Huai Sun, Yi Luo and Yi Lu
Department of Ophthalmology, Eye and ENT Hospital of Fudan University, Shanghai, People's Republic of China

Guo-Rui Dou and Yu-Sheng Wang
Department of Ophthalmology, Xijing Hospital, Fourth Military Medical University, Xi'an, People's Republic of China

Hannah Kuper
Department of Epidemiology and Population Health, London School of Hygiene and Tropical Medicine, London, United Kingdom

Sarah Polack, Wanjiku Mathenge and Allen Foster
Department of Infectious and Tropical Diseases, London School of Hygiene and Tropical Medicine, London, United Kingdom

Cristina Eusebio
Cataract Foundation of the Philippines, Bacolod, Negros Occidental, Philippines

Zakia Wadud
Child Sight Foundation, Dhaka, Bangladesh

Mamunur Rashid
CSS Rawm Hospital, Khulna, Bangladesh

Nicky Cockburn, Karin Lecuona, Francois Joubert, Graeme Rogers and Colin Cook
Department of Ophthalmology, Groote Schuur Hospital, Cape Town, South Africa

David Steven
Eerste River Hospital, Cape Town, South Africa

Sarah Polack
London School of Hygiene and Tropical Medicine, London, United Kingdom

Rohit C. Khanna, Padmaja Kumari Rani and Subhabrata Chakrabarti
Brien Holden Eye Research Centre, L.V. Prasad Eye Institute, Banjara Hills, Hyderabad, India

Rohit C. Khanna and Padmaja Kumari Rani
Allen Foster Research Centre for Community Eye Health, International Centre for Advancement of Rural Eyecare, L.V. Prasad Eye Institute, Hyderabad, India

Srinivasa Reddy Pallerla, Shiva Shankar Eeda and Bala Krishna Gudapati
Andhra Pradesh Right to Sight Society, Hyderabad, India

Sandra D. Cassard and Oliver D. Schein
Wilmer Eye Institute, Johns Hopkins University, Baltimore, Maryland, United States of America

Ghanshyam Palamaner Subash Shantha and Oliver D. Schein
Johns Hopkins Bloomberg School of Public Health, Baltimore, Maryland, United States of America

Line Kessel, Lars Eskildsen and Michael Larsen
Department of Ophthalmology, Glostrup Hospital, University of Copenhagen, Glostrup, Denmark

Lars Eskildsen and Mike van der Poel
Department of Photonics Engineering, Technical University of Denmark, Kgs. Lyngby, Denmark

Robert P. Finger, David G. Kupitz and Frank G. Holz
Department of Ophthalmology, University of Bonn, Bonn, Germany

Robert P. Finger and Eva Fenwick
Centre for Eye Research Australia, Royal Victorian Eye and Ear Hospital, University of Melbourne, Melbourne, Australia

Bharath Balasubramaniam and Ramanathan V. Ramani
Sankara Eye Care Institutions, Coimbatore, India

Clare E. Gilbert
International Centre for Eye Health, London School for Hygiene and Tropical Medicine, London, United Kingdom

Xiao-feng Zhu, Hai-dong Zou and Qian Sun
Department of Ophthalmology, Shanghai First People's Hospital Affiliated Shanghai Jiao Tong University, Shanghai, China

Yong-fu Yu and Nai-qing Zhao
Department of Biostatistics, School of Public Health, Fudan University, Shanghai, China

Gergely Losonczy, Attila Vajas, Lili Takács, Éva Márhoffer and András Berta
Department of Ophthalmology, University of Debrecen, Debrecen

Erika Dzsudzsák
Department of Laboratory Medicine, University of Debrecen, Debrecen, Hungary

Ágnes Fekete
Department of Anesthesiology and Intensive Care, University of Debrecen, Debrecen, Hungary

László Kardos
Hygiene and Infection Control Services, Kenézy Gyula County Hospital, Debrecen, Hungary

Éva Ajzner
Central Laboratory, Jósa András Teaching Hospital, Nyíregyháza, Hungary

Begoña Hurtado and Pablo Garcia de Frutos
Department of Cell Death and Proliferation, Institute of Biomedical Research of Barcelona (IIBB-CSIC, IDIBAPS), Barcelona, Spain

Pablo Artal, Antonio Benito, Guillermo M. Pérez, Encarna Alcón
Laboratorio de Óptica, Universidad de Murcia, Murcia, Spain

Álvaro De Casas and José M. Marín
Hospital Universitario Virgen de la Arrixaca, Murcia, Spain

Jaume Pujol
Centre de Desenvolupament de Sensors, Instrumentacióі Sistemes (CD6), Universidad Politécnica de Cataluña, Tarrasa, Barcelona, Spain

Yuki Fujimichi and Nobuyuki Hamada
Radiation Safety Research Center, Nuclear Technology Research Laboratory, Central Research Institute of Electric Power Industry (CRIEPI), Komae, Tokyo, Japan

Xingjun Fan, Xiaoqin Liu, Shuyu Hao and Vincent M. Monnier
Department of Pathology, Case Western Reserve University, Cleveland, Ohio, United States of America

Benlian Wang
Case Center for Proteomics and Mass Spectrometry, Case Western Reserve University, Cleveland, Ohio, United States of America

Michael L. Robinson
Department of Zoology, Miami University, Oxford, Ohio, United States of America

Vincent M. Monnier
Department of Biochemistry, Case Western Reserve University, Cleveland, Ohio, United States of America

Khumbo Kalua
Department of Ophthalmology, College of Medicine, University of Malawi, Blantyre, Malawi

Khumbo Kalua and Robert Lindfield
International Centre for Eye Health, London School of Hygiene and Tropical Medicine, London, United Kingdom

Maxwell Mtupanyama
Ministry of Health, Chiradzulu District Hospital, Chiradzulu, Malawi

Davie Mtumodzi
Ministry of Health, Thyolo District Hospital, Thyolo, Malawi

Vincent Msiska
Ministry of Health, Mzuzu Central Hospital, Mzuzu, Malawi

Sarah Polack, Allen Foster and Hannah Kuper
Department of Infectious and Tropical Diseases, London School of Hygiene and Tropical Medicine, Keppel Street, London, United Kingdom

Christina Eusebio
Cataract Foundation of the Philippines, Bacolod, Philippines

Wanjiku Mathenge
Eye Unit, Rift Valley Provincial Hospital, Nakuru, Kenya

Zazkia Wadud
Child Sight Foundation, Dhaka, Bangladesh

Mamunur Rashid
CSS Rawm Hospital, Khulna, Bangladesh

Robert Lindfield
International Centre for Eye Health, London School of Hygiene and Tropical Medicine (LSHTM), London, United Kingdom

Ulla Griffiths and Fiammetta Bozzani
Department of Global Health and Development, London School of Hygiene and Tropical Medicine (LSHTM), London, United Kingdom

Musonda Mumba
Lusaka Eye Hospital, Lusaka, Zambia

Joseph Munsanje
S and S Development Consultants, Lusaka, Zambia

Far Chiang, Nasrallah Khalilia, Habes Batta and Nicholas Sargent
St. John Eye Hospital, Jerusalem, Occupied Palestinian Territories

Hannah Kuper and Robert Lindfield
London School of Hygiene and Tropical Medicine, London, United Kingdom

Tiarnan Keenan
Manchester Royal Eye Hospital, Manchester, United Kingdom

Náel Seyam
Military Medical Services, Gaza, Occupied Palestinian Territories

Denise Magauran
Epsom and St. Helier University Hospitals NHS Trust, Sutton, United Kingdom

Ziad Abdeen
Al-Quds Nutrition and Health Research Institute, Al Quds University, Jerusalem, Occupied Palestinian Territories

Yang Wang, Qian Gao, Liwen Hu, Na Gao, Huizhi Gong and Yang Liu
School of Public Health, China Medical University, Shenyang, People's Republic of China

Jiaming Yu
Ophthalmology Department, The Fourth Affiliated Hospital of China Medical University, Shenyang, People's Republic of China

Zhuhuang Zhou and Shuicai Wu
Biomedical Engineering Center, College of Life Science and Bioengineering, Beijing University of Technology, Beijing, China

Chih-Chung Huang
Department of Biomedical Engineering, National Cheng Kung University, Tainan, Taiwan

K. Kirk Shung
NIH Resource on Medical Ultrasonic Transducer Technology, Department of Biomedical Engineering, University of Southern California, Los Angeles, California, United States of America

Po-Hsiang Tsui and Yang Ma
Department of Medical Imaging and Radiological Sciences, College of Medicine, Chang Gung University, Taoyuan, Taiwan

Po-Hsiang Tsui
Institute for Radiological Research, Chang Gung University and Chang Gung Memorial Hospital, Taoyuan, Taiwan

Jui Fang
Ph.D. Program in Biomedical Engineering, Chang Gung University, Taoyuan, Taiwan

Hsiang-Yang Ma
Graduate Institute of Clinical Medical Sciences, College of Medicine, Chang Gung University, Taoyuan, Taiwan

Chung-Chih Lin
Department of Computer Science and Information Engineering, Chang Gung University, Taoyuan, Taiwan

Wei Shen, Yongming Yang, Juanjuan Li, Xiaodan Su, Hua Zhong and Yuansheng Yuan
The First Affiliated Hospital of Kunming Medical University, Kunming, China

Wei Shen and Jun Li
Yunnan Red Cross Hospital, Kunming, China

Minbin Yu
State Key Laboratory of Ophthalmology, Zhongshan Ophthalmic Center, Sun Yat-sen University, Guangzhou, China

Tao Wei and Xun Li
Kunming Medical University, Kunming, China

Juan Ye, Li-Xia Lou, Jin-Jing He and Yu-Feng Xu
Department of Ophthalmology, the Second Affiliated Hospital of Zhejiang University, College of Medicine, Hangzhou, Zhejiang, China

Jong-Hyun Oh, Jae Rock Do and Choul Yong Park
Department of Ophthalmology, Dongguk University Ilsan Hospital, Goyang, South Korea

Roy S. Chuck
Department of Ophthalmology and Visual Sciences, Montefiore Medical Center, Albert Einstein College of Medicine, Bronx, New York, United States of America

Yangfan Yang, Yiming Ye, Xianchai Lin, Kaili Wu and Minbin Yu
State Key Laboratory of Ophthalmology, Zhongshan Ophthalmic Center, Sun Yat-sen University, Guangzhou, China

Sushma Tejwani and Shoruba Dinakaran
Glaucoma Service, Narayana Nethralaya, Bangalore, Karnataka, India

Rohit Shetty
Refractive Surgery, Narayana Nethralaya, Bangalore, Karnataka, India

Mathew Kurien
Cataract Surgery, Narayana Nethralaya, Bangalore, Karnataka, India

Arkasubhra Ghosh
Gene, Repair and Regeneration in Ocular Workstation (GROW research lab), Narayana Nethralaya, Bangalore, Karnataka, India

Abhijit Sinha Roy
Imaging, Biomechanics and Mathematical Modeling Solutions (IBMS) lab, Narayana Nethralaya, Bangalore, Karnataka, India

Lisa Danquah, Hannah Kuper, Liza Bowen, Allen Foster and Sarah Polack
Faculty of Infectious and Tropical Diseases, London School of Hygiene and Tropical Medicine, London, United Kingdom

Cristina Eusebio
Cataract Foundation of the Philippines, Bacolod, Philippines

Mamunur Akm Rashid
Dhaka Community Medical College, Dhaka, Bangladesh

Wei Wang and Xiulan Zhang
Zhongshan Ophthalmic Center, State Key Laboratory of Ophthalmology, Sun Yat-Sen University, Guangzhou, People's Republic of China

Lixia Luo, Haotian Lin, Weirong Chen, Chunxiao Wang, Xinyu Zhang, Xiangchen Tang, Jianping Liu, Nathan Congdon, Jingjing Chen, Zhuoling Lin and Yizhi Liu
State Key Laboratory of Ophthalmology, Zhongshan Ophthalmic Center, Sun Yat-sen University, Guangzhou, China

Xiao-feng Zhu, Jin-juan Peng, Hai-dong Zou, Xun Xu and Xi Zhang
Department of Ophthalmology, Shanghai First People's Hospital, Affiliated Shanghai Jiaotong University, Shanghai, China

Jiong Fu and Wei-wei Wang
Beixinjing Community Health Service Center, Shanghai, China

Wan Chen, Haotian Lin, Xiaojian Zhong, Zhaochuan Liu, Yu Geng, Chufang Xie and Weirong Chen
State Key Laboratory of Ophthalmology, Zhongshan Ophthalmic Center, Sun Yat-sen University, Guangzhou, Guangdong, China

Young-Hoon Park and Jeong Ah Shin
Department of Ophthalmology and Visual Science, College of Medicine, The Catholic University of Korea, Seoul, Korea

Kyungdo Han
Department of Biostatistics, College of Medicine, The Catholic University of Korea, Seoul, Korea

Kyungdo Han, Hyeon Woo Yim, Won-Chul Lee and Yong-Moon Park
Department of Preventive Medicine, College of Medicine, The Catholic University of Korea, Seoul, Korea

Yong-Moon Park
Department of Epidemiology and Biostatistics, Arnold School of Public Health, University of South Carolina, Columbia, South Carolina, United States of America

Lei Shao and Wen Bin Wei
Beijing Tongren Eye Center, Beijing Tongren Hospital, Capital Medical University, Beijing, China

Liang Xu, Qi Sheng You, Ya Xing Wang, Chang Xi Chen, Hua Yang, Jin Qiong Zhou and Jost B. Jonas
Beijing Institute of Ophthalmology, Beijing Tongren Hospital, Capital Medical University, Beijing, China

Jost B. Jonas
Department of Ophthalmology, Medical Faculty Mannheim of the Ruprecht-Karls-University, Heidelberg, Germany

Jacquelyn Gerhart, Victoria Scheinfeld, Mitchell Crawford, Arturo Bravo-Nuevo, Meghan Pitts and Mindy George-Weinstein
Lankenau Institute for Medical Research, Wynnewood, Pennsylvania, United States of America

Marvin Greenbaum
Lankenau Medical Center, Wynnewood, Pennsylvania, United States of America

Paul FitzGerald
Department of Cell Biology and Human Anatomy, School of Medicine, University of California Davis, Davis, California, United States of America

Dongmei Su, Qian Li, Lina Guan, Huiling Zhang, Dandan E, Lei Zhang and Xu Ma
Department of Genetics, National Research Institute for Family Planning, Beiing, China

Zhenfei Yang and Siquan Zhu
Capital Medical University, Beijing Ophthalmology and Visual Sciences Key Lab, Beijing, China

E Song
Lixiang Eye Hospital of Soochow University, Suzhou, China

Hongpeng Sun, Yong Xu, Yana Ma, Hong Zhu and Chen-Wei Pan
School of Public Health, Medical College of Soochow University, Suzhou, China

Index